Deep Learning in Medical
Image Analysis

Deep Learning in Medical Image Analysis

Editors

Yudong Zhang
Juan Manuel Gorriz
Zhengchao Dong

MDPI • Basel • Beijing • Wuhan • Barcelona • Belgrade • Manchester • Tokyo • Cluj • Tianjin

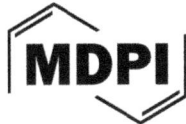

Editors
Yudong Zhang
University of Leicester
UK

Juan Manuel Gorriz
University of Granada
Spain

Zhengchao Dong
Columbia University,
USA

Editorial Office
MDPI
St. Alban-Anlage 66
4052 Basel, Switzerland

This is a reprint of articles from the Special Issue published online in the open access journal *Journal of Imaging* (ISSN 2313-433X) (available at: https://www.mdpi.com/journal/jimaging/special_issues/dlmia).

For citation purposes, cite each article independently as indicated on the article page online and as indicated below:

LastName, A.A.; LastName, B.B.; LastName, C.C. Article Title. *Journal Name* **Year**, *Volume Number*, Page Range.

ISBN 978-3-0365-1469-7 (Hbk)
ISBN 978-3-0365-1470-3 (PDF)

© 2021 by the authors. Articles in this book are Open Access and distributed under the Creative Commons Attribution (CC BY) license, which allows users to download, copy and build upon published articles, as long as the author and publisher are properly credited, which ensures maximum dissemination and a wider impact of our publications.

The book as a whole is distributed by MDPI under the terms and conditions of the Creative Commons license CC BY-NC-ND.

Contents

About the Editors ix

Preface to "Deep Learning in Medical Image Analysis" xi

Yudong Zhang, Juan Manuel Gorriz and Zhengchao Dong
Deep Learning in Medical Image Analysis
Reprinted from: *J. Imaging* 2021, 7, 74, doi:10.3390/jimaging7040074 1

Johannes Leuschner, Maximilian Schmidt, Poulami Somanya Ganguly, Vladyslav Andriiashen, Sophia Bethany Coban, Alexander Denker, Dominik Bauer, Amir Hadjifaradji, Kees Joost Batenburg, Peter Maass and Maureen van Eijnatten
Quantitative Comparison of Deep Learning-Based Image Reconstruction Methods for Low-Dose and Sparse-Angle CT Applications
Reprinted from: *J. Imaging* 2021, 7, 44, doi:10.3390/jimaging7030044 5

Boris Shirokikh, Alexey Shevtsov, Alexandra Dalechina, Egor Krivov, Valery Kostjuchenko, Andrey Golanov, Victor Gombolevskiy, Sergey Morozov and Mikhail Belyaev
Accelerating 3D Medical Image Segmentation by Adaptive Small-Scale Target Localization
Reprinted from: *J. Imaging* 2021, 7, 35, doi:10.3390/jimaging7020035 55

Penghao Zhang, Jiayue Li, Yining Wang and Judong Pan
Domain Adaptation for Medical Image Segmentation:
A Meta-Learning Method
Reprinted from: *J. Imaging* 2021, 7, 31, doi:10.3390/jimaging7020031 65

Antonella Nannavecchia, Francesco Girardi, Pio Raffaele Fina, Michele Scalera and Giovanni Dimauro
Personal Heart Health Monitoring Based on 1D Convolutional Neural Network
Reprinted from: *J. Imaging* 2021, 7, 26, doi:10.3390/jimaging7020026 79

Pedro Furtado
Testing Segmentation Popular Loss and Variations in Three Multiclass Medical Imaging Problems
Reprinted from: *J. Imaging* 2021, 7, 16, doi:10.3390/jimaging7020016 97

Tomohiro Shimizu, Ryo hachiuma, Hiroki Kajita, Yoshifumi Takatsume, and Hideo Saito
Hand Motion-Aware Surgical Tool Localization and Classification from an Egocentric Camera
Reprinted from: *J. Imaging* 2021, 7, 15, doi:10.3390/jimaging7020015 113

Sami Bourouis, Abdullah Alharbi and Nizar Bouguila
Bayesian Learning of Shifted-Scaled Dirichlet Mixture Models and Its Application to Early COVID-19 Detection in Chest X-ray Images
Reprinted from: *J. Imaging* 2021, 7, 7, doi:10.3390/jimaging7010007 127

Catarina Andrade, Luís F. Teixeira, Maria João M. Vasconcelos and Luís Rosado
Data Augmentation Using Adversarial Image-to-Image Translation for the Segmentation of Mobile-Acquired Dermatological Images
Reprinted from: *J. Imaging* 2021, 7, 2, doi:10.3390/jimaging7010002 141

Ibrahem Kandel, Mauro Castelli and Aleš Popovič
Musculoskeletal Images Classification for Detection of Fractures Using Transfer Learning
Reprinted from: *J. Imaging* 2020, 6, 127, doi:10.3390/jimaging6110127 157

Albert Comelli
Fully 3D Active Surface with Machine Learning for PET Image Segmentation
Reprinted from: *J. Imaging* **2020**, 6, 113, doi:10.3390/jimaging6110113 . . . . **171**

Mauricio Alberto Ortega-Ruiz, Cefa Karabağ, Victor García Garduño and Constantino Carlos Reyes-Aldasoro
Morphological Estimation of Cellularity on Neo-Adjuvant Treated Breast Cancer Histological Images
Reprinted from: *J. Imaging* **2020**, 6, 101, doi:10.3390/jimaging6100101 . . . . **183**

Ibrahem Kandel, Mauro Castelli and Aleš Popovič
Comparative Study of First Order Optimizers for Image Classification Using Convolutional Neural Networks on Histopathology Images
Reprinted from: *J. Imaging* **2020**, 6, 92, doi:10.3390/jimaging6090092 . . . . **201**

David La Barbera, António Polónia, Kevin Roitero Eduardo Conde-Sousa and Vincenzo Della Mea
Detection of HER2 from Haematoxylin-Eosin Slides Through a Cascade of Deep Learning Classifiers via Multi-Instance Learning
Reprinted from: *J. Imaging* **2020**, 6, 82, doi:10.3390/jimaging6090082 . . . . **219**

Vahab Khoshdel, Mohammad Asefi, Ahmed Ashraf, Joe LoVetri
Full 3D Microwave Breast Imaging Using a Deep-Learning Technique
Reprinted from: *J. Imaging* **2020**, 6, 80, doi:10.3390/jimaging6080080 . . . . **233**

Guillaume Dupont, Ekaterina Kalinicheva, Jérémie Sublime, Florence Rossant and Michel Pâques
Analyzing Age-Related Macular Degeneration Progression in Patients with Geographic Atrophy Using Joint Autoencoders for Unsupervised Change Detection
Reprinted from: *J. Imaging* **2020**, 6, 57, doi:10.3390/jimaging6070057 . . . . **251**

Marcos A. M. Almeida and Iury A. X. Santos
Classification Models for Skin Tumor Detection Using Texture Analysis in Medical Images
Reprinted from: *J. Imaging* **2020**, 6, 51, doi:10.3390/jimaging6060051 . . . . **273**

Michelle Tang, Pulkit Kumar, Hao Chen and Abhinav Shrivastava
Deep Multimodal Learning for the Diagnosis of Autism Spectrum Disorder
Reprinted from: *J. Imaging* **2020**, 6, 47, doi:10.3390/jimaging6060047 . . . . **289**

Emmanuel Pintelas, Meletis Liaskos, Ioannis E. Livieris, Sotiris Kotsiantis and Panagiotis Pintelas
Explainable Machine Learning Framework for Image Classification Problems: Case Study on Glioma Cancer Prediction
Reprinted from: *J. Imaging* **2020**, 6, 37, doi:10.3390/jimaging6060037 . . . . **301**

Stefanus Tao Hwa Kieu, Abdullah Bade, Mohd Hanafi Ahmad Hijazi and Hoshang Kolivand
A Survey of Deep Learning for Lung Disease Detection on Medical Images: State-of-the-Art, Taxonomy, Issues and Future Directions
Reprinted from: *J. Imaging* **2020**, 6, 131, doi:10.3390/jimaging6120131 . . . . **323**

Taye Girma Debelee, Samuel Rahimeto Kebede, Friedhelm Schwenker and Zemene Matewos
Deep Learning in Selected Cancers' Image Analysis—A Survey
Reprinted from: *J. Imaging* **2020**, 6, 121, doi:10.3390/jimaging6110121 . . . . **361**

Kehinde Aruleba, George Obaido, Blessing Ogbuokiri, Adewale Oluwaseun Fadaka, Ashwil Klein, Tayo Alex Adekiya and Raphael Taiwo Aruleba
Applications of Computational Methods in Biomedical Breast Cancer Imaging Diagnostics: A Review
Reprinted from: *J. Imaging* **2020**, *6*, 105, doi:10.3390/jimaging6100105 . . . . **401**

Amitojdeep Singh, Sourya Sengupta and Vasudevan Lakshminarayanan
Explainable Deep Learning Models in Medical Image Analysis
Reprinted from: *J. Imaging* **2020**, *6*, 52, doi:10.3390/jimaging6060052 . . . . **425**

About the Editors

Yudong Zhang completed his PhD degree in Signal and Information Processing at Southeast University in 2010. He worked as a postdoc from 2010 to 2012 at Columbia University, USA; and as an assistant research scientist from 2012 to 2013, with Research Foundation of Mental Hygiene (RFMH), USA. He served as a Full Professor from 2013 to 2017 with Nanjing Normal University. Now, he serves as a Professor at School of Informatics, University of Leicester, UK. His research interests include deep learning and medical image analysis. He is the Fellow of IET (FIET), and Senior Members of IEEE, IES, and ACM. He was included in "Most Cited Chinese researchers (Computer Science)" by Elsevier from 2014 to 2018. He was the 2019 recipient of "Web of Science Highly Cited Researcher". He won "Emerald Citation of Excellence 2017" and "MDPI Top 10 Most Cited Papers 2015". He is included in "Top Scientist" in Guide2Research. He is the author of over 250 peer-reviewed articles, including more than 40 "ESI Highly Cited Papers", and 3 "ESI Hot Papers". His citation reached 15,235 in Google Scholar (h-index 68), and 8947 in Web of Science (h-index 53). He has partaken in many successful industrial projects and academic grants at NIH, Royal Society, GCRF, EPSRC, MRC, British Council, and NSFC.

Juan Manuel Gorriz completed the BSc degree in Physics and BSc degree in electronic engineering at the University of Granada, Spain, in 2000 and 2001, respectively. He completed his PhD degree at the University of Cádiz, Spain, in 2003, and PhD degree from the University of Granada in 2006, both with honors. He is currently a Full Professor (2012) at the Department of Signal Theory, Networking and Communications, University of Granada and a Visiting Professor (2017) at the Department of Psychiatry at the University of Cambridge, UK. He has co-authored over 400 technical journals and conference papers in these areas. His current interests include statistical signal processing and its application to biosignal and medical image processing. He received the National Academy of Engineering Medal in 2015. He has served as an Editor for several journals and books.

Zhengchao Dong is an MR physicist specialized in Nuclear Magnetic Resonance (NMR) and MR imaging/spectroscopy in his MSc and Dr. rer. nat. studies, respectively. He is currently an associate professor at Columbia University and a research scientist at the New York State Psychiatric Institute, USA. His research experiences include design of NMR probes and MRI coils, design of NMR and MRI sequences, development of MRI/MR spectroscopy postprocessing methods, and applications of MR techniques in biomedical sciences. His current interests include MR spectroscopy, and MR-based thermometry, and their applications in psychiatric disorders.

Preface to "Deep Learning in Medical Image Analysis"

In recent years, deep learning (DL) has established itself as a powerful tool across a broad spectrum of domains in imaging, e.g., classification, prediction, detection, segmentation, diagnosis, interpretation, reconstruction, etc. While deep neural networks initially found their place in the computer vision community, they have quickly spread over medical imaging applications.

The purpose of this book "Deep Learning in Medical Image Analysis" is to present and highlight novel algorithms, architectures, techniques, and applications of DL for medical image analysis. This book is a reliable resource for researchers, teachers, PhD students, and clinicians.

This book called for papers from April/2020. It received more than 60 submissions from over 30 different countries. After strict peer reviews, only 22 papers from 19 different countries were accepted and published. Eighteen papers are research articles and the other 4 are review papers.

All the three Book Editors—Yu-Dong Zhang, Juan M Gorriz, Zhengchao Dong—hope that this book "Deep Learning in Medical Image Analysis" will benefit the scientific community and contribute to the knowledge base, and would like to take this opportunity to applaud the contributions of all the authors of this book. The contributions and efforts of the reviewers to enhance the quality of the manuscripts are also much appreciated. It is also necessary to acknowledge the assistance given by the MDPI editorial team who make our editors' tasks much easier.

Yudong Zhang, Juan Manuel Gorriz, Zhengchao Dong
Editors

Journal of Imaging

Editorial
Deep Learning in Medical Image Analysis

Yudong Zhang [1,*], Juan Manuel Gorriz [2] and Zhengchao Dong [3]

1. School of Informatics, University of Leicester, Leicester LE1 7RH, UK
2. Department of Signal Theory, Telematics and Communications, University of Granada, 18071 Granada, Spain; gorriz@ugr.es
3. Molecular Imaging and Neuropathology Division, Columbia University and New York State Psychiatric Institute, New York, NY 10032, USA; zhengchao.dong@nyspi.columbia.edu
* Correspondence: yudongzhang@ieee.org

Citation: Zhang, Y.; Gorriz, J.M.; Dong, Z. Deep Learning in Medical Image Analysis. *J. Imaging* **2021**, *7*, 74. https://doi.org/10.3390/jimaging7040074

Received: 12 April 2021
Accepted: 16 April 2021
Published: 20 April 2021

Publisher's Note: MDPI stays neutral with regard to jurisdictional claims in published maps and institutional affiliations.

Copyright: © 2021 by the authors. Licensee MDPI, Basel, Switzerland. This article is an open access article distributed under the terms and conditions of the Creative Commons Attribution (CC BY) license (https://creativecommons.org/licenses/by/4.0/).

Over recent years, deep learning (DL) has established itself as a powerful tool across a broad spectrum of domains in imaging—e.g., classification, prediction, detection, segmentation, diagnosis, interpretation, reconstruction, etc. While deep neural networks were initially nurtured in the computer vision community, they have quickly spread over medical imaging applications.

The accelerating power of DL in diagnosing diseases will empower physicians and speed-up decision making in clinical environments. Applications of modern medical instruments and digitalization of medical care have led to enormous amounts of medical images being generated in recent years. In the big data arena, new DL methods and computational models for efficient data processing, analysis, and modeling of the generated data are crucial for clinical applications and understanding the underlying biological process.

The purpose of this Special Issue (SI) "Deep Learning in Medical Image Analysis" is to present and highlight novel algorithms, architectures, techniques, and applications of DL for medical image analysis.

This SI called for papers in April 2020. It received more than 60 submissions from over 30 different countries. After strict peer reviews, only 22 papers were accepted and published. A total of 18 papers are research articles and the remaining 4 are review papers.

Leuschner and Schmidt (2021) [1] from Germany, the Netherlands, and Canada present the results of a data challenge that the authors organized, bringing together algorithm experts from different institutes to jointly work on quantitative evaluation of several data-driven methods on two large, public datasets during a ten-day sprint.

Shirokikh and Shevtsov (2021) [2] from Russia propose a new segmentation method with a human-like technique to segment a 3D study. Their method not only reduces the inference time from 10min to 15s, but also preserves state-of-the-art segmentation quality.

Zhang and Li (2021) [3] from China and the USA propose a meta-learning algorithm to augment the existing algorithms with the capability to learn from diverse segmentation tasks across the entire task distribution. The authors conduct experiments using a diverse set of segmentation tasks from the Medical Segmentation Decathlon and two meta-learning benchmarks.

Nannavecchia and Girardi (2021) [4] from Italy present a system able to automatically detect the causes of cardiac pathologies in electrocardiogram (ECG) signals from personal monitoring devices, with the aim to alert the patient to send the ECG to the medical specialist for a correct diagnosis and proper therapy.

Furtado (2021) [5] from Portugal takes on three different medical image segmentation problems: (i) segmentation of organs in magnetic resonance images, (ii) liver in computer tomography images, and (iii) diabetic retinopathy lesions in eye fundus images. The author quantifies loss functions and variations, as well as segmentation scores of different targets. The author concludes that dice is the best.

Shimizu and Hachiuma (2021) [6] from Japan combine three modules for localization, selection, and classification for the detection of the two surgical tools. In the localization module, the authors employ the Faster R-CNN to detect surgical tools and target hands, and in the classification module, the authors extract hand movement information by combining ResNet-18 and long short-term memory (LSTM) to classify two tools.

Bourouis and Alharbi (2021) [7] from Saudi Arabia and Canada introduce a new statistical framework to discriminate patients who are either negative or positive for certain kinds of virus and pneumonia. The authors tackle the current problem via a fully Bayesian approach based on a flexible statistical model named shifted-scaled Dirichlet mixture models.

Andrade and Teixeira (2021) [8] from Portugal present a technique to efficiently utilize the sizable number of dermoscopic images to improve the segmentation capacity of macroscopic skin lesion images. The quantitative segmentation results are demonstrated on the available macroscopic segmentation databases, SMARTSKINS and Dermofit Image Library.

Kandel and Castelli (2020) [9] from Portugal and Slovenia study an appropriate method to classify musculoskeletal images by transfer learning and by training from scratch. The authors apply six state-of-the-art architectures and compare their performances with transfer learning and with a network trained from scratch.

Comelli (2020) [10] from Italy presents an algorithm capable of achieving the volume reconstruction directly in 3D by leveraging an active surface algorithm. The results confirm that the active surface algorithm is superior to the active contour algorithm, outperforming an earlier approach on all the investigated anatomical districts with a dice similarity coefficient of $90.47 \pm 2.36\%$ for lung cancer, $88.30 \pm 2.89\%$ for head and neck cancer, and $90.29 \pm 2.52\%$ for brain cancer.

The methodology proposed by Ortega-Ruiz and Karabağ (2020) [11] from Mexico and the United Kingdom is based on traditional computer vision methods (K-means, watershed segmentation, Otsu's binarization, and morphological operations), implementing color separation, segmentation, and feature extraction. The methodology is validated with the score assigned by two pathologists through the intraclass correlation coefficient.

The main aim of Kandel and Castelli (2020) [12] from Portugal and Slovenia is to improve the robustness of the classifier used by comparing six different first-order stochastic gradient-based optimizers to select the best for this particular dataset. Their results show that the adaptative-based optimizers achieved the highest results, except for AdaGrad, which achieved the lowest results.

La Barbera and Polónia (2020) [13] from Italy and Portugal employ a pipeline based on a cascade of deep neural network classifiers and multi-instance learning to detect the presence of HER2 from haematoxylin–eosin slides, which partly mimics the pathologist's behavior by first recognizing cancer and then evaluating HER2.

Khoshdel and Asefi (2020) [14] from Canada employ a 3D convolutional neural network, based on the U-Net architecture, that takes in 3D images obtained using the contrast-source inversion method and attempts to produce the true 3D image of the permittivity.

Dupont and Kalinicheva (2020) [15] from France proposes a DL architecture that can detect changes in the eye fundus images and assess the progression of the disease. Their method is based on joint autoencoders and is fully unsupervised. Their algorithm has been applied to pairs of images from time series of different eye fundus images of 24 age-related macular degeneration patients.

Almeida and Santos (2020) [16] from Brazil propose a strategy for the analysis of skin images, aiming to choose the best mathematical classifier model for the identification of melanoma, with the objective of assisting the dermatologist in the identification of melanomas, especially towards an early diagnosis.

Tang and Kumar (2020) [17] from the USA propose a deep multimodal model that learns a joint representation from two types of connectomic data offered by fMRI scans. Their multimodal training strategy achieves a classification accuracy of 74% and a recall of

95%, as well as an F1 score of 0.805, and its overall performance is superior to that of using only one type of functional data.

In the work of Pintelas and Liaskos (2020) [18] from Greece, an accurate and interpretable machine learning framework is proposed for image classification problems able to make high quality explanations. Their results demonstrate the efficiency of the proposed model since it managed to achieve sufficient prediction accuracy, which is also interpretable and explainable in simple human terms.

Kieu and Bade (2020) [19] from Malaysia and the United Kingdom present a taxonomy of the state-of-the-art DL-based lung disease detection systems, visualize the trends of recent work on the domain and identify the remaining issues and potential future directions in this domain.

In the survey of Debelee and Kebede (2020) [20] from Ethiopia and Germany, several DL-based approaches applied to breast cancer, cervical cancer, brain tumor, colon and lung cancers are studied and reviewed. The result of the review process indicates that DL methods are the state-of-the-art in tumor detection, segmentation, feature extraction and classification.

Aruleba and Obaido (2020) [21] from South Africa provide a concise overview of past and present conventional diagnostics approaches in breast cancer detection. Further, the authors give an account of several computational models (machine learning, deep learning, and robotics), which have been developed and can serve as alternative techniques for breast cancer diagnostics imaging.

Singh and Sengupta (2020) [22] from Canada present a review of the current applications of explainable deep learning for different medical imaging tasks. The various approaches, challenges for clinical deployment, and the areas requiring further research are discussed in this review from a practical standpoint of a deep learning researcher designing a system for the clinical end-users.

The 22 accepted papers in this SI are from 19 countries: Brazil, Canada, China, Ethiopia, France, Germany, Greece, Italy, Japan, Malaysia, Mexico, Netherlands, Portugal, Russia, Saudi Arabia, Slovenia, South Africa, the UK, and the USA.

All the three Guest Editors hope that this Special Issue "Deep Learning in Medical Image Analysis" will benefit the scientific community and contribute to the knowledge base, and would like to take this opportunity to applaud the contributions of all the authors in this Special Issue. The contributions and efforts of the reviewers to enhance the quality of the manuscripts are also much appreciated. It is also necessary to acknowledge the assistance provided by the MDPI editorial team who make our GE tasks much easier.

Conflicts of Interest: The authors declare no conflict of interest.

References

1. Leuschner, J.; Schmidt, M.; Ganguly, P.; Andriiashen, V.; Coban, S.; Denker, A.; Bauer, D.; Hadjifaradji, A.; Batenburg, K.; Maass, P.; et al. Quantitative Comparison of Deep Learning-Based Image Reconstruction Methods for Low-Dose and Sparse-Angle CT Applications. *J. Imaging* **2021**, *7*, 44. [CrossRef]
2. Shirokikh, B.; Shevtsov, A.; Dalechina, A.; Krivov, E.; Kostjuchenko, V.; Golanov, A.; Gombolevskiy, V.; Morozov, S.; Belyaev, M. Accelerating 3D Medical Image Segmentation by Adaptive Small-Scale Target Localization. *J. Imaging* **2021**, *7*, 35. [CrossRef]
3. Zhang, P.; Li, J.; Wang, Y.; Pan, J. Domain Adaptation for Medical Image Segmentation: A Meta-Learning Method. *J. Imaging* **2021**, *7*, 31. [CrossRef]
4. Nannavecchia, A.; Girardi, F.; Fina, P.; Scalera, M.; DiMauro, G. Personal Heart Health Monitoring Based on 1D Convolutional Neural Network. *J. Imaging* **2021**, *7*, 26. [CrossRef]
5. Furtado, P. Testing Segmentation Popular Loss and Variations in Three Multiclass Medical Imaging Problems. *J. Imaging* **2021**, *7*, 16. [CrossRef]
6. Shimizu, T.; Hachiuma, R.; Kajita, H.; Takatsume, Y.; Saito, H. Hand Motion-Aware Surgical Tool Localization and Classification from an Egocentric Camera. *J. Imaging* **2021**, *7*, 15. [CrossRef]
7. Bourouis, S.; Alharbi, A.; Bouguila, N. Bayesian Learning of Shifted-Scaled Dirichlet Mixture Models and Its Application to Early COVID-19 Detection in Chest X-ray Images. *J. Imaging* **2021**, *7*, 7. [CrossRef]
8. Andrade, C.; Teixeira, L.F.; Vasconcelos, M.J.M.; Rosado, L. Data Augmentation Using Adversarial Image-to-Image Translation for the Segmentation of Mobile-Acquired Dermatological Images. *J. Imaging* **2021**, *7*, 2. [CrossRef]

9. Kandel, I.; Castelli, M.; Popovič, A. Musculoskeletal Images Classification for Detection of Fractures Using Transfer Learning. *J. Imaging* **2020**, *6*, 127. [CrossRef]
10. Comelli, A. Fully 3D Active Surface with Machine Learning for PET Image Segmentation. *J. Imaging* **2020**, *6*, 113. [CrossRef]
11. Ortega-Ruiz, M.A.; Karabağ, C.; Garduño, V.G.; Reyes-Aldasoro, C.C. Morphological Estimation of Cellularity on Neo-Adjuvant Treated Breast Cancer Histological Images. *J. Imaging* **2020**, *6*, 101. [CrossRef]
12. Kandel, I.; Castelli, M.; Popovič, A. Comparative Study of First Order Optimizers for Image Classification Using Convolutional Neural Networks on Histopathology Images. *J. Imaging* **2020**, *6*, 92. [CrossRef]
13. La Barbera, D.; Polónia, A.; Roitero, K.; Conde-Sousa, E.; Della Mea, V. Detection of HER2 from Haematoxylin-Eosin Slides Through a Cascade of Deep Learning Classifiers via Multi-Instance Learning. *J. Imaging* **2020**, *6*, 82. [CrossRef]
14. Khoshdel, V.; Asefi, M.; Ashraf, A.; LoVetri, J. Full 3D Microwave Breast Imaging Using a Deep-Learning Technique. *J. Imaging* **2020**, *6*, 80. [CrossRef]
15. Dupont, G.; Kalinicheva, E.; Sublime, J.; Rossant, F.; Pâques, M. Analyzing Age-Related Macular Degeneration Progression in Patients with Geographic Atrophy Using Joint Autoencoders for Unsupervised Change Detection. *J. Imaging* **2020**, *6*, 57. [CrossRef]
16. Almeida, M.A.M.; Santos, I.A.X. Classification Models for Skin Tumor Detection Using Texture Analysis in Medical Images. *J. Imaging* **2020**, *6*, 51. [CrossRef]
17. Tang, M.; Kumar, P.; Chen, H.; Shrivastava, A. Deep Multimodal Learning for the Diagnosis of Autism Spectrum Disorder. *J. Imaging* **2020**, *6*, 47. [CrossRef]
18. Pintelas, E.; Liaskos, M.; Livieris, I.E.; Kotsiantis, S.; Pintelas, P. Explainable Machine Learning Framework for Image Classification Problems: Case Study on Glioma Cancer Prediction. *J. Imaging* **2020**, *6*, 37. [CrossRef]
19. Kieu, S.T.H.; Bade, A.; Hijazi, M.H.A.; Kolivand, H. A Survey of Deep Learning for Lung Disease Detection on Medical Images: State-of-the-Art, Taxonomy, Issues and Future Directions. *J. Imaging* **2020**, *6*, 131. [CrossRef]
20. Debelee, T.G.; Kebede, S.R.; Schwenker, F.; Shewarega, Z.M. Deep Learning in Selected Cancers' Image Analysis—A Survey. *J. Imaging* **2020**, *6*, 121. [CrossRef]
21. Aruleba, K.; Obaido, G.; Ogbuokiri, B.; Fadaka, A.O.; Klein, A.; Adekiya, T.A.; Aruleba, R.T. Applications of Computational Methods in Biomedical Breast Cancer Imaging Diagnostics: A Review. *J. Imaging* **2020**, *6*, 105. [CrossRef]
22. Singh, A.; Sengupta, S.; Lakshminarayanan, V. Explainable Deep Learning Models in Medical Image Analysis. *J. Imaging* **2020**, *6*, 52. [CrossRef]

Article

Quantitative Comparison of Deep Learning-Based Image Reconstruction Methods for Low-Dose and Sparse-Angle CT Applications

Johannes Leuschner [1,*,†], Maximilian Schmidt [1,†], Poulami Somanya Ganguly [2,3], Vladyslav Andriiashen [2], Sophia Bethany Coban [2], Alexander Denker [1], Dominik Bauer [4], Amir Hadjifaradji [5], Kees Joost Batenburg [2,6], Peter Maass [1] and Maureen van Eijnatten [2,7,*]

1. Center for Industrial Mathematics, University of Bremen, Bibliothekstr. 5, 28359 Bremen, Germany; maximilian.schmidt@uni-bremen.de (M.S.); adenker@uni-bremen.de (A.D.); pmaass@uni-bremen.de (P.M.)
2. Centrum Wiskunde & Informatica, Science Park 123, 1098 XG Amsterdam, The Netherlands; poulami.ganguly@cwi.nl (P.S.G.); vladyslav.andriiashen@cwi.nl (V.A.); sophia.coban@cwi.nl (S.B.C.); k.j.batenburg@cwi.nl (K.J.B.)
3. The Mathematical Institute, Leiden University, Niels Bohrweg 1, 2333 CA Leiden, The Netherlands
4. Computer Assisted Clinical Medicine, Heidelberg University, Theodor-Kutzer-Ufer 1-3, 68167 Mannheim, Germany; dominik.bauer@medma.uni-heidelberg.de
5. School of Biomedical Engineering, University of British Columbia, 2222 Health Sciences Mall, Vancouver, BC V6T 1Z3, Canada; ahadji@student.ubc.ca
6. Leiden Institute of Advanced Computer Science, Niels Bohrweg 1, 2333 CA Leiden, The Netherlands
7. Department of Biomedical Engineering, Eindhoven University of Technology, Groene Loper 3, 5612 AE Eindhoven, The Netherlands
* Correspondence: jleuschn@uni-bremen.de (J.L.); m.a.j.m.v.eijnatten@tue.nl (M.v.E.)
† These authors contributed equally to this work.

Abstract: The reconstruction of computed tomography (CT) images is an active area of research. Following the rise of deep learning methods, many data-driven models have been proposed in recent years. In this work, we present the results of a *data challenge* that we organized, bringing together algorithm experts from different institutes to jointly work on quantitative evaluation of several data-driven methods on two large, public datasets during a ten day sprint. We focus on two applications of CT, namely, low-dose CT and sparse-angle CT. This enables us to fairly compare different methods using standardized settings. As a general result, we observe that the deep learning-based methods are able to improve the reconstruction quality metrics in both CT applications while the top performing methods show only minor differences in terms of peak signal-to-noise ratio (PSNR) and structural similarity (SSIM). We further discuss a number of other important criteria that should be taken into account when selecting a method, such as the availability of training data, the knowledge of the physical measurement model and the reconstruction speed.

Keywords: computed tomography (CT); image reconstruction; low-dose; sparse-angle; deep learning; quantitative comparison

1. Introduction

Computed tomography (CT) is a widely used (bio)medical imaging modality, with various applications in clinical settings, such as diagnostics [1], screening [2] and virtual treatment planning [3,4], as well as in industrial [5] and scientific [6–8] settings. One of the fundamental aspects of this modality is the reconstruction of images from multiple X-ray measurements taken from different angles. Because each X-ray measurement exposes the sample or patient to harmful ionizing radiation, minimizing this exposure remains an active area of research [9]. The challenge is to either minimize the dose per measurement or the total number of measurements while maintaining sufficient image quality to perform subsequent diagnostic or analytic tasks.

To date, the most common classical methods used for CT image reconstruction are filtered back-projection (FBP) and iterative reconstruction (IR) techniques. FBP is a stabilized and discretized version of the inverse Radon transform, in which 1D projections are filtered by the 1D Radon kernel (back-projected) in order to obtain a 2D signal [10,11]. FBP is very fast, but is not suitable for limited-data or sparse-angle setups, resulting in various imaging artifacts, such as streaking, stretching, blurring, partial volume effects, or noise [12]. Iterative reconstruction methods, on the other hand, are computationally intensive but are able to incorporate *a priori* information about the system during reconstruction. Many iterative techniques are based on statistical methods such as Markov random fields or regularization methods where the regularizers are designed and incorporated into the problem of reconstruction mathematically [13]. A popular choice for the regularizer is total variation (TV) [14,15]. Another well-known iterative method suitable for large-scale tomography problems is the conjugate gradient method applied to solve the least squares problem (CGLS) [16].

When classical techniques such as FBP or IR are used to reconstruct low-dose CT images, the image quality often deteriorates significantly in the presence of increased noise. Therefore, the focus is shifting towards developing reconstruction methods in which a single or multiple component(s), or even the entire reconstruction process is performed using deep learning [17]. Generally data-driven approaches promise fast and/or accurate image reconstruction by taking advantage of a large number of examples, that is, training data.

The methods that learn parts of the reconstruction process can be roughly divided into learned regularizers, unrolled iterative schemes, and post-processing of reconstructed CT images. Methods based on learned regularizers work on the basis of learning convolutional filters from the training data that can subsequently be used to regularize the reconstruction problem by plugging into a classical iterative optimization scheme [18]. Unrolled iterative schemes go a step further in the sense that they "unroll" the steps of the iterative scheme into a sequence of operations where the operators are replaced with convolutional neural networks (CNNs). A recent example is the learned primal-dual algorithm proposed by Adler et al. [19]. Finally, various post-processing methods have been proposed that correct noisy images or those with severe artifacts in the image domain [20]. Examples are improving tomographic reconstruction from limited data using a mixed-scale dense (MS-D) CNN [21], U-Net [22] or residual encoder-decoder CNN (RED-CNN) [23], as well as CT image denoising techniques [24,25]. Somewhat similar are the methods that can be trained in a supervised manner to improve the measurement data in the sinogram domain [26].

The first fully end-to-end learned reconstruction method was the automated transform by the manifold approximation (AUTOMAP) algorithm [27] developed for magnetic resonance (MR) image reconstruction. This method directly learns the (global) relation between the measurement data and the image, that is, it replaces the Radon or Fourier transform with a neural network. The disadvantages of this approach are the large memory requirements, as well as the fact that it might not be necessary to learn the entire transformation from scratch because an efficient analytical transform is already available. A similar approach for CT reconstruction was iRadonMAP proposed by He et al. [28], who developed an interpretable framework for Radon inversion in medical X-ray CT. In addition, Li et al. [29] proposed an end-to-end reconstruction framework for Radon inversion called iCT-Net, and demonstrated its advantages in solving sparse-view CT reconstruction problems.

The aforementioned deep learning-based CT image reconstruction methods differ greatly in terms of which component of the reconstruction task is learned and in which domain the method operates (image or sinogram domain), as well as the computational and data-related requirements. As a result, it remains difficult to compare the performance of deep learning-based reconstruction methods across different imaging domains and applications. Thorough comparisons between different reconstruction methods are further complicated by the lack of sufficiently large benchmarking datasets, including ground truth reconstructions, for training, validation, and testing. CT manufacturers are typically very reluctant in making raw measurement data available for research purposes, and privacy regulations for making medical imaging data publicly available are becoming increasingly strict [30,31].

1.1. Goal of This Study

The aim of this study is to quantitatively compare the performance of classical and deep learning-based CT image reconstruction methods on two large, two-dimensional (2D) parallel-beam CT datasets that were specifically created for this purpose. We opted for a 2D parallel-beam CT setup to facilitate large-scale experiments with many example images, whereas the underlying operators in the algorithms have straightforward generalizations to other geometries. We focus on two reconstruction tasks with high relevance and impact—the first task is the reconstruction of low-dose medical CT images, and the second is the reconstruction of sparse-angle CT images.

1.1.1. Reconstruction of Low-Dose Medical CT Images

In order to compare (learned) reconstruction techniques in a low-dose CT setup, we use the low-dose parallel beam (LoDoPaB) CT dataset [32]. This dataset contains 42,895 two-dimensional CT images and corresponding simulated low-intensity measurements. The ground truth images of this dataset are human chest CT reconstructions taken from the LIDC/IDRI database [33]. These scans had been acquired with a wide range of scanners and models. The initial image reconstruction for creating the LIDC/IDRI database was performed with different convolution kernels, depending on the manufacturer. Poisson noise is applied to the simulated projection data to model the low intensity setup. A more detailed description can be found in Section 2.1.

1.1.2. Reconstruction of Sparse-Angle CT Images

When using X-ray tomography in high-throughput settings (i.e., scanning multiple objects per second) such as quality control, luggage scanning or inspection of products on conveyor belts, very few X-ray projections can be acquired for each object. In such settings, it is essential to incorporate *a priori* information about the object being scanned during image reconstruction. In order to compare (learned) reconstruction techniques for this application, we reconstruct parallel-beam CT images of apples with internal defects using as few measurements as possible. We experimented with three different noise settings: noise-free, Gaussian noise, and scattering noise. The generation of the datasets is described in Section 2.2.

2. Dataset Description

For both datasets, the simulation model uses a 2D parallel beam geometry for the creation of the measurements. The attenuation of the X-rays is simulated using the Radon transform [10]

$$\mathcal{A}x(s,\varphi) := \int_{\mathbb{R}} x\left(s\begin{bmatrix}\cos(\varphi)\\ \sin(\varphi)\end{bmatrix} + t\begin{bmatrix}-\sin(\varphi)\\ \cos(\varphi)\end{bmatrix}\right) dt, \qquad (1)$$

where $s \in \mathbb{R}$ is the distance from the origin and $\varphi \in [0, \pi)$ the angle of the beam (cf. Figure 1). Mathematically, the image is transformed into a function of (s, φ). For each fixed angle φ the 2D image x is projected onto a line parameterized by s, namely the X-ray detector.

A detailed description of both datasets is given below. Their basic properties are also summarized in Table 1.

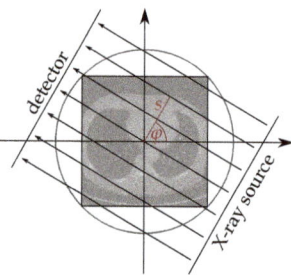

Figure 1. Parallel beam geometry. Adopted from [34].

Table 1. Settings of the low-dose parallel beam computed tomography (LoDoPaB-CT) and Apple CT datasets.

Property	LoDoPaB-CT	Apple CT
Subject	Human thorax	Apples
Scenario	low photon count	sparse-angle
Challenge	3678 reconstructions	100 reconstructions
Image size	362 px × 362 px	972 px × 972 px
Angles	1000	50, 10, 5, 2
Detector bins	513	1377
Sampling ratio	≈3.9	≈0.07–0.003

2.1. LoDoPaB-CT Dataset

The LoDoPaB-CT dataset [32] is a comprehensive collection of reference reconstructions and simulated low-dose measurements. It builds upon normal-dose thoracic CT scans from the LIDC/IDRI Database [33,35], whereby quality-assessed and processed 2D reconstructions are used as a ground truth. LoDoPaB features more than 40,000 scan slices from around 800 different patients. The dataset can be used for the training and evaluation of all kinds of reconstruction methods. LoDoPaB-CT has a predefined division into four parts, where each subset contains images from a distinct and randomly chosen set of patients. Three parts were used for training, validation and testing, respectively. It also contains a special challenge set with scans from 60 different patients. The ground truth images are undisclosed, and the patients are only included in this set. The challenge set is used for the evaluation of the model performance in this paper. Overall, the dataset contains 35,820 training images, 3522 validation images, 3553 test images and 3678 challenge images.

Low-intensity measurements suffer from an increased noise level. The main reason is so called quantum noise. It stems from the process of photon generation, attenuation and detection. The influence on the number of detected photons $\tilde{N}_1$ can be modeled, based on the mean photon count without attenuation N_0 and the Radon transform (1), by a Poisson distribution [36]

$$\tilde{N}_1(s, \varphi) \sim \text{Pois}(N_0 \exp(-\mathcal{A}x(s, \varphi))). \tag{2}$$

The model has to be discretized concerning s and φ for the simulation process. In this case, the Radon transform (1) becomes a finite-dimensional linear map $A : \mathbb{R}^n \to \mathbb{R}^m$, where n is the number of image pixels and m is the product of the number of detector pixels and the number of discrete angles. Together with the Poisson noise, the discrete simulation model is given by

$$Ax + \mathrm{e}(Ax) = y_\delta, \quad \mathrm{e}(Ax) = -Ax - \ln(\tilde{N}_1/N_0), \quad \tilde{N}_1 \sim \text{Pois}(N_0 \exp(-Ax)). \tag{3}$$

A single realization $y_\delta \in \mathbb{R}^m$ of y_δ is observed for each ground truth image, $x = x^\dagger \in \mathbb{R}^n$. After the simulation according to (3), all data pairs $(y_\delta, x^\dagger)$ have been divided by

$\mu_{\max} = 81.35858$ to normalize the image values to the range $[0, 1]$. In the following sections, y_θ, y_δ and $x^\dagger$ denote the normalized values.

The LoDoPaB ground truth images have a resolution of 362 px × 362 px on a domain of size 26 cm × 26 cm. The scanning setup consists of 513 equidistant detector pixels s spanning the image diameter and 1000 equidistant angles φ between 0 and π. The mean photon count per detector pixel without attenuation is $N_0 = 4096$. The sampling ratio between the size of the measurements and the images is around 3.9 (oversampling case).

2.2. Apple CT Datasets

The Apple CT datasets [37] are a collection of ground truth reconstructions and simulated parallel beam data with various noise types and angular range sampling. The data is intended for benchmarking different algorithms and is particularly suited for use in deep learning settings due to the large number of slices available.

A total of 94 apples were scanned at the Flex-Ray Laboratory [8] using a point-source circular cone-beam acquisition setup. High quality ground truth reconstructions were obtained using a full rotation with an angular resolution of 0.005 rad and a spatial resolution of 54.2 μm. A collection of 1D parallel beam data for more than 70,000 slices were generated using the simulation model in Equation (1). A total of 50 projections were generated over an angular range of $[0, \pi)$, each of size 1 × 1377. The Apple CT ground truth images have a resolution of 972 px × 972 px. In order to make the angular sampling even sparser, we also reduced the data to include only 10, 5 and 2 angles. The angular sampling ranges are shown in Figure 2.

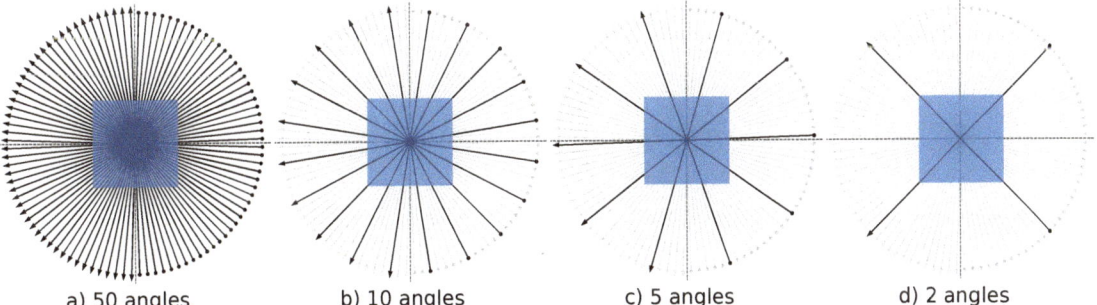

Figure 2. The angular sampling ranges employed for sparse image reconstructions for (**a**) 50 (full), (**b**) 10 (subset of 50 angles), (**c**) 5 (subset of 50 angles) and (**d**) 2 angles (subset of 10 angles). The black arrows show the position of the X-ray source (dot) and the position of the detector (arrowhead). For the sparse-angle scenario, the unused angles are shown in light gray.

The noise-free simulated data (henceforth Dataset A) were corrupted with 5% Gaussian noise to create Dataset B. Dataset C was generated by adding an imitation of scattering to Dataset A. Scattering intensity in a pixel u' is computed according to the formula

$$S(u') = \int_{u \in \mathbb{R}^2} G(u) \exp\left[-\frac{(u-u')^2}{2\sigma_1(u)^2}\right] + H(u) \exp\left[-\frac{(u-u')^2}{2\sigma_2(u)^2}\right], \quad (4)$$

where $|u - u'|$ is a distance between pixels, and scattering is approximated as a combination of Gaussian blurs with scaling factors G and H, standard deviations σ_1 and σ_2. Scattering noise in the target pixel u' contains contributions from all image pixels u as sources of scattering. Gaussian blur parameters depend on the X-ray absorption in the source pixel. To sample functions $G(u)$, $H(u)$, $\sigma_1(u)$ and $\sigma_2(u)$, a Monte Carlo simulation was performed for different thicknesses of water that was chosen as a material close to apple flesh. Furthermore, scaling factors $G(u)$ and $H(u)$ were increased to create a more challenging problem. We note that due to the computational complexity required, the number of slices on which the scattering model is applied is limited to 7520 (80 slices per apple), meaning the scattering training subset is smaller.

The Apple CT datasets consist of apple slices with and without internal defects. Internal defects were observed to be of four main types: bitter pit, holes, rot and browning. A reconstruction of a healthy apple slice and one with bitter pit is shown in Figure 3 as examples. Each Apple CT dataset was divided into training and test subsets using an empirical bias elimination method to ensure that apples in both subsets had similar defect statistics. This process is detailed in [38].

For the network training, the noise-free and Gaussian noise training subsets are further split into 44,647 training and 5429 validation samples, and the scattering training subset is split into 5280 training and 640 validation samples.

From the test subsets, 100 test slices were extracted in a similar manner like for the split in training and test subsets. All evaluations in this paper refer to these 100 test slices in order to keep the reconstruction time and storage volume within reasonable limits. Five slices were extracted from each of the 20 test apples such that in total each defect type is occurring with a pixel count ratio similar to its ratio on the full test subset. Additionally, the extracted slices have a pairwise distance of at least 15 slices in order to improve the image diversity. The selected list of slices is specified in the supplementing repository [39] as file supp_material/apples/test_samples_ids.csv.

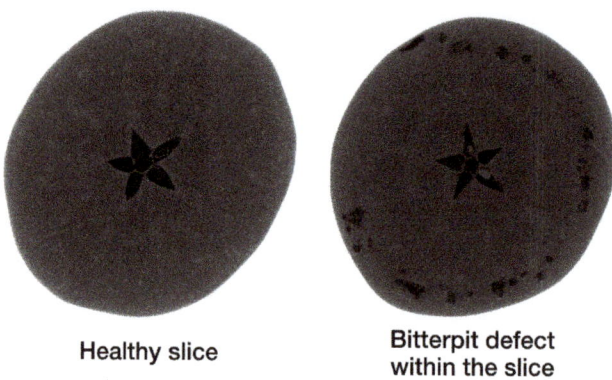

Healthy slice

Bitterpit defect within the slice

Figure 3. A horizontal cross-section of a healthy slice in an apple is shown on the **left**, and another cross-section with the bitter pit defects in the same apple on the **right**.

3. Algorithms

A variety of learned reconstruction methods were used to create a benchmark. The selection is based on methods submitted by participants for the data challenge on the LoDoPaB-CT and Apple CT datasets. The reconstruction methods include unrolled architectures, post-processing approaches, and fully-learned methods. Furthermore, classical methods such as FBP, TV regularization and CGLS were used as a baseline.

3.1. Learned Reconstruction Methods

In this section, the learned methods included in the benchmark are presented. An overview of the hyperparameters and pseudocode can be found in Appendix A. All methods utilize artificial neural networks F_Θ, each in different roles, for the reconstruction process.

Learning refers to the adaption of the parameters Θ for the reconstruction process in a data-driven manner. In general, one can divide this process into supervised and unsupervised learning. Almost all methods in this comparison are trained in a supervised way. This means that sample pairs $(y_\delta, x^\dagger)$ of noisy measurements and ground truth data are used for the optimization of the parameters, for example, by minimizing some discrepancy $\mathcal{D}_X : X \times X \to \mathbb{R}$ between the output of the reconstruction model $\mathcal{T}_{F_\Theta}$ and the ground truth

$$\min_{\Theta} \mathcal{D}_X\left(\mathcal{T}_{F_\Theta}(y_\delta), x^\dagger\right). \qquad (5)$$

Supervised methods often provide excellent results, but the number of required ground truth data can be high [34]. While the acquisition of ground truth images is infeasible in many applications, this is not a problem in the low-dose and sparse-angle case. Here, reconstructions of regular (normal-dose, full-angle) scans play the role of the reference.

3.1.1. Post-Processing

Post-processing approaches aim to improve the reconstruction quality of an existing method. When used in computed tomography, FBP (cf. Appendix B.1) is often used to obtain an initial reconstruction. Depending on the scan scenario, the FBP reconstruction can be noisy or contain artifacts. Therefore, it functions as an input for a learned post-processing method. This setting simplifies the task because the post-processing network $F_\Theta : X \to X$ maps directly from the target domain into the target domain

$$\hat{x} := [F_\Theta \circ \mathcal{T}_{\text{FBP}}](y_\delta).$$

Convolutional neural networks (CNN) have successfully been used in recent works to remove artifacts and noise from FBP reconstructions. Four of these CNN post-processing approaches were used for the benchmark. The U-Net architecture [40] is a popular choice in many different applications and was also used for CT reconstruction [20]. The details of the network used in the comparison can be found in Appendix A.2. The U-Net++ [41] (cf. Appendix A.3) and ISTA U-Net [42] (cf. Appendix A.6) represent modifications of this approach. In addition, a mixed-scale dense (MS-D)-CNN [21] is included, which has a different architecture (cf. Appendix A.4). Like for the U-Net, one can consider to adapt other architectures originally used for segmentation, for example, the ENET [43], for the post-processing task.

3.1.2. Fully Learned

The goal of fully learned methods is to extract the structure of the inversion process from data. In this case, the neural network $F_\Theta : Y \to X$ directly maps from the measurement space Y to the target domain X. A prominent example is the AUTOMAP architecture [27], which was successfully used for reconstruction in magnetic resonance imaging (MRI). The main building blocks consist of fully-connected layers. This makes the network design very general, but the number of parameters can grow quickly with the data dimension. For example, a single fully-connected layer mapping from Y to X on the LoDoPaB-CT dataset (cf. Section 2.1) would require over $1000 \times 513 \times 362^2 \approx 67 \times 10^9$ parameters.

Adapted model designs exist for large CT data. They include knowledge about the inversion process in the structure of the network. He et al. [28] introduced an adapted two-part approach, called iRadonMap. The first part uses small fully-connected layers with parameter sharing to reproduce the structure of the FBP. This is followed by a post-processing network in the second part. Another approach is the iCT-Net [29], which uses convolutions in combination with fully-connected layers for the inversion. An extended version of the iCT-Net, called iCTU-Net, is part of our comparison and a detailed description can be found in Appendix A.8.

3.1.3. Learned Iterative Schemes

Similar to the fully learned approach, learned iterative methods also define a mapping directly from the measurement space Y to the target domain X. The idea in this case is that the network architecture is inspired by an analytic reconstruction operator $\mathcal{T} : Y \to X$ implicitly defined by an iterative scheme. The basic principle of unrolling can be explained by the example of learned gradient descent (see e.g., [17]). Let $J(\cdot, y_\delta) : X \to \mathbb{R}$ be a smooth data discrepancy term and, possibly an additional regularization term. For an initial value $x^{[0]}$ the gradient descent is defined via the iteration

$$x^{[k+1]} = x^{[k]} - \omega_k \nabla_x J\left(x^{[k]}, y_\delta\right),$$

with a step size ω_k. Unrolling these iteration and stopping after K iterations, we can write the K-th iteration as

$$\mathcal{T}(y_\delta) := (\Lambda_{\omega_K} \circ \ldots \circ \Lambda_{\omega_1})(x^{[0]})$$

with $\Lambda_{\omega_k} := \mathrm{id} - \omega_k \nabla_x J(\cdot, y_\delta)$. In a learned iteration scheme, the operators Λ_{ω_k} are replaced by neural networks. As an example of a learned iterative procedure, learned primal-dual [19] was included in the comparison. A description of this method can be found in the Appendix A.1.

3.1.4. Generative Approach

The goal of the statistical approach to inverse problems is to determine the conditional distribution of the parameters given measured data. This statistical approach is often linked to Bayes' theorem [44]. In this Bayesian approach to inverse problems, the conditional distribution $p(x|y_\delta)$, called the posterior distribution, is supposed to be estimated. Based on this posterior distribution, different estimators, such as the maximum a posterior solution or the conditional mean, can be used as a reconstruction for the CT image. This theory provides a natural way to model the noise behavior and to integrate prior information into the reconstruction process. There are two different approaches that have been used for CT. Adler et al. [45] use a conditional variant of a generative adversarial network (GAN, [46]) to generate samples from the posterior. In contrast to this likelihood free approach, Ardizzone et al. [47] designed a conditional variant of invertible neural networks to directly estimate the posterior distribution. These conditional invertible neural networks (CINN) were also applied to the reconstruction of CT images [48]. The CINN was included for this benchmark. For a more detailed description, see Appendix A.5.

3.1.5. Unsupervised Methods

Unsupervised reconstruction methods just make use of the noisy measurements. They are favorable in applications where ground truth data is not available. The parameters of the model are chosen based on some discrepancy $\mathcal{D}_Y : Y \times Y \to \mathbb{R}$ between the output of the method and the measurements, for example,

$$\min_{\Theta} \mathcal{D}_Y\left(\mathcal{A} \mathcal{T}_{F_\Theta}(\cdot), y_\delta\right). \tag{6}$$

In this example, the output of $\mathcal{T}_{F_\Theta}$ plays the role of the reconstruction $\hat{x}$. However, comparing the distance just in the measurement domain can be problematic. This applies in particular to ill-posed reconstruction problems. For example, if the forward operator $\mathcal{A}$ is not bijective, no/multiple reconstruction(s) might match the measurement perfectly (ill-posed in the sense of Hadamard [49]). Another problem can occur for forward operators with an unstable inversion, where small differences in the measurement space, for example, due to noise, can result in arbitrary deviations in the reconstruction domain (ill-posed in the sense of Nashed [50]). In general, the minimization problem (6) is combined with some kind of regularization to mitigate these problems.

The optimization Formulation (6) is also used for the deep image prior (DIP) approach. DIP takes a special role among all neural network methods. The parameters are not determined on a dedicated training set, but during the reconstruction on the challenge data. This is done for each reconstruction separately. One could argue that the DIP approach is therefore not a learned method in the classical sense. The DIP approach, in combination with total variation regularization, was successfully used for CT reconstruction [34]. It is part of the comparison on the LoDoPaB dataset in this paper. A detailed description is given in Appendix A.7.

3.2. Classical Reconstruction Methods

In addition to the learned methods, we implemented the popularly used direct and iterative reconstruction methods, henceforth referred to as classical methods. They can often be described as a variational approach

$$\mathcal{T}(y_\delta) \in \arg\min_x \mathcal{D}_Y(\mathcal{A}x, y_\delta) + \alpha \mathcal{R}(x),$$

where $\mathcal{D}_Y : Y \times Y \to \mathbb{R}$ is a data discrepancy and $\mathcal{R} : X \to \mathbb{R}$ is a regularizer. In this context $\mathcal{T} : Y \to X$ defines the reconstruction operator. The included methods in the benchmark are filtered back-projection (FBP) [10,51], conjugate gradient least squares (CGLS) [52,53] and anisotropic total variation minimization (TV) [54]. Detailed description of each classical method along with pseudocode are given in Appendix B.

4. Evaluation Methodology

4.1. Evaluation Metrics

Two widely used evaluation metrics were used to assess the performance of the methods.

4.1.1. Peak Signal-to-Noise Ratio

The peak signal-to-noise ratio (PSNR) is measured by a log-scaled version of the mean squared error (MSE) between the reconstruction $\hat{x}$ and the ground truth image $x^\dagger$. PSNR expresses the ratio between the maximum possible image intensity and the distorting noise

$$\text{PSNR}\left(\hat{x}, x^\dagger\right) := 10 \log_{10}\left(\frac{L^2}{\text{MSE}(\hat{x}, x^\dagger)}\right), \quad \text{MSE}\left(\hat{x}, x^\dagger\right) := \frac{1}{n}\sum_{i=1}^{n}\left|\hat{x}_i - x_i^\dagger\right|^2. \quad (7)$$

In general, higher PSNR values are an indication of a better reconstruction. The maximum image value L can be chosen in different ways. In our study, we report two different values that are commonly used:

- **PSNR**: In this case $L = \max(x^\dagger) - \min(x^\dagger)$, that is, the difference between the highest and lowest entry in $x^\dagger$. This allows for a PSNR value that is adapted to the range of the current ground truth image. The disadvantage is that the PSNR is image-dependent in this case.
- **PSNR-FR**: The same fixed L is chosen for all images. It is determined as the maximum entry computed over all training ground truth images, that is, $L = 1.0$ for LoDoPaB-CT and $L = 0.0129353$ for the Apple CT datasets. This can be seen as an (empirical) upper limit of the intensity range in the ground truth. In general, a fixed L is preferable because the scaling of the metric is image-independent in this case. This allows for a direct comparison of PSNR values calculated on different images. The downside for most CT applications is, that high values ($\hat{=}$ dense material) are not present in every scan. Therefore, the results can be too optimistic for these scans. However, based on Equation (7), all mean PSNR-FR values can be directly converted for another fixed choice of L.

4.1.2. Structural Similarity

The structural similarity (SSIM) [55] compares the overall image structure of ground truth and reconstruction. It is based on assumptions about the human visual perception.

Results lie in the range $[0,1]$, with higher values being better. The SSIM is computed through a sliding window at M locations

$$\text{SSIM}(\hat{x}, x^\dagger) := \frac{1}{M} \sum_{j=1}^{M} \frac{(2\hat{\mu}_j \mu_j + C_1)(2\Sigma_j + C_2)}{(\hat{\mu}_j^2 + \mu_j^2 + C_1)(\hat{\sigma}_j^2 + \sigma_j^2 + C_2)}. \tag{8}$$

In the formula above $\hat{\mu}_j$ and μ_j are the average pixel intensities, $\hat{\sigma}_j$ and σ_j the variances and Σ_j the covariance of $\hat{x}$ and $x^\dagger$ at the j-th local window. Constants $C_1 = (K_1 L)^2$ and $C_2 = (K_2 L)^2$ stabilize the division. Following Wang et al. [55] we choose $K_1 = 0.01$ and $K_2 = 0.03$ and a window size of 7×7. In accordance with the PSNR metric, results for the two different choices for L are reported as SSIM and SSIM-FR (cf. Section 4.1.1).

4.1.3. Data Discrepancy

Checking data consistency, that is, the discrepancy $\mathcal{D}_Y(A\hat{x}, y_\delta)$ between the forward-projected reconstruction and the measurement, can provide additional insight into the performance of the reconstruction methods. Since noisy data is used for the comparison, an ideal method would yield a data discrepancy that is close to the present noise level.

Poisson Regression Loss on LoDoPaB-CT Dataset

For the Poisson noise model used by LoDoPaB-CT, an equivalent to the negative log-likelihood is calculated to evaluate the data consistency. It is conventional to employ the negative log-likelihood for this task, since minimizing the data discrepancy is equivalent to determining a maximum likelihood (ML) estimate (cf. Section 5.5 in [56] or Section 2.4 in [17]). Each element $y_{\delta,j}$, $j = 1, \ldots, m$, of a measurement y_δ, obtained according to (3) and subsequently normalized by μ_max, is associated with an independent Poisson model of a photon count $\tilde{N}_{1,j}$ with

$$\mathbb{E}(\tilde{N}_{1,j}) = \mathbb{E}(N_0 \exp(-y_{\delta,j} \mu_\text{max})) = N_0 \exp(-y_j \mu_\text{max}),$$

where y_j is a parameter that should be estimated [36]. A Poisson regression loss for y is obtained by summing the negative log-likelihoods for all measurement elements and omitting constant parts,

$$-\ell_\text{Pois}(y \mid y_\delta) = -\sum_{j=1}^{m} N_0 \exp(-y_{\delta,j} \mu_\text{max})(-y_j \mu_\text{max} + \ln(N_0)) - N_0 \exp(-y_j \mu_\text{max}), \tag{9}$$

with each $y_{\delta,j}$ being the only available realization of $y_{\delta,j}$. In order to evaluate the likelihood-based loss (9) for a reconstructed image $\hat{x}$ given y_δ, the forward projection $A\hat{x}$ is passed for y.

Mean Squared Error on Apple CT Data

On the Apple CT datasets we consider the mean squared error (MSE) data discrepancy,

$$\text{MSE}_Y(y, y_\delta) = \frac{1}{m} \|y - y_\delta\|_2^2. \tag{10}$$

For an observation y_δ with Gaussian noise (Dataset B), this data discrepancy term is natural, as it is a scaled and shifted version of the negative log-likelihood of y given y_δ. In this noise setting, a good reconstruction usually should not achieve an MSE less than the variance of the Gaussian noise, that is, $\text{MSE}_Y(A\hat{x}, y_\delta) \geq [0.05 \frac{1}{m} \sum_{j=1}^{m} (Ax^\dagger)_j]^2$. This can be motivated intuitively by the conception that a reconstruction that achieves a smaller MSE than the expected MSE of the ground truth probably fits the noise rather than the actual data of interest.

In the setting of y_δ being noise-free (Dataset A), the MSE of ideal reconstructions would be zero. On the other hand the MSE being zero does not imply that the reconstruction matches the ground truth image because of the sparse-angle setting. Further, the MSE can not be used to judge reconstruction quality directly, as crucial differences in image domain may not be equally pronounced in the sinogram domain.

For the scattering observations (Dataset C), the MSE data discrepancy is considered, too, for simplicity.

4.2. Training Procedure

While the reconstruction process with learned methods usually is efficient, their training is more resource consuming. This limits the practicability of large hyperparameter searches. It can therefore be seen as a drawback of a learned reconstruction method if they require very specific hyperparameter choices for different tasks. As a result, it benefits a fair comparison to minimize the amount of hyperparameter searches. In general, default parameters, for example, from the original publications of the respective method, were used as a starting point. For some of the methods, good choices had been determined for the LoDoPaB-CT dataset first (cf. [34]) and were kept similar for the experiments on the Apple CT datasets. Further searches were only performed if required to obtain reasonable results. More details regarding the individual methods can be found in Appendix A. For the classical methods, hyperparameters were optimized individually for each setting of the Apple CT datasets (cf. Appendix B).

Most learned methods are trained using the mean squared error (MSE) loss. The exceptions are the U-Net++ using a loss combining MSE and SSIM, the iCTU-Net using an SSIM loss for the Apple CT datasets, and the CINN for which negative log-likelihood (NLL) and an MSE term are combined (see Appendix A for more details). Training curves for the trainings on the Apple CT datasets are shown in Appendix D. While we consider the convergence to be sufficient, continuing some of the trainings arguably would slightly improve the network. However, this mainly can be expected for those methods which are comparably time consuming to train (approximately 2 weeks for 20 epochs), in which case the limited number of epochs can be considered a fair regulation of resource usage.

Early stopping based on the validation performance is used for all trainings except for the ISTA U-Net on LoDoPaB-CT and for the iCTU-Net.

Source code is publicly available in a supplementing github repository [39]. Further records hosted by Zenodo provide the trained network parameters for the experiments on the Apple CT Datasets [57], as well as the submitted LoDoPaB-CT Challenge reconstructions [58] and the Apple CT test reconstructions of the 100 selected slices in all considered settings [59]. Source code and network parameters for some of the LoDoPaB-CT experiments are included in the DIVαℓ library [60], for others the original authors provide public repositories containing source code and/or parameters.

5. Results

5.1. LoDoPaB-CT Dataset

Ten different reconstruction methods were evaluated on the challenge set of the LoDoPaB-CT dataset. Reconstructions from these methods were either submitted as part of the CT Code Sprint 2020 (http://dival.math.uni-bremen.de/code_sprint_2020/, last accessed: 1 March 2021) (15 June–31 August 2020) or in the period after the event (1 September–31 December 2020).

5.1.1. Reconstruction Performance

In order to assess the quality of the reconstructions, the PSNR and the SSIM were calculated. The results from the official challenge website (https://lodopab.grand-challenge.org/, last accessed: 1 March 2021) are shown in Table 2. The differences between the learned methods are generally small. Notably, learned primal-dual yields the best performance with respect to both the PSNR and the SSIM. The following places are occupied by post-processing approaches, also with only minor differences in terms of the metrics. Of the other methods, DIP + TV stands out, with relatively good results for an unsupervised method. DIP + TV is able to beat the supervised method iCTU-Net. The classical reconstruction models perform the worst of all methods. In particular, the performance of FBP shows a clear gap with the other methods. While learned primal-dual performs slightly better than the post-processing methods, the difference is not as significant as one could expect, considering that it incorporates the forward operator directly in the network. This could be explained by the beneficial combination of the convolutional architectures used for the post-processing, which are observed to perform well on a number of image processing tasks, and a sufficient number of available training samples. Otero et al. [34] investigated the influence of the size of the training dataset on the performance of different learned procedures on the LoDoPaB-CT dataset. Here, a significant difference is seen between learned primal-dual and other learned procedures when only a small subset of the training data is used.

Table 2. Results on the LoDoPaB-CT challenge set. Methods are ranked by their overall performance. The highest value for each metric is highlighted. All values are taken from the official challenge leaderboard https://lodopab.grand-challenge.org/evaluation/challenge/leaderboard/ (accessed on 4 January 2021).

Model	PSNR	PSNR-FR	SSIM	SSIM-FR	Number of Parameters
Learned P.-D.	36.25 ± 3.70	40.52 ± 3.64	0.866 ± 0.115	0.926 ± 0.076	874,980
ISTA U-Net	36.09 ± 3.69	40.36 ± 3.65	0.862 ± 0.120	0.924 ± 0.080	83,396,865
U-Net	36.00 ± 3.63	40.28 ± 3.59	0.862 ± 0.119	0.923 ± 0.079	613,322
MS-D-CNN	35.85 ± 3.60	40.12 ± 3.56	0.858 ± 0.122	0.921 ± 0.082	181,306
U-Net++	35.37 ± 3.36	39.64 ± 3.40	0.861 ± 0.119	0.923 ± 0.080	9,170,079
CINN	35.54 ± 3.51	39.81 ± 3.48	0.854 ± 0.122	0.919 ± 0.081	6,438,332
DIP + TV	34.41 ± 3.29	38.68 ± 3.29	0.845 ± 0.121	0.913 ± 0.082	hyperp.
iCTU-Net	33.70 ± 2.82	37.97 ± 2.79	0.844 ± 0.120	0.911 ± 0.081	147,116,792
TV	33.36 ± 2.74	37.63 ± 2.70	0.830 ± 0.121	0.903 ± 0.082	(hyperp.)
FBP	30.19 ± 2.55	34.46 ± 2.18	0.727 ± 0.127	0.836 ± 0.085	(hyperp.)

5.1.2. Visual Comparison

A representative reconstruction of all learned methods and the classical baseline is shown in Figure 4 to enable a qualitative comparison of the methods. An area of interest around the spine is magnified to compare the reproduction of small details and the sharpness of edges in the image. Some visual differences can be observed between the reconstructions. The learned methods produce somewhat smoother reconstructions in comparison to the ground truth. A possible explanations for the smoothness is the minimization of the empirical risk with respect to some variant of the $L2$-loss during the training of most learned methods, which has an averaging effect. The convolutional architecture of the networks can also have an impact. Adequate regularization during training and/or inference can be beneficial in this case (cf. Section 6.2.2 for a suitable class of regularizers). Additionally, the DIP + TV reconstruction appears blurry, which can be explained by the fact that it is the only unsupervised method in this comparison and thus has no access to ground truth data. The U-Net and the two modifications, U-Net++ and ISTA U-Net, show only slight visual differences on this example image.

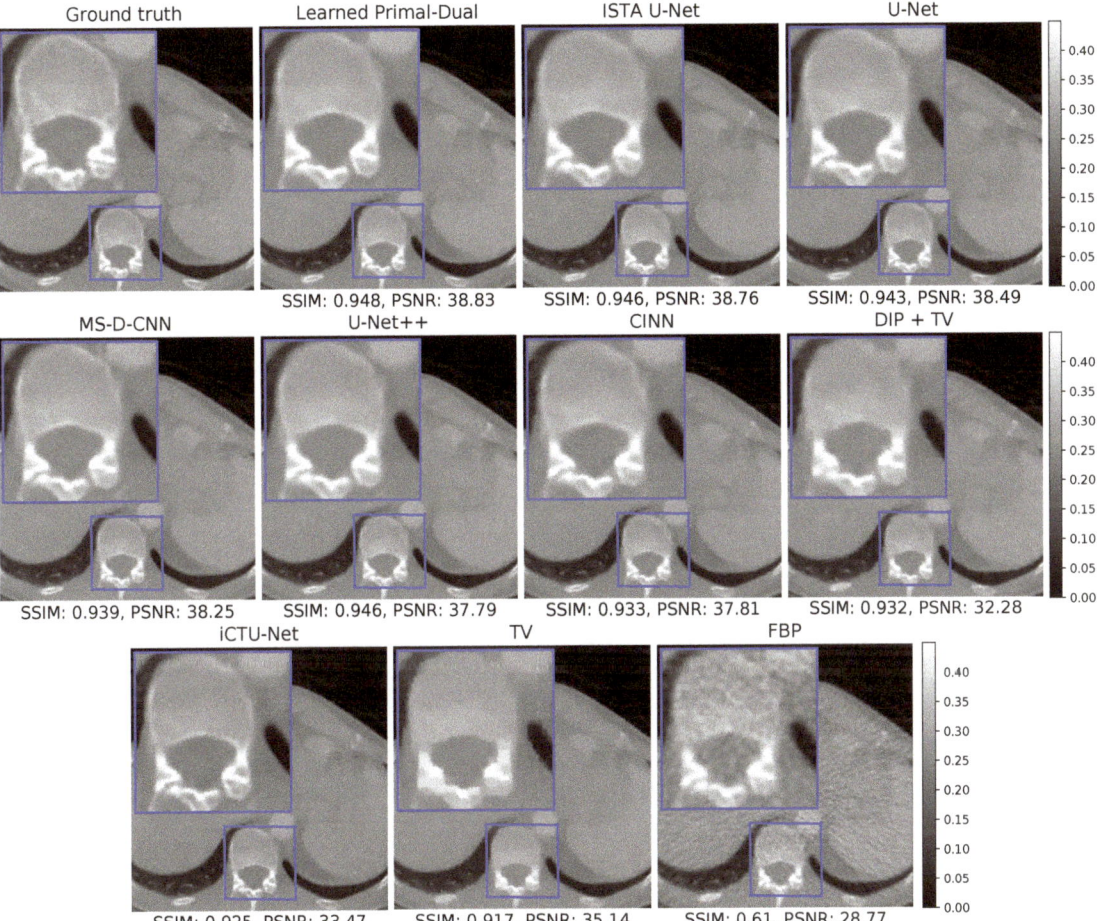

Figure 4. Reconstructions on the challenge set from the LoDoPaB-CT dataset. The window [0, 0.45] corresponds to a HU range of ≈ [−1001, 831].

5.1.3. Data Consistency

The mean data discrepancy of all methods is shown in Figure 5, plotted against their reconstruction performance. The mean difference between the noise-free and noisy measurements is included as a reference. Good-performing models should be close to this empirical noise level. Values above the mean can indicate a sub-optimal data consistency, while values below can be a sign of overfitting to the noise. A data consistency term is only explicitly used in the TV and DIP + TV model. Nevertheless, the mean data discrepancy for most of the methods is close to the empirical noise level. The only visible outliers are the FBP and the iCTU-Net. A list of all mean data discrepancy values, including standard deviations, can be found in Table 3.

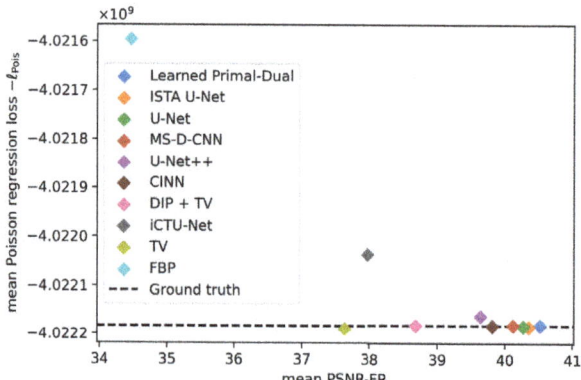

Figure 5. Mean data discrepancy $-\ell_{\text{Pois}}$ between the noisy measurements and the forward-projected reconstructions, respectively the noise-free measurements. Evaluation is done on the LoDoPaB challenge images.

Table 3. Mean and standard deviation of data discrepancy $-\ell_{\text{Pois}}$. Evaluation is done on the LoDoPaB challenge images.

Method	$-\ell_{\text{Pois}}(A\hat{x}\,|\,y_\delta)/10^9$
Learned Primal-Dual	-4.022182 ± 0.699460
ISTA U-Net	-4.022185 ± 0.699461
U-Net	-4.022185 ± 0.699460
MS-D-CNN	-4.022182 ± 0.699460
U-Net++	-4.022163 ± 0.699461
CINN	-4.022184 ± 0.699460
DIP + TV	-4.022183 ± 0.699466
iCTU-Net	-4.022038 ± 0.699430
TV	-4.022189 ± 0.699463
FBP	-4.021595 ± 0.699282
	$-\ell_{\text{Pois}}(Ax^\dagger\,|\,y_\delta)/10^9$
Ground truth	-4.022184 ± 0.699461

5.2. Apple CT Datasets

A total of 6 different learned methods were evaluated on the Apple CT data. This set included post-processing methods (MS-D-CNN, U-Net, ISTA U-Net), learned iterative methods (learned primal-dual), fully learned approaches (iCTU-Net), and generative models (CINN). As described in Section 2.2, different noise cases (noise-free, Gaussian noise and scattering noise) and different numbers of angles (50, 10, 5, 2) were used. In total, each model was trained on the 12 different settings of the Apple CT dataset. In addition to the learned methods, three classical techniques, namely CGLS, TV, and FBP, have been included as a baseline.

5.2.1. Reconstruction Performance

A subset of 100 data samples from the test set was selected for the evaluation (cf. Section 2.2). The mean PSNR and SSIM values for all experiments can be found in Table 4. Additionally, Tables A3–A5 in the appendix provide standard deviations and PSNR-FR and SSIM-FR values.

Table 4. Peak signal-to-noise ratio (PSNR) and structural similarity (SSIM) (adapted to the data range of each ground truth image) for the different noise settings on the Apple CT datasets. Best results are highlighted in gray. See Figures A7 and A8 for a visualization.

Noise-Free	PSNR				SSIM			
Number of Angles	50	10	5	2	50	10	5	2
Learned Primal-Dual	38.72	35.85	30.79	22.00	0.901	0.870	0.827	0.740
ISTA U-Net	38.86	34.54	28.31	20.48	0.897	0.854	0.797	0.686
U-Net	39.62	33.51	27.77	19.78	0.913	0.803	0.803	0.676
MS-D-CNN	39.85	34.38	28.45	20.55	0.913	0.837	0.776	0.646
CINN	39.59	34.84	27.81	19.46	0.913	0.871	0.762	0.674
iCTU-Net	36.07	29.95	25.63	19.28	0.878	0.847	0.824	0.741
TV	39.27	29.00	22.04	15.95	0.915	0.783	0.607	0.661
CGLS	33.05	21.81	12.60	15.25	0.780	0.619	0.537	0.615
FBP	30.39	17.09	15.51	13.97	0.714	0.584	0.480	0.438

Gaussian Noise	PSNR				SSIM			
Number of Angles	50	10	5	2	50	10	5	2
Learned Primal-Dual	36.62	33.76	29.92	21.41	0.878	0.850	0.821	0.674
ISTA U-Net	36.04	33.55	28.48	20.71	0.871	0.851	0.811	0.690
U-Net	36.48	32.83	27.80	19.86	0.882	0.818	0.789	0.706
MS-D-CNN	36.67	33.20	27.98	19.88	0.883	0.831	0.748	0.633
CINN	36.77	31.88	26.57	19.99	0.888	0.771	0.722	0.637
iCTU-Net	32.90	29.76	24.67	19.44	0.848	0.837	0.801	0.747
TV	32.36	27.12	21.83	16.08	0.833	0.752	0.622	0.637
CGLS	27.36	21.09	14.90	15.11	0.767	0.624	0.553	0.616
FBP	27.88	17.09	15.51	13.97	0.695	0.583	0.480	0.438

Scattering Noise	PSNR				SSIM			
Number of Angles	50	10	5	2	50	10	5	2
Learned Primal-Dual	37.80	34.19	27.08	20.98	0.892	0.866	0.796	0.540
ISTA U-Net	35.94	32.33	27.41	19.95	0.881	0.820	0.763	0.676
U-Net	34.96	32.91	26.93	18.94	0.830	0.784	0.736	0.688
MS-D-CNN	38.04	33.51	27.73	20.19	0.899	0.818	0.757	0.635
CINN	38.56	34.08	28.04	19.14	0.915	0.863	0.839	0.754
iCTU-Net	26.26	22.85	21.25	18.32	0.838	0.796	0.792	0.765
TV	21.09	20.14	17.86	14.53	0.789	0.649	0.531	0.611
CGLS	20.84	18.28	14.02	14.18	0.789	0.618	0.547	0.625
FBP	21.01	15.80	14.26	13.06	0.754	0.573	0.475	0.433

The biggest challenge with the noise-free dataset is that the measurements become increasingly undersampled as the number of angles decreases. As expected, the reconstruction quality in terms of PSNR and SSIM deteriorates significantly as the number of angles decreases. In comparison with LoDoPaB-CT, no model performs best in all scenarios. Furthermore, most methods were trained to minimize the MSE between the output image and ground truth. The MSE is directly related to the PSNR. However, minimizing the MSE does not necessarily translate into a high SSIM. In many cases, the best method in terms of PSNR does not result in the best SSIM. These observations are also evident in the two noisy datasets. Noteworthy is the performance of the classical TV method on the noise-free dataset for 50 angles. This result is comparable to the best-performing learned methods, while the other classical approaches show a clear gap.

Noisy measurements, in addition to undersampling, present an additional difficulty on the Gaussian and scattering datasets. Intuitively, one would therefore expect a worse performance compared to the noise-free case. In general, a decrease in performance can be observed. However, this effect depends on the method and the noise itself. For example, the negative impact on classical methods is much more substantial for the scattering noise. In contrast, the learned methods often perform slightly worse on the Gaussian noise. There are also some outliers with higher values than on the noise-free set. Possible explanations are the hyperparameter choices and the stochastic nature of the model training. Overall, the learned approaches can reach similar performances on the noisy data, while the performance of classical methods drops significantly. An additional observation can be made when comparing the results between Gaussian and scattering noise. For Gaussian noise with 50 angles, all learned methods, except for the iCTU net, achieve a PSNR of at least 36 dB. In contrast, the variation on scattering noise with 50 angles is much larger. The CINN obtains a much higher PSNR of 38.56 dB than the post-processing U-Net with 34.96 dB.

As already observed on the LoDoPaB dataset, the post-processing methods (MS-D-CNN, U-Net and ISTA U-Net) show only minor differences in all noise cases. This could be explained by the fact that these methods are all trained with the same objective function and differ only in their architecture.

5.2.2. Visual Comparison

Figure 6 shows reconstructions from all learned methods for an apple slice with bitter pit. The decrease in quality with the decrease in the number of angles is clearly visible. For 2 angles, none of the methods are able to accurately recover the shape of the apple. The iCTU-Net reconstruction has sharp edges for the 2-angle case, while the other methods produce blurry reconstructions.

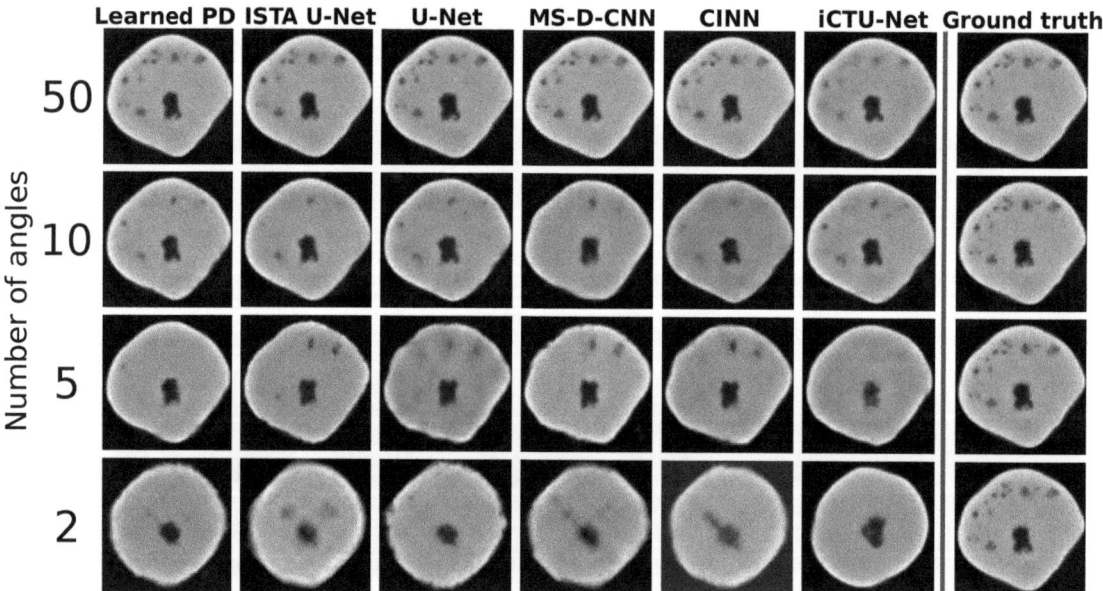

Figure 6. Visual overview of one apple slice with bitter pit for different learned methods. Evaluated on Gaussian noise. The quality of the reconstruction deteriorates very quickly for a reduced number of angles. For the 2-angle case, none of the methods can reconstruct the exact shape of the apple.

The inner structure, including the defects, is accurately reconstructed for 50 angles by all methods. The only exception is the iCTU-Net. Reconstructions from this network show a smooth interior of the apple. The other methods also result in the disappearance of smaller defects with fewer measurement angles. Nonetheless, a defect-detection system might still be able to sort out the apple based on the 5-angle reconstructions. The 2-angle case can be used to assess failure modes of the different approaches. The undersampling case is so severe that a lot of information is lost. However, the iCTU-Net is able to produce a smooth image of an apple, but it has few similarities with the ground truth apple. It appears that the models have memorized the roundness of an apple and produce a round apple that has little in common with the real apple except for its size and core.

5.2.3. Data Consistency

The data consistency is evaluated for all three Apple CT datasets. The MSE is used to measure the discrepancy. It is the canonical choice for measurements with Gaussian noise (cf. Section 4.1.3). Table A6 in the appendix contains all MSE values and standard deviations. Figure 7 shows the results depending on the number of angles for the noise-free and Gaussian noise dataset.

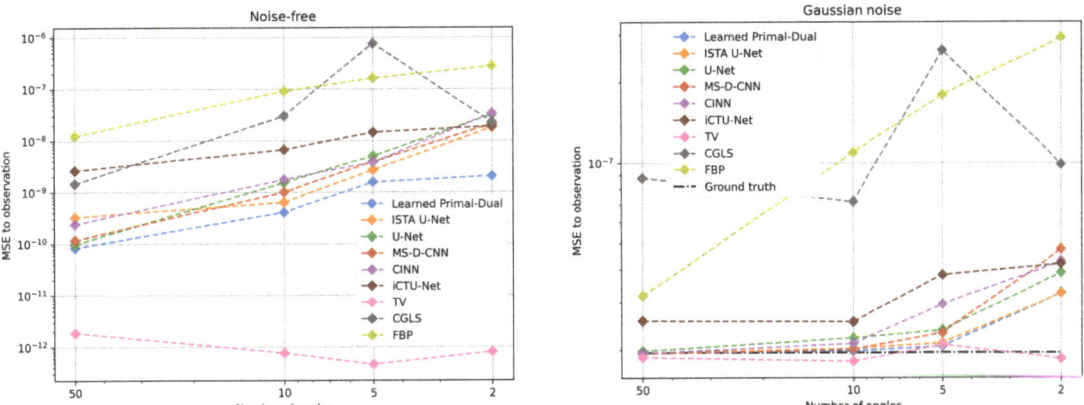

Figure 7. Mean squared error (MSE) data discrepancy between the measurements and the forward-projected reconstructions for the noise-free (**left**) and Gaussian noise (**right**) dataset. The MSE values are plotted against the number of angles used for the reconstruction. For the Gaussian dataset, the mean data discrepancy between noisy and noise-free measurements is given for reference. Evaluation is done on 100 Apple CT test images. See Table A6 for the exact values.

In the noise-free setup, the optimal MSE value is zero. Nonetheless, an optimal data consistency does not correspond to perfect reconstructions in this case. Due to the undersampling of the measurements, the discretized linear forward operator A has a non-trivial null space, that is, $\tilde{x} \in X$, apart from $\tilde{x} = 0$, for which $A\tilde{x} = 0$. Any element from the null space can be added to the true solution $x^\dagger$ without changing the data discrepancy

$$A\left(x^\dagger + \tilde{x}\right) = Ax^\dagger + A\tilde{x} = Ax^\dagger + 0 = Ax^\dagger = y.$$

In the Gaussian setup, the MSE between noise-free and noisy measurements is used as a reference for a good data discrepancy. The problem from the undersampling is also relevant in this setting.

Both setups show an increase in the data discrepancy with fewer measurement angles. The reason for the increase is presumably the growing number of deviations in the reconstructions. In the Gaussian noise setup, the high data discrepancy of all learned methods for 2 angles coincides with the poor reconstructions of the apple slice in Figure 6. Only the TV method, which enforces data consistency during the reconstruction, keeps a constant level. The main problem for this approach are the ambiguous solutions due to the undersampling. The TV method is not able to identify the correct solution given by the ground truth. Therefore, the PSNR and SSIM values are also decreasing.

Likewise, the data consistency was analyzed for the dataset with scattering noise. The MSE values of all learned methods are close to the empirical noise level. In contrast, FBP and TV have a much smaller discrepancy. Therefore, their reconstructions are most likely influenced by the scattering noise. An effect that is also reflected in the PSNR and SSIM values in Table 4.

6. Discussion

Among all the methods we compared, there is no definite winner that is the best on both LoDoPaB-CT and Apple CT. Learned primal-dual, as an example of a learned iterative method, is the best method on LoDoPaB-CT, in terms of both PSNR and SSIM, and also gives promising results on Apple CT. However, it should be noted that the differences in performance between the learned methods are relatively small. The ISTA U-Net, second place in terms of PSNR on LoDoPaB-CT, scores only 0.14 dB less than learned primal-dual. The performance in terms of SSIM is even closer on LoDoPaB-CT. The best performing learned method resulted in an SSIM that was only 0.022 higher than the last placed learned method. The observation that the top scoring learned methods did not differ greatly in terms of performance has also been noted in the fastMRI challenge [61]. In addition to the performance of the learned methods, other characteristics are also of interest.

6.1. Computational Requirements and Reconstruction Speed

When discussing the computational requirements of deep learning methods, it is important to distinguish between training and inference. Training usually requires significantly more processing power and memory. All outputs of intermediate layers have to be stored for the determination of the gradients during backpropagation. Inference is much faster and less resource-intensive. In both cases, the requirements are directly influenced by image size, network architecture and batch size.

A key feature and advantage of the learned iterative methods, post-processing methods and fully-learned approaches is the speed of reconstruction. Once the network is trained, the reconstruction can be obtained by a simple forward pass of the model. Since the CINN, being a generative model, draws samples from the posterior distribution, many forward passes are necessary to well approximate the mean or other moments. Therefore, the quality of the reconstruction may depend on the number of forward passes [48]. The DIP + TV method requires a separate model to be trained to obtain a reconstruction. As a result, reconstruction is very time-consuming and resource-intensive, especially on the 972 px × 972 px images in the Apple CT datasets. However, DIP + TV does not rely on a large, well-curated dataset of ground truth images and measurements. As an unsupervised method, only measurement data is necessary. The large size of the Apple CT images is also an issue for the other methods. In comparison to LoDoPaB-CT, the batch size had to be reduced significantly in order to train the learned models. This small batch size can cause instability in the training process, especially for CINN (cf. Figure A14).

Transfer to 3D Reconstruction

The reconstruction methods included in this study were evaluated based on the reconstruction of individual 2D slices. In real applications, however, the goal is often to obtain a 3D reconstruction of the volume. This can be realized with separate reconstructions of 2D slices, but (learned) methods might benefit from additional spatial information. On the other hand, a direct 3D reconstruction can have a high demand on the required computing power. This is especially valid when training neural networks.

One way to significantly reduce the memory consumption of backpropagation is to use invertible neural networks (INN). Due to the invertibility, the intermediate activations can be calculated directly and do not have to be stored in memory. INNs were successfully applied to 3D reconstructions tasks in MRI [62] and CT [63]. The CINN approach from our comparison can be adapted in a similar way for 3D data. In most post-processing methods, the U-Net can be replaced by an invertible iUnet, as proposed by Etmann et al. [63].

Another option is the simultaneous reconstruction of only a part of the volume. The information from multiple neighboring slices is used in this case, which is also referred to as 2.5D reconstruction. Networks that operate on this scenario usually have a mixture of 2D and 3D convolutional layers [64]. The goal is to strike a balance between the speed and memory advantage of the 2D scenario and the additional information from the third dimension. All deep learning methods included in this study would be suitable for 2.5D reconstruction with slight modifications to their network architecture.

Overall, 2.5D reconstruction can be seen as an intermediate step that can already be realized with many learned methods. The pure 3D case, on the other hand, requires specially adapted deep learning approaches. Technical innovations such as mixed floating point precision and increasing computing power may facilitate the transition in the coming years.

6.2. Impact of the Datasets

The type, composition and size of a dataset can have direct impact on the performance of the models. The observed effects can provide insight into how the models can be improved or how the results translate to other datasets.

6.2.1. Number of Training Samples

A large dataset is often required to successfully train deep learning methods. In order to assess the impact of the number of data pairs on the performance of the methods, we consider the Apple CT datasets. The scattering noise dataset (Dataset C), with 5280 training images, is only about 10% as large as the noise free dataset (Dataset A) and the Gaussian noise dataset (Dataset B). Here it can be noted that the iCTU net, as an example of a fully learned approach, performs significantly worse on this smaller dataset than on dataset A and dataset B (26.26 dB PSNR on Dataset C with 50 angles, 36.07 dB and 32.90 dB on Dataset A and Dataset B with 50 angles, respectively). This drop in performance could also be caused by the noise case. However, Baguer et al. [34] have already noted in their work that the performance of fully learned approaches heavily depends on the number of training images. This could be explained by the fact that fully learned methods need to infer most of the information about the inversion process purely from data. Unlike learned iterative methods, such as learned primal-dual, fully learned approaches do not incorporate the physical model. A drop in performance due to a smaller training set was not observed for the other learned methods. However, 5280 training images is still comprehensive. Baguer et al. [34] also investigated the low-data regime on LoDoPaB-CT, down to around 30 training samples. In their experiments, learned primal-dual worked well in this scenario, but was surpassed by the DIP + TV approach. The U-Net post-processing lined up between learned Primal-Dual and the fully learned method. Therefore, the amount of available training data should be considered when choosing a model. To enlarge the training set, the DIP + TV approach can also be used to generate pseudo ground truth data. Afterwards, a supervised method with a fast reconstruction speed can be trained to mimic the behavior of DIP + TV.

6.2.2. Observations on LoDoPaB-CT and Apple CT

The samples and CT setups differ greatly between the two datasets. The reconstructions obtained using the methods compared in this study reflect these differences to some extent, but there were also some effects that were observed for both datasets.

The sample reconstructions in Figures 4 and 6 show that most learned methods produce smooth images. The same observation can be made for TV, where smoothness is an integral part of the modeling. An extension by a suitable regularization can help to preserve edges in the reconstruction without the loss of small details, or the introduction of additional noise. One possibility is to use diffusion filtering [65], for example, variants of the Perona-Malik diffusion [66] in this role. Diffusion filtering was also successfully applied as a post-processing step for CT [67]. Whether smoothness of reconstructions is desired depends on the application and further use of the images, for example, visual or computer-aided diagnosis, screening, treatment planning, or abnormality detection. For the apple scans, a subsequent task could be the detection of internal defects for sorting them into different grades. The quality of the reconstructions deteriorates with the decreasing number of measurement angles. Due to increasing undersampling, the methods have to interpolate more and more information to find an adequate solution. The model output is thereby influenced by the training dataset.

The effects of severe undersampling can be observed in the 2-angle setup in Figure 6. All reconstructions of the test sample show a prototypical apple with a round shape and a core in the center. The internal defects are not reproduced. One explanation is that supervised training aims to minimize the empirical risk on the ground truth images. Therefore, only memorizing and reconstructing common features in the dataset, like the roundness and the core, can be optimal in some ways to minimize the empirical risk on severely undersampled training data. Abnormalities in the data, such as internal defects, are not captured in this case. This effect is subsequently transferred to the reconstruction of test data. Hence, special attention should be paid to the composition of the training data. As shown in the next Section 6.2.3, this is particularly important when the specific features of interest are not well represented in the training set.

In the 5-angle setup, all methods are able to accurately reconstruct the shape of the apple. Internal defects are partially recovered only by the post-processing methods and the CINN. These approaches all use FBP reconstructions as a starting point. Therefore, they rely on the information that is extracted by the FBP. This can be useful in the case of defects but aggravating for artifacts in the FBP reconstruction. The CINN approach has the advantage of sampling from the space of possible solutions and the evaluability of the likelihood under the model. This information can help to decide whether objects in the reconstruction are really present.

In contrast, Learned Primal-Dual and the iCTU-Net work directly on the measurements. They are more flexible with respect to the extraction of information. However, this also means that the training objective strongly influences which aspects of the measurements are important for the model. Tweaking the objective or combining the training of a reconstruction and a detection model, that is, end-to-end learning or task-driven reconstruction, might be able to increase the model performance in certain applications [68,69].

6.2.3. Robustness to Changes in the Scanning Setup

A known attribute of learned methods is that they can often only be applied to data similar to the training data. It is often unclear how a method trained in one setting generalizes to a different setting. In CT, such a situation could for example arise due to altered scan acquisition settings or application to other body regions. Switching between CT devices from different manufacturers can also have an impact.

As an example, we evaluated the U-Net on a different number of angles than it was trained on. The results of this experiment are shown in Table 5. In most setups the PSNR drops by at least 10 dB when evaluated on a different setting. In practice, the angular sampling pattern may change and it would be cumbersome to train a separate model for each pattern.

Table 5. Performance of a U-Net trained on the Apple CT dataset (scattering noise) and evaluated on different angular samplings. In general, a U-Net trained on a specific number of angles fails to produce good results on a different number of angles. PSNR and SSIM are calculated with image-dependent data range.

Training \ Evaluation	50 Angles		10 Angles		5 Angles		2 Angles	
	PSNR	SSIM	PSNR	SSIM	PSNR	SSIM	PSNR	SSIM
50 angles	39.62	0.913	16.39	0.457	11.93	0.359	8.760	0.252
10 angles	27.59	0.689	33.51	0.803	18.44	0.607	9.220	0.394
5 angles	24.51	0.708	26.19	0.736	27.77	0.803	11.85	0.549
2 angles	15.57	0.487	14.59	0.440	15.94	0.514	19.78	0.676

6.2.4. Generalization to Other CT Setups

The LoDoPaB-CT and Apple CT datasets were acquired by simulating parallel-beam measurements, based on the Radon transform. This setup facilitates large-scale experiments with many example images, whereas the underlying operators in the algorithms have straightforward generalizations to other geometries. Real-world applications of CT are typically more complex. For example, the standard scanning geometries in medical applications are helical fan-beam or cone-beam [36]. In addition, the simulation model does not cover all physical effects that may occur during scanning. For this reason, the results can only be indicative of performance on real data.

However, learned methods are known to adapt well to other setups when retrained from scratch on new samples. It is often not necessary to adjust the architecture for this purpose, other than by replacing the forward operator and its adjoint where they are involved. For example, most learned methods show good performance on the scattering observations, whereas the classical methods perform worse compared to the Gaussian noise setup. This can be explained by the fact that the effect of scattering is structured, which, although adding to the instability of the reconstruction problem, can be learned to be (partially) compensated for. In contrast, classical methods require the reconstruction model to be manually adjusted in order to incorporate knowledge about the scattering. If scattering is treated like an unknown distortion (i.e., a kind of noise), such as in our comparison, the classical assumption of pixel-wise independence of the noise is violated by the non-local structure of the scattering. Convolutional neural networks are able to capture these non-local effects.

6.3. Conformance of Image Quality Scores and Requirements in Real Applications

The goal in tomographic imaging is to provide the expert with adequate information through a clearly interpretable reconstructed image. In a medical setting, this can be an accurate diagnosis or plan for an operation; and in an industrial setting, the image may be used for detection and identification of faults or defects as part of quality control.

PSNR and SSIM, among other image quality metrics, are commonly used in publications and data challenges [61] to evaluate the quality of reconstructed medical images [70]. However, there can be cases in which PSNR and SSIM are in a disagreement. Although not a huge difference, the results given in Table 4 are a good example of this. This often leads to the discussion of which metric is better suited for a certain application. The PSNR expresses a pixel-wise difference between the reconstructed image and its ground truth, whereas the SSIM checks for local structural similarities (cf. Section 4.1). A common issue with both metrics is that a local inaccuracy in the reconstructed image, such as a small artifact, would only have a minor influence on the final assessment. The effect of the artifact is further downplayed when the PSNR or SSIM values are averaged over the test samples. This is evident in some reconstructions from the DIP + TV approach, where an artifact was observed on multiple LoDoPaB-CT reconstructions whereas this is not reflected in the metrics. This artifact is highlighted with a red circle in the DIP + TV reconstruction in Figure A9.

An alternative or supporting metric to PSNR and SSIM is visual inspection of the reconstructions. A visual evaluation can be done, for example, through a blind study with assessments and rating of reconstructions by (medical) experts. However, due to the large amount of work involved, the scope of such an evaluation is often limited. The 2016 Low Dose CT Grand Challenge [9] based their comparison on the visibility of liver lesions, as evaluated by a group of physicians. Each physician had to rate 20 different cases. The fastMRI Challenge [61] employed radiologists to rank MRI reconstructions. The authors were able to draw parallels between the quantitative and blind study results, which revealed that, in their data challenge, SSIM was a reasonable estimate for the radiologists' ranking of the images. In contrast, Mason et al. [71] found differences in their study between several image metrics and experts' opinions on reconstructed MRI images.

In industrial settings, PSNR or related pixel-based image quality metrics fall short on assessing the accuracy or performance of a reconstruction method when physical and hardware-related factors in data acquisition play a role in the final reconstruction. These factors are not accurately reflected in the image quality metrics, and therefore the conclusions drawn may not always be applicable. An alternative practice is suggested in [72], in which reconstructions of a pack of glass beads are evaluated using pixel-based metrics, such as contrast-to-noise ratio (CNR), and pre-determined physical quantification techniques. The physical quantification is object-specific, and assessment is done by extracting a physical quality of the object and comparing this to a reference size or shape. In one of the case studies, the CNR values of iterated reconstructions suggest an earlier stopping for the best contrast in the image, whereas a visual inspection reveals the image with the "best contrast" to be too blurry and the bead un-segmentable. The Apple CT reconstructions can be assessed in a similar fashion, where we look at the overall shape of a healthy apple, as well as the shape and position of its pit.

6.4. Impact of Data Consistency

Checking the discrepancy between measurement and forward-projected reconstruction can provide additional insight into the quality of the reconstruction. Ground truth data is not needed in this case. However, an accurate model $\mathcal{A}$ of the measurement process must be known. Additionally, the evaluation must take into account the noise type and level, as well as the sampling ratio.

Out of all tested methods, only the TV, CGLS and DIP + TV approach use the discrepancy to the measurements as (part of) their minimization objective for the reconstruction process. Still, the experiments on LoDoPaB-CT and Apple CT showed data consistency on the test samples for most of the methods. Based on these observations, data consistency does not appear to be a problem with test samples coming from a comparable distribution to the training data. However, altering the scan setup can significantly reduce the reconstruction performance of learned methods (cf. Section 6.2.3). Verification of the data consistency can serve as an indicator without the need for ground truth data or continuous visual inspection.

Another problem can be the instability of some learned methods, which is also known under the generic term of adversarial attacks [73]. Recent works [74,75] show that some methods, for example, fully learned and post-processing approaches, can be unstable. Tiny perturbations in the measurements may result in severe artifacts in the reconstructions. Checking the data discrepancy may also help in this case. Nonetheless, severe artifacts were also found in some reconstructions from the DIP + TV method on LoDoPaB-CT.

All in all, including a data consistency objective in training (bi-directional loss), could further improve the results from learned approaches. Checking the discrepancy during the application of trained models can also provide additional confidence about the reconstructions' accuracy.

6.5. Recommendations and Future Work

As many learned methods demonstrated similar performance in both low-dose CT and sparse-angle CT setups, further attributes have to be considered when selecting a learned method for a specific application. As discussed above, consideration should also be given to reconstruction speed, availability of training data, knowledge of the physical process, data consistency, and subsequent image analysis tasks. An overview can be found in Table 6. From the results of our comparison, some recommendations for the choice and further investigation of deep learning methods for CT reconstruction emerge.

Table 6. Summary of selected reconstruction method features. The reconstruction error ratings reflect the average performance improvement in terms of the evaluated metrics PSNR and SSIM compared to filtered back-projection (FBP). Specifically, for LoDoPaB-CT improvement quotients are calculated for PSNR and SSIM, and the two are averaged; for the Apple CT experiments the quotients are determined by first averaging PSNR and SSIM values within each noise setting over the four angular sampling cases, next computing improvement quotients independently for all three noise settings and for PSNR and SSIM, and finally averaging over these six quotients. GPU memory values are compared for 1-sample batches.

Model	Reconstruction Error (Image Metrics)		Training Time	Reconstruction Time	GPU Memory	Learned Parameters	Uses $\mathcal{D}_Y$ Discrepancy	Operator Required
Learned P.-D.	★★	★	★★★★	★★	★★★★	★★	no	★★★
ISTA U-Net	★★	★	★★★	★★	★★★	★★★	no	★★
U-Net	★★	★	★★	★★	★★	★★	no	★★
MS-D-CNN	★★	★	★★★★	★★	★★	★	no	★★
U-Net++	★★	-	★★	★★	★★★	★★★	no	★★
CINN	★★	★	★★	★★★	★★★	★★★	no	★★
DIP + TV	★★★	-	-	★★★★	★★	3+	yes	★★★★
iCTU-Net	★★★	★★	★★	★★	★★★	★★★★	no	★
TV	★★★	★★★	-	★★★	★	3	yes	★★★★
CGLS	-	★★★★	-	★	★	1	yes	★★★★
FBP	★★★★	★★★★	-	★	★	2	no	★★★★

Legend	LoDoPaB Avg. improv. over FBP	Apple CT	Rough values for Apple CT Dataset B (varying for different setups and datasets)					
★★★★	0%	0–15%	>2 weeks	>10 min	>10 GiB	>10^8		Direct
★★★	12–16%	25–30%	>5 days	>30 s	>3 GiB	>10^6		In network
★★	17–20%	40–45%	>1 day	>0.1 s	>1.5 GiB	>10^5		For input
★		50–60%		≤0.02 s	≤1 GiB	≤10^5		Only concept

Overall, the learned primal-dual approach proved to be a solid choice on the tested low photon count and sparse-angle datasets. The applicability of the method depends on the availability and fast evaluation of the forward and the adjoint operators. Both requirements were met for the 2D parallel beam simulation setup considered. However, without adjustments to the architecture, more complicated measurement procedures and especially 3D reconstruction could prove challenging. In contrast, the post-processing methods are more flexible, as they only rely on some (fast) initial reconstruction method. The performance of the included post-processing models was comparable to learned primal-dual. A disadvantage is the dependence on the information provided by the initial reconstruction.

The other methods included in this study are best suited for specific applications due to their characteristics. Fully learned methods do not require knowledge about the forward operator, but the necessary amount of training data is not available in many cases. The DIP + TV approach is on the other side of the spectrum, as it does not need any ground truth data. One downside is the slow reconstruction speed. However, faster reconstruction methods can be trained based on pseudo ground truth data created by DIP + TV. The CINN method allows for the evaluation of the likelihood of a reconstruction and can provide additional statistics from the sampling process. The invertible network architecture also enables the model to be trained in a memory-efficient way. The observed performance for 1000 samples per reconstruction was comparable to the post-processing methods. For time-critical applications, the number of samples would need to be lowered considerably, which can deteriorate the image quality.

In addition to the choice of model, the composition and amount of the training data also plays a significant role for supervised deep learning methods. The general difficulty of application to data that deviate from the training scenario was also observed in our comparison. Therefore, the training set should either contain examples of all expected cases or the model must be modified to include guarantees to work in divergent scenarios, such as different noise levels or number of angles. Special attention should also be directed to subsequent tasks. Adjusting the training objective or combining training with successive detection models can further increase the value of the reconstruction. Additionally, incorporating checks for the data consistency during training and/or reconstruction can help to detect and potentially prevent deviations in reconstruction quality. This potential is currently underutilized by many methods and could be a future improvement. Furthermore, the potential of additional regularization techniques to reduce the smoothness of reconstructions from learned methods should be investigated.

Our comparison lays the foundation for further research that is closer to real-world applications. Important points are the refinement of the simulation model, the use of real measurement data and the transition to fan-beam/cone-beam geometries. The move to 3D reconstruction techniques and the study of the influence of the additional spatial information is also an interesting aspect. Besides the refinement of the low photon count and sparse-angle setup, a future comparison should include limited-angle CT. A first application of this setting to Apple CT can be found in the dataset descriptor [38].

An important aspect of the comparison was the use of PSNR and SSIM image quality metrics to rate the produced reconstructions. In the future, this assessment should be supplemented by an additional evaluation of the reconstruction quality of some samples by (medical) professionals. A multi-stage blind study for the evaluation of unmarked reconstructions, including or excluding the (un)marked ground truth image, may provide additional insights.

Finally, a comparison is directly influenced by the selection of the included models. While we tested a broad range of different methods, there are still many missing types, for example, learned regularization [18] and null space networks [76]. We encourage readers to test additional reconstruction methods on the datasets from our comparison and submit reconstructions to the respective data challenge websites: (https://lodopab.grand-challenge.org/, last accessed: 1 March 2021) and (https://apples-ct.grand-challenge.org/, last accessed: 1 March 2021).

7. Conclusions

The goal of this work is to quantitatively compare learned, data-driven methods for image reconstruction. For this purpose, we organized two online data challenges, including a 10-day *kick-off event*, to give experts in this field the opportunity to benchmark their methods. In addition to this event, we evaluated some popular learned models independently. The appendix includes a thorough explanation and references to the methods used. We focused on two important applications of CT. With the LoDoPaB-CT dataset we simulated low-dose measurements and with the Apple CT datasets we included several sparse-angle setups. In order to ensure reproducibility, the source code of the methods, network parameters and the individual reconstruction are released. In comparison to the classical baseline (FBP and TV regularization) the data-driven methods are able to improve the quality of the CT reconstruction in both sparse-angle and low-dose settings. We observe that the top scoring methods, namely learned primal-dual and different post-processing approaches, perform similarly well in a variety of settings. Besides that, the applicability of deep learning-based models depends on the availability of training examples, prior knowledge about the physical system and requirements for the reconstruction speed.

Supplementary Materials: The following are available online at https://zenodo.org/record/4460055#.YD9IiIsRVPZ; https://zenodo.org/record/4459962#.YD9IqIsRVPZ; https://zenodo.org/record/4459250#.YD9GtU5xdPY.

Author Contributions: Conceptualization, J.L., M.S., P.S.G., P.M. and M.v.E.; Data curation, J.L., V.A. and S.B.C.; Formal analysis, J.L., M.S., P.S.G., V.A., S.B.C. and A.D.; Funding acquisition, K.J.B. and P.M.; Investigation, J.L., M.S., V.A., S.B.C. and A.D.; Project administration, M.S.; Software, J.L., M.S., P.S.G., V.A., S.B.C., A.D., D.B., A.H. and M.v.E.; Supervision, K.J.B., P.M. and M.v.E.; Validation, J.L. and M.S.; Visualization, J.L. and A.D.; Writing—original draft, J.L., M.S., P.S.G., V.A., S.B.C., A.D., D.B., A.H. and M.v.E.; Writing—review & editing, J.L., M.S., P.S.G., V.A., S.B.C., A.D., D.B., A.H., K.J.B., P.M. and M.v.E. All authors have read and agreed to the published version of the manuscript.

Funding: J.L., M.S., A.D. and P.M. were funded by the German Research Foundation (DFG; GRK 2224/1). J.L. and M.S. additionally acknowledge support by the project DELETO funded by the Federal Ministry of Education and Research (BMBF, project number 05M20LBB). A.D. further acknowledges support by the Klaus Tschira Stiftung via the project MALDISTAR (project number 00.010.2019). P.S.G. was funded by The Marie Skłodowska-Curie Innovative Training Network MUMMERING (Grant Agreement No. 765604). S.B.C. was funded by The Netherlands Organisation for Scientific Research (NWO; project number 639.073.506). M.v.E. and K.J.B. acknowledge the financial support by Holland High Tech through the PPP allowance for research and development in the HTSM topsector.

Institutional Review Board Statement: Not applicable.

Informed Consent Statement: Not applicable.

Data Availability Statement: The two datasets used in this study are the LoDoPaB-CT dataset [32], and the AppleCT dataset [37], both publicly available on Zenodo. The reconstructions discussed in Section 5 are provided as supplementary materials to this submission. These are shared via Zenodo through [57–59].

Acknowledgments: We are grateful for the help of GREEFA b.v. and the FleX-ray Laboratory of CWI for making CT scans of apples with internal defects available for the Code Sprint. The Code Sprint was supported by the DFG and the European Commission's MUMMERING ITN. We would like to thank Jens Behrmann for fruitful discussions. Finally, we would like to thank all participants of the Code Sprint 2020 for contributing to the general ideas and algorithms discussed in this paper.

Conflicts of Interest: The authors declare no conflict of interest, financial or otherwise.

Appendix A. Learned Reconstruction Methods

Appendix A.1. Learned Primal-Dual

The *Learned Primal-Dual* algorithm is a learned iterative procedure to solve inverse problems [19]. A primal-dual scheme [77] is unrolled for a fixed number of steps and the proximal operators are replaced by neural networks (cf. Figure A1). This unrolled architecture is then trained using data pairs from measurements and ground truth reconstructions. The forward pass is given in Algorithm A1. In contrast to the regular primal-dual algorithm, the primal and the dual space are extended to allow memory between iterations:

$$x = [x_{(1)}, \ldots, x_{(N_{\text{primal}})}] \in X^{N_{\text{primal}}},$$

$$h = [h_{(1)}, \ldots, h_{(N_{\text{dual}})}] \in Y^{N_{\text{dual}}}.$$

For the benchmark $N_{\text{primal}} = 5$ and $N_{\text{dual}} = 5$ was used. Both the primal and dual operators were parameterized as convolutional neural networks with 3 layers and 64 intermediate convolution channels. The primal-dual algorithm was unrolled for $K = 10$ iterations. Training was performed by minimizing the mean squared error loss using the Adam optimizer [78] with a learning rate of 0.0001. The model was trained for 10 epochs on LoDoPaB-CT and for at most 50 epochs on the apple data, whereby the model with the highest PSNR on the validation set was selected. Batch size 1 was used. Given a learned primal-dual algorithm the reconstruction can be obtained using Algorithm A1.

Algorithm A1 Learned Primal-Dual.

Given learned proximal dual and primal operators $\Gamma_{\theta_k^d}, \Lambda_{\theta_k^p}$ for $k = 1, \ldots, K$ the reconstruction from noisy measurements y_δ is calculated as follows.

1. Initialize $x^{[0]} \in X^{N_{\text{primal}}}, h^{[0]} \in Y^{N_{\text{dual}}}$
2. **for** $k = 1 : K$
3. $\quad h^{[k]} = \Gamma_{\theta_k^d}\left(h^{[k-1]}, \mathcal{A}(x_{(2)}^{[k-1]}), y_\delta\right)$
4. $\quad x^{[k]} = \Lambda_{\theta_k^p}\left(x^{[k-1]}, \left[\mathcal{A}(x_{(1)}^{[k-1]})\right]^*(h_{(1)}^{[m]})\right)$
5. **end**
6. **return** $\hat{x} = x_{(1)}^{[K]}$

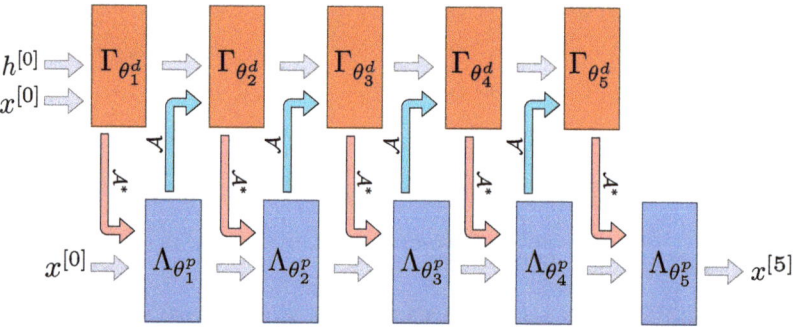

Figure A1. Architecture of the learned primal dual algorithm unrolled for $K = 5$ iterations. We used a zero initialization for $h^{[0]}$ and the FBP reconstruction for $x^{[0]}$. Adapted from [19].

Appendix A.2. U-Net

The goal of post-processing methods is to improve a pre-computed reconstruction. For CT, the FBP is used to obtain an initial reconstruction. This reconstruction is then used as an input to a post-processing network. For the enhancement of CT reconstructions, the post-processing network is implemented as a U-Net [20]. The U-Net architecture, as proposed by Ronneberger et al. [40], was originally designed for the task of semantic segmentation, but has many properties that are also beneficial for denoising. The general architecture is shown in Figure A2. In our implementation we used 5 scales (4 up- and downsampling blocks each) both for the LoDoPaB-CT and the Apple CT datasets. The skip connection between same scale levels mitigates the vanishing gradient problem so that deeper networks can be trained. In addition, the multi-scale architecture can be considered as a decomposition of the input image, in which an optimal filtering can be learned for each scale. There are many extensions to this basic architecture. For example, the U-Net++ (cf. Appendix A.3) extends the skip connections to different pathways.

The used numbers of channels at the different scales are 32, 32, 64, 64, and 128. For all skip connections 4 channels were used. The input FBPs were computed with Hann filtering and no frequency scaling. Linear activation (i.e., no sigmoid or ReLU activation) was used for the network output. Training was performed by minimizing the mean squared error loss using the Adam optimizer. For each training, the model with the highest PSNR on the validation set was selected. Due to the different memory requirements imposed by the image sizes of LoDoPaB-CT and the Apple CT data, different batch sizes were used. While for LoDoPaB-CT the batch size was 32 and standard batch normalization was applied, for the Apple CT data a batch size of 4 was used and layer normalization was applied instead of batch normalization. On LoDoPaB-CT, the model was trained for 250 epochs with learning rate starting from 0.001, reduced to 0.0001 by cosine annealing. On the Apple CT datasets, the model was trained for at most 50 epochs with fixed learning rate 0.001.

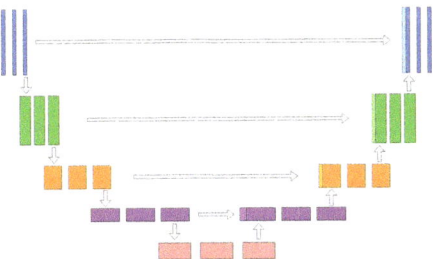

Figure A2. Architecture of the mutli-scale, post-processing U-Net. The general architecture of a U-Net consists on a downsampling path on the left and a upsampling path on the right with intermediate connection between similar scales. Adapted from [40].

Appendix A.3. U-Net++

The U-Net++ was introduced by Zhou et al. [41], the network improves on the original U-Net [40] architecture by incorporating nested and dense convolution blocks between skip connections. In U-Net, the down-sample block outputs of the encoder are directly input into the decoder's up-sample block at the same resolution. In U-Net++, the up-sampling block receives a concatenated input of a series of dense convolutional blocks at the same resolution. The input to these dense convolutional blocks is the concatenation of all previous dense convolutional blocks and the corresponding up-sample of a lower convolutional block.

The design is intended to convey similar semantic information across the skip-pathway. Zhou et al. suggest that U-Net's drawback is that the skip connections combine semantically dissimilar feature maps from the encoder and decoder. The results of these dissimilar semantic feature maps can limit the learning of the network. As a result, they proposed U-Net++ to address this drawback in the U-Net architecture. The purpose of the network is to progressively gain more fine-grained details from the nested dense convolutional blocks. Once these feature maps are combined with the decoder feature maps, it should, in theory, reduce the dissimilarity between the feature maps [41]. U-Net++ has shown to be successful in nodule segmentation of low-dose CT scans.

For our comparison on the LoDoPaB-CT dataset, we adopted a U-Net++ architecture with five levels, four down-samples reduced by a factor of 2 and four up-samples. The numbers of filters per convolutional block were 32, 64, 128, 256, 512 for the different levels, respectively. Each convolutional block contained two convolutional layers, each followed by batch normalization and ReLU activation. Input FBPs computed with Hann filtering and no frequency scaling were used. Linear activation (i.e., no sigmoid or ReLU activation) was used for the network output.

The loss function was chosen as a combination of MSE and SSIM,

$$\alpha \operatorname{MSE}(\hat{x}, x^\dagger) + (1 - \alpha)(1 - \operatorname{SSIM}(\hat{x}, x^\dagger)).$$

Empirically, the mixed loss function with weighting of 0.35 and 0.65 for MSE and SSIM, respectively, provided the best results.

The optimizer used for this task was RMSprop [79] with a weight decay of 1×10^{-8} and momentum of 0.9. The model was trained for 8 epochs with a learning rate of 1×10^{-5} using a batch size of 4, and the model with the lowest loss on the validation set was selected.

Source code and model weights are publicly available in a github repository (https://github.com/amirfaraji/LowDoseCTPytorch, last accessed: 1 March 2021).

Appendix A.4. Mixed-Scale Dense Convolutional Neural Network

The Mixed-Scale Dense (MS-D) network architecture was introduced by Pelt & Sethian [21]. The main properties of the MS-D architecture are mixing scales in every layer and dense connection of all feature maps. Instead of downscaling and upscaling, features at different scales are captured with dilated convolutions, and multiple scales are used in each layer. All feature maps have the same size, and every layer can use all previously computed feature maps as an input. Thus, feature maps are maximally reused, and features do not have to be replicated in multiple layers to be used deeper in the network. The output image is computed based on all layers instead of only the last one.

The authors show that MS-D architecture can achieve results comparable to typical DCNN with fewer feature maps and trainable parameters. This enables training with smaller datasets, which is highly important for CT. Furthermore, accurate results can usually be achieved without fine-tuning hyperparameters, and the same network architecture can often be used for different problems. A small number of feature maps leads to less memory usage in comparison with typical DCNN and enables training with larger images.

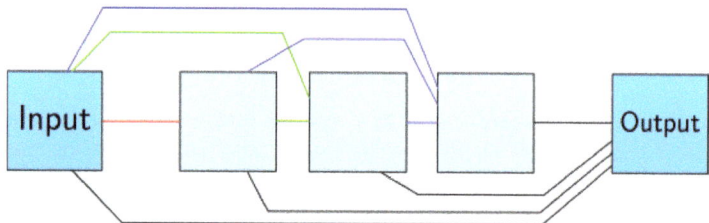

Figure A3. Architecture of the MS-D neural network for width of 1 and depth of 3, feature maps are drawn as light blue squares. Colored lines represent dilated convolutions, different colors correspond to different dilation values. Black lines represent 1×1 convolutions that connect the input and all feature maps to the output image. Adapted from [21].

The networks used equally distributed dilations with intervals from 1 to 10. The depth was 200 layers for the LoDoPaB-CT dataset and 100 layers for the Apple CT datasets. For the input FBPs, Hann filtering and no frequency scaling were used. The training was performed by minimizing MSE loss using the Adam optimizer with a learning rate of 0.001, using batch size 1. The model was trained for 15 epochs on LoDoPaB-CT and for at most 50 epochs on the apple data, whereby the model with the highest PSNR on the validation set was selected. Data augmentation consisting of rotations and flips was used for the apple data, but not for LoDoPaB-CT.

Appendix A.5. Conditional Invertible Neural Networks

Conditional invertible neural networks (CINN) are a relatively new approach for solving inverse problems [47,80]. Models of this type consist of two network parts (cf. Figure A4). An invertible network F represents a learned transformation between the (unknown) distribution $\mathcal{X}$ of the ground truth data and a standard probability distribution $\mathcal{Z}$, e.g., a Gaussian distribution. The second building block is a conditioning network C, which includes physical knowledge about the problem and encodes information from the measured data as an additional input to F.

A CINN was successfully applied to the task of low-dose CT reconstruction by Denker et al. [48]. Their model uses a multi-scale convolutional architecture as proposed in [81] and is built upon the FrEIA (https://github.com/VLL-HD/FrEIA, last accessed: 1 March 2021) python library. For the experiments in this paper, several improvements over the design in [48] are incorporated. The structure of the invertible network F and the conditioning network C are simplified. Using additive coupling layers [82] with Activation Normalization [83] improves stability of the training. Replacing downsampling operations with a learned version from Etmann et al. [63] prevents checkerboard artifacts and enhances the overall reconstruction quality. In addition, the negative log-likelihood (NLL) loss is combined with a weighted mean-squared error (MSE) term

$$\min_{\Theta} \left[\log p_Z \left(F_{\Theta}(x^\dagger, C_{\Theta}(y_\delta)) \right) + \log \left| \det \left(J_{F_{\Theta}}(x^\dagger, C_{\Theta}(y_\delta)) \right) \right| + \alpha \, \mathrm{MSE}\left(F_{\Theta}^{-1}(z, C_{\Theta}(y_\delta)), x^\dagger \right) \right].$$

The applied network has 5 different downsampling scales, where both spatial dimensions are reduced by factor 2. Simultaneously, the number of channels increases by a factor of 4, making the operation invertible. After each downsampling step, half the channels are split of and send directly to the output layer. In total, the network has around 6.5 million parameters. It is trained with the Adam optimizer and a learning rate of 0.0005 for at most 200 epochs using batch size 4 (per GPU) on LoDoPaB-CT and for at most 32 epochs using batch size 3 on the apple data. The best model according to the validation loss is selected. A Gaussian distribution is chosen for Z. The MSE weight is set to $\alpha = 1.0$. After training, the reconstructions are generated as a conditioned mean over $K = 1000$ sample reconstructions from the Gaussian distribution (cf. Algorithm A2).

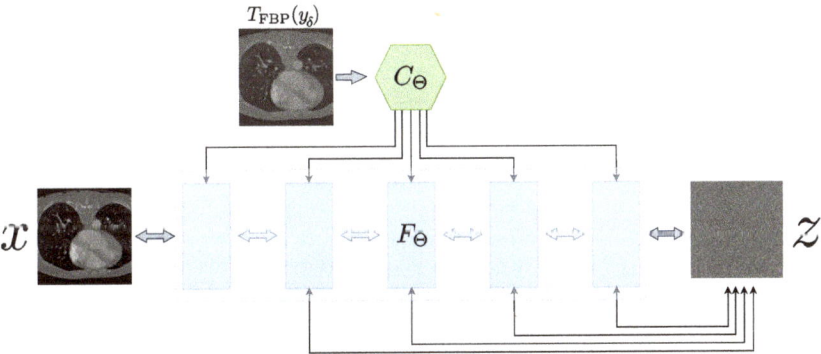

Figure A4. Architecture of the conditional invertible neural network. The ground truth image x is transformed by F_{Θ} to a Gaussian distributed z. Adapted from [48].

Algorithm A2 Conditional Invertible Neural Network (CINN).

Given a noisy measurement, y_δ, an invertible neural network F and a conditioning network C. Let $K \in \mathbb{N}$ be the number of random samples that should be drawn from a normal distribution $\mathcal{N}(0, \mathbb{I})$. The algorithm calculates the mean and variance of the conditioned reconstructions.

1. Calculate FBP: $c_0 = \mathcal{T}_{\mathrm{FBP}}(y_\delta)$.
2. Calculate outputs of the conditioning: $c = C_{\Theta}(c_0)$
3. for $k = 1 : K$
4. $\quad z^{[k]} \sim \mathcal{N}(0, \mathbb{I})$
5. $\quad \hat{x}^{[k]} = F^{-1}\left(z^{[k]}, c \right)$
6. end
7. Calculate mean: $\hat{x} = \frac{1}{K} \sum_k \hat{x}^{[k]}$
8. Calculate variance: $\hat{\sigma} = \frac{1}{K} \sum_k \left(\hat{x}^{[k]} - \hat{x} \right)^2$

Appendix A.6. ISTA U-Net

The ISTA U-Net [42] is a relatively new approach based on the encoder-decoder structure of the original U-Net. The authors draw parallels from the supervised training of U-Nets to task-driven dictionary learning and sparse coding. For the ISTA U-Net the encoder is replaced by a sparse representation of the input vector and the decoder is linearized by removing all non-linearities, batch normalization and additive biases (cf. Figure A5). Given a data set of measurements and ground truth pairs $\{y_{\delta i}, x_i^\dagger\}_{i=1}^M$ the training problem can be formulated as a bi-level optimization problem

$$\min_{\{\theta,\gamma\},\lambda>0} \frac{1}{M}\sum_{i=1}^M \frac{1}{2}\|D_\gamma \alpha_{y_{\delta i},\theta} - x_i^\dagger\|_2^2$$

$$\text{where } \alpha_{y_{\delta i},\theta} = \arg\min_{\alpha\geq 0} \frac{1}{2}\|D_\theta \alpha - y_{\delta i}\|_2^2 + \|\lambda \odot \alpha\|_1,$$

where $\odot$ denotes the Hadamard product. Using an encoder dictionary D_θ the corresponding sparse code α_θ can be determined with the iterative thresholding algorithm (ISTA, [84]) with an additional non-negativity constraint for the sparse code. Liu et al. [42] use a learned variant of ISTA, called LISTA [85], to compute the sparse code. LISTA works by unrolling ISTA for a fixed number of K iterations

$$\alpha_{y_\delta,\theta}^{[k]} = \text{ReLU}\left(\alpha_{y_\delta,\theta}^{[k-1]} + \eta D_K^T\left(y_\delta - D_\theta \alpha_{y_\delta,\theta}^{[k-1]}\right) - \eta\lambda\right),$$

with $k = 1,\ldots,K$. In their framework they additionally untie the parameters for D_K and D_θ, although both dictionaries have the same structure. The forward pass of the network is given in Algorithm A3.

For all experiments, $K = 5$ unrolled ISTA iterations were used. On LoDoPaB-CT, five scales with hidden layer widths 1024, 512, 256, 128, 64 were used and the lasso parameters λ were initialized with 10^{-3}. For the Apple CT datasets, the network appeared to be relatively sensitive with respect to the hyperparameter choices. For the noise-free data (Dataset A), five scales with hidden layer widths 512, 256, 128, 64, 32 were used and λ was initialized with 10^{-5}. For Datasets B and C, six scales, but less wide hidden layers, namely 512, 256, 128, 64, 32, 16, were used and λ was initialized with 10^{-4}. In all experiments, input FBPs computed with Hann filtering and no frequency scaling were used. A ReLU activation was applied to the network output. The network was trained by minimizing the mean squared error loss using the Adam optimizer. For LoDoPaB-CT, the network was trained for 20 epochs with a learning rate starting from 2×10^{-4}, reduced by cosine annealing to 1×10^{-5}, using batch size 2. For the Apple CT datasets, the network was trained for at most 80 epochs with a learning rate starting from 1×10^{-4}, reduced by cosine annealing to 1×10^{-5}, using batch size 1, whereby the model with the highest PSNR on the validation set was selected.

Source code is publicly available in a github repository (https://github.com/liutianlin0121/ISTA-U-Net, last accessed: 1 March 2021). A slightly modified copy of the code used for training on the Apple CT datasets is also contained in our github repository (https://github.com/jleuschn/learned_ct_reco_comparison_paper, last accessed: 1 March 2021).

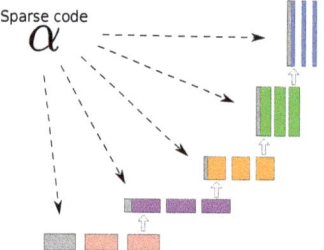

Figure A5. Architecture of the ISTA U-Net adapted from [42]. The sparse code α replaces the downsampling part in the standard U-Net (cf. Figure A2).

Algorithm A3 ISTA U-Net.

Given a noisy input y_δ, learned dictionaries $D_\kappa, D_\theta, D_\gamma$ and learned step sizes η and λ the reconstruction using the ISTA U-Net can be computed as follows.

1. Calculate FBP: $\hat{x} = \mathcal{T}_{\mathrm{FBP}}(y_\delta)$
2. Initialize $\alpha_{y_\delta}^{[0]} = 0$
3. **for** $k = 1 : K$
4. $\quad \alpha_{y_\delta}^{[k]} = \mathrm{ReLU}\left(\alpha_{y_\delta}^{[k-1]} + \eta D_\kappa^T\left(\hat{x} - D_\theta \alpha_{y_\delta}^{[i-1]}\right) - \eta\lambda\right)$
5. **end**
6. **return** $\hat{x} = D_\gamma \alpha_{y_\delta}^{[K]}$

Appendix A.7. Deep Image Prior with TV Denoising

The deep image prior (DIP) [86] takes a special role among the listed neural network approaches. In general, a DIP network F is not previously trained and, therefore, omits the problem of ground truth acquisition. Instead, the parameters Θ are adjusted iteratively during the reconstruction process by gradient descent steps (cf. Algorithm A4). The main objective is to minimize the data discrepancy of the output of the network for a fixed random input z

$$\min_\Theta \mathcal{D}_Y(\mathcal{A}F_\Theta(z), y_\delta). \quad (A1)$$

The number of iterations have a great influence on the reconstruction quality: While too few can result in an overall bad image, too many can cause overfitting to the noise of the measurement. The general regularization strategy for this problem is a combination of early stopping and the architecture itself [87], where the prior is related to the implicit structural bias of the network. Especially convolutional networks, in combination with gradient descent, fit natural images faster than noise and learn to construct them from low to high frequencies [86,88,89].

The loss function (A1) can also be combined with classical regularization. Baguer et al. [34] add a weighted anisotropic total variation (TV) term and apply their approach to low-dose CT measurements. The method DIP + TV is also used for this comparison. The network architecture is based on the same U-Net as for the FBP U-Net post-processing (cf. Appendix A.2). It has 6 different scales with 128 channels each and a skip-channel setup of $(0,0,0,0,4,4)$. The data discrepancy $\mathcal{D}_Y$ was measured with a Poisson loss (see Equation (9)) and the weight for TV was chosen as $\alpha = 7.0$. Gradient descent was performed for $K = 17,000$ iterations with a stepsize of 5×10^{-4}.

Algorithm A4 Deep Image Prior + Total Variation (DIP + TV).

Given a noisy measurement y_δ, a neural network F_Θ with initial parameterization $\Theta^{[0]}$, forward operator $\mathcal{A}$ and a fixed random input z. The reconstruction $\hat{x}$ is calculated iteratively over a number of $K \in \mathbb{N}$ iterations:

1. **for** $k = 1 : K$
2. $\quad$ Evaluate loss: $L = \mathcal{D}\left(\mathcal{A}F_{\Theta^{[k-1]}}(z), y_\delta\right) + \alpha\,\mathrm{TV}\left(F_{\Theta^{[k-1]}}(z)\right)$
3. $\quad$ Calculate gradients: $\nabla_{\Theta^{[k-1]}} = \nabla_\Theta L$
4. $\quad$ Update parameters: $\Theta^{[k]} = \mathrm{Optimizer}\left(\Theta^{[k-1]}, \nabla_{\Theta^{[k-1]}}\right)$
5. $\quad$ Current reconstruction: $\hat{x}^{[k]} = F_{\Theta^{[k]}}(z)$
6. **end**

Appendix A.8. iCTU-Net

The iCTU-Net is based on the iCT-Net by Li et al. [29], which in turn is inspired by the common filtered back-projection. The reconstruction process is learned end-to-end, that is, the sinogram is the input of the network and the output is the reconstructed image. The full network architecture is shown in Figure A6.

First, disturbances in the raw measurement data, such as excessive noise, are suppressed as much as possible via 3 × 3 convolutions (refining layers). The corrected sinogram is then filtered using 10 × 1 convolutions (filtering layers). The filtered sinogram maintains the size of the input sinogram. Afterwards, the sinogram is back-projected into the image space. This is realized by a $d \times 1$ convolution with N^2 output channels without padding, where d is the number of detectors in the sinogram and N is the output image size. This convolution corresponds to a fully connected layer for each viewing angle, as it connects every detector element with every pixel in the image space. The results for each view are reshaped to $N \times N$ sized images and rotated according to the acquisition angle. A 1×1 convolution combines all views into the back projected image. Finally, a U-Net further refines the image output.

To significantly lower the GPU memory requirements, an initial convolutional layer with stride 1 × 2 was added, to downsample the LoDoPaB sinograms from 1000 to 500 projection angles. For the apple reconstruction the number of detector elements d and the output image size N were halved. After reconstruction the image size was doubled again using linear interpolation. Training was performed using the Adam optimizer with a learning rate of 0.001 and batch size 1. For LoDoPaB-CT the mean squared error loss and for Apple CT the SSIM loss function was used. The network was trained for 2 epochs on LoDoPaB-CT and for at most 60 epochs on the Apple CT datasets, without validation based model selection (i.e., no automated early stopping).

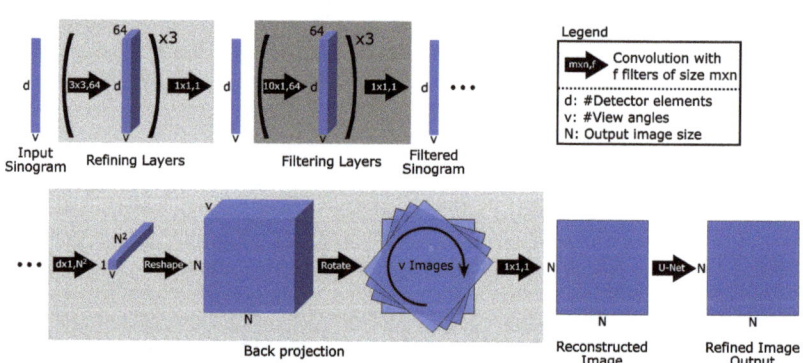

Figure A6. Architecture of the iCTU-Net.

Appendix B. Classical Reconstruction Methods

Appendix B.1. Filtered Back-Projection (FBP)

The Radon transform [10] maps (or projects) a function $x(u)$, $u = (u_1, u_2)$, defined on a two-dimensional plane to a function $\mathcal{A}x(s, \varphi)$ defined on a two-dimensional space of lines, which are parameterized by distance to the origin, s and the angle φ of the normal. The Radon transform is given by

$$\mathcal{A}x(s, \varphi) := \int_{\mathbb{R}} x\left(s \begin{bmatrix} \cos(\varphi) \\ \sin(\varphi) \end{bmatrix} + t \begin{bmatrix} -\sin(\varphi) \\ \cos(\varphi) \end{bmatrix}\right) dt,$$

A simple inversion idea consists in back-projecting the intensities $\mathcal{A}x(s, \varphi)$ to those positions u in the image $x(u)$ that lie on the corresponding lines parameterized by s and φ, that is, those positions that contribute to the respective measured intensity. Mathematically, the back-projection is described by the adjoint Radon transform $\mathcal{A}^*$, also provided in [10]. To obtain an inversion formula, the projections $\mathcal{A}x$ need to be filtered before the back-projection (see e.g., [36] for a derivation and an alternative formula applying a filter after obtaining the back-projection $\mathcal{A}^*\mathcal{A}x$). A generic FBP reconstruction formula reads

$$\hat{x} = \frac{1}{2}\mathcal{A}^*\mathcal{F}^{-1}|\cdot|W\mathcal{F}y_\delta,$$

where $\mathcal{F}$ denotes the one-dimensional Fourier transform along the detector pixel dimension s, $|\cdot|$ denotes the Ram-Lak filter, which multiplies each frequency component with the absolute value of the frequency, and W is a low-pass filter (applying a window function). While from perfect projections $\mathcal{A}x(s,\varphi)$ exact recovery of $x(u)$ is possible by choosing a rectangular window function for W, in practice W is also used to reduce high frequency components. This stabilizes the inversion by reducing the impact of noise present in higher frequencies. Typical choices for W are the Hann or the Cosine window. Sometimes the resulting weighting function is additionally shrunk along the frequency axis with a frequency scaling factor, which leads to removal of all frequency components above a threshold frequency.

For all experiments the implementation of ODL [90] was used in conjunction with the ASTRA toolbox [91]. Suitable hyperparameters have been determined based on the performance on validation samples and are listed in Table A1. The FBPs used for post-processing networks were computed with the Hann window and without frequency scaling. The Hann window thereby serves as a pre-processing step for the network and the frequency scaling was omitted in order to keep all information available.

Table A1. Hyperparameters for filtered back-projection (FBP).

		Window	Frequency Scaling
LoDoPaB-CT Dataset		Hann	0.641
Apple CT Dataset A (Noise-free)	50 angles	Cosine	0.11
	10 angles	Cosine	0.013
	5 angles	Hann	0.011
	2 angles	Hann	0.011
Apple CT Dataset B (Gaussian noise)	50 angles	Cosine	0.08
	10 angles	Cosine	0.013
	5 angles	Hann	0.011
	2 angles	Hann	0.011
Apple CT Dataset C (Scattering)	50 angles	Cosine	0.09
	10 angles	Hann	0.018
	5 angles	Hann	0.011
	2 angles	Hann	0.009

Appendix B.2. Conjugate Gradient Least Squares

The Conjugate Gradient Least Squares (CGLS) method is the modification of the well-known Conjugate Gradient [52] where the CG method is applied to solve the least squares problem $A^T A\hat{x} = A^T y_\delta$. Here, $A \in \mathbb{R}^{m \times n}$ is the geometry matrix, $y_\delta \in \mathbb{R}^{m \times 1}$ is the measured data and $\hat{x} \in \mathbb{R}^{n \times 1}$ is the reconstruction. CGLS is a popular method in signal and image processing for its simple and computationally inexpensive implementation and fast convergence. The method is given in Algorithm A5, codes from [92].

Our implementation also includes a non-negativity step (negative pixel values equal to zero), applied to the final iterated solution. There is no parameter-tuning done for this implementation since the only user-defined parameter is the maximum number of iterations, K.

Algorithm A5 Conjugate Gradient Least Squares (CGLS).

Given a geometry matrix, A, a data vector y_δ and a zero solution vector $\hat{x}^{[0]} = 0$ (a black image) as the starting point, the algorithm below gives the solution at k^{th} iteration.

1. Initialise the direction vector as $d^{[0]} = A^T y_\delta$.
2. **for** $k = 1 : K$
3. $\quad q^{[k-1]} = A d^{[k-1]}, \alpha = \|d^{[k-1]}\|_2^2 / \|q^{[k-1]}\|_2^2$
4. $\quad$ Update: $\hat{x}^{[k]} = \hat{x}^{[k-1]} + \alpha d^{[k-1]}, b^{[k]} = b^{[k-1]} - \alpha q^{[k-1]}$
5. $\quad$ Reinitialise: $q^{[k]} = A^T q^{[k-1]}, \beta = \|q^{[k]}\|_2^2 / \|d^{[k-1]}\|_2^2, d^{[k]} = q^{[k]} + \beta d^{[k-1]}$
6. **end**

Appendix B.3. Total Variation Regularization

Regularizing the reconstruction process with anisotropic total variation (TV) is a common approach for CT [93]. In addition to the data discrepancy $\mathcal{D}$, a weighted regularization term is added to the minimization problem

$$\mathcal{T}_{TV}(y_\delta) \in \arg\min_x \mathcal{D}(\mathcal{A}x, y_\delta) + \alpha(\|\nabla_h x\|_1 + \|\nabla_v x\|_1), \tag{A2}$$

where ∇_h and ∇_v denote gradients in horizontal and vertical image direction, respectively, and can be approximated by finite differences in the discrete setting. TV penalizes variations in the image, e.g., from noise. Therefore, it is often applied in a denoising role. A number of optimization algorithms exist for minimizing (A2) [54]. The choice and exact formulation depend on the properties of the data discrepancy term.

For our comparison, we use the standard DIVαℓ implementation of TV. Adam gradient descent minimizes (A2), whereby the gradients are calculated by automatic differentiation in PyTorch [94] (cf. Algorithm A6).

Algorithm A6 Total Variation Regularization (TV).

Given a noisy measurement y_δ, an initial reconstruction $\hat{x}^{[0]}$, a weight $\alpha > 0$ and a maximum number of iterations K.

1. **for** $k = 1 : K$
2. $\quad$ Evaluate loss: $L = \mathcal{D}\left(A\hat{x}^{[k-1]}, y_\delta\right) + \alpha\left(\left\|\nabla_h \hat{x}^{[k-1]}\right\|_1 + \left\|\nabla_v \hat{x}^{[k-1]}\right\|_1\right)$
3. $\quad$ Calculate gradients: $\nabla_{\hat{x}^{[k-1]}} = \nabla_x L$
4. $\quad$ Update: $\hat{x}^{[k]} = \text{Optimizer}\left(\hat{x}^{[k-1]}, \nabla_{\hat{x}^{[k-1]}}\right)$
5. **end**

For the data discrepancy $\mathcal{D}$, a Poisson loss (see (9)) was used for LoDoPaB-CT, while the MSE was used for the Apple CT datasets. Suitable hyperparameters have been determined based on the performance on validation samples and are listed in Table A2. For lower numbers of angles, a very high number of iterations was found to be beneficial, leading to very slow reconstruction ($\approx$17 min per image for $K = 150{,}000$ iterations, which we chose to be the maximum). In all cases an FBP with Hann window and frequency scaling factor 0.1 was used as initial reconstruction.

Table A2. Hyperparameters for total variation regularization (TV).

		Discrepancy	Iterations	Step Size	α
LoDoPaB-CT Dataset		$-\ell_{\text{Pois}}$	5000	0.001	20.56
Apple CT Dataset A (Noise-free)	50 angles	MSE	600	3×10^{-2}	2×10^{-12}
	10 angles	MSE	75,000	3×10^{-3}	6×10^{-12}
	5 angles	MSE	146,000	1.5×10^{-3}	1×10^{-11}
	2 angles	MSE	150,000	1×10^{-3}	2×10^{-11}
Apple CT Dataset B (Gaussian noise)	50 angles	MSE	900	3×10^{-4}	2×10^{-10}
	10 angles	MSE	66,000	2×10^{-5}	6×10^{-10}
	5 angles	MSE	100,000	1×10^{-5}	3×10^{-9}
	2 angles	MSE	149,000	1×10^{-5}	4×10^{-9}
Apple CT Dataset C (Scattering)	50 angles	MSE	400	5×10^{-3}	1×10^{-11}
	10 angles	MSE	13,000	2×10^{-3}	4×10^{-11}
	5 angles	MSE	149,000	1×10^{-3}	4×10^{-11}
	2 angles	MSE	150,000	4×10^{-4}	6×10^{-11}

Appendix C. Further Results

Table A3. Standard deviation of PSNR and SSIM (adapted to the data range of each ground truth image) for the different noise settings on the 100 selected Apple CT test images.

Noise-Free	Standard Deviation of PSNR				Standard Deviation of SSIM			
Number of Angles	50	10	5	2	50	10	5	2
Learned Primal-Dual	1.51	1.63	1.97	2.58	0.022	0.016	0.014	0.022
ISTA U-Net	1.40	1.77	2.12	2.13	0.018	0.018	0.022	0.037
U-Net	1.56	1.61	2.28	1.63	0.021	0.019	0.025	0.031
MS-D-CNN	1.51	1.65	1.81	2.09	0.021	0.020	0.024	0.022
CINN	1.40	1.64	1.99	2.17	0.016	0.019	0.023	0.027
iCTU-Net	1.68	2.45	1.92	1.93	0.024	0.027	0.030	0.028
TV	1.60	1.29	1.21	1.49	0.022	0.041	0.029	0.023
CGLS	0.69	0.48	2.94	0.70	0.014	0.027	0.029	0.039
FBP	0.80	0.58	0.54	0.50	0.021	0.023	0.028	0.067
Gaussian Noise	Standard Deviation of PSNR				Standard Deviation of SSIM			
Number of Angles	50	10	5	2	50	10	5	2
Learned Primal-Dual	1.56	1.63	2.00	2.79	0.021	0.018	0.021	0.022
ISTA U-Net	1.70	1.76	2.27	2.12	0.025	0.021	0.022	0.038
U-Net	1.66	1.59	1.99	2.22	0.023	0.020	0.025	0.026
MS-D-CNN	1.66	1.75	1.79	1.79	0.025	0.024	0.019	0.022
CINN	1.53	1.51	1.62	2.06	0.023	0.017	0.017	0.020
iCTU-Net	1.98	2.06	1.89	1.91	0.031	0.032	0.039	0.027
TV	1.38	1.26	1.09	1.62	0.036	0.047	0.039	0.030
CGLS	0.78	0.49	1.76	0.68	0.014	0.026	0.029	0.037
FBP	0.91	0.58	0.54	0.50	0.028	0.023	0.028	0.067

Table A3. *Cont.*

Scattering Noise	Standard Deviation of PSNR				Standard Deviation of SSIM			
Number of Angles	50	10	5	2	50	10	5	2
Learned Primal-Dual	1.91	1.80	1.71	2.47	0.017	0.016	0.016	0.060
ISTA U-Net	1.48	1.59	2.05	1.81	0.023	0.019	0.019	0.038
U-Net	1.76	1.56	1.81	1.47	0.015	0.021	0.027	0.024
MS-D-CNN	2.04	1.78	1.85	2.03	0.023	0.022	0.015	0.020
CINN	1.82	1.92	2.32	2.25	0.019	0.024	0.029	0.030
iCTU-Net	1.91	2.09	1.78	2.29	0.030	0.031	0.033	0.040
TV	2.53	2.44	1.86	1.59	0.067	0.076	0.035	0.062
CGLS	2.38	1.32	1.71	0.95	0.020	0.020	0.026	0.032
FBP	2.23	0.97	0.80	0.68	0.044	0.025	0.023	0.058

Table A4. PSNR-FR and SSIM-FR (computed with fixed data range 0.0129353 for all images) for the different noise settings on the 100 selected Apple CT test images. Best results are highlighted in gray.

Noise-Free	PSNR-FR				SSIM-FR			
Number of Angles	50	10	5	2	50	10	5	2
Learned Primal-Dual	45.33	42.47	37.41	28.61	0.971	0.957	0.935	0.872
ISTA U-Net	45.48	41.15	34.93	27.10	0.967	0.944	0.907	0.823
U-Net	46.24	40.13	34.38	26.39	0.975	0.917	0.911	0.830
MS-D-CNN	46.47	41.00	35.06	27.17	0.975	0.936	0.898	0.808
CINN	46.20	41.46	34.43	26.07	0.975	0.958	0.896	0.838
iCTU-Net	42.69	36.57	32.24	25.90	0.957	0.938	0.920	0.861
TV	45.89	35.61	28.66	22.57	0.976	0.904	0.746	0.786
CGLS	39.66	28.43	19.22	21.87	0.901	0.744	0.654	0.733
FBP	37.01	23.71	22.12	20.58	0.856	0.711	0.596	0.538
Gaussian Noise	**PSNR-FR**				**SSIM-FR**			
Number of Angles	50	10	5	2	50	10	5	2
Learned Primal-Dual	43.24	40.38	36.54	28.03	0.961	0.944	0.927	0.823
ISTA U-Net	42.65	40.17	35.09	27.32	0.956	0.942	0.916	0.826
U-Net	43.09	39.45	34.42	26.47	0.961	0.924	0.904	0.843
MS-D-CNN	43.28	39.82	34.60	26.50	0.962	0.932	0.886	0.797
CINN	43.39	38.50	33.19	26.60	0.966	0.904	0.878	0.816
iCTU-Net	39.51	36.38	31.29	26.06	0.939	0.932	0.905	0.867
TV	38.98	33.73	28.45	22.70	0.939	0.883	0.770	0.772
CGLS	33.98	27.71	21.52	21.73	0.884	0.748	0.668	0.734
FBP	34.50	23.70	22.12	20.58	0.839	0.711	0.596	0.538
Scattering Noise	**PSNR-FR**				**SSIM-FR**			
Number of Angles	50	10	5	2	50	10	5	2
Learned Primal-Dual	44.42	40.80	33.69	27.60	0.967	0.954	0.912	0.760
ISTA U-Net	42.55	38.95	34.03	26.57	0.959	0.922	0.887	0.816
U-Net	41.58	39.52	33.55	25.56	0.932	0.910	0.877	0.828
MS-D-CNN	44.66	40.13	34.34	26.81	0.969	0.927	0.889	0.796
CINN	45.18	40.69	34.66	25.76	0.976	0.952	0.936	0.878
iCTU-Net	32.88	29.46	27.86	24.93	0.931	0.901	0.896	0.873
TV	27.71	26.76	24.48	21.15	0.903	0.799	0.674	0.743
CGLS	27.46	24.89	20.64	20.80	0.896	0.738	0.659	0.736
FBP	27.63	22.42	20.88	19.68	0.878	0.701	0.589	0.529

Table A5. Standard deviation of PSNR-FR and SSIM-FR (computed with fixed data range 0.0129353 for all images) for the different noise settings on the 100 selected Apple CT test images.

Noise-Free	Standard Deviation of PSNR-FR				Standard Deviation of SSIM-FR			
Number of Angles	50	10	5	2	50	10	5	2
Learned Primal-Dual	1.49	1.67	2.03	2.54	0.007	0.006	0.010	0.019
ISTA U-Net	1.37	1.82	2.21	2.21	0.005	0.010	0.020	0.034
U-Net	1.53	1.66	2.33	1.68	0.006	0.012	0.019	0.026
MS-D-CNN	1.46	1.71	1.90	2.15	0.006	0.011	0.021	0.015
CINN	1.35	1.65	2.09	2.21	0.004	0.007	0.023	0.025
iCTU-Net	1.82	2.54	2.03	1.91	0.014	0.017	0.020	0.023
TV	1.54	1.32	1.28	1.36	0.006	0.023	0.026	0.018
CGLS	0.71	0.51	2.96	0.56	0.009	0.029	0.033	0.045
FBP	0.77	0.46	0.38	0.41	0.011	0.015	0.029	0.088
Gaussian Noise	Standard Deviation of PSNR-FR				Standard Deviation of SSIM-FR			
Number of Angles	50	10	5	2	50	10	5	2
Learned Primal-Dual	1.52	1.68	2.04	2.83	0.006	0.008	0.013	0.016
ISTA U-Net	1.65	1.78	2.36	2.17	0.008	0.010	0.018	0.034
U-Net	1.61	1.62	2.05	2.24	0.007	0.012	0.019	0.024
MS-D-CNN	1.62	1.80	1.84	1.84	0.008	0.011	0.015	0.014
CINN	1.50	1.59	1.65	2.09	0.007	0.016	0.017	0.019
iCTU-Net	2.07	2.12	1.93	1.90	0.020	0.021	0.026	0.024
TV	1.30	1.26	1.15	1.50	0.014	0.027	0.030	0.019
CGLS	0.63	0.45	1.76	0.53	0.012	0.028	0.034	0.043
FBP	0.83	0.46	0.38	0.41	0.014	0.015	0.029	0.088
Scattering Noise	Standard Deviation of PSNR-FR				Standard Deviation of SSIM-FR			
Number of Angles	50	10	5	2	50	10	5	2
Learned Primal-Dual	1.92	1.85	1.81	2.51	0.005	0.007	0.014	0.038
ISTA U-Net	1.56	1.68	2.17	1.89	0.010	0.014	0.014	0.035
U-Net	1.72	1.63	1.91	1.59	0.010	0.012	0.024	0.024
MS-D-CNN	2.02	1.84	1.96	2.08	0.008	0.012	0.016	0.019
CINN	1.74	1.97	2.41	2.21	0.005	0.011	0.016	0.022
iCTU-Net	1.96	2.14	1.79	2.32	0.016	0.023	0.022	0.030
TV	2.43	2.35	1.80	1.49	0.048	0.074	0.040	0.051
CGLS	2.28	1.24	1.67	0.83	0.016	0.021	0.030	0.035
FBP	2.14	0.87	0.66	0.55	0.028	0.016	0.020	0.078

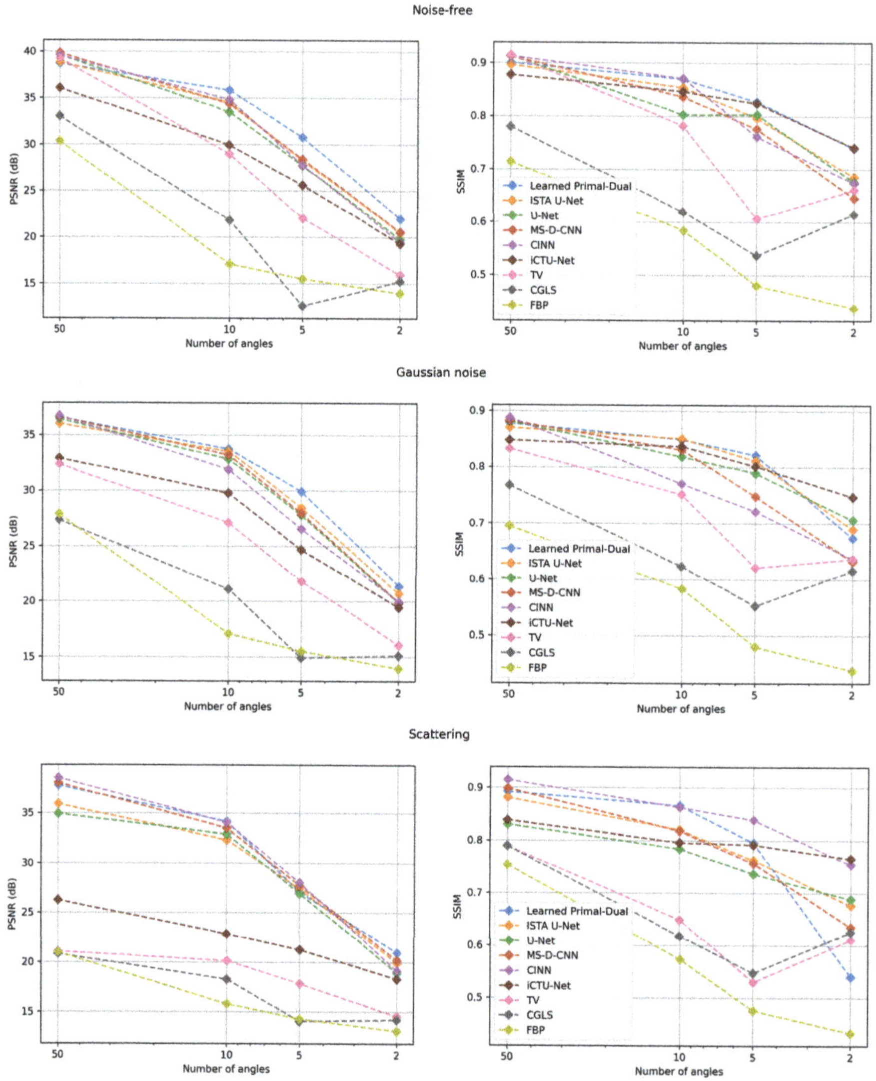

Figure A7. PSNR and SSIM depending on the number of angles on the Apple CT datasets.

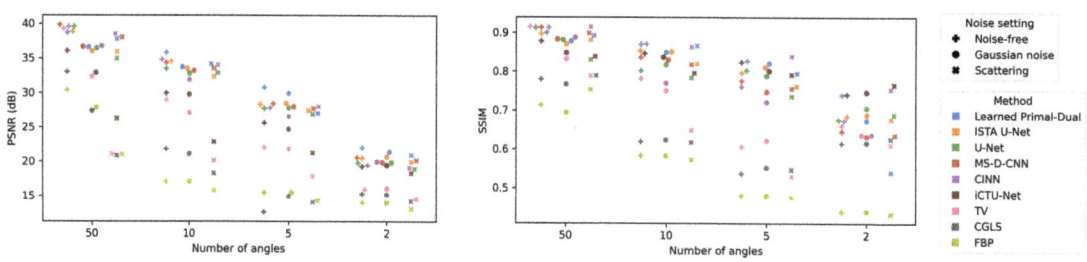

Figure A8. PSNR and SSIM compared for all noise settings and numbers of angles.

Table A6. Mean and standard deviation of the mean squared difference between the noisy measurements and the forward-projected reconstructions, respectively the noise-free measurements, on the 100 selected Apple CT test images.

Noise Free	MSE $\times 10^9$			
Number of Angles	50	10	5	2
Learned Primal-Dual	0.083 ± 0.027	0.405 ± 0.156	1.559 ± 0.543	2.044 ± 1.177
ISTA U-Net	0.323 ± 0.240	0.633 ± 0.339	2.672 ± 1.636	17.840 ± 12.125
U-Net	0.097 ± 0.093	1.518 ± 0.707	5.011 ± 3.218	31.885 ± 17.219
MS-D-CNN	0.117 ± 0.088	0.996 ± 0.595	3.874 ± 2.567	20.879 ± 12.038
CINN	0.237 ± 0.259	1.759 ± 0.348	3.798 ± 2.176	33.676 ± 16.747
iCTU-Net	2.599 ± 3.505	6.686 ± 8.469	14.508 ± 16.694	18.876 ± 12.553
TV	0.002 ± 0.000	0.001 ± 0.000	0.000 ± 0.000	0.001 ± 0.000
CGLS	1.449 ± 0.299	29.921 ± 6.173	752.997 ± 722.151	22.507 ± 13.748
FBP	12.229 ± 3.723	89.958 ± 9.295	159.746 ± 15.596	273.054 ± 114.552
Ground truth	0.000 ± 0.000	0.000 ± 0.000	0.000 ± 0.000	0.000 ± 0.000
Gaussian Noise	MSE $\times 10^9$			
Number of Angles	50	10	5	2
Learned Primal-Dual	19.488 ± 5.923	19.813 ± 5.851	20.582 ± 5.690	32.518 ± 4.286
ISTA U-Net	19.438 ± 5.943	20.178 ± 6.060	21.167 ± 6.052	32.435 ± 9.782
U-Net	19.802 ± 6.247	22.114 ± 6.364	23.645 ± 6.527	38.895 ± 17.211
MS-D-CNN	19.348 ± 5.921	20.056 ± 5.930	23.080 ± 5.959	47.625 ± 18.133
CINN	19.429 ± 5.891	21.069 ± 5.663	29.517 ± 7.296	42.876 ± 15.471
iCTU-Net	25.645 ± 9.602	25.421 ± 9.976	38.179 ± 22.887	41.956 ± 15.942
TV	18.760 ± 5.674	18.107 ± 5.395	20.837 ± 5.510	18.514 ± 5.688
CGLS	87.892 ± 23.312	71.526 ± 17.600	262.616 ± 151.655	98.520 ± 18.245
FBP	31.803 ± 9.558	109.430 ± 14.107	179.260 ± 19.744	292.692 ± 109.223
Ground truth	19.538 ± 6.029	19.505 ± 6.019	19.551 ± 6.028	19.483 ± 6.086
Scattering Noise	MSE $\times 10^9$			
Number of Angles	50	10	5	2
Learned Primal-Dual	541.30 ± 311.82	579.14 ± 317.59	549.30 ± 328.41	435.07 ± 260.02
ISTA U-Net	553.64 ± 355.14	557.03 ± 342.67	575.94 ± 338.82	522.33 ± 365.58
U-Net	629.62 ± 353.54	635.91 ± 343.31	550.54 ± 340.27	642.20 ± 295.46
MS-D-CNN	579.86 ± 332.39	585.18 ± 331.93	533.35 ± 331.21	606.55 ± 365.25
CINN	638.80 ± 355.24	619.47 ± 353.47	603.53 ± 362.96	649.30 ± 409.83
iCTU-Net	622.51 ± 348.32	622.63 ± 335.28	652.18 ± 359.00	573.46 ± 324.00
TV	3.35 ± 5.02	3.19 ± 4.83	2.96 ± 4.47	2.55 ± 6.33
CGLS	6.40 ± 6.39	34.71 ± 8.16	286.20 ± 205.42	19.92 ± 14.01
FBP	12.48 ± 6.88	73.53 ± 10.19	144.70 ± 15.82	221.79 ± 59.71
Ground truth	610.47 ± 355.25	610.40 ± 355.16	611.23 ± 354.51	620.11 ± 386.79

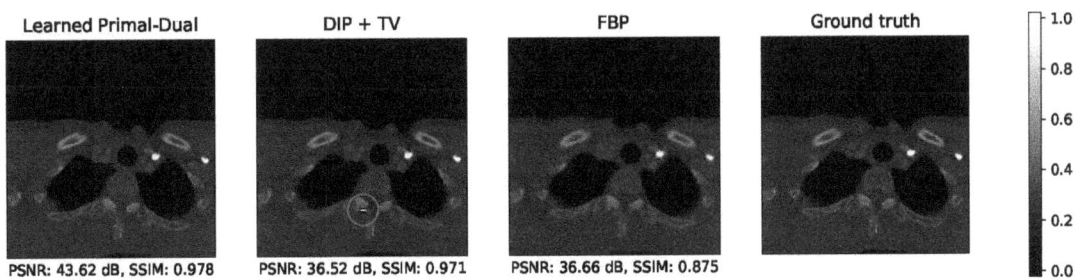

Figure A9. Example of an artifact produced by DIP + TV, which has only minor impact on the evaluated metrics (especially the SSIM). The area containing the artifact is marked with a red circle.

Appendix D. Training Curves

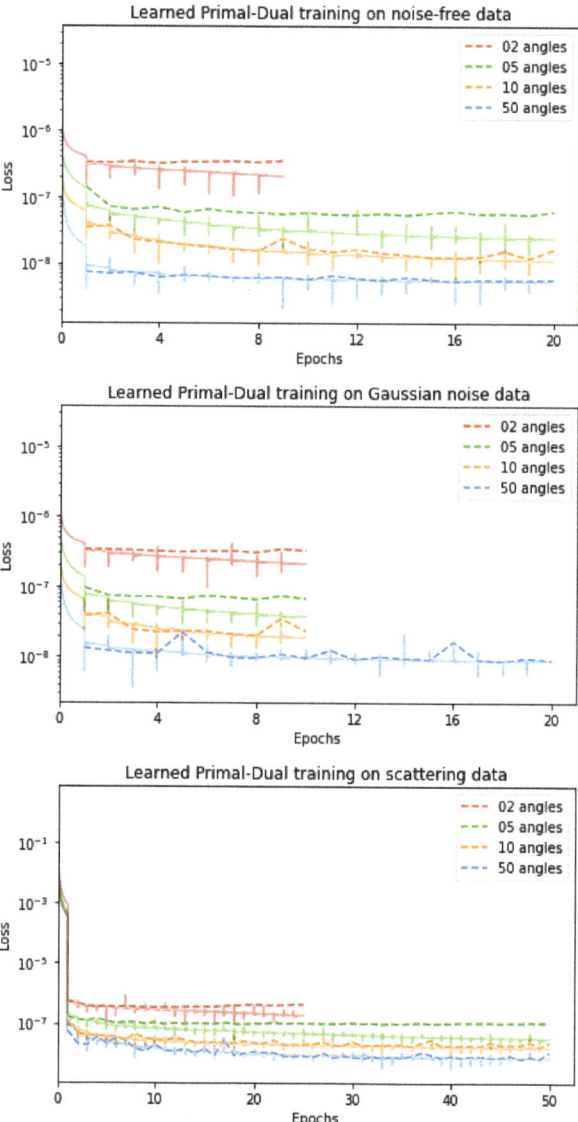

Figure A10. Training curves of Learned Primal-Dual on the Apple CT dataset. Dashed lines: average validation loss computed after every full training epoch; solid lines: running average of training loss since start of epoch. Duration of 20 epochs on full dataset: ≈10–17 days, varying with the number of angles.

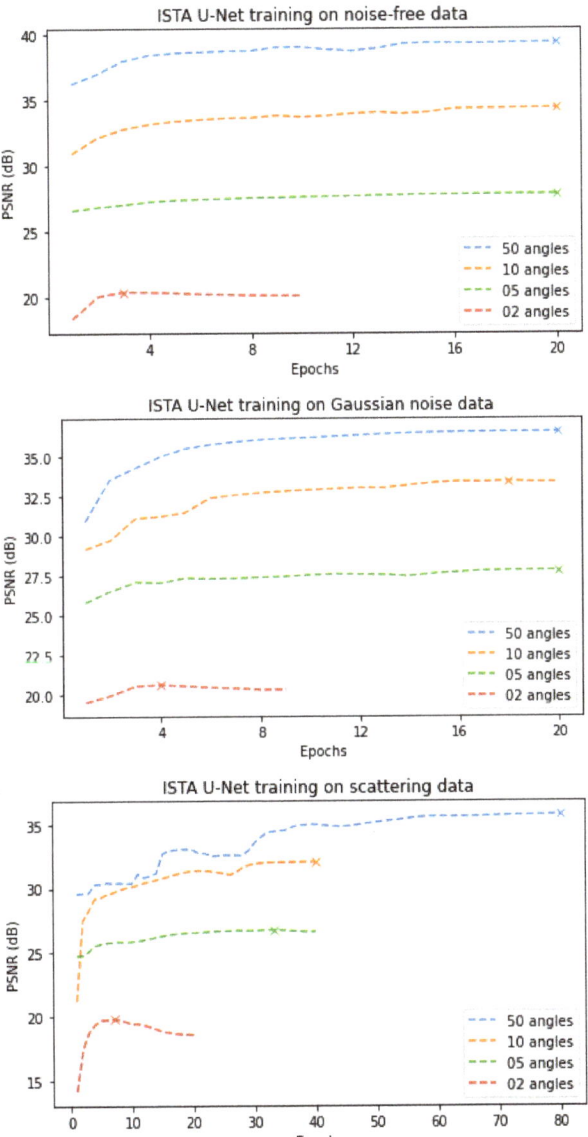

Figure A11. Training curves of ISTA U-Net on the Apple CT dataset. Dashed lines: average validation PSNR in decibel computed after every full training epoch; marks: selected model. Duration of 20 epochs on full dataset: ≈10 days for hidden layer width 32+ and 5 scales, respectively ≈5.5 days for hidden layer width 16+ and 6 scales.

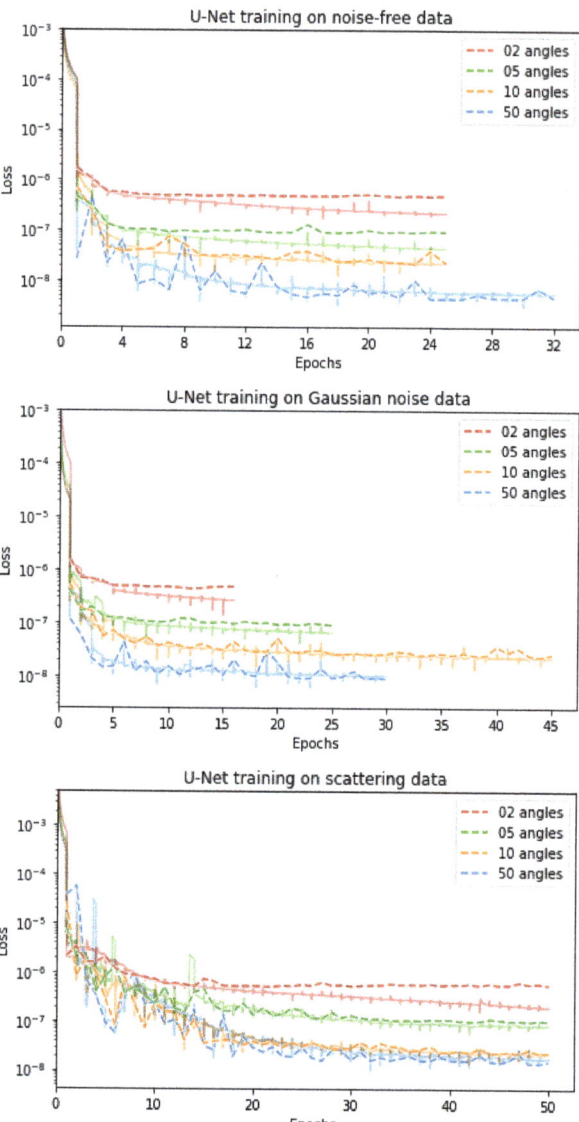

Figure A12. Training curves of U-Net on the Apple CT dataset. Dashed lines: average validation loss computed after every full training epoch; solid lines: running average of training loss since start of epoch. Duration of 20 epochs on full dataset: ≈1.5 days.

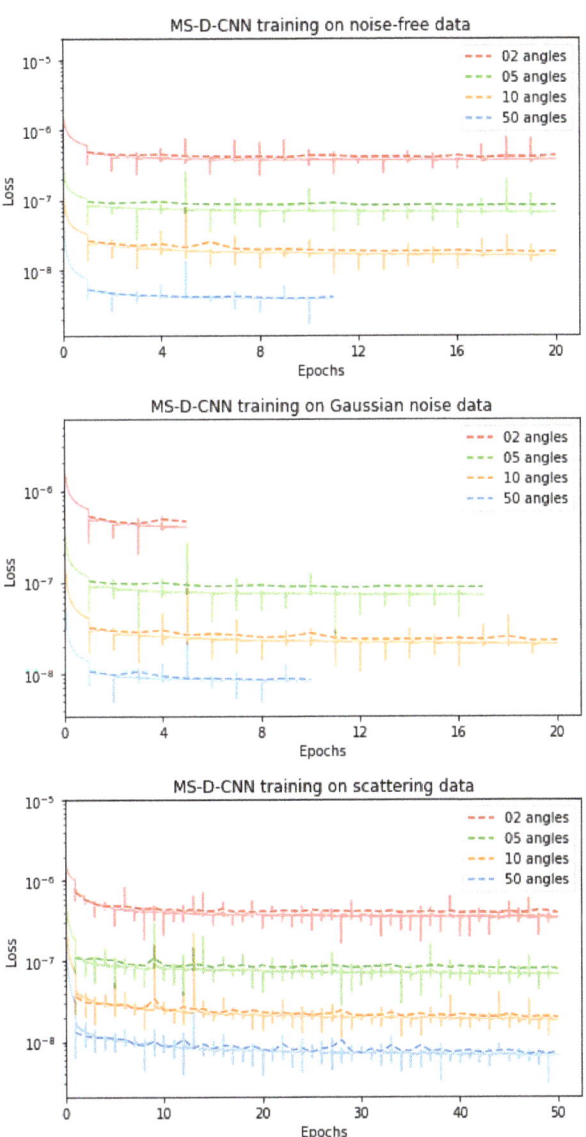

Figure A13. Training curves of MS-D-CNN on the Apple CT dataset. Dashed lines: average validation loss computed after every full training epoch; solid lines: running average of training loss since start of epoch. Duration of 20 epochs on full dataset: ≈20 days.

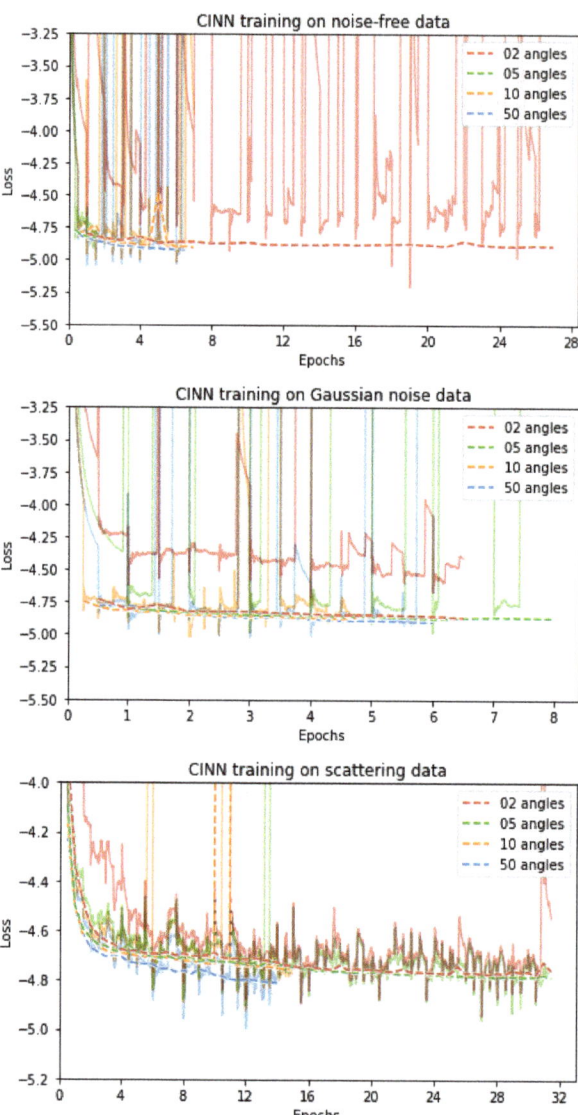

Figure A14. Training curves of CINN on the Apple CT dataset. Dashed lines: average validation loss computed after every full training epoch; solid lines: running average of training loss (at every 50-th step) since start of epoch. For some of the trainings, the epochs were divided into multiple shorter ones. Duration of 20 epochs on full dataset: ≈2.5 days (using 2 GPUs).

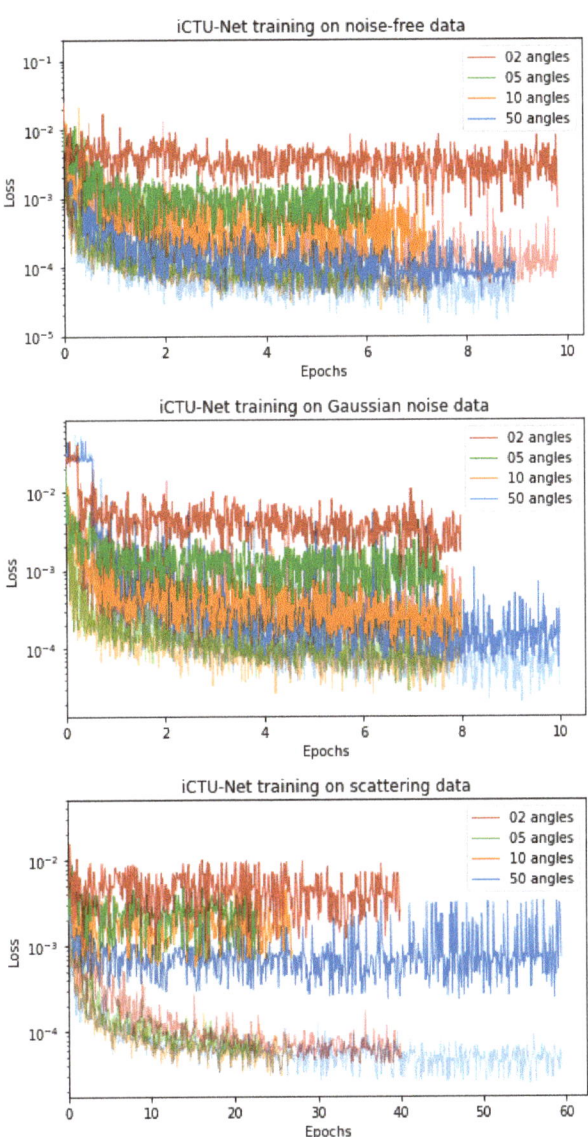

Figure A15. Training curves of iCTU-Net on the Apple CT dataset. Opaque lines: loss for a validation sample (after every 500-th step); semi-transparent lines: training loss (at every 500-th step). Duration of 20 epochs on full dataset: ≈3 days.

References

1. Liguori, C.; Frauenfelder, G.; Massaroni, C.; Saccomandi, P.; Giurazza, F.; Pitocco, F.; Marano, R.; Schena, E. Emerging clinical applications of computed tomography. *Med. Devices* **2015**, *8*, 265.
2. National Lung Screening Trial Research Team. Reduced lung-cancer mortality with low-dose computed tomographic screening. *N. Engl. J. Med.* **2011**, *365*, 395–409. [CrossRef]
3. Yoo, S.; Yin, F.F. Dosimetric feasibility of cone-beam CT-based treatment planning compared to CT-based treatment planning. *Int. J. Radiat. Oncol. Biol. Phys.* **2006**, *66*, 1553–1561. [CrossRef]
4. Swennen, G.R.; Mollemans, W.; Schutyser, F. Three-dimensional treatment planning of orthognathic surgery in the era of virtual imaging. *J. Oral Maxillofac. Surg.* **2009**, *67*, 2080–2092. [CrossRef]

5. De Chiffre, L.; Carmignato, S.; Kruth, J.P.; Schmitt, R.; Weckenmann, A. Industrial applications of computed tomography. *CIRP Ann.* **2014**, *63*, 655–677. [CrossRef]
6. Mees, F.; Swennen, R.; Van Geet, M.; Jacobs, P. *Applications of X-ray Computed Tomography in the Geosciences*; Special Publications; Geological Society: London, UK, 2003; Volume 215, pp. 1–6.
7. Morigi, M.; Casali, F.; Bettuzzi, M.; Brancaccio, R.; d'Errico, V. Application of X-ray computed tomography to cultural heritage diagnostics. *Appl. Phys. A* **2010**, *100*, 653–661. [CrossRef]
8. Coban, S.B.; Lucka, F.; Palenstijn, W.J.; Van Loo, D.; Batenburg, K.J. Explorative Imaging and Its Implementation at the FleX-ray Laboratory. *J. Imaging* **2020**, *6*, 18. [CrossRef]
9. McCollough, C.H.; Bartley, A.C.; Carter, R.E.; Chen, B.; Drees, T.A.; Edwards, P.; Holmes, D.R., III; Huang, A.E.; Khan, F.; Leng, S.; et al. Low-dose CT for the detection and classification of metastatic liver lesions: Results of the 2016 Low Dose CT Grand Challenge. *Med Phys.* **2017**, *44*, e339–e352. [CrossRef] [PubMed]
10. Radon, J. On the determination of functions from their integral values along certain manifolds. *IEEE Trans. Med Imaging* **1986**, *5*, 170–176. [CrossRef]
11. Natterer, F. The mathematics of computerized tomography (classics in applied mathematics, vol. 32). *Inverse Probl.* **2001**, *18*, 283–284.
12. Boas, F.E.; Fleischmann, D. CT artifacts: Causes and reduction techniques. *Imaging Med.* **2012**, *4*, 229–240. [CrossRef]
13. Wang, G.; Ye, J.C.; Mueller, K.; Fessler, J.A. Image Reconstruction is a New Frontier of Machine Learning. *IEEE Trans. Med. Imaging* **2018**, *37*, 1289–1296. [CrossRef] [PubMed]
14. Sidky, E.Y.; Pan, X. Image reconstruction in circular cone-beam computed tomography by constrained, total-variation minimization. *Phys. Med. Biol.* **2008**, *53*, 4777. [CrossRef]
15. Niu, S.; Gao, Y.; Bian, Z.; Huang, J.; Chen, W.; Yu, G.; Liang, Z.; Ma, J. Sparse-view X-ray CT reconstruction via total generalized variation regularization. *Phys. Med. Biol.* **2014**, *59*, 2997. [CrossRef] [PubMed]
16. Hestenes, M.R.; Stiefel, E. Methods of conjugate gradients for solving linear systems. *J. Res. Natl. Bur. Stand.* **1952**, *49*, 409–436. [CrossRef]
17. Arridge, S.; Maass, P.; Öktem, O.; Schönlieb, C.B. Solving inverse problems using data-driven models. *Acta Numer.* **2019**, *28*, 1–174. [CrossRef]
18. Lunz, S.; Öktem, O.; Schönlieb, C.B. Adversarial Regularizers in Inverse Problems. In *Advances in Neural Information Processing Systems*; Bengio, S., Wallach, H., Larochelle, H., Grauman, K., Cesa-Bianchi, N., Garnett, R., Eds.; Curran Associates, Inc.: Red Hook, NY, USA, 2018; Volume 31, pp. 8507–8516.
19. Adler, J.; Öktem, O. Learned Primal-Dual Reconstruction. *IEEE Trans. Med. Imaging* **2018**, *37*, 1322–1332. TMI.2018.2799231. [CrossRef]
20. Jin, K.H.; McCann, M.T.; Froustey, E.; Unser, M. Deep Convolutional Neural Network for Inverse Problems in Imaging. *IEEE Trans. Image Process.* **2017**, *26*, 4509–4522. [CrossRef]
21. Pelt, D.M.; Batenburg, K.J.; Sethian, J.A. Improving Tomographic Reconstruction from Limited Data Using Mixed-Scale Dense Convolutional Neural Networks. *J. Imaging* **2018**, *4*, 128. [CrossRef]
22. Chen, H.; Zhang, Y.; Zhang, W.; Liao, P.; Li, K.; Zhou, J.; Wang, G. Low-dose CT via convolutional neural network. *Biomed. Opt. Express* **2017**, *8*, 679–694. [CrossRef]
23. Chen, H.; Zhang, Y.; Kalra, M.K.; Lin, F.; Chen, Y.; Liao, P.; Zhou, J.; Wang, G. Low-dose CT with a residual encoder-decoder convolutional neural network. *IEEE Trans. Med. Imaging* **2017**, *36*, 2524–2535. [CrossRef]
24. Yang, Q.; Yan, P.; Kalra, M.K.; Wang, G. CT image denoising with perceptive deep neural networks. *arXiv* **2017**, arXiv:1702.07019.
25. Yang, Q.; Yan, P.; Zhang, Y.; Yu, H.; Shi, Y.; Mou, X.; Kalra, M.K.; Zhang, Y.; Sun, L.; Wang, G. Low-dose CT image denoising using a generative adversarial network with Wasserstein distance and perceptual loss. *IEEE Trans. Med. Imaging* **2018**, *37*, 1348–1357. [CrossRef]
26. Feng, R.; Rundle, D.; Wang, G. Neural-networks-based Photon-Counting Data Correction: Pulse Pileup Effect. *arXiv* **2018**, arXiv:1804.10980.
27. Zhu, B.; Liu, J.Z.; Cauley, S.F.; Rosen, B.R.; Rosen, M.S. Image reconstruction by domain-transform manifold learning. *Nature* **2018**, *555*, 487–492. [CrossRef]
28. He, J.; Ma, J. Radon inversion via deep learning. *IEEE Trans. Med. Imaging* **2020**, *39*, 2076–2087. [CrossRef] [PubMed]
29. Li, Y.; Li, K.; Zhang, C.; Montoya, J.; Chen, G.H. Learning to reconstruct computed tomography images directly from sinogram data under a variety of data acquisition conditions. *IEEE Trans. Med Imaging* **2019**, *38*, 2469–2481. [CrossRef]
30. European Society of Radiology (ESR). The new EU General Data Protection Regulation: What the radiologist should know. *Insights Imaging* **2017**, *8*, 295–299. [CrossRef] [PubMed]
31. Kaissis, G.A.; Makowski, M.R.; Rückert, D.; Braren, R.F. Secure, privacy-preserving and federated machine learning in medical imaging. *Nat. Mach. Intell.* **2020**, *2*, 305–311. [CrossRef]
32. Leuschner, J.; Schmidt, M.; Baguer, D.O.; Maass, P. The LoDoPaB-CT Dataset: A Benchmark Dataset for Low-Dose CT Reconstruction Methods. *arXiv* **2020**, arXiv:1910.01113.
33. Armato, S.G., III; McLennan, G.; Bidaut, L.; McNitt-Gray, M.F.; Meyer, C.R.; Reeves, A.P.; Zhao, B.; Aberle, D.R.; Henschke, C.I.; Hoffman, E.A.; et al. The Lung Image Database Consortium (LIDC) and Image Database Resource Initiative (IDRI): A Completed Reference Database of Lung Nodules on CT Scans. *Med. Phys.* **2011**, *38*, 915–931. [CrossRef]

34. Baguer, D.O.; Leuschner, J.; Schmidt, M. Computed tomography reconstruction using deep image prior and learned reconstruction methods. *Inverse Probl.* **2020**, *36*, 094004. [CrossRef]
35. Armato, S.G., III; McLennan, G.; Bidaut, L.; McNitt-Gray, M.F.; Meyer, C.R.; Reeves, A.P.; Zhao, B.; Aberle, D.R.; Henschke, C.I.; Hoffman, E.A.; et al. *Data From LIDC-IDRI*; The Cancer Imaging Archive: Frederick, MD, USA, 2015.10.7937/K9/TCIA.2015.LO9QL9SX. [CrossRef]
36. Buzug, T. *Computed Tomography: From Photon Statistics to Modern Cone-Beam CT*; Springer: Berlin/Heidelberg, Germany, 2008. [CrossRef]
37. Coban, S.B.; Andriiashen, V.; Ganguly, P.S. *Apple CT Data: Simulated Parallel-Beam Tomographic Datasets*; Zenodo: Geneva, Switzerland, 2020. [CrossRef]
38. Coban, S.B.; Andriiashen, V.; Ganguly, P.S.; van Eijnatten, M.; Batenburg, K.J. Parallel-beam X-ray CT datasets of apples with internal defects and label balancing for machine learning. *arXiv* **2020**, arXiv:2012.13346.
39. Leuschner, J.; Schmidt, M.; Ganguly, P.S.; Andriiashen, V.; Coban, S.B.; Denker, A.; van Eijnatten, M. Source Code and Supplementary Material for "Quantitative comparison of deep learning-based image reconstruction methods for low-dose and sparse-angle CT applications". *Zenodo* **2021**. [CrossRef]
40. Ronneberger, O.; Fischer, P.; Brox, T. U-net: Convolutional networks for biomedical image segmentation. In *International Conference on Medical Image Computing and Computer-Assisted Intervention*; Springer: Heidelberg, Germany, 2015; pp. 234–241.
41. Zhou, Z.; Siddiquee, M.M.R.; Tajbakhsh, N.; Liang, J. Unet++: A nested u-net architecture for medical image segmentation. In *Deep Learning in Medical Image Analysis and Multimodal Learning for Clinical Decision Support*; Springer: Heidelberg, Germany, 2018; pp. 3–11.
42. Liu, T.; Chaman, A.; Belius, D.; Dokmanić, I. Interpreting U-Nets via Task-Driven Multiscale Dictionary Learning. *arXiv* **2020**, arXiv:2011.12815.
43. Comelli, A.; Dahiya, N.; Stefano, A.; Benfante, V.; Gentile, G.; Agnese, V.; Raffa, G.M.; Pilato, M.; Yezzi, A.; Petrucci, G.; et al. Deep learning approach for the segmentation of aneurysmal ascending aorta. *Biomed. Eng. Lett.* **2020**, 1–10.
44. Dashti, M.; Stuart, A.M. The Bayesian Approach to Inverse Problems. In *Handbook of Uncertainty Quantification*; Springer International Publishing: Cham, Switzerland, 2017; pp. 311–428. [CrossRef]
45. Adler, J.; Öktem, O. Deep Bayesian Inversion. *arXiv* **2018**, arXiv:1811.05910.
46. Goodfellow, I.; Pouget-Abadie, J.; Mirza, M.; Xu, B.; Warde-Farley, D.; Ozair, S.; Courville, A.; Bengio, Y. Generative adversarial nets. *arXiv* **2014**, arXiv:1406.2661.
47. Ardizzone, L.; Lüth, C.; Kruse, J.; Rother, C.; Köthe, U. Guided image generation with conditional invertible neural networks. *arXiv* **2019**, arXiv:1907.02392.
48. Denker, A.; Schmidt, M.; Leuschner, J.; Maass, P.; Behrmann, J. Conditional Normalizing Flows for Low-Dose Computed Tomography Image Reconstruction. *arXiv* **2020**, arXiv:2006.06270.
49. Hadamard, J. *Lectures on Cauchy's Problem in Linear Partial Differential Equations*; Dover: New York, NY, USA, 1952.
50. Nashed, M. A new approach to classification and regularization of ill-posed operator equations. In *Inverse and Ill-Posed Problems*; Engl, H.W., Groetsch, C., Eds.; Academic Press: Cambridge, MA, USA, 1987; pp. 53–75. [CrossRef]
51. Natterer, F.; Wübbeling, F. *Mathematical Methods in Image Reconstruction*; Society for Industrial and Applied Mathematics: Philadelphia, PA, USA, 2001.
52. Saad, Y. *Iterative Methods for Sparse Linear Systems*, 2nd ed.; Society for Industrial and Applied Mathematics: Philadelphia, PA, USA, 2003.
53. Björck, Å.; Elfving, T.; Strakos, Z. Stability of conjugate gradient and Lanczos methods for linear least squares problems. *SIAM J. Matrix Anal. Appl.* **1998**, *19*, 720–736. [CrossRef]
54. Chen, H.; Wang, C.; Song, Y.; Li, Z. Split Bregmanized anisotropic total variation model for image deblurring. *J. Vis. Commun. Image Represent.* **2015**, *31*, 282–293. [CrossRef]
55. Wang, Z.; Bovik, A.C.; Sheikh, H.R.; Simoncelli, E.P. Image quality assessment: From error visibility to structural similarity. *IEEE Trans. Image Process.* **2004**, *13*, 600–612. [CrossRef] [PubMed]
56. Goodfellow, I.; Bengio, Y.; Courville, A. *Deep Learning*; MIT Press: Cambridge, MA, USA, 2016. Available online: http://www.deeplearningbook.org (accessed on 1 March 2021).
57. Leuschner, J.; Schmidt, M.; Ganguly, P.S.; Andriiashen, V.; Coban, S.B.; Denker, A.; van Eijnatten, M. Supplementary Material for Experiments in "Quantitative comparison of deep learning-based image reconstruction methods for low-dose and sparse-angle CT applications". *Zenodo* **2021**. [CrossRef]
58. Leuschner, J.; Schmidt, M.; Baguer, D.O.; Bauer, D.; Denker, A.; Hadjifaradji, A.; Liu, T. LoDoPaB-CT Challenge Reconstructions compared in "Quantitative comparison of deep learning-based image reconstruction methods for low-dose and sparse-angle CT applications". *Zenodo* **2021**. [CrossRef]
59. Leuschner, J.; Schmidt, M.; Ganguly, P.S.; Andriiashen, V.; Coban, S.B.; Denker, A.; van Eijnatten, M. Apple CT Test Reconstructions compared in "Quantitative comparison of deep learning-based image reconstruction methods for low-dose and sparse-angle CT applications". *Zenodo* **2021**. [CrossRef]
60. Leuschner, J.; Schmidt, M.; Otero Baguer, D.; Erzmann, D.; Baltazar, M. DIVal Library. *Zenodo* **2021**. [CrossRef]

61. Knoll, F.; Murrell, T.; Sriram, A.; Yakubova, N.; Zbontar, J.; Rabbat, M.; Defazio, A.; Muckley, M.J.; Sodickson, D.K.; Zitnick, C.L.; et al. Advancing machine learning for MR image reconstruction with an open competition: Overview of the 2019 fastMRI challenge. *Magn. Reson. Med.* **2020**, *84*, 3054–3070. [CrossRef]
62. Putzky, P.; Welling, M. Invert to Learn to Invert. In *Advances in Neural Information Processing Systems*; Wallach, H., Larochelle, H., Beygelzimer, A., dAlch'e-Buc, F., Fox, E., Garnett, R., Eds.; Curran Associates, Inc.: Red Hook, NY, USA, 2019; Volume 32, pp. 446–456.
63. Etmann, C.; Ke, R.; Schönlieb, C. iUNets: Learnable Invertible Up- and Downsampling for Large-Scale Inverse Problems. In Proceedings of the 30th IEEE International Workshop on Machine Learning for Signal Processing (MLSP 2020), Espoo, Finland, 21–24 September 2020; pp. 1–6. [CrossRef]
64. Ziabari, A.; Ye, D.H.; Srivastava, S.; Sauer, K.D.; Thibault, J.; Bouman, C.A. 2.5D Deep Learning For CT Image Reconstruction Using A Multi-GPU Implementation. In Proceedings of the 2018 52nd Asilomar Conference on Signals, Systems, and Computers, Pacific Grove, CA, USA, 28–31 October 2018; pp. 2044–2049. [CrossRef]
65. Scherzer, O.; Weickert, J. Relations Between Regularization and Diffusion Filtering. *J. Math. Imaging Vis.* **2000**, *12*, 43–63. [CrossRef]
66. Perona, P.; Malik, J. Scale-space and edge detection using anisotropic diffusion. *IEEE Trans. Pattern Anal. Mach. Intell.* **1990**, *12*, 629–639. [CrossRef]
67. Mendrik, A.M.; Vonken, E.; Rutten, A.; Viergever, M.A.; van Ginneken, B. Noise Reduction in Computed Tomography Scans Using 3-D Anisotropic Hybrid Diffusion With Continuous Switch. *IEEE Trans. Med Imaging* **2009**, *28*, 1585–1594. [CrossRef] [PubMed]
68. Adler, J.; Lunz, S.; Verdier, O.; Schönlieb, C.B.; Öktem, O. Task adapted reconstruction for inverse problems. *arXiv* **2018**, arXiv:1809.00948.
69. Boink, Y.E.; Manohar, S.; Brune, C. A partially-learned algorithm for joint photo-acoustic reconstruction and segmentation. *IEEE Trans. Med. Imaging* **2019**, *39*, 129–139. [CrossRef]
70. Handels, H.; Deserno, T.M.; Maier, A.; Maier-Hein, K.H.; Palm, C.; Tolxdorff, T. (Eds.) *Bildverarbeitung für die Medizin 2019*; Springer Fachmedien Wiesbaden: Wiesbaden, Germany, 2019. [CrossRef]
71. Mason, A.; Rioux, J.; Clarke, S.E.; Costa, A.; Schmidt, M.; Keough, V.; Huynh, T.; Beyea, S. Comparison of objective image quality metrics to expert radiologists' scoring of diagnostic quality of MR images. *IEEE Trans. Med. Imaging* **2019**, *39*, 1064–1072. [CrossRef] [PubMed]
72. Coban, S.B.; Lionheart, W.R.B.; Withers, P.J. Assessing the efficacy of tomographic reconstruction methods through physical quantification techniques. *Meas. Sci. Technol.* **2021**. [CrossRef]
73. Goodfellow, I.J.; Shlens, J.; Szegedy, C. Explaining and Harnessing Adversarial Examples. In Proceedings of the 3rd International Conference on Learning Representations (ICLR 2015), San Diego, CA, USA, 7–9 May 2015.
74. Antun, V.; Renna, F.; Poon, C.; Adcock, B.; Hansen, A.C. On instabilities of deep learning in image reconstruction and the potential costs of AI. *Proc. Natl. Acad. Sci. USA* **2020**. [CrossRef]
75. Gottschling, N.M.; Antun, V.; Adcock, B.; Hansen, A.C. The troublesome kernel: Why deep learning for inverse problems is typically unstable. *arXiv* **2020**, arXiv:2001.01258.
76. Schwab, J.; Antholzer, S.; Haltmeier, M. Deep null space learning for inverse problems: Convergence analysis and rates. *Inverse Probl.* **2019**, *35*, 025008. [CrossRef]
77. Chambolle, A.; Pock, T. A first-order primal-dual algorithm for convex problems with applications to imaging. *J. Math. Imaging Vis.* **2011**, *40*, 120–145. [CrossRef]
78. Kingma, D.P.; Ba, J. Adam: A Method for Stochastic Optimization. In Proceedings of the 3rd International Conference on Learning Representations (ICLR 2015), San Diego, CA, USA, 7–9 May 2015.
79. Hinton, G.; Srivastava, N.; Swersky, K. Neural networks for machine learning lecture 6a overview of mini-batch gradient descent. *Lect. Notes* **2012**, *14*, 1–31.
80. Winkler, C.; Worrall, D.; Hoogeboom, E.; Welling, M. Learning likelihoods with conditional normalizing flows. *arXiv* **2019**, arXiv:1912.00042.
81. Dinh, L.; Sohl-Dickstein, J.; Bengio, S. Density estimation using Real NVP. In Proceedings of the 5th International Conference on Learning Representations (ICLR 2017), Toulon, France, 24–26 April 2017.
82. Dinh, L.; Krueger, D.; Bengio, Y. NICE: Non-linear Independent Components Estimation. In Proceedings of the 3rd International Conference on Learning Representations (ICLR 2015), San Diego, CA, USA, 7–9 May 2015.
83. Kingma, D.P.; Dhariwal, P. Glow: Generative Flow with Invertible 1x1 Convolutions. In Proceedings of the Advances in Neural Information Processing Systems 31: Annual Conference on Neural Information Processing Systems 2018 (NeurIPS 2018), Montréal, QC, Canada, 3–8 December 2018; Bengio, S., Wallach, H.M., Larochelle, H., Grauman, K., Cesa-Bianchi, N., Garnett, R., Eds.; 2018; pp. 10236–10245.
84. Daubechies, I.; Defrise, M.; De Mol, C. An iterative thresholding algorithm for linear inverse problems with a sparsity constraint. *Commun. Pure Appl. Math.* **2004**, *57*, 1413–1457. [CrossRef]
85. Gregor, K.; LeCun, Y. Learning fast approximations of sparse coding. In Proceedings of the 27th International Conference on International Conference on Machine Learning, Haifa, Israel, 21–24 June 2010; pp. 399–406.

86. Lempitsky, V.; Vedaldi, A.; Ulyanov, D. Deep Image Prior. In Proceedings of the 2018 IEEE/CVF Conference on Computer Vision and Pattern Recognition, Salt Lake City, UT, USA, 18–23 June 2018; pp. 9446–9454. [CrossRef]
87. Dittmer, S.; Kluth, T.; Maass, P.; Otero Baguer, D. Regularization by Architecture: A Deep Prior Approach for Inverse Problems. *J. Math. Imaging Vis.* **2019**, *62*, 456–470. [CrossRef]
88. Chakrabarty, P.; Maji, S. The Spectral Bias of the Deep Image Prior. *arXiv* **2019**, arXiv:1912.08905.
89. Heckel, R.; Soltanolkotabi, M. Denoising and Regularization via Exploiting the Structural Bias of Convolutional Generators. *Int. Conf. Learn. Represent.* **2020**.
90. Adler, J.; Kohr, H.; Ringh, A.; Moosmann, J.; Banert, S.; Ehrhardt, M.J.; Lee, G.R.; Niinimäki, K.; Gris, B.; Verdier, O.; et al. Operator Discretization Library (ODL). *Zenodo* **2018**. [CrossRef]
91. Van Aarle, W.; Palenstijn, W.J.; De Beenhouwer, J.; Altantzis, T.; Bals, S.; Batenburg, K.J.; Sijbers, J. The ASTRA Toolbox: A platform for advanced algorithm development in electron tomography. *Ultramicroscopy* **2015**, *157*, 35–47. [CrossRef] [PubMed]
92. Coban, S. SophiaBeads Dataset Project Codes. Zenodo. 2015. Available online: http://sophilyplum.github.io/sophiabeads-datasets/ (accessed on 10 June 2020)
93. Wang, T.; Nakamoto, K.; Zhang, H.; Liu, H. Reweighted Anisotropic Total Variation Minimization for Limited-Angle CT Reconstruction. *IEEE Trans. Nucl. Sci.* **2017**, *64*, 2742–2760. [CrossRef]
94. Paszke, A.; Gross, S.; Massa, F.; Lerer, A.; Bradbury, J.; Chanan, G.; Killeen, T.; Lin, Z.; Gimelshein, N.; Antiga, L.; et al. PyTorch: An Imperative Style, High-Performance Deep Learning Library. In *Advances in Neural Information Processing Systems 32*; Wallach, H., Larochelle, H., Beygelzimer, A., dAlch'e-Buc, F., Fox, E., Garnett, R., Eds.; Curran Associates, Inc.: Red Hook, NY, USA, 2019; pp. 8024–8035.

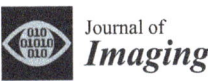

Article

Accelerating 3D Medical Image Segmentation by Adaptive Small-Scale Target Localization

Boris Shirokikh [1,*,†], Alexey Shevtsov [1,2,3,†], Alexandra Dalechina [4], Egor Krivov [2,3], Valery Kostjuchenko [4], Andrey Golanov [5], Victor Gombolevskiy [6], Sergey Morozov [6] and Mikhail Belyaev [1]

1. Center for Neurobiology and Brain Restoration, Skolkovo Institute of Science and Technology, 121205 Moscow, Russia; Alexey.Shevtsov@skoltech.ru (A.S.); m.belyaev@skoltech.ru (M.B.)
2. Sector of Data Analysis for Neuroscience, Kharkevich Institute for Information Transmission Problems, 127051 Moscow, Russia; Egor.Krivov@frtk.ru
3. Department of Radio Engineering and Cybernetics, Moscow Institute of Physics and Technology, 141701 Moscow, Russia
4. Moscow Gamma-Knife Center, 125047 Moscow, Russia; adalechina@nsi.ru (A.D.); VKostjuchenko@nsi.ru (V.K.)
5. Department of Radiosurgery and Radiation, Burdenko Neurosurgery Institute, 125047 Moscow, Russia; Golanov@nsi.ru
6. Medical Research Department, Research and Practical Clinical Center of Diagnostics and Telemedicine Technologies of the Department of Health Care of Moscow, 127051 Moscow, Russia; gombolevskiy@npcmr.ru (V.G.); morozov@npcmr.ru (S.M.)
* Correspondence: Boris.Shirokikh@skoltech.ru
† These authors contributed equally to this work.

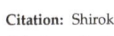

Citation: Shirokikh, B.; Shevtsov, A.; Dalechina, A.; Krivov, E.; Kostjuchenko, V.; Golanov, A.; Gombolevskiy, V.; Morozov, S.; Belyaev, M. Accelerating 3D Medical Image Segmentation by Adaptive Small-Scale Target Localization. J. Imaging 2021, 7, 35. https://doi.org/10.3390/jimaging7020035

Academic Editors: Yudong Zhang, Juan Manuel Gorriz and Zhengchao Dong

Received: 31 December 2020
Accepted: 5 February 2021
Published: 13 February 2021

Publisher's Note: MDPI stays neutral with regard to jurisdictional claims in published maps and institutional affiliations.

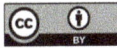

Copyright: © 2021 by the authors. Licensee MDPI, Basel, Switzerland. This article is an open access article distributed under the terms and conditions of the Creative Commons Attribution (CC BY) license (https://creativecommons.org/licenses/by/4.0/).

Abstract: The prevailing approach for three-dimensional (3D) medical image segmentation is to use convolutional networks. Recently, deep learning methods have achieved human-level performance in several important applied problems, such as volumetry for lung-cancer diagnosis or delineation for radiation therapy planning. However, state-of-the-art architectures, such as U-Net and DeepMedic, are computationally heavy and require workstations accelerated with graphics processing units for fast inference. However, scarce research has been conducted concerning enabling fast central processing unit computations for such networks. Our paper fills this gap. We propose a new segmentation method with a human-like technique to segment a 3D study. First, we analyze the image at a small scale to identify areas of interest and then process only relevant feature-map patches. Our method not only reduces the inference time from 10 min to 15 s but also preserves state-of-the-art segmentation quality, as we illustrate in the set of experiments with two large datasets.

Keywords: deep learning; medical image segmentation; computed tomography (CT); magnetic resonance imaging (MRI)

1. Introduction

Segmentation plays a vital role in many medical image analysis applications [1]. For example, the volume of lung nodules must be measured to diagnose lung cancer [2], or brain lesions must be accurately delineated before stereotactic radiosurgery [3] on Magnetic Resonance Imaging (MRI) or Positron Emission Tomography [4]. The academic community has extensively explored automatic segmentation methods and has achieved massive progress in algorithmic development [5]. The widely accepted current state-of-the-art methods are based on convolutional neural networks (CNNs), as shown by the results of major competitions, such as Lung Nodule Analysis 2016 (LUNA16) [6] and Multimodal Brain Tumor Segmentation (BraTS) [7]. Although a gap exists between computer science research and medical requirements [8], several promising clinical-ready results have been achieved (e.g., [9]). We assume that the number of validated applications and subsequent clinical installations will soon grow exponentially.

The majority of the current segmentation methods, such as DeepMedic [10] and 3D U-Net [11], rely on heavy 3D convolutional networks and require substantial computational resources. Currently, radiological departments are not typically equipped with graphics processing units (GPUs) [12]. Even when deep-learning-based tools are eligible for clinical installation and are highly demanded by radiologists, the typically slow hardware renewal cycle [13] is likely to limit the adoption of these new technologies. The critical issue is low processing time on the central processing unit (CPU) because modern networks require more than 10 min to segment large 3D images, such as a Computed Tomography (CT) chest scan. Cloud services may potentially resolve the problem, but privacy-related concerns hinder this solution in many countries. Moreover, the current workload of radiologists is more than 16.1 images per minute and continues to increase [14]. Though slow background processing is an acceptable solution for some situations, in many cases, nearly real-time performance is crucial even for diagnostics [15].

Scarce research has been conducted on evaluating the current limitations and accelerating 3D convolutional networks on a CPU (see the existing examples in Section 2). The nonmedical computer vision community actively explores different methods to increase the inference speed of the deep learning methods (e.g., mobile networks [16] that provide substantial acceleration at the cost of a moderate decrease in quality). This paper fills this gap and investigates the computational limitations of popular 3D convolutional networks in medical image segmentation using two large MRI and CT databases.

Our main contribution is a new acceleration method that adaptively processes regions of the input image. The concept is intuitive and similar to the way humans analyze 3D studies. First, we roughly process the whole image to identify areas of interest, such as lung nodules or brain metastases, and then locally segment each small part independently. As a result, our method processes 3D medical images 50 times faster than DeepMedic and 3D U-Net with the same quality and requires 15 s or less on a CPU (see Figure 1). Our idea is simple and can be jointly applied with other acceleration techniques for additional acceleration and with other architecture improvements for quality increase. We have released (https://github.com/neuro-ml/low-resolution, accessed on 29 December 2020) our code for the proposed model and the experiments with the LUNA16 dataset to facilitate future research.

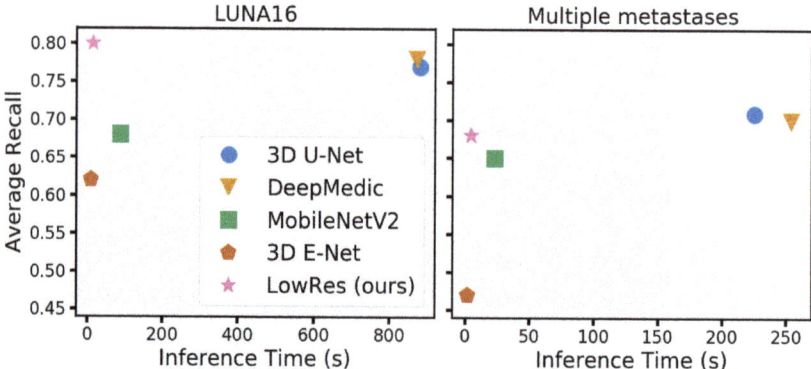

Figure 1. Time-performance trade-off for different convolutional neural network models under 8 GB of RAM and eight central processing unit thread restrictions. We evaluate models on two clinically relevant datasets with lung nodules (LUNA16) and brain metastases in terms of the average object-wise recall (LUNA16 competition metric [17]). Our model spends less than 15 s per study on processing time while preserving or even surpassing the performance of the state-of-the-art models.

2. Related Work

Many different CNN architectures have been introduced in the past to solve the semantic segmentation of volumetric medical images. Popular models, such as 3D U-Net [11] or DeepMedic [10], provide convincing results on public medical datasets [7,18]. Here, we aim to validate the effective and well-known models without diving into architecture details. Following the suggestion of [19], we mainly focus on building a state-of-the-art deep learning pipeline arguing that the architecture tweaks will have a minor contribution. Moreover, we address that the majority of the architecture tweaks could be applied to benefit our method as well (see Section 7). However, all of these methods are based on 3D convolutional layers and have numerous parameters. Therefore, the inference time could be severely affected by the absence of GPU-accelerated workstations.

2.1. Medical Imaging

Several researchers have recently studied ways to accelerate CNNs for 3D medical imaging segmentation. The authors of [20] proposed a CPU-GPU data swapping approach that allows for training a neural network on the full-size images instead of the patches. Consequently, their approach reduces the number of iterations on training, hence it reduces the total training time. However, the design of their method can hardly be used to reduce the inference time. The design does not change the number of network's parameters and moreover introduces additional time costs on the CPU-GPU data swapping process in the forward step alone. In [21], the authors developed the M-Net model for faster segmentation of brain extraction from MRI scans. The M-Net model aggregates volumetric information with a large initial 3D convolution and then processes data with a 2D CNN; hence, the resulting network has fewer parameters than the 3D analogies. However, the inference time on the CPU is 5 min for a $256 \times 256 \times 128$ volume, which is comparable to that of DeepMedic and 3D U-Net. The authors of [22] proposed a TernaryNet with sparse and binary convolutions for medical image segmentation. It tremendously reduces the inference time on the CPU from 80 s for the original 2D U-Net [23] to 7 s. The additional use of proposed weight quantization can significantly reduce the segmentation quality. In general, 2D networks perform worse than their 3D analogous in segmentation tasks with volumetric images [11,24]. The simple and natural reason for it is the inability of 2D networks to capture the objects' given volumetric information. Hence, in our work, we focus the attention on the 3D architectures.

Within our model, we use a natural two-stage method of regional localization and detailed segmentation (see Section 3). The similar approaches were proposed by [25,26]. In both papers, the first part of the method roughly localized the target anatomical region in the study. Then, the second part provided the detailed segmentation. However, the authors did not focus on the inference time and suggested using the methods to improve the segmentation quality. In addition, these architectures use independent networks, whereas we propose using weight-sharing between the first and second stages to achieve more effective inference. A similar idea of increasing the segmentation quality using multiple resolutions was studied by [27].

2.2. Nonmedical Imaging

The most common way to reduce the model size and thus increase inference speed is to use *mobile neural network architectures* [16], which are designed to run on low-power devices. For example, *E-Net* [28] replaces the standard convolutional blocks with asymmetric convolutions that could be especially effective in our 3D tasks. Additionally, *MobileNetV2* [29] uses inverted residual blocks with separable convolutions to reduce the computationally expensive convolutions. Unfortunately, most mobile architectures suffer from a loss in quality due to the achieved speed gain, which could be crucial for medical tasks.

3. Method

The current state-of-the-art segmentation models spend equal computational resources on all parts of the input image. However, the fraction of the target on the images is often very low (e.g., 10^{-2} or even 10^{-3}) for lung-nodule segmentation (see the distribution of the lesions diameters in the Figure 2). Moreover, these multiple small targets are distinct. With our architecture, *LowRes* (Figure 3), we aim to use the human-like approach to delineate the image. First, we solve the simpler task of *target localization*, modeling a human expert's quick review of the whole image. Then, we apply *detailed segmentation* to the proposed regions, incorporating features from the first step. A similar idea was proposed in [30] where low resolution image was used to localize a large object prior to further segmentation to reduce GPU memory consumption.

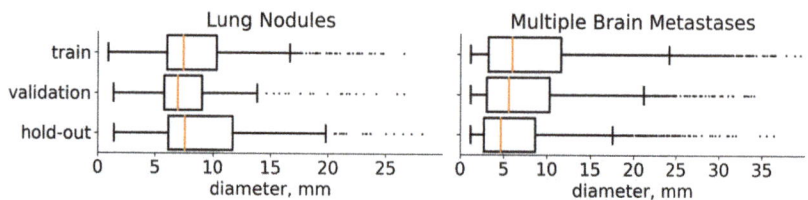

Figure 2. Diameter distribution of tumors in the chosen datasets. On both plots, the distribution is presented separately for each subset for which we split the data. The median value is highlighted with orange. In addition, medical studies [31,32] recommend choosing a 10 mm threshold for the data that contain lung nodules and 5 mm threshold for multiple brain metastases, when classifying the particular component of a target as small.

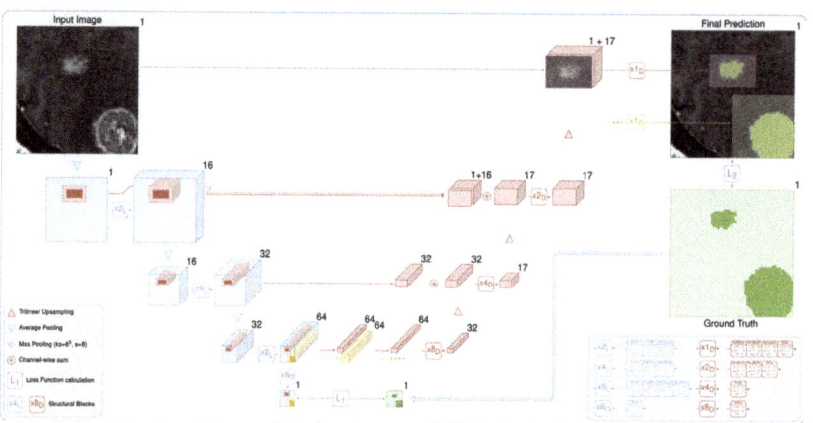

Figure 3. The proposed architecture is a two-stage fully convolutional neural network. It includes *low-resolution segmentation* (blue), which predicts the 8^3 times downsampled mask, and *detailed segmentation* (red), which *iteratively* and *locally* aggregates features from the first stage and predicts the segmentation map in the original resolution. Speedup comes from two main factors: the lighter network with early downsampling in the first stage and the heavier second part that typically processes only 5% of the image.

We demonstrate the effectiveness of the method without delving into the architecture details. Our architecture is the de-facto 3D implementation of U-Net [23]. We use residual blocks (ResBlocks) [33], apply batch normalization, and ReLU activation [34] after every convolution except the output convolution. The number of input and output channels is shown for every convolution and ResBlock in the legend of Figure 3. We apply the sigmoid function to the one-channel output logits to obtain the probabilities of the foreground class. Note that our architecture could be trivially extended to solve the multiclass segmentation task by changing the number of output layers and replacing the sigmoid function with softmax.

3.1. Target Localization

The current approach to localizing targets is neural networks for object detection [35]. Nevertheless, classical object detection tasks often include multi-label classification and overlapping bounding box detection and are sensitive to a set of hyperparameters: intersection over union threshold, anchor sizes, and so on. We consider it to be overly complicated for our problem of semantic segmentation. Hence, we use the CNN segmentation model to predict the $8 \times 8 \times 8$ times downsampled probability map ($x8_O$ output in Figure 3). Processing an image in the initial resolution is the main bottleneck of the standard segmentation CNNs. We avoid this by downsampling an image before passing it to the model. For our tasks, we downsample an input image only twice in every spatial dimension. Applying downsampling with a factor of 4 gives us significantly worse results. We train the low-resolution part of our model via standard backpropagation, minimizing the loss function between the output probability map and the ground truth downsampled with $8 \times 8 \times 8$ kernels of max pooling. It is detailed in Figure 3 in green.

Early downsampling and lighter modeling allow us to process a 3D image much faster. Moreover, the model can solve a "simpler" task of object localization with higher object-wise recall than the standard segmentation models. The U-Net-like architecture allows us to efficiently aggregate features and pass them to the next stage of detailed segmentation.

3.2. Detailed Segmentation

The pretrained first part of our model predicts the downsampled probability map, which we use to localize the regions of interest. We binarize the downsampled prediction using the standard probability threshold of 0.5. We do not use any fine-tuning of the threshold and also use this standard value to obtain a binary segmentation map for every model. After binarization, we divide the segmentation map into the connected components. Then, we create bounding boxes with a margin of 1 voxel (in low resolution) for every component. We apply the margin to correct the possible drawbacks of the previous rough segmentation step in detecting boundaries. The larger margins will sufficiently increase the inference time, hence we use the minimum possible margin.

The detailed part of our model predicts every bounding box in the original resolution. It processes, aggregates, and upsamples features from the first stage, similar to the original U-Net, but with two major differences: (i) the model uses features corresponding only to the selected bounding box and (ii) iteratively predicts every proposed component. The process is detailed in Figure 3 in red. The outputs are finally inserted into the prediction map with the original resolution, which is initially filled with zeros. Although the detailed part is heavier than the low-resolution path, it preserves the fast inference speed because it typically processes only 5% of the image.

We train the model through the standard backpropagation procedure, simply minimizing the loss function between the full prediction map and the corresponding ground truth. We use the pretrained first part of our model and freeze its weights while training the second part. The same training set is used for both stages to ensure no leak in validation or hold-out data, which could lead to overfitting.

4. Data

We report our results based on two large datasets: a private MRI dataset with multiple brain metastases and a publicly available CT chest scan from LUNA16 [17]. The dataset with multiple brain metastases consists of 1952 unique T1-weighted MRI of the head with a $0.94 \times 0.94 \times 1$ mm image resolution and $211 \times 198 \times 164$ typical shape. We do not perform any brain-specific preprocessing, such as template registration or skull stripping.

LUNA16 includes 888 3D chest scans from the LIDC/IDRI database [18] with the typical shape $432 \times 306 \times 214$ and the largest at $512 \times 512 \times 652$. To preprocess the image, we apply the provided lung masks (excluding the aorta component). In addition, we exclude all cases with nodules located outside of the lung mask (72 cases). Then, we clip the intensities to between -1000 and 300 Hounsfield units. We average four given annotations [18] to generate the mean mask for the subsequent training. Finally, we scale the images from both datasets to reach values between 0 and 1.

We use the *train-validation* setup to select hyperparameters and then merge these subsets to retrain the final model. The results are reported on a previously unseen *hold-out* set. Furthermore, LUNA16 is presented as 10 approximately equal subsets [17] so we use the first six for *training* (534 images), the next two for *validation* (178 images), and the last two as *hold-out* (174 images). Multiple metastases datasets are randomly divided into *training* (1250 images), *validation* (402 images), and *hold-out* (300 images). The diameters distribution of the tumors on these three sets for both datasets is given in Figure 2.

5. Experiments and Results

5.1. Training

We minimize Dice Loss [36] because it provides consistently better results on the validation data for all models. The only exception is the first stage of LowRes—we use weighted cross-entropy [23] to train it. We train all models for 100 epochs consisting of 100 iterations of stochastic gradient descent with Nesterov momentum (0.9). The training starts with a learning rate of 10^{-2}, and it is reduced to 10^{-3} at epoch 80. During the preliminary experiments, we ensure that both training loss and validation score reach a plateau for all models. Therefore, we assume this training policy to be enough for the representative performance and the further fine-tuning will result only in the minor score changes.

We also use validation scores of the preliminary experiments to determine the best combination of patch size and batch size for every model. The latter represents a memory trade-off between a larger batch size for the better generalization and a sufficient patch size to capture enough contextual information. We set the patch size of $64 \times 64 \times 64$ for all models except the DeepMedic. DeepMedic has a patch size of $39 \times 39 \times 39$. The batch size is 12 for the 3D U-Net, 16 for DeepMedic, and 32 for the LowRes and mobile networks. Sampled patch contains a ground truth object with the probability of 0.5, otherwise it is sampled randomly. This sampling strategy is suggested to efficiently alleviate class-imbalance [10].

We use the DeepMedic and 3D U-Net architectures without any adjustments. Mobile network architectures [28,29] are designed for 2D image processing, hence we add an extra dimension. Apart from the 3D generalization, we use the vanilla E-Net architecture. However, MobileNetV2 is a feature extractor by the design, thus we complete it with a U-Net-like decoder preserving the speedup ideas.

5.2. Experimental Setup

We highlight two main characteristics of all methods: *inference time* and *segmentation quality*. We measure the average inference time for 10 randomly chosen images for each dataset. To ensure broad coverage of the possible hardware setups, we report time at 4, 8, and 16 threads on an Intel(R) Xeon(R) CPU E5-2690 v4 @ 2.60 GHz. Models running on a standard workstation have random-access memory (RAM) usage constraints. Hence, during the inference step, we divide an image into patches to iteratively predict them and combine them back into the full segmentation map. We operate under the upper boundary of 16 GB of RAM. We also noted that the inference time does not heavily depend on the partition sizes and strides, except the cases with a huge overlap of predicting patches.

The most common method to measure segmentation performance is the Dice Score [7]. However, averaging the Dice Score over images has a serious drawback in the case of multiple targets because large objects overshadow small ones. Hence, we report the average Dice Score per unique object. We use the Free-response Receiver Operating Characteristic (FROC) analysis [37] to assess the detection quality. Such a curve illustrates the trade-off between the model's object-wise recall and average false positives (FPs) per image. The authors of [37] also extracted a single score from these curves—the *average recall* at seven predefined FP rates: 1/8, 1/4, 1/2, 1, 2, 4, and 8 FPs per scan. We report more robust values averaged over FP points from 0 to 5 with a step of 0.01. Hence, the detection quality is measured similarly to the LUNA16 challenge [17]. This is our main quality metric because the fraction of detected lesions per case is an important clinical characteristic, especially for lung-cancer screening [38].

5.3. Results

The final evaluation of the hold-out data of the inference time and segmentation quality is given in Table 1 for LUNA16 and in Table 2 for multiple metastase datasets. Moreover, LowRes achieves a comparable inference speed with the fastest 3D mobile network E-Net. The maximum inference time is 23 s with four CPU threads on LUNA16 data. Our model achieves the same detection quality using the state-of-the-art DeepMedic and 3D U-Net models, outperforming them in terms of speed by approximately 60 times. The visual representation of the time-performance trade-off is given in Figure 1.

Table 1. Comparative performance of segmentation models on LUNA16 data. Standard deviation for every measurement is given in brackets. The best values for each column are emphasized in bold. The quality metrics definitions are given in the last paragraph of Section 5.2.

	Inference Time * (CPU Threads)			Quality Metrics	
	4 Threads	8 Threads	16 Threads	Avg Recall	Obj DSC
3D U-Net	1293 (100)	880 (61)	828 (62)	0.77 (0.02)	**0.82 (0.16)**
DeepMedic	1139 (162)	872 (138)	840 (127)	0.78 (0.02)	0.78 (0.20)
3D MobileNetV2	108 (14)	89 (12)	74 (10)	0.68 (0.02)	0.75 (0.22)
3D E-Net	**11 (1.2)**	**9.5 (1.2)**	**9.2 (1.0)**	0.62 (0.02)	0.70 (0.22)
LowRes	23 (2.9)	15 (1.9)	13 (1.7)	**0.80 (0.02)**	0.75 (.18)

* in seconds.

Table 2. Comparative performance of segmentation models on Multiple Metastases data. Standard deviation for every measurement is given in brackets. The best values for each column are emphasized in bold. The quality metrics definitions are given in the last paragraph of Section 5.2.

	Inference Time * (CPU Threads)			Quality Metrics	
	4 Threads	8 Threads	16 Threads	Avg Recall	Obj DSC
3D U-Net	342 (36)	225 (20)	202 (16)	**0.71 (0.01)**	**0.72 (0.21)**
DeepMedic	381 (74)	254 (50)	226 (46)	0.70 (0.02)	0.69 (0.23)
3D MobileNetV2	33 (4.6)	23 (3.0)	21 (2.4)	0.65 (0.01)	0.69 (0.22)
3D E-Net	**3.2 (0.3)**	**1.7 (0.2)**	**1.9 (0.3)**	0.47 (0.01)	0.59 (0.23)
LowRes	6.1 (0.7)	4.3 (0.6)	3.7 (0.6)	0.68 (0.01)	0.64 (0.22)

* in seconds.

6. Discussion

To our knowledge, the proposed method is the first two-stage network that utilizes local feature representation from the first network to accelerate a heavy second network. We carefully combined well studied DL techniques with the new final goal to speed up CPU processing time significantly without minor quality loss (see Section 1, the last paragraph). De-facto, our method can indeed be considered two separate networks as far as they are trained separately. However, we highlight that our work is one of the first accelerated DL methods for medical images, so it opens up a curious research direction of simultaneous learning of both CNN parts, among other ideas.

The "other ideas" mean the key concepts proposed to reduce the inference time or increase the segmentation and detection quality in many recent papers, which can be applied to our method. However, the research direction for medical image segmentation is naturally biased towards addressing the segmentation and detection quality, so these papers' results are of particular interest. We can not address all of them here and provide comparison only to the well-known baseline methods like 3D U-Net and DeepMedic on the open-source LUNA16 dataset for the two main reasons. First, researchers can easily compare their great methods with ours and elaborate on this curious research direction. Second, most of the best practices from the recent methods can be adapted to ours without restriction. For example, one can modify skip connections by adding Bi-Directional ConvLSTM [39] or add a residual path with deconvolution and activation operations [40]. However, applying these improvements will likely preserve the time gap between the particular method and ours, modified correspondingly. Note that our pioneer work proposes the general idea of the speed up on CPU, so we treat such experiments as a possible way to work on in future, which is a common practice.

7. Conclusions

We proposed a two-stage CNN called LowRes (Figure 3) to solve 3D medical image segmentation tasks on a CPU workstation within 15 s for a single case. Our network uses a human-like approach of a quick review of the image to detect regions of interest and then processes these regions locally (see Section 3). The proposed model achieves an inference speed close to that of mobile networks and preserves or even increases the performance of the state-of-the-art segmentation networks (Tables 1 and 2).

Author Contributions: B.S.: methodology, investigation, software, formal analysis, data curation, writing—original draft preparation, visualization; A.S.: investigation, software, formal analysis, data curation, visualization, writing—original draft; A.D.: conceptualization; data curation; E.K.: methodology, software; V.K.: data curation; A.G.: supervision, data curation; V.G.: conceptualization; S.M.: supervision, conceptualization; M.B.: conceptualization, methodology, writing—review and editing, supervision, funding acquisition. All authors have read and agreed to the published version of the manuscript.

Funding: This research was supported by the Russian Science Foundation grant 20-71-10134.

Institutional Review Board Statement: Ethical review and approval were waived for this study due to the full anonymization of the utilized data.

Informed Consent Statement: Patient consent was waived due to the full anonymization of the utilized data.

Data Availability Statement: The CT chest scan dataset from LUNA16 competition presented in this study is openly available [17]. The MRI dataset with multiple brain metastasis presented in this study is not available publicly due to the privacy reasons.

Acknowledgments: The authors acknowledge the National Cancer Institute and the Foundation for the National Institutes of Health, and their critical role in the creation of the free publicly available LIDC/IDRI Database used in this study.

Conflicts of Interest: The authors declare no conflict of interest.

Abbreviations

The following abbreviations are used in this manuscript:

MDPI	Multidisciplinary Digital Publishing Institute
BraTS	Multimodal Brain Tumor Segmentation
CNN	Convolutional Neural Network
CPU	Central Processing Unit

CT	Computed Tomography
DSC	Dice Score
FP	False Positive
FROC	Free-response Receiver Operating Characteristic
GPU	Graphics Processing Unit
LUNA16	Lung Nodule Analysis 2016
MRI	Magnetic Resonance Imaging
RAM	Random Access Memory
ReLU	Rectified Linear Unit

References

1. Pham, D.L.; Xu, C.; Prince, J.L. Current methods in medical image segmentation. *Annu. Rev. Biomed. Eng.* **2000**, *2*, 315–337. [CrossRef]
2. The Lancet Digital Health. Leaving cancer diagnosis to the computers. *Lancet Digit. Health* **2020**, *2*, e49. [CrossRef]
3. Meyer, P.; Noblet, V.; Mazzara, C.; Lallement, A. Survey on deep learning for radiotherapy. *Comput. Biol. Med.* **2018**, *98*, 126–146. [CrossRef] [PubMed]
4. Comelli, A. Fully 3D Active Surface with Machine Learning for PET Image Segmentation. *J. Imaging* **2020**, *6*, 113. [CrossRef]
5. Greenspan, H.; Van Ginneken, B.; Summers, R.M. Guest editorial deep learning in medical imaging: Overview and future promise of an exciting new technique. *IEEE Trans. Med. Imaging* **2016**, *35*, 1153–1159. [CrossRef]
6. Setio, A.A.A.; Traverso, A.; De Bel, T.; Berens, M.S.; van den Bogaard, C.; Cerello, P.; Chen, H.; Dou, Q.; Fantacci, M.E.; Geurts, B.; et al. Validation, comparison, and combination of algorithms for automatic detection of pulmonary nodules in computed tomography images: The LUNA16 challenge. *Med. Image Anal.* **2017**, *42*, 1–13. [CrossRef]
7. Bakas, S.; Reyes, M.; Jakab, A.; Bauer, S.; Rempfler, M.; Crimi, A.; Shinohara, R.T.; Berger, C.; Ha, S.M.; Rozycki, M.; et al. Identifying the best machine learning algorithms for brain tumor segmentation, progression assessment, and overall survival prediction in the BRATS challenge. *arXiv* **2018**, arXiv:1811.02629.
8. Liu, X.; Faes, L.; Kale, A.U.; Wagner, S.K.; Fu, D.J.; Bruynseels, A.; Mahendiran, T.; Moraes, G.; Shamdas, M.; Kern, C.; et al. A comparison of deep learning performance against health-care professionals in detecting diseases from medical imaging. A systematic review and meta-analysis. *Lancet Digit. Health* **2019**, *1*, e271–e297. [CrossRef]
9. Ardila, D.; Kiraly, A.P.; Bharadwaj, S.; Choi, B.; Reicher, J.J.; Peng, L.; Tse, D.; Etemadi, M.; Ye, W.; Corrado, G.; et al. End-to-end lung cancer screening with three-dimensional deep learning on low-dose chest computed tomography. *Nat. Med.* **2019**, *25*, 954–961. [CrossRef]
10. Kamnitsas, K.; Ledig, C.; Newcombe, V.F.; Simpson, J.P.; Kane, A.D.; Menon, D.K.; Rueckert, D.; Glocker, B. Efficient multi-scale 3D CNN with fully connected CRF for accurate brain lesion segmentation. *Med. Image Anal.* **2017**, *36*, 61–78. [CrossRef]
11. Çiçek, Ö.; Abdulkadir, A.; Lienkamp, S.S.; Brox, T.; Ronneberger, O. 3D U-Net: Learning dense volumetric segmentation from sparse annotation. In *International Conference on Medical Image Computing and Computer-Assisted Intervention*; Springer: Berlin, Germany, 2016; pp. 424–432.
12. Chen, D.; Liu, S.; Kingsbury, P.; Sohn, S.; Storlie, C.B.; Habermann, E.B.; Naessens, J.M.; Larson, D.W.; Liu, H. Deep learning and alternative learning strategies for retrospective real-world clinical data. *NPJ Digit. Med.* **2019**, *2*, 1–5. [CrossRef]
13. European Society of Radiology. Renewal of radiological equipment. *Insights Imaging* **2014**, *5*, 543–546. [CrossRef]
14. McDonald, R.J.; Schwartz, K.M.; Eckel, L.J.; Diehn, F.E.; Hunt, C.H.; Bartholmai, B.J.; Erickson, B.J.; Kallmes, D.F. The effects of changes in utilization and technological advancements of cross-sectional imaging on radiologist workload. *Acad. Radiol.* **2015**, *22*, 1191–1198. [CrossRef]
15. Lindfors, K.K.; O'Connor, J.; Parker, R.A. False-positive screening mammograms: Effect of immediate versus later work-up on patient stress. *Radiology* **2001**, *218*, 247–253. [CrossRef] [PubMed]
16. Howard, A.G.; Zhu, M.; Chen, B.; Kalenichenko, D.; Wang, W.; Weyand, T.; Andreetto, M.; Adam, H. Mobilenets: Efficient convolutional neural networks for mobile vision applications. *arXiv* **2017**, arXiv:1704.04861.
17. Jacobs, C.; Setio, A.A.A.; Traverso, A.; van Ginneken, B. LUng Nodule Analysis 2016. Available online: https://luna16.grand-challenge.org (accessed on 9 December 2019).
18. Armato, S.G., III; McLennan, G.; Bidaut, L.; McNitt-Gray, M.F.; Meyer, C.R.; Reeves, A.P.; Zhao, B.; Aberle, D.R.; Henschke, C.I.; Hoffman, E.A.; et al. The lung image database consortium (LIDC) and image database resource initiative (IDRI): A completed reference database of lung nodules on CT scans. *Med. Phys.* **2011**, *38*, 915–931.
19. Isensee, F.; Kickingereder, P.; Wick, W.; Bendszus, M.; Maier-Hein, K.H. No new-net. In *International MICCAI Brainlesion Workshop*; Springer: Berlin, Germany, 2018; pp. 234–244.
20. Imai, H.; Matzek, S.; Le, T.D.; Negishi, Y.; Kawachiya, K. Fast and accurate 3d medical image segmentation with data-swapping method. *arXiv* **2018**, arXiv:1812.07816.
21. Mehta, R.; Sivaswamy, J. M-net: A convolutional neural network for deep brain structure segmentation. In Proceedings of the 2017 IEEE 14th International Symposium on Biomedical Imaging (ISBI 2017), Melbourne, VIC, Australia, 18–21 April 2017; pp. 437–440.

22. Heinrich, M.P.; Blendowski, M.; Oktay, O. TernaryNet: Faster deep model inference without GPUs for medical 3D segmentation using sparse and binary convolutions. *Int. J. Comput. Assist. Radiol. Surg.* **2018**, *13*, 1311–1320. [CrossRef]
23. Ronneberger, O.; Fischer, P.; Brox, T. U-net: Convolutional networks for biomedical image segmentation. In *International Conference on Medical Image Computing and Computer-Assisted Intervention*; Springer: Berlin, Germany, 2015; pp. 234–241.
24. Lai, M. Deep learning for medical image segmentation. *arXiv* **2015**, arXiv:1505.02000.
25. Zhao, N.; Tong, N.; Ruan, D.; Sheng, K. Fully Automated Pancreas Segmentation with Two-Stage 3D Convolutional Neural Networks. In *International Conference on Medical Image Computing and Computer-Assisted Intervention*; Springer: Berlin, Germany, 2019; pp. 201–209.
26. Wang, C.; MacGillivray, T.; Macnaught, G.; Yang, G.; Newby, D. A two-stage 3D Unet framework for multi-class segmentation on full resolution image. *arXiv* **2018**, arXiv:1804.04341.
27. Gerard, S.E.; Herrmann, J.; Kaczka, D.W.; Musch, G.; Fernandez-Bustamante, A.; Reinhardt, J.M. Multi-resolution convolutional neural networks for fully automated segmentation of acutely injured lungs in multiple species. *Med. Image Anal.* **2020**, *60*, 101592. [CrossRef] [PubMed]
28. Paszke, A.; Chaurasia, A.; Kim, S.; Culurciello, E. Enet: A deep neural network architecture for real-time semantic segmentation. *arXiv* **2016**, arXiv:1606.02147.
29. Sandler, M.; Howard, A.; Zhu, M.; Zhmoginov, A.; Chen, L.C. Mobilenetv2: Inverted residuals and linear bottlenecks. In Proceedings of the IEEE Conference on Computer Vision and Pattern Recognition, Salt Lake City, UT, USA, 18–23 June 2018; pp. 4510–4520.
30. Vesal, S.; Maier, A.; Ravikumar, N. Fully Automated 3D Cardiac MRI Localisation and Segmentation Using Deep Neural Networks. *J. Imaging* **2020**, *6*, 65. [CrossRef]
31. Lin, N.U.; Lee, E.Q.; Aoyama, H.; Barani, I.J.; Barboriak, D.P.; Baumert, B.G.; Bendszus, M.; Brown, P.D.; Camidge, D.R.; Chang, S.M.; et al. Response assessment criteria for brain metastases: Proposal from the RANO group. *Lancet Oncol.* **2015**, *16*, e270–e278. [CrossRef]
32. Bankier, A.A.; MacMahon, H.; Goo, J.M.; Rubin, G.D.; Schaefer-Prokop, C.M.; Naidich, D.P. Recommendations for measuring pulmonary nodules at CT: A statement from the Fleischner Society. *Radiology* **2017**, *285*, 584–600. [CrossRef] [PubMed]
33. He, K.; Zhang, X.; Ren, S.; Sun, J. Deep residual learning for image recognition. In Proceedings of the IEEE Conference on Computer Vision and Pattern Recognition, Las Vegas, NV, USA, 27–30 June 2016; pp. 770–778.
34. Nair, V.; Hinton, G.E. Rectified linear units improve restricted boltzmann machines. In Proceedings of the 27th International Conference on Machine Learning (ICML-10), Haifa, Israel, 21–24 June 2010; pp. 807–814.
35. Zhao, Z.Q.; Zheng, P.; Xu, S.t.; Wu, X. Object detection with deep learning: A review. *IEEE Trans. Neural Netw. Learn. Syst.* **2019**, *30*, 3212–3232. [CrossRef]
36. Milletari, F.; Navab, N.; Ahmadi, S.A. V-net: Fully convolutional neural networks for volumetric medical image segmentation. In Proceedings of the 2016 Fourth International Conference on 3D Vision (3DV), Stanford, CA, USA, 25–28 October 2016; pp. 565–571.
37. Van Ginneken, B.; Armato, S.G., III; de Hoop, B.; van Amelsvoort-van de Vorst, S.; Duindam, T.; Niemeijer, M.; Murphy, K.; Schilham, A.; Retico, A.; Fantacci, M.E.; et al. Comparing and combining algorithms for computer-aided detection of pulmonary nodules in computed tomography scans: The ANODE09 study. *Med. Image Anal.* **2010**, *14*, 707–722.
38. Quekel, L.G.; Kessels, A.G.; Goei, R.; van Engelshoven, J.M. Miss rate of lung cancer on the chest radiograph in clinical practice. *Chest* **1999**, *115*, 720–724. [CrossRef] [PubMed]
39. Azad, R.; Asadi-Aghbolaghi, M.; Fathy, M.; Escalera, S. Bi-directional convlstm u-net with densley connected convolutions. In Proceedings of the IEEE/CVF International Conference on Computer Vision Workshops, Seoul, Korea, 27–28 October 2019.
40. Seo, H.; Huang, C.; Bassenne, M.; Xiao, R.; Xing, L. Modified U-Net (mU-Net) with incorporation of object-dependent high level features for improved liver and liver-tumor segmentation in CT images. *IEEE Trans. Med. Imaging* **2019**, *39*, 1316–1325. [CrossRef]

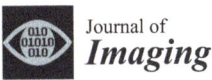

Article

Domain Adaptation for Medical Image Segmentation: A Meta-Learning Method

Penghao Zhang [1,†], Jiayue Li [2,*,†], Yining Wang [3] and Judong Pan [4]

1. School of Information and Communication Engineering, Beijing University of Posts and Telecommunications, Beijing 100876, China; zphbupt@bupt.edu.cn
2. School of Computing, Informatics, and Decision Systems Engineering, Arizona State University, Tempe, AZ 85281, USA
3. Department of Radiology, State Key Laboratory of Complex Severe and Rare Diseases, Peking Union Medical College Hospital, Chinese Academy of Medical Sciences and Peking Union Medical College, Beijing 100730, China; WangYiNing@pumch.cn
4. Department of Radiology and Biomedical Imaging, University of California San Francisco, San Francisco, CA 94143, USA; judong.pan@ucsf.edu
* Correspondence: jiayuel1@asu.edu
† These authors contributed equally to this work.

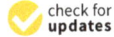

Citation: Zhang, P.; Li, J.; Wang, Y.; Pan, J. Domain Adaptation for Medical Image Segmentation: A Meta-Learning Method. *J. Imaging* **2021**, *7*, 31. https://doi.org/10.3390/jimaging7020031

Academic Editor: Yudong Zhang
Received: 30 December 2020
Accepted: 4 February 2021
Published: 10 February 2021

Publisher's Note: MDPI stays neutral with regard to jurisdictional claims in published maps and institutional affiliations.

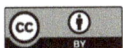

Copyright: © 2021 by the authors. Licensee MDPI, Basel, Switzerland. This article is an open access article distributed under the terms and conditions of the Creative Commons Attribution (CC BY) license (https://creativecommons.org/licenses/by/4.0/).

Abstract: Convolutional neural networks (CNNs) have demonstrated great achievement in increasing the accuracy and stability of medical image segmentation. However, existing CNNs are limited by the problem of dependency on the availability of training data owing to high manual annotation costs and privacy issues. To counter this limitation, domain adaptation (DA) and few-shot learning have been extensively studied. Inspired by these two categories of approaches, we propose an optimization-based meta-learning method for segmentation tasks. Even though existing meta-learning methods use prior knowledge to choose parameters that generalize well from few examples, these methods limit the diversity of the task distribution that they can learn from in medical image segmentation. In this paper, we propose a meta-learning algorithm to augment the existing algorithms with the capability to learn from diverse segmentation tasks across the entire task distribution. Specifically, our algorithm aims to learn from the diversity of image features which characterize a specific tissue type while showing diverse signal intensities. To demonstrate the effectiveness of the proposed algorithm, we conducted experiments using a diverse set of segmentation tasks from the Medical Segmentation Decathlon and two meta-learning benchmarks: model-agnostic meta-learning (MAML) and Reptile. U-Net and Dice similarity coefficient (DSC) were selected as the baseline model and the main performance metric, respectively. The experimental results show that our algorithm maximally surpasses MAML and Reptile by 2% and 2.4% respectively, in terms of the DSC. By showing a consistent improvement in subjective measures, we can also infer that our algorithm can produce a better generalization of a target task that has few examples.

Keywords: medical image segmentation; domain adaptation; meta-learning; U-Net

1. Introduction

Image segmentation is often the first and the most critical step in the analysis of medical images for computer-aided diagnosis and therapy. Medical image segmentation is a challenging and complex task due to the intrinsic nature of images. For instance, it is difficult for experienced experts to accurately identify multiple sclerosis lesions in MRIs due to the variability in lesion location, size, and shape, and the anatomical variability across patients [1]. Manual segmentation has been gradually replaced by automatic segmentation because of the high costs and time consumption [2]. Among existing automatic segmentation methods, Convolutional neural networks (CNNs) have demonstrated great achievement in increasing segmentation accuracy and stability [3–8]. However, existing

CNNs are limited by the problem of dependency on the availability of training data owing to high manual annotation costs and privacy issues.

To counter that limitation, domain adaptation (DA) and few-shot learning have been extensively studied in semantic segmentation. DA focuses on using some data from the target domain to quickly adapt a model trained in the source domain [9–14]. Few-shot learning aims to learn the patterns of new concepts unseen in the training data, given only a few labeled examples [15–19]. Inspired by previous works on DA and few-shot learning, we have a question: can we adjust an optimization algorithm so that the segmentation model can be good at learning with only a few examples? In order to solve this question, we take an optimization-based meta-learning method to DA. The meta-learning method learns to align source and target data in a domain-invariant discriminative feature space [20–22]. Existing optimization-based meta-learning algorithms such as model-agnostic meta-learning (MAML) [23] and Reptile [24] aim to search for the optimal initialization state to quickly adapt a base-learner to a new task. MAML is compatible with any model trained with gradient descent. It is also applicable to a variety of different learning problems, including classification, regression, and reinforcement learning. MAML provides a good initialization of model parameters which achieve optimal fast learning toward a new task with only a small number of gradient steps. In the meantime, MAML can avoid the overfitting that may happen when using a small dataset. In MAML, source tasks are split into support and query sets for support-training and query-testing purposes, respectively. In the inner loop of MAML, a model is trained to solve each support set in turn based on a few examples and gradient steps. Fast domain adaptation is achieved by training the source model with the query set in the outer loop. Unlike MAML, which uses a support-query scheme to quickly adapt a model to a new task, in the inner loop of Reptile, the model is iteratively trained on a sampled task by multiple gradient steps. The model is then updated towards the gradients learned from the sampled task in the outer loop. Reptile does not require differentiating through the optimization process, making it more suitable for optimization problems where many update steps are required.

Even though MAML and Reptile use prior knowledge to choose parameters that generalize well from few examples, both algorithms limit the diversity of the task distribution that they can learn from in medical image segmentation. Specifically, MAML updates the initial parameter vector towards the direction of a query-testing phase, which limits the capability of updating the initial parameter vector by learning from the tasks in the support-training phase. Reptile limits the ability of updating the model parameters since it does not learn from diverse tasks in the inner loop. In order to counter the limitations in MAML and Reptile, we propose to augment both algorithms with the capability to learn from diverse segmentation tasks across the entire task distribution. Specifically, our algorithm aims to learn from the diversity of image features which characterize a specific tissue type while showing diverse signal intensities. The reason that the proposed idea can benefit from signal intensities is described as follows. In MRI, the terms low, intermediate, and high signal intensities are used. Depending on the scan protocol, a tissue type is imaged as white if it has high signal intensities, as gray if it has intermediate signal intensities, and as dark gray/black if it has low signal intensities. We focus on a class of tissue types which move often: the heart is moving as it beats, the colon is moving as it digests, etc. Due to the movement, these tissue types show diverse image features regarding location, size, shape, and impact on the surrounding area. The image features are described by diverse signal intensities, such as high, intermediate, and low. The learning capability is therefore enhanced if we can learn from the diversity of image features which characterize a specific tissue type while showing diverse signal intensities. Figure 1 displays two example tissue types; each one shows diverse image features regarding location, size, shape, and impact on the surrounding area.

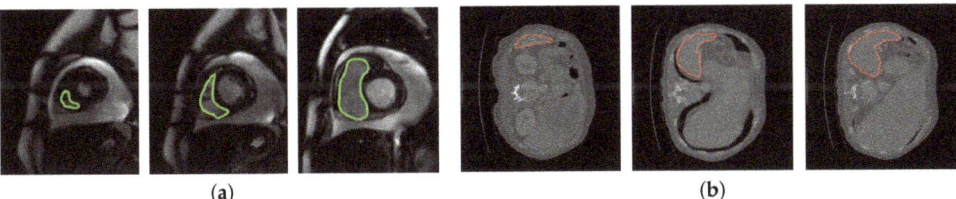

Figure 1. The diversity of image features in two example tissue types: heart (**left**) and spleen (**right**). The image features are segmented by green and red lines in the heart and spleen, respectively. (**a**) Heart; (**b**) spleen.

Our algorithm is briefly introduced as follows: In the inner loop, we first iteratively train the initial parameter vector on a batch of support sets via multiple gradient steps. Based on the parameter vector learned from the support batch, we then adapt the parameter vector to a batch of query sets via one gradient step in the outer loop. After that, we update the model towards the parameter vector learned from the query batch. Both support and query batches are sampled from the entire task distribution. To demonstrate the effectiveness of our method, we conducted experiments using a diverse set of segmentation tasks from the Medical Segmentation Decathlon and two meta-learning benchmarks: MAML and Reptile. U-Net [25] and Dice similarity coefficient (DSC) were selected as the baseline model and the main performance metric, respectively. The experimental result shows that our algorithm maximally surpasses MAML and Reptile by 2% and 2.4% respectively, in terms of the DSC. By showing a consistent improvement in subjective measures, we can also infer that our algorithm can produce a better generalization of a target task that has few examples. The contributions of our algorithm focus on two points:

- Unlike existing meta-learning algorithms which limit the capability of learning from diverse task distributions, we studied the feasibility of learning from the diversity of image features which characterizes a specific tissue type while showing diverse signal intensities.
- We propose an algorithm which can nicely learn from diverse segmentation tasks across the entire task distribution. The effectiveness of our algorithm is illustrated by showing consistent improvements in DSC and subjective measures.

2. Related Work

2.1. Convolutional Neural Networks

The concept of deep learning originates from the research of hierarchical artificial neural networks. Unlike traditional segmentation methods that only utilize low-level information such as pixel color, brightness, and texture, deep learning methods perform better on extracting semantic information. One of the deep learning methods is CNN. CNN is a kind of neural network with a special connective structure in hidden layers. With its rich feature extractors, some classic models such as AlexNet [26], VGG [27], GoogleNet [28], and ResNet [29] have been widely used in most computer vision tasks.

In the field of medical image processing, the fully convolutional network (FCN) [30] and U-Net [25] are commonly used. Since FCN is a pixel-wise classification model, it does not perform as well as U-Net for exploiting the relationship between pixels and boundary information of the up-sampling results. U-Net consists of a contraction path (encoder) and a symmetrical extension path (decoder) connected by a bottleneck. The encoder gradually reduces the spatial size of feature maps, which captures the context information and transmits it to the decoder. The decoder recovers the image details and spatial dimensions of the object through up-sampling and skip connections. Even though there has been a collection of variations of U-Net produced to improve segmentation accuracy, it still appears to be inadequate for a segmentation task which needs to learn from a limited amount of training data. Considering its satisfactory performance in medical image segmentation, we selected U-Net as the baseline model and applied the proposed meta-learning method to it.

2.2. Optimization-Based Meta-Learning Methods

The inspiration of meta-learning comes from the human learning process, which can adapt new tasks quickly according to a few examples [31]. The proposed meta-learning method in this paper is optimization-based. This category of methods like MAML [23] and Reptile are closely related to our method.

MAML aims to learn from a number of tasks $\mathcal{T}$ sampled from a distribution $p(\mathcal{T})$. These tasks are composed of a support set τ^s and a query set τ^q. MAML requires that τ^s and τ^q do not have any overlapping class. The algorithm attempts to find a desirable parameter vector θ for a given model. In each inner loop of MAML, as shown in Figure 2a, the model is learned from a support batch τ^s sampled from $\mathcal{T}^s$ with a loss function $\mathcal{L}_{\tau^s}(\theta, \tau^s)$. A transitional parameter vector θ^s is obtained by updating θ through a number of gradient steps. In the outer loop of MAML, a query batch τ^q sampled from $\mathcal{T}^q$ is then used to update θ^s to θ^q based on a query loss $\mathcal{L}_{\tau^q}(\theta^s, \tau^q)$. After that, θ^q is applied to the update of θ. In Figure 2a, we use arrows to represent the direction of update. The arrow directed from θ^s to θ^q is parallel to the arrow directed from θ to θ^*, where the entire updating process ends with θ^*.

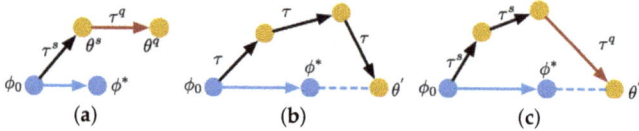

Figure 2. Optimization-based meta-learning algorithms. We use black and red arrows to represent the gradient steps in the inner loop and the outer loop, respectively. The blue arrow represents the direction of model update. (a) MAML; (b) Reptile; (c) our algorithm.

Instead of using a support-query scheme, as shown in Figure 2b, in each inner loop, Reptile updates θ by learning from the same batch τ through multiple gradient descent steps. The direction of update in the outer loop is determined by θ and θ', where θ' is the transitional parameter vector obtained from the inner loop. Reptile focuses on learning from the same batch and improving generalization with a particular number of gradient descent steps. The entire updating process ends with θ^*.

Differently from MAML and Reptile, as shown in Figure 2c, in the inner loop of our algorithm, we first train the model parameters on a support batch τ^s with multiple gradient steps. In the outer loop, we then adapt the model parameters to a query batch τ^q by one gradient step. In Figure 2c, both τ^s and τ^q are sampled from the entire task distribution. Figure 3 displays how MAML and our algorithm select τ^s and τ^q in the meta-training phase. Each training task (1 or 2) mimics the few-shot scenario, which includes three classes with two support examples and one query example. Each example in either the support set or the query set is randomly selected from a set of training examples, which is displayed in different colors. Each example includes three classes: H, S, and P which represent the MRI images from THE heart, spleen, and prostate, respectively. We can observe from Figure 3a that the examples for support and query purposes are split into two partitions. in our algorithm, as shown in Figure 3b, the examples in each training task are selected from diverse examples across the entire example distribution. MAML updates the initial parameter vector towards the direction of query-testing phase, which limits the capability of updating the initial parameter vector by learning from the examples in the support-training phase. Unlike MAML, our algorithm avoids the limitation by removing the boundary between support and query examples. By doing so, the parameter vector is updated by learning from the diversity of support and query examples. The capability of learning is therefore enhanced. The diversity can be interpreted as: for any tissue type in a set of examples, this tissue type shows diverse image features over location, size, shape, and impact on the surrounding area (as shown in Figure 1). The direction of update in the outer loop is determined by θ and θ'. The entire updating process ends with θ^*.

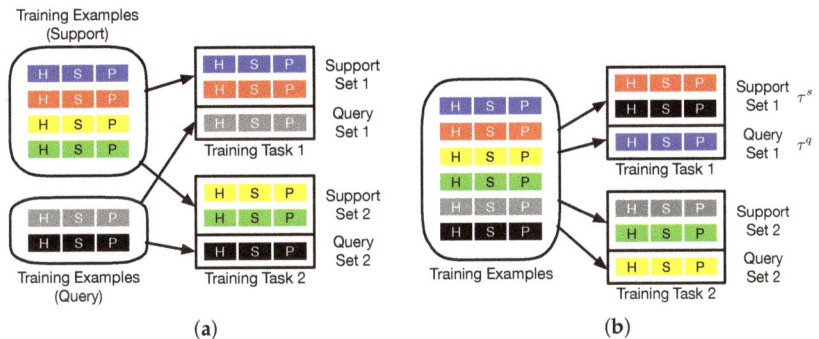

Figure 3. The selection of examples in the meta-training phase. Left: MAML. Right: Our algorithm. H, S, and P represent the MRI images from the heart, spleen, and prostate, respectively. Each example is displayed by a particular color. (**a**) MAML; (**b**) ours.

3. Methodology

In this study, we used U-Net [25] as the baseline model and learned the initialization of U-Net from multiple source tasks. Based on the parameter vector learned from the source tasks, we fine-tuned the model on the target task. We aimed to train a U-Net that can produce good generalization performance on the target task. In this section, we first present the general form of our algorithm. After that, we provide some theoretical analysis to better explain why the proposed algorithm works.

3.1. Meta-Learning Domain Adaptation

As shown in Algorithm 1, let θ denote the initial parameter vector, and we use a parametrized function f_θ to represent the baseline model. For any batch of tasks τ^s sampled from $p(\mathcal{T})$, when f_θ adapts to τ^s, the parameter vector θ becomes θ'_i. The updated parameter vector θ'_i is computed using i gradient steps on τ^s. Let $f_{\theta'_i}$ denote the updated model; the update on the gradient at the ith step is described as

$$\theta'_i = \theta'_{i-1} - \alpha \nabla_{\theta'_{i-1}} \mathcal{L}_{\tau^s}(f_{\theta'_{i-1}}), \tag{1}$$

where α is a fixed hyper-parameter and represents the learning-rate in the inner loop. $\mathcal{L}_{\tau^s}(f_{\theta'_{i-1}})$ represents the loss function of model $f_{\theta'_{i-1}}$ on τ^s. θ'_i can be obtained by optimizing $f_{\theta'_{i-1}}$ with respect to θ'_{i-1} on the same batch of tasks sampled from $p(\mathcal{T})$. The meta-objective can be described as

$$\min_{\theta'_i} \mathcal{L}_{\tau^s}(f_{\theta'_i}) = \mathcal{L}_{\tau^s}(f_{\theta'_{i-1} - \alpha \nabla_{\theta'_{i-1}} \mathcal{L}_{\tau^s}(f_{\theta'_{i-1}})}). \tag{2}$$

The optimization on the entire meta-learning process is performed over parameters θ. We can obtain θ' by updating θ'_i based on another batch of tasks τ^q which is also sampled from $p(\mathcal{T})$. The optimization process is therefore described as

$$\theta \leftarrow \theta + \beta [\theta'_i - \alpha \nabla_{\theta'_i} \mathcal{L}_{\tau^q}(f_{\theta'_i}) - \theta], \tag{3}$$

where β is a fixed hyper-parameter on step size in the outer loop. Table 1 shows all the symbols associated with the proposed algorithm.

Algorithm 1 Our meta-learning algorithm.

Require: $p(\mathcal{T})$: distribution over tasks
Parameter: α, β: step size hyperparameters
1: Initialize θ randomly
2: **while** not done **do**
3:     Sample a batch of tasks $\tau^s \sim p(\mathcal{T})$
4:     $\theta'_0 = \theta$
5:     **for** $i = 1, 2, .., k$ **do**
6:         Compute $\theta'_i = \theta'_{i-1} - \alpha \nabla_{\theta'_{i-1}} \mathcal{L}_{\tau^s}(f_{\theta'_{i-1}})$
7:     **end for**
8:     Sample another batch of tasks $\tau^q \sim p(\mathcal{T})$
9:     Compute $\theta' = \theta'_k - \alpha \nabla_{\theta'_k} \mathcal{L}_{\tau^q}(f_{\theta'_k})$
10:     Update $\theta \leftarrow \theta + \beta(\theta' - \theta)$
11: **end while**

3.2. Algorithm Analysis

In this subsection, we provide some analysis to better understand why the proposed algorithm works. We first used a Taylor series to approximate the update performed by our algorithm. Then, the effectiveness of our algorithm is shown via the computation of the expected gradient over task and batch sampling.

Table 1. All the symbols associated with the proposed algorithm.

Symbol	Description
θ	The initial parameter vector
θ'	Updated parameter vector (out loop)
α	Learning rate (inner loop)
β	Step size (outer loop)
$p(\mathcal{T})$	The source training set
τ^s	Support batch
τ^q	Query batch
$\mathcal{L}$	Loss function
f	The parametrized function
∇	Gradient descent steps

Suppose we perform two stochastic gradient descent (SGD) steps on $\mathcal{L}_{\tau^s}$ and one step on $\mathcal{L}_{\tau^q}$. Let ϕ_0 denote the initial parameter vector. The updated parameter after two steps can be described as

$$\phi_0 = \theta \tag{4}$$

$$\phi_1 = \phi_0 - \alpha \mathcal{L}'_{\tau^s}(\phi_0) \tag{5}$$

$$\phi_2 = \phi_0 - \alpha \mathcal{L}'_{\tau^s}(\phi_0) - \alpha \mathcal{L}'_{\tau^q}(\phi_1) \tag{6}$$

The Taylor expansion of $\mathcal{L}'_{\tau^q}(\phi_1)$ can be described as

$$\mathcal{L}'_{\tau^q}(\phi_1) = \mathcal{L}'_{\tau^q}(\phi_0) + \mathcal{L}''_{\tau^q}(\phi_0)(\phi_1 - \phi_0) + O(\alpha^2) \tag{7}$$

$$= \mathcal{L}'_{\tau^q}(\phi_0) - \alpha \mathcal{L}''_{\tau^q}(\phi_0) \mathcal{L}'_{\tau^s}(\phi_0) + O(\alpha^2). \tag{8}$$

The gradient of our algorithm after two gradient steps is defined as

$$g_{ours} = (\phi_0 - \phi_2)/\beta = \mathcal{L}'_{\tau^s}(\phi_0) + \mathcal{L}'_{\tau^q}(\phi_1) \tag{9}$$

$$= \alpha/\beta \mathcal{L}'_{\tau^s}(\phi_0) + \alpha/\beta \mathcal{L}'_{\tau^q}(\phi_0) - \alpha^2/\beta \mathcal{L}''_{\tau^q}(\phi_0) \mathcal{L}'_{\tau^s}(\phi_0) + O(\alpha^2). \tag{10}$$

For any sampled task τ, let $\mathbb{E}_{\tau,\tau^s}[\mathcal{L}'_{\tau^s}(\theta)]$ and $\mathbb{E}_{\tau,\tau^q}[\mathcal{L}'_{\tau^q}(\theta)]$ denote the expected losses with $\mathcal{L}_{\tau^s}$ and $\mathcal{L}_{\tau^s}$, respectively. The expected losses with $\mathcal{L}_{\tau^q}$ after the generalization on τ^s is denoted as $\mathbb{E}_{\tau,\tau_s,\tau_q}[\mathcal{L}''_{\tau^s}(\theta)\mathcal{L}'_{\tau^q}(\theta)]$. The expectation of g_{ours} is therefore described as

$$\mathbb{E}[g_{ours}] = \mathbb{E}_{\tau,\tau^s}[\mathcal{L}'_{\tau^s}(\theta)] + \mathbb{E}_{\tau,\tau^q}[\mathcal{L}'_{\tau^q}(\theta)] - \alpha \cdot \mathbb{E}_{\tau,\tau_s,\tau_q}[\mathcal{L}''_{\tau^s}(\theta)\mathcal{L}'_{\tau^q}(\theta)] + O(\alpha^2), \qquad (11)$$

if the ratio between α and β is a constant. From Equation (11), we could find out that the expected loss is minimized over tasks; then the higher-order $\mathbb{E}_{\tau,\tau_s,\tau_q}[\mathcal{L}''_{\tau^s}(\theta)\mathcal{L}'_{\tau^q}(\theta)]$ enables fast learning.

4. Experiments

In this section, we evaluate the proposed meta-learning algorithm by establishing two medical image segmentation scenarios. We first introduce the dataset for evaluation and the architecture of the baseline model. Then, we discuss the setup for implementation. After that, we compare the proposed algorithm with two existing meta-learning benchmarks: MAML and Reptile. In the final subsection, we study the hyper-parameter.

4.1. Dataset and the Baseline Model

We evaluated the proposed algorithm based on a public dataset from the Medical Segmentation Decathlon. This dataset contains ten segmentation tasks, and each task contains diverse scans on a specific tissue type. All the scans have been labeled and verified by an expert human rater, and with his best attempt to mimic the accuracy required for clinical use. We reshaped each scan to 256 × 256 and simplified the multi-value annotation to a binary segmentation task. Among all the tasks, we randomly selected eight tasks for evaluation owing to computational overheads and memory issues. Six tasks are randomly selected as source tasks, which were the heart from King's College London, the liver from IRCAD, the prostate from Nijmegen Medical Centre, and the pancreas, spleen, and colon from the Memorial Sloan Kettering Cancer Center. The remaining two tasks, colon and liver, were selected as target tasks. Two medical image segmentation scenarios were established based on these two tasks. For comparison purposes, the scans related to the source tasks were divided into two groups. The source training set of the first group contained 2611 scans of prostate, pancreas, and spleen. The target training set of the first group consisted of 214 scans which were randomly sampled for the task of the colon. The target testing set contained the remaining 1070 scans. The source training set of the second group contained 2877 scans which were of the prostate, heart, and spleen. The target training set of the second group consisted of 191 scans which were randomly sampled for the tasks of liver. The target testing set contained the remaining 18,791 scans.

U-Net was selected as the baseline model, which is illustrated in Figure 4. This model is composed of three partitions, which are the encoder, skip connections, and decoder. The encoder consists of four down-sampling blocks. Each block consists of the repeated application of two 3 × 3 convolutions, each followed by batch normalization (BN), a rectified linear unit (ReLU), and a 2 × 2 max-pooling operation with stride 2 for down-sampling. The 2 × 2 max-pooling operations are replaced with 2 × 2 transposed convolutions in the decoder. Skip connections concatenate the feature maps before the max-pooling operation in down-sampling blocks with the output of the transposed convolution in up-sampling blocks, which corresponds to the associated depth.

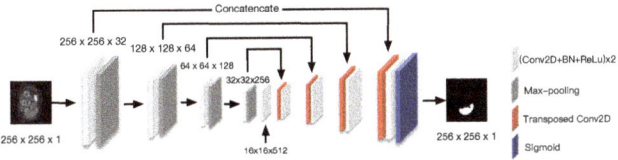

Figure 4. U-Net architecture.

4.2. Implementation

We used cross validation to randomly split either the target training set or the source training set into two subsets. One was for training. The other one was for validation. The volume of the training subset was four times that of the validation subset. Each training set was shuffled in each epoch. We utilized data augmentation to reduce the risk of overfitting. The data augmentation included 0~180 degree random angle flipping, image moving, cross cutting transformation, and image stretching. We applied the cross-entropy function as a loss function. The batch size and the number of epochs were set to 8 and 300, respectively. The batch size in the meta-training phase was set to 6. During meta-training phase, we adopted SGD for each batch with category equipartitioning. The initial learning rate α in algorithm 1 was set as 1×10^{-3}. The step size β and the gradient step k were set as 0.4 and 3, respectively. We implemented the experiment with Keras. The implementation was performed with an Ubuntu system which employed an NVIDIA GeForce 1080 Ti graphics card which had an 11 Gigabyte memory.

The implementation of the proposed meta-learning algorithm and the two benchmarks relates to pipeline III which is depicted in Figure 5c. In pipeline I, the baseline model is trained directly on the target training set with random initialized parameters. The training phase of pipeline II starts from the parameter vector obtained from the pre-training phase on source domains. Pipeline III applies meta-learning algorithms on source training set.

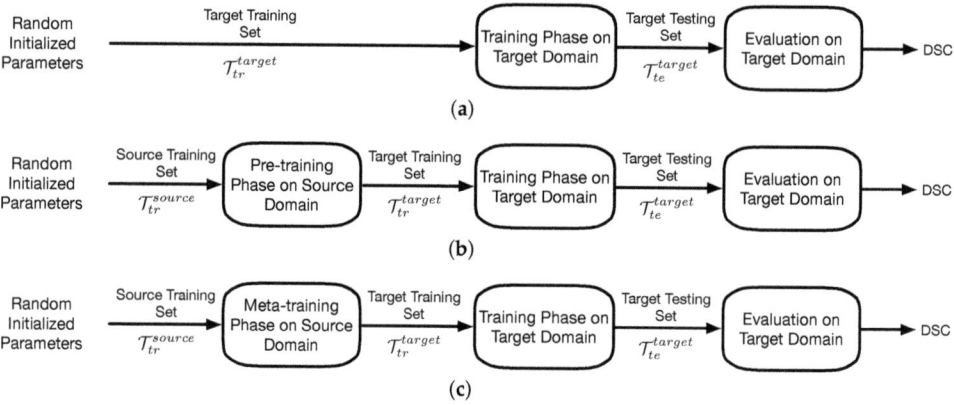

Figure 5. The three pipelines. (a) Pipeline I; (b) pipeline II; (c) pipeline III.

For MAML, in either the colon or the liver task, we first equally split the source tasks into two partitions where each partition contained all the three classes. The two partitions were used for either support or query purposes. The support and query batches were randomly selected from the support and the query sets, respectively. Each batch contained two examples with three classes. For Reptile, in either the colon or the liver task, each batch was randomly selected from the source tasks, which included two examples with three classes. In our approach, we bring in the layer-freezing technique to optimize the whole feature space. Specifically, when we transfer the initialized parameter vector generated by source domain to target domain, we first train the baseline model on the target training set T_{tr}^{target} with the first two down-sampling blocks which has been frozen. We set the learning rate at this phase as 1×10^{-3}. Then, the second block is unfrozen and the target training set T_{tr}^{target} is utilized again. We set the learning rate and the decay rate at this phase as 1×10^{-3} and 0.0077, respectively. For the third time, the target training set T_{tr}^{target} will be applied to the optimization process with entire trainable parameters adjustable. The learning rate at this phase is set as 1×10^{-4}.

4.3. Experimental Results

Table 2 shows the experimental results of the established two segmentation scenarios. The segmentation performance is described with Dice score (DSC), precision, and recall. DSC is a method which measures the overlap between any two images. DSC has been widely used to evaluate the performance of medical image segmentation when ground truth is available. For binary segmentation of medical images, we set the ratio on target area as 0.9. The ratio on background is 0.1.

Table 2. The results from two few-shot scenarios.

Source Domain		Target Domain		Dice Coefficient	Δ	Precision	Recall
Task (s)	Method	Task (s)	Method				
Null	Null		SST	0.537 ± 0.356	-	0.573 ± 0.362	0.573 ± 0.396
Prostate	Pre-training		SST	0.591 ± 0.332	0.054	0.595 ± 0.326	0.655 ± 0.377
Pancreas	Pre-training		SST	0.590 ± 0.347	0.053	0.634 ± 0.338	0.622 ± 0.384
Slpeen	Pre-training		SST	0.591 ± 0.318	0.054	0.594 ± 0.313	0.663 ± 0.362
	Pre-training	Colon	SST	0.611 ± 0.325	0.074	0.629 ± 0.318	0.661 ± 0.362
			Layer-freezing	0.652 ± 0.303	0.115	0.653 ± 0.296	0.717 ± 0.335
Multi-source I	MAML		SST	0.615 ± 0.323	0.078	0.655 ± 0.327	0.659 ± 0.342
			Layer-freezing	0.655 ± 0.306	0.118	0.658 ± 0.301	0.716 ± 0.308
	Reptile		SST	0.608 ± 0.336	0.071	0.652 ± 0.332	0.637 ± 0.367
			Layer-freezing	0.651 ± 0.308	0.114	0.652 ± 0.305	0.714 ± 0.341
	Our Algorithm		SST	0.628 ± 0.323	0.091	0.644 ± 0.319	0.673 ± 0.358
			Layer-freezing	**0.675 ± 0.292**	**0.138**	**0.669 ± 0.288**	**0.741 ± 0.322**
Null	Null		SST	0.904 ± 0.169	-	0.891 ± 0.165	0.934 ± 0.172
Prostate	Pre-training		SST	0.903 ± 0.176	−0.001	0.902 ± 0.163	0.923 ± 0.184
Heart	Pre-training		SST	0.902 ± 0.176	−0.002	0.894 ± 0.172	0.928 ± 0.175
Slpeen	Pre-training		SST	0.905 ± 0.163	0.001	0.892 ± 0.174	0.935 ± 0.170
	Pre-training	Liver	SST	0.905 ± 0.168	0.001	0.888 ± 0.170	0.942 ± 0.157
			Layer-freezing	0.916 ± 0.157	0.012	0.904 ± 0.156	0.944 ± 0.152
Multi-source II	MAML		SST	0.905 ± 0.167	0.001	0.895 ± 0.172	0.936 ± 0.168
			Layer-freezing	0.916 ± 0.158	0.012	0.905 ± 0.154	0.943 ± 0.160
	Reptile		SST	0.904 ± 0.175	0	0.896 ± 0.172	0.927 ± 0.190
			Layer-freezing	0.917 ± 0.158	0.013	0.907 ± 0.156	0.943 ± 0.158
	Our Algorithm		SST	0.912 ± 0.159	0.008	0.896 ± 0.161	0.944 ± 0.150
			Layer-freezing	**0.926 ± 0.141**	**0.022**	**0.914 ± 0.143**	**0.952 ± 0.133**

DSC can be calculated with the bottom equation

$$DSC = \sum_k^K \frac{2\omega_k \sum_i^N p_{(k,i)} g_{(k,i)}}{\sum_i^N p_{(k,i)}^2 + \sum_i^N g_{(k,i)}^2}, \quad (12)$$

where N represents the pixel number. $p_{(k,i)} \in [0,1]$ and $g_{(k,i)} \in \{0,1\}$ denote the predicted probability and the ground truth label of class k, respectively. K is the number of class and ω_k denotes the weight of class k. The task of semantic segmentation is to predict the class of each pixel in an image. Precision effectively describes the purity of our positive predictions relative to the ground truth. Recall describes the completeness of our positive predictions relative to the ground truth. The bold values in Table 2 indicate that the most suitable freezing depth is 2, since the DSC achieved by this setting is the best.

As shown in Table 2, in the segmentation scenario of colon, we first implemented pipeline I, where the baseline model is trained on the target training set with standard supervised training (SST) without the use of any source training sets. The DSC achieved by this method was 0.537. Then, we implemented pipeline II by respectively pre-training the baseline model on three different source training sets which were the tasks on the prostate, pancreas, and spleen. After the pre-training phase on each task, we trained on the target training set with the SST method. The DSCs of the three tasks were 0.591, 0.590, and 0.591, respectively. We use Δ to represent the DSC improved upon the baseline method. We also implemented pipeline II by pre-training on a batch that contained all the three tissue types; we name this case multi-source I. The DSC achieved by this case was 0.611. The DSCs achieved by MAML, Reptile, and our proposed algorithm were 0.615, 0.608, and 0.628, respectively. We also evaluated the performance of each method when the layer-freezing technique was combined. On average, the layer-freezing technique improved DSC by approximately 4.5% for pipeline II in the cases of multi-source I, MAML, Reptile, and our proposed algorithm. Our proposed algorithm performed the best in terms of DSC, which respectively surpassed pipeline II, MAML, and Reptile by 2.3%, 2%, and 2.4%. The bold values in Table 2 represent the results achieved by our algorithm combined with the layer-freezing technique. The DSC achieved is 0.675, which is an improvement of 0.138 upon the baseline method, and it performed the best among all the methods.

In the segmentation scenario of liver, the DSC achieved by pipeline I was 0.904. The DSCs achieved by pipeline II with single-source pre-training were 0.903, 0.902, and 0.905, respectively. The DSC achieved by pipeline II with the case of multi-source II was 0.905. The DSCs achieved by MAML, Reptile, and our proposed algorithm were 0.904 and 0.912, respectively. On average, the layer-freezing technique improved DSC by approximately 1.2% for pipeline II in the case of multi-source II, MAML, Reptile, and our proposed algorithm. Our proposed algorithm performed the best in terms of DSC, which respectively surpassed pipeline II, MAML, and Reptile by 1%, 1%, and 0.9%. The DSC achieved by our algorithm that used the layer-freezing technique was 0.926, which is 0.022 better than the baseline method.

Figure 6 displays the convergence of loss function on the three approaches under the segmentation scenario of colon. We use red, blue, purple, and green lines to represent our algorithm, pipeline II with the case of multi-source I, MAML + layer-freezing, and Reptile + layer-freezing, respectively. The three approaches all trained on the target training set of colon in the last phase of layer-freezing transfer. We found that all the methods were almost converged in approximately 300 epochs. The computational cost of the proposed framework is introduced by the number of Giga-bytes Floating-point Operations per second (GFLOPs). We estimated the number of GFLOPs and parameters by calling the THOP library function. The number of GFLOPs of the CNN model was 10.112532480. The number of parameters was 4,320,609.

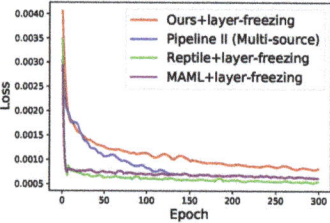

Figure 6. The convergence of three different approaches under the few-shot scenario of colon.

We also calculated the GFLOPs of the CNN model (U-Net) to introduce the computational costs behind the proposed framework. We called the THOP library function to estimate the number of FLOPs and parameters. The GFLOPs of the model was 10.112532480. The number of parameters was 4,320,609.

Figure 7 shows the subjective measures of different approaches in the two established segmentation scenarios. We use green and red contours to represent the image features of ground truth and generated images. For each tissue type, we selected the sample where its segmented image feature was the most visually similar to the ground truth label. From a subjective view, the image produced by our algorithm is visually more similar to the ground truth label and more accurate than the images produced by the other three approaches. For example, in the segmentation task of colon, pipeline II significantly under-estimated the sizes of both the lumen and walls of colon compared to the ground truth labels, while our algorithm reproduced ground truth labels reliably. Even though contour drawing using MAML produced grossly similar results as ground truth, there is an apparent fusion of two adjacent bowel loops. In the segmentation task of the liver, the portal vein (the area circled by an orange circle in raw scans) was mistakenly included as part of the liver parenchyma in (c), (d), and (e), while the ground truth labels in (b) and our algorithm correctly excluded it from liver parenchyma. MAML also generated sharp edges around the gallbladder.

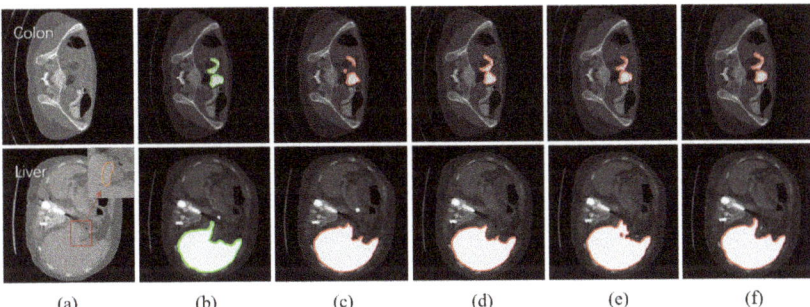

Figure 7. Subjective measures of different approaches in the established segmentation scenarios (top: colon, bottom: liver). Each row presents one typical task, from left to right: (**a**) raw scans; (**b**) ground truth labels; (**c**) pipeline II (multi-source Training); (**d**) MAML + layer-freezing; (**e**) Reptile + layer-freezing; (**f**) ours + layer-freezing. White areas represent the image features of colon and liver.

4.4. An Ablation Study on the Hyper-Parameter

The initial freezing depth is an important hyper-parameter in layer-freezing, which determines how many layers to be frozen during the training on the target domain. A shallow model will lead to a catastrophic forgetting problem which may destroy the experience learned by meta-learning algorithms. More and more experiences could be obtained and fine-tuned by using a deeper model, but this still cannot guarantee one to achieve a better performance on segmentation, not to mention a higher computational cost. To address this problem, we studied the initial freezing depth under the two few-shot segmentation tasks with an ablation study.

In this study, we investigate the DSCs achieved under three different initial freezing depths. The results are displayed in Table 3. In the case that the depth is one, the learning rates of the first stage and the second stage are 1×10^{-3} and 1×10^{-4}, respectively. In the case that the depth is two, the learning rates of the first two stages and the third stage are 1×10^{-3} and 1×10^{-4}, respectively. We set the decay rate of the second stage as 0.0077. In the case that the depth is three, the learning rates of the first three stages and the fourth stage are 1×10^{-3} and 1×10^{-4}, respectively. We set the decay rate of the third stage as 0.0077. By observing the results shown in Table 3, in the two established segmentation scenarios, we found that the segmentation performance was the best when the depth was set as 2. Although the DSC in the case that the depth was three was better than the case when the depth was one, a deeper depth leads to a higher computational cost.

Table 3. The results on the two established segmentation scenarios under different initial freezing depths. The bold values represent the most suitable depths that achieve the best DSCs.

DSC Depths \ Target Domain	Colon	Liver
1	0.660 ± 0.306	0.920 ± 0.160
2	**0.675 ± 0.292**	**0.926 ± 0.141**
3	0.671 ± 0.298	0.924 ± 0.148

In [24], the authors point out that using only one gradient descent is not effective during the learning process. The reason is that it optimizes the expected loss over all tasks. It turns out that the performance achieved by the two-step Reptile is worse than the performance achieved by two-step standard supervised learning. However, with more inner loop steps, the performance of Reptile can be further improved and surpass the standard supervised learning. The authors also show that the learning performance is the best when the number of inner loops is four. We therefore set the number of inner loops as four when we implemented Reptile. We set the number of inner loops as three for our algorithm such that the number of gradient descent calculations was the same for each time the parameter was updated.

5. Discussion

By observing the results shown in Table 2, we could find out that DSC can be improved when pre-knowledge is used. In the meantime, a better DSC can be achieved when the source training set is sampled from a diverse task distribution. The DSCs achieved by MAML and Reptile are almost same as the result achieved by pipeline II with multi-source training. What is more, the combination of our proposed algorithm and the layer-freezing technique achieved the best performance in the two established scenarios among pipeline I, pipeline II with single-source training, pipeline II with multi-source training, MAML, and Reptile. Specifically, our algorithm achieved 13.8% and 2.4% better DSCs than pipeline I and Reptile, respectively. All our results are reported as averages over five independent runs and with 95% confidence intervals.

In Figure 6, we can see that the losses in the three approaches can be converged to a smaller value in contrast to our algorithm. However, our algorithm achieved a higher DSC than the other three approaches. This observation implies that our algorithm can do a better job of alleviating the overfitting problem for few-shot segmentation tasks.

6. Conclusions

This paper proposes a novel meta-learning algorithm to adjust the optimization algorithm so that the segmentation model is nicely learned from a target task which has few examples. Specifically, this algorithm can learn from diverse segmentation tasks across the entire task distribution. In contrast to existing meta-learning algorithms, the proposed algorithm augments the capability to learn from the diversity of image features which characterize a specific tissue type while showing diverse signal intensities. To demonstrate the effectiveness of the proposed algorithm, extensive experiments were conducted by using a diverse set of segmentation tasks on two optimization-based meta-learning benchmarks. The experimental results show that our algorithm surpasses the two benchmarks and brings consistent improvements to both DSC and subjective measures, which implies that the proposed algorithm can produce a better generalization of the target task which has few examples.

Author Contributions: Conceptualization, P.Z. and J.L.; methodology, P.Z. and J.L.; software, P.Z.; validation, P.Z. and J.L.; formal analysis, J.L.; investigation, P.Z. and J.L.; resources, P.Z. and J.L.; data curation, P.Z.; writing—original draft preparation, P.Z. and J.L.; writing—review and editing, J.L., Y.W. and J.P.; visualization, J.L.; supervision, Y.W. and J.P.; project administration, Y.W. and J.P.; funding acquisition, Y.W. All authors have read and agreed to the published version of the manuscript.

Funding: This research was partially supported by the National Natural Science Foundation of China, 2019, grant number 81873891, in part supported by the Major International (Regional) Joint Research Project of China, 2021, grant number 82020108018, and in part supported by China International Medical Foundation SKY Image Research Fund Project, 2019, grant number Z-2014-07-1912-01.

Institutional Review Board Statement: Not applicable.

Informed Consent Statement: Not applicable.

Data Availability Statement: The proposed algorithm was tested on the Medical Segmentation Decathlon, see http://medicaldecathlon.com/ (accessed on 8 February 2020).

Conflicts of Interest: The authors declare no conflict of interest.

References

1. Zhang, H.; Valcarcel, A.M.; Bakshi, R.; Chu, R.; Bagnato, F.; Shinohara, R.T.; Hett, K.; Oguz, I. Multiple Sclerosis Lesion Segmentation with Tiramisu and 2.5 D Stacked Slices. In *International Conference on Medical Image Computing and Computer-Assisted Intervention (MICCAI)*; Springer: Berlin/Heidelberg, Germany, 2019; pp. 338–346.
2. Chiu, S.J.; Li, X.T.; Nicholas, P.; Toth, C.A.; Izatt, J.A.; Farsiu, S. Automatic segmentation of seven retinal layers in SDOCT images congruent with expert manual segmentation. *Opt. Express* **2010**, *18*, 19413–19428. [CrossRef] [PubMed]
3. Cheng, F.; Chen, C.; Wang, Y.; Shi, H.; Cao, Y.; Tu, D.; Zhang, C.; Xu, Y. Learning directional feature maps for cardiac mri segmentation. In *International Conference on Medical Image Computing and Computer-Assisted Intervention (MICCAI)*; Springer: Berlin/Heidelberg, Germany, 2020; pp. 108–117.
4. Zhou, Z.; Siddiquee, M.M.R.; Tajbakhsh, N.; Liang, J. Unet++: Redesigning skip connections to exploit multiscale features in image segmentation. *IEEE Trans. Med. Imaging* **2019**, *39*, 1856–1867. [CrossRef] [PubMed]
5. Dou, Q.; de Castro, D.C.; Kamnitsas, K.; Glocker, B. Domain generalization via model-agnostic learning of semantic features. *arXiv* **2019**, arXiv:1910.13580.
6. Chen, L.C.; Zhu, Y.; Papandreou, G.; Schroff, F.; Adam, H. Encoder-decoder with atrous separable convolution for semantic image segmentation. In Proceedings of the European Conference on Computer Vision (ECCV), Munich, Germany, 8–14 September 2018; pp. 801–818.
7. Litjens, G.; Kooi, T.; Bejnordi, B.E.; Setio, A.A.A.; Ciompi, F.; Ghafoorian, M.; Van Der Laak, J.A.; Van Ginneken, B.; Sánchez, C.I. A survey on deep learning in medical image analysis. *Med. Image Anal.* **2017**, *42*, 60–88. [CrossRef] [PubMed]
8. Esteva, A.; Kuprel, B.; Novoa, R.A.; Ko, J.; Swetter, S.M.; Blau, H.M.; Thrun, S. Dermatologist-level classification of skin cancer with deep neural networks. *Nature* **2017**, *542*, 115. [CrossRef] [PubMed]
9. Ouyang, C.; Kamnitsas, K.; Biffi, C.; Duan, J.; Rueckert, D. Data efficient unsupervised domain adaptation for cross-modality image segmentation. In *International Conference on Medical Image Computing and Computer-Assisted Intervention (MICCAI)*; Springer: Berlin/Heidelberg, Germany, 2019; pp. 669–677.
10. Jiang, X.; Ding, L.; Havaei, M.; Jesson, A.; Matwin, S. Task Adaptive Metric Space for Medium-Shot Medical Image Classification. In *International Conference on Medical Image Computing and Computer-Assisted Intervention (MICCAI)*; Springer: Berlin/Heidelberg, Germany, 2019; pp. 147–155.
11. Maicas, G.; Bradley, A.P.; Nascimento, J.C.; Reid, I.; Carneiro, G. Training medical image analysis systems like radiologists. In *International Conference on Medical Image Computing and Computer-Assisted Intervention (MICCAI)*; Springer: Berlin/Heidelberg, Germany, 2018; pp. 546–554.
12. Tzeng, E.; Hoffman, J.; Saenko, K.; Darrell, T. Adversarial discriminative domain adaptation. In Proceedings of the IEEE Conference on Computer Vision and Pattern Recognition (CVPR), Honolulu, HI, USA, 21–26 July 2017; pp. 7167–7176.
13. Kumar, A.; Saha, A.; Daume, H. Co-regularization based semi-supervised domain adaptation. *Adv. Neural Inf. Process. Syst.* **2010**, *23*, 478–486.
14. Saenko, K.; Kulis, B.; Fritz, M.; Darrell, T. Adapting visual category models to new domains. In *European Conference on Computer Vision (ECCV)*; Springer: Berlin/Heidelberg, Germany, 2010; pp. 213–226.
15. Roy, A.G.; Siddiqui, S.; Pölsterl, S.; Navab, N.; Wachinger, C. 'Squeeze & excite' guided few-shot segmentation of volumetric images. *Med. Image Anal.* **2020**, *59*, 101587.
16. Wang, K.; Liew, J.H.; Zou, Y.; Zhou, D.; Feng, J. Panet: Few-shot image semantic segmentation with prototype alignment. In Proceedings of the IEEE International Conference on Computer Vision (ICCV), Seoul, Korea, 27–28 October 2019; pp. 9197–9206.
17. Rakelly, K.; Shelhamer, E.; Darrell, T.; Efros, A.; Levine, S. Conditional networks for few-shot semantic segmentation. In Proceedings of the 6th International Conference on Learning Representations (ICLR) Workshop, Vancouver, BC, Canada, 30 April–3 May 2018.
18. Dong, N.; Xing, E.P. Few-Shot Semantic Segmentation with Prototype Learning. In Proceedings of the BMVC, Newcastle, UK, 3–6 September 2018; Volume 3.
19. Shaban, A.; Bansal, S.; Liu, Z.; Essa, I.; Boots, B. One-shot learning for semantic segmentation. *arXiv* **2017**, arXiv:1709.03410.
20. Hospedales, T.; Antoniou, A.; Micaelli, P.; Storkey, A. Meta-learning in neural networks: A survey. *arXiv* **2020**, arXiv:2004.05439.
21. Andrychowicz, M.; Denil, M.; Gomez, S.; Hoffman, M.W.; Pfau, D.; Schaul, T.; Shillingford, B.; De Freitas, N. Learning to learn by gradient descent by gradient descent. *arXiv* **2016**, arXiv:1606.04474.
22. Schmidhuber, J. Evolutionary Principles in Self-Referential Learning, or on Learning How to Learn: The Meta-Meta-... Hook. Ph.D. Thesis, Technische Universität München, Munich, Germany, 1987.
23. Finn, C.; Abbeel, P.; Levine, S. Model-Agnostic Meta-Learning for Fast Adaptation of Deep Networks. In Proceedings of the 34th International Conference on Machine Learning (ICML), JMLR.org, Sydney, Australia, 6–11 August 2017; pp. 1126–1135.
24. Nichol, A.; Schulman, J. Reptile: A scalable metalearning algorithm. *arXiv* **2018**, arXiv:1803.02999.
25. Ronneberger, O.; Fischer, P.; Brox, T. U-Net: Convolutional Networks for Biomedical Image Segmentation. In *Medical Image Computing and Computer-Assisted Intervention (MICCAI)*; Navab, N., Hornegger, J., Wells, W.M., Frangi, A.F., Eds.; Springer International Publishing: Cham, Switzerland, 2015; pp. 234–241.
26. Krizhevsky, A.; Sutskever, I.; Hinton, G.E. Imagenet classification with deep convolutional neural networks. *Adv. Neural Inf. Process. Syst.* **2012**, *25*, 1097–1105. [CrossRef]

27. Simonyan, K.; Zisserman, A. Very deep convolutional networks for large-scale image recognition. *arXiv* **2014**, arXiv:1409.1556.
28. Szegedy, C.; Liu, W.; Jia, Y.; Sermanet, P.; Reed, S.; Anguelov, D.; Erhan, D.; Vanhoucke, V.; Rabinovich, A. Going deeper with convolutions. In Proceedings of the IEEE Conference on Computer Vision and Pattern Recognition (CVPR), Boston, MA, USA, 7–12 June 2015; pp. 1–9.
29. Szegedy, C.; Ioffe, S.; Vanhoucke, V.; Alemi, A. Inception-v4, inception-resnet and the impact of residual connections on learning. *arXiv* **2016**, arXiv:1602.07261.
30. Long, J.; Shelhamer, E.; Darrell, T. Fully convolutional networks for semantic segmentation. In Proceedings of the IEEE Conference on Computer Vision and Pattern Recognition (CVPR), Boston, MA, USA, 7–12 June 2015; pp. 3431–3440.
31. Naik, D.K.; Mammone, R.J. Meta-neural networks that learn by learning. In Proceedings of the International Joint Conference on Neural Networks, Baltimore, MD, USA, 7–11 June 1992; IEEE: New York, NY, USA, 1992; Volume 1, pp. 437–442.

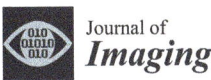

Article

Personal Heart Health Monitoring Based on 1D Convolutional Neural Network

Antonella Nannavecchia [1], Francesco Girardi [2], Pio Raffaele Fina [3], Michele Scalera [4] and Giovanni Dimauro [4,*]

- [1] Department of Management, Finance and Technology, University LUM Jean Monnet, 70010 Casamassima, Italy; nannavecchia@lum.it
- [2] UVARP Azienda Sanitaria Locale, 70132 Bari, Italy; francesco.girardi@asl.bari.it
- [3] Department of Computer Science, University of Torino, 10124 Torino, Italy; pio.fina@edu.unito.it
- [4] Department of Computer Science, University of Bari, 70125 Bari, Italy; michele.scalera@uniba.it
- * Correspondence: giovanni.dimauro@uniba.it

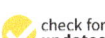

Citation: Nannavecchia, A.; Girardi, F.; Fina, P.R.; Scalera, M.; Dimauro, G. Personal Heart Health Monitoring Based on 1D Convolutional Neural Network. *J. Imaging* **2021**, *7*, 26. https://doi.org/10.3390/jimaging7020026

Academic Editor: Yudong Zhang
Received: 27 November 2020
Accepted: 2 February 2021
Published: 5 February 2021

Publisher's Note: MDPI stays neutral with regard to jurisdictional claims in published maps and institutional affiliations.

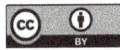

Copyright: © 2021 by the authors. Licensee MDPI, Basel, Switzerland. This article is an open access article distributed under the terms and conditions of the Creative Commons Attribution (CC BY) license (https://creativecommons.org/licenses/by/4.0/).

Abstract: The automated detection of suspicious anomalies in electrocardiogram (ECG) recordings allows frequent personal heart health monitoring and can drastically reduce the number of ECGs that need to be manually examined by the cardiologists, excluding those classified as normal, facilitating healthcare decision-making and reducing a considerable amount of time and money. In this paper, we present a system able to automatically detect the suspect of cardiac pathologies in ECG signals from personal monitoring devices, with the aim to alert the patient to send the ECG to the medical specialist for a correct diagnosis and a proper therapy. The main contributes of this work are: (a) the implementation of a binary classifier based on a 1D-CNN architecture for detecting the suspect of anomalies in ECGs, regardless of the kind of cardiac pathology; (b) the analysis was carried out on 21 classes of different cardiac pathologies classified as anomalous; and (c) the possibility to classify anomalies even in ECG segments containing, at the same time, more than one class of cardiac pathologies. Moreover, 1D-CNN based architectures can allow an implementation of the system on cheap smart devices with low computational complexity. The system was tested on the ECG signals from the MIT-BIH ECG Arrhythmia Database for the MLII derivation. Two different experiments were carried out, showing remarkable performance compared to other similar systems. The best result showed high accuracy and recall, computed in terms of ECG segments and even higher accuracy and recall in terms of patients alerted, therefore considering the detection of anomalies with respect to entire ECG recordings.

Keywords: ECG signal detection; portable monitoring devices; 1D-convolutional neural network; deep learning

1. Introduction

The aging of the population is leading to an increase in patients suffering from cardiac pathologies, therefore requiring electrocardiographic monitoring. An electrocardiogram (ECG) is an easy, rapid, and non-invasive tool that traces the electrical activity of the heart [1] revealing the presence of cardiac pathologies such as conduction disease, channelopathies, structural heart disease, and previous ischemic injury [2]. On the other hand, investigating the altered acoustic characteristics of the cardiac tones, as an example, may allow the early identification of valve malfunction [3].

Systems able to support the doctors' work in the diagnosis of pathologies can facilitate health care decision making reducing considerably expenditure of time and money [4–12]. The ECG has become the diagnostic procedure most commonly performed in clinical cardiology [13–15] and the diffusion of wearable and portable devices has been enabling patients to constantly monitor the cardiac activity, for example of elder people through wireless sensor networks [16]. Cardiologists cannot examine millions of ECGs daily recorded from portable devices. Thus, systems able to automatically detect suspicious anomalies in ECGs are required, in order to reduce the number of ECGs that need to be manually examined by the cardiologists, identifying those that need a further examination and also the urgency of such examination. For this reason, systems require high detection performance in order to avoid that normal ECGs incorrectly detected as anomalous should be examined by a medical professional, and, even more important, that the presence of an electrocardiographic alteration, which could be the indicator of cardiac pathology, is recognized and does not escape the observation of the cardiologist. To make the anomalous ECGs be examined by the medical specialist and that the proper therapy is administered, the detection system should maximize recall for anomalous ECGs, which is to maximize the number of ECGs correctly classified as anomalous, even losing accuracy.

The future of quick and efficient disease diagnosis lays in the development of reliable non-invasive methods [17] also through the use of artificial intelligence techniques. Artificial neural networks and deep learning architectures have recently found broad application [18] achieving striking success in different domains such as image classification [19–24], speech recognition [25], intrusion detection systems [26,27], smart city [28], or biological studies [29,30].

Therefore, high expectations are placed in the use of such techniques also for the improvement of health care and clinical practice [31–36]. Furthermore, numerous portable devices for personal and frequent monitoring of cardiac activity, such as Kardia [37], D-hearth [38], and eKuore [39], are spreading.

The goal of this paper is to implement a system able to automatically detect the suspect of cardiac pathologies in ECG signals to support personal monitoring devices. We propose a 1D-CNN architecture optimized to detect anomalous ECG recordings, regardless of the kind of cardiac pathology, including in the analysis 21 classes of anomalies.

The system here presented was designed to be implemented on devices for personal use and with the aim to only send to the cardiologist ECGs detected with the suspect of a cardiac alteration for further examination, thus no information about the specific class of anomaly is detected. The proposed system is based on a binary classification model.

In fact, as of now, we want to make it clear that the main goal of our study is not to classify different cardiac pathologies, but to make sure that the suspect of a pathology can be detected and that patients are alarmed: then a correct diagnosis can be carried on with specific tests and the intervention of medical staff. The cardiologist will examine all ECGs detected as anomalous identifying the pathology and prescribing the proper treatment. The system has been implemented with the aim to achieve high levels of recall for anomalous ECGs in order to minimize the possibility that the presence of any kind of cardiac alteration could escape the observation of the cardiologist.

This paper is organized as follows: Section 2 reports a wide background, Section 3 describes ECG signals; Section 4 illustrates material and methods; in Section 5 are pointed out results and discussions; and Section 6 sets out conclusions.

2. Background

Many studies have proposed the implementation of artificial neural networks and deep learning architectures for the development of automatic systems able to recognize the suspect of cardiac anomalies [40–42]. In the literature the detection of cardiac anomalies has been investigated analyzing both heart sounds acquired by digital stethoscopes and ECG signals from portable devices.

Meintjes et al. [43] implemented continuous wavelet transform (CWT) scalograms and convolutional neural networks for the correct classification of the fundamental heart sounds in recordings of normal and pathological heart sounds. They implemented a methodology in order to distinguish between the first and second heart sounds using CWT decomposition and convolutional neural network (CNN) features. Results show the high potential in the use of CWT and CNN in the analysis of heart sounds compared to support vector machine (SVM), and k-nearest neighbors (kNN) classifiers. In [44] authors propose the classification of heart sounds on short, unsegmented recordings and normalized spectral amplitude of 5 s duration phonocardiogram segments was determined by fast Fourier transform and wavelet entropy by wavelet analysis. Spectral amplitude and wavelet entropy features were then combined in a classification tree. They achieved accuracy comparable to other algorithms obtained without the complexity of segmentation. Redlarski et al. [17] presented a new heart sound classification technique combining linear predictive coding coefficients, used for feature extraction, with a classifier built upon combining support vector machine and the modified cuckoo search algorithm. It showed good performance of the diagnostic system, in terms of accuracy, complexity [45–47] and range of distinguishable heart sounds.

With the application of deep learning architectures, also the accuracy of ECG diagnostic analysis has achieved new high levels. The systems implemented using such techniques allow the automated interpretation of ECG signals from portable devices in real time. The common deep learning networks for the analysis of ECG signals are mainly based on recurrent neural networks (RNNs), convolutional neural networks (CNNs), and some other architectures [1].

Chauhan et al. [48] investigated the applicability of deep recurrent neural network architectures with long short term memory (LSTM) for detecting cardiac arrhythmias in ECG signals. This approach is quite fast, does not require preprocessing of the data [49] or hand coded features and do not need prior information about the abnormal signal. The network was tested on the MIT-BIH Arrhythmia Database for the classification of four different types of Arrhythmias showing that LSTMs may be a viable candidate for anomaly detection in ECG signals.

Saadatnejad et al. [50] proposed an LSTM-based ECG classification algorithm for continuous cardiac monitoring on wearable devices. They preprocessed data extracting RR interval and wavelet features from ECG samples The ECG signal along with the extracted features were fed into multiple LSTM recurrent neural networks. The MIT-BIH ECG Arrhythmia Database was used for the classification of six different types of anomalies. The proposed algorithm achieved accurate LSTM-based ECG classification to wearable devices with low computational costs.

Thill et al. [51] presented an unsupervised time series anomaly detection algorithm to detect anomalies in ECG readings. They performed a recurrent LSTM network to predict the normal time series behavior without the usage of the anomaly class labels building a multivariate normal error model for the nominal data. Anomalous events were detected with a high probability through a high Mahalanobis distance. They classified six anomaly classes and obtained good performance achieving high levels of precision and recall.

Although RNN architectures are suitable to process time series data, they present some limitations. The major drawbacks of RNNs are the vanishing gradient and gradient exploding problems that make their training difficult, not allowing the processing of very long sequences. Moreover, due to its recurrent nature, the computation is slow. For this reason, some studies investigated the implementation of 1D-CNNs, with the main aim to design low computational complexity systems to support portable devices. In fact, Kiranyaz et al. [52] revised the state of the art techniques used in signal processing applications such as patient-specific ECG classification, structural health monitoring, anomaly detection in power electronics circuitry, and motor-fault detection. In particular, they highlighted how the implementation of adaptive and compact 1D-CNN can achieve higher performance than deep conventional 2D with low computational complexity. Adaptive and compact 1D-CNNs can be efficiently trained with a limited data set of 1D signals instead of massive size data sets required by deep 2D CNNs. It can be performed directly to the raw signal without any pre or post processing, such as features extraction, selection, dimensionality reduction, etc., and it is able to extract features from shorter segments of the overall data set. Moreover, due to the low computational requirements, 1D-CNNs are well suited for real-time and low-cost applications, especially on smart mobile devices that can be the proper tools for personal health monitoring [52,53]. Yıldırım et al. [54] proposed a new 1D-convolutional neural network approach for the automatic classification of cardiac arrhythmia on long-duration electrocardiography (ECG) signal analysis. The model was performed on 10-s fragments of ECG signals including 17 different classes of cardiac arrhythmia. The model showed remarkable performance and could be implemented with low computational complexity on mobile devices and cloud computing for tele-medicine, e.g., patient self-monitoring and preventive health. Li et al. [55] proposed a 1D-CNN based model to classify ECG signals. The model consisted of five layers and realized the classification of five typical kinds of arrhythmia signals. It achieved promising classification accuracy and significantly outperformed several typical ECG classification methods. Zubair et al. [56] propose an ECG beat classification system using a 1D-CNN model. The proposed classification system efficiently classified ECG beats into five different classes. Results showed that the model achieved a significant classification accuracy and superior computational efficiency than most of the state-of-the-art methods for ECG signal classification. Avanzato et al. [57] proposed a new neural architecture based on 1D-CNN for the development of automatic heart disease diagnosis systems using ECG signals. The model was performed on 30 s segments and classified three different classes of anomalies. It showed high performance and low complexity implementation. Kamaleswaran et al. [58] introduced a novel deep learning architecture for detection of normal sinus rhythm, AF, other abnormal rhythms, and noise. They proposed an optimal 13-layer 1D-CNN model with identified normal, AF and other rhythms using single lead short ECG recordings. The architecture was computationally fast and could also be used in real-time cardiac arrhythmia detection applications.

3. ECG Signal

The mechanical pumping activity of the heart muscle is determined by the rhythmic generation of an electrical impulse that originates at the level of the sinoatrial node and, through specialized conduction pathways, spreads to all cardiac muscle cells causing cycles of depolarization and repolarization underlying the contraction of single cells.

ECG is the graphic reproduction of the electrical activity of the heart during its functioning, recorded at the surface of the body. The doctor, usually a cardiologist specialist, interprets the electrocardiographic recording by detecting the presence of cardiac arrhythmias, structural changes in the cardiac cavities, atria and/or ventricles, ischemia, myocardial infarction, and other cardiopathies, characterized by an alteration of electrical conduction. A beat of ECG signals can be observed by five characteristic waves—P, Q, R, S, and T [59], where each wave is related to a specific interval of the polarization–depolarization cycle. The characteristic of the normal ECG is that varies only in the presence of problems. The fundamental morphology of the ECG is given by three deflections (P, QRS, and T), which represent the formation and diffusion of the cardiac electrical impulse along the pathways of the conduction system (Figure 1).

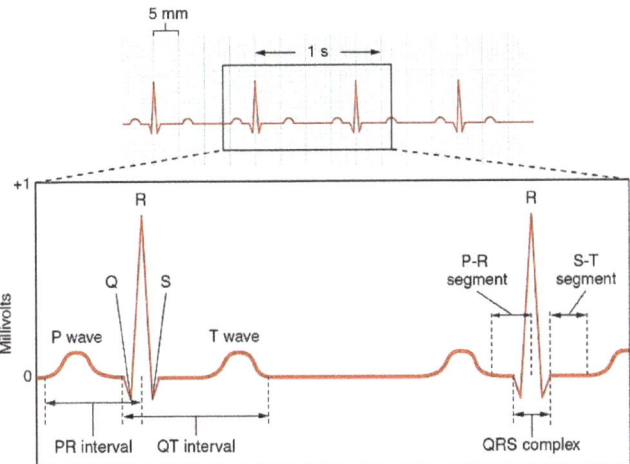

Figure 1. Tracing of a normal electrocardiogram (ECG) including P wave, QRS complex, and T wave. Reproduced with permission from Gordon Betts et al., Anatomy and Physiology, Connexions Website. http://cnx.org/content/col11496/1.6/; published by OpenStax, 19 June 2013.

4. Materials and Methods

4.1. Dataset

The proposed method was tested on the MIT-BIH Arrhythmia Database supplied by PhysioNet, a web resource for complex physiologic signals databases [60]. The MIT-BIH Arrhythmia Database contains 48 half-hour extracts of two-channel ambulatory ECG recordings, obtained from 47 subjects: 25 males aged between 32 and 89 years and 22 females aged between 23 and 89 years. As described by the authors in [60], the database consists of 23 recordings randomly selected by a set of 4000 24-h ambulatory ECG recordings collected from a mixed population of hospitalized (approximately 60%) and ambulatory (approximately 40%) patients at Beth Israel Hospital in Boston. The remaining 25 recordings were selected from the same set in order to include less common but clinically significant arrhythmias that would not be well represented in a small random sample. The recordings were digitized at 360 samples per second per channel with an 11-bit resolution over a 10-mV range. For our analysis, we used the same data published by Kaggle in txt and csv format, since they were easier to process [61].

The database contains 22 classes, 1 for normal beat, and 21 for various kinds of anomalies in ECG recordings.

4.2. Data Organization

Data were structured in a tabular form in order to be processed by the neural network. The ECGs are two-channel recordings including main derivations, varied among subjects. In most ECGs one channel is a Modified-Lead II (MLII) and the other channel is generally V1, sometimes V2, V4, or V5, depending on the subject. For this reason, since the MLII is almost present in every ECGs, we only considered this lead. Four ECG recordings, only containing leads V1 and V5, were excluded from the analysis. The 30-min ECG recordings were fragmented into segments of 15 s. Since the recordings were digitized at 360 samples per second, each segment consisted of 5400 samples (Tables 1 and 2). Each segment was included in the analysis and no data cleaning process was executed.

Table 1. Example of one 30-min ECG recording digitized at 360 samples per second provided by Kaggle. (**a**) Each row is a sample of Modified-Lead II MLII and V5 lead signals quantized with 11-bit resolution over a ±5 mV range. Sample values thus range from 0 to 2047 inclusive, with a value of 1024 corresponding to zero volts; (**b**) only includes annotated samples f(N = normal or A = anomalous) with a timestamp.

Sample	MLII	V5	Time	Sample	Type
0	995	1011	0:00.214	77	N
1	1000	1008	0:01.028	370	N
2	997	1008	0:01.839	662	N
...	...	...	...	...	...
648,000	969	997	30:00.564	648,203	A
648,000	969	1003	30:01.325	648,477	N
(a)				(b)	

Table 2. Data organization of one 30-min ECG recording fragmented into segments. Columns from MLII_0 to MLII_539 represent samples contained in 15 s fragment. Each row is a different and consecutive fragment. Type N = normal, A = anomaly.

MLII_0	MLII_1	MLII_2	MLII_3	...	MLII_5396	MLII_5397	MLII_5398	MLII_5399	Type
995	1000	997	995	...	977	979	975	974	N
...	...	...	...	...	...	...	...	...	...
989	988	986	990	...	974	972	969	969	A

Based on the annotations assigned to the peaks present, each segment was labeled as follows: if in the segment all peaks were annotated as normal then the entire segment was labeled as normal; if in the segment at least one peak was annotated as anomalous, presenting any kind of anomalies, then the entire segment was labeled as anomalous.

In the dataset, each row represented a segment of 15 s labeled as normal or anomalous. Labeled as normal were 2105 segments and 3175 as anomalous. Since the dataset presented clearly imbalanced classes showing a proportion bias, we undersampled the segments labeled as anomalous in order to keep only a part of these data, thus balancing the training set. The anomalous segments in excess were included in the test set.

As will be detailed later, we carried out two distinct experiments, preprocessing data in different ways. In the first experimentation, segments were randomly included in the training set, using an equal proportion of segments for the two classes. The training set consisted of 2930 segments, 1465 labeled as normal, and 1465 labeled as anomalous. The training set was split in 70% for training and 30% for validation, keeping the same proportion of normal and anomalous segments. Segments contained in the test set presented a different proportion of the two classes, including 640 labeled as normal (60%) and 426 as anomalous (40%). Examples of normal and anomalous ECG recording are shown in Figure 2. Table 3 shows the number of ECG segments for each normal or anomalous class. The segments classified as anomalous can include one or more types of anomalies.

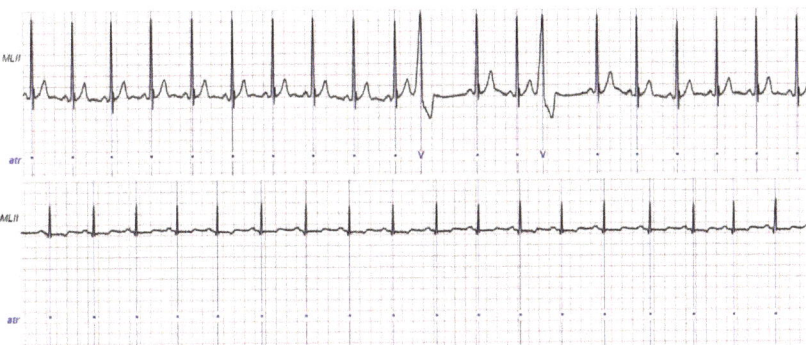

Figure 2. Examples of ECG recordings. (**Top**) Premature ventricular contraction (V). (**Bottom**) Normal record.

In the first experiment, as a widespread procedure used in literature and in the studies we compared to our work, we randomly assigned segments extracted from the same ECG recordings into training and test set. In the second experiment, we carried out a patient-oriented analysis, assigning to the training set only segments extracted from the same ECG recordings. This procedure was carried out for ECGs from 28 patients, since each ECG is related to a single patient. Segments extracted from the remaining 16 ECGs were assigned to the test set. In this way, segments of the same patient ECG recording are not interleaved between the training and test set. The training set consisted of 3360 segments, 1594 normal, and 1766 anomalous and the test set included 1800 segments, 435 normal, and 1365 anomalous. With this selection procedure, every segment of ECG recordings included in the test set had never been presented to the network during the training phase. Thus, the evaluation is only done on ECG recordings of patients never seen by the model.

4.3. Model Architecture

Convolutional neural network is a special kind of artificial neural network developed for image classification in which the model normally processes two-dimensional spatial input data representing an image's pixels, in a process called feature learning. The same model can be used for one-dimensional sequence of data, such as an analysis of time series data, signal data, or natural language processing. The architecture of the model is described in [62]. The electrocardiogram signal is a time series data sequence that represents electrical impulses from the myocardium [63]. Thus, we propose a 1D convolutional neural network consisting of four convolutional blocks and one output block for the analysis of ECG signal data, in order to automatically identify normal and anomalous ECG recordings.

The convolutional block, as represented in Figure 3, consists of a 1D convolutional layer, a batch normalization layer, a 1D max pooling layer, and a rectified linear unit (ReLU) layer, while the output contains a 1D average pooling, a flatten layer, a dense layer, and a Softmax layer. We chose a four convolutional blocks architecture, since it showed a right tradeoff between computational efficiency and results accuracy.

The 1D convolutional layer creates a convolution kernel that is convolved with the input layer over a single dimension to produce a tensor of output. The kernel size was set to 80 in the first layer and decreased to 4 in the subsequent layers, in order to reduce computational costs (Table 4). The batch normalization standardized the input and it was applied after each convolutional layer and before the level of pooling, in order to improve performance and stabilize the learning process of the deep neural network [59]. The output of the batch normalization layer was downsampled by means of a 1D max pooling layer with a pool size of 4.

Table 3. ECG segments for each ECG class in train and test sets for the first experimentation. Since our goal is to detect any kind of anomaly, we considered both rhythm and beat alterations with no difference. We also considered signal related annotations since a low quality noise signal could represent an issue to medical diagnosis.

Type	Class	Train	Test
Normal	Normal beat	1465	640
Anomalous	Left bundle branch block beat	331	123
	Right bundle branch block beat	330	131
	Atrial premature beat	406	150
	Aberrated atrial premature beat	49	29
	Nodal (junctional) premature beat	5	2
	Supraventricular premature beat	1	0
	Premature ventricular contraction	1236	520
	Fusion of ventricular and normal beat	165	74
	Ventricular flutter wave	12	2
	Atrial escape beat	12	4
	Nodal (junctional) escape beat	45	14
	Ventricular escape beat	5	4
	Paced beat	151	86
	Fusion of paced and normal beat	46	30
	Non-conducted P-wave (blocked APB)	26	16
	Unclassifiable beat	6	4
	Isolated QRS-like artifact	55	30
	Change in signal quality (qq)	253	115
	Rhythm change	432	189
	Start of ventricular flutter/fibrillation	5	1
	End of ventricular flutter/fibrillation	5	1

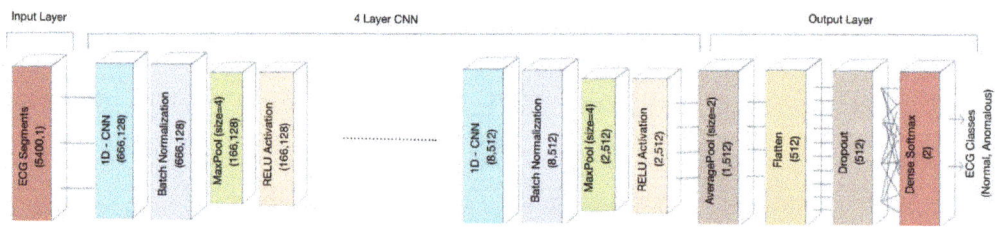

Figure 3. Architecture of the proposed 1D-convolutional neural network (CNN) model.

The 1D max pooling resizes the input representation by taking the maximum value on the window defined by pool size. The strides specify how much the pooling window moved for each pooling step. The pooling level was placed before ReLU to reduce overfitting.

Table 4. Detailed parameters of the proposed 1D-CNN model.

	Input Shape (5400;1)–Sample of 5400 Samples	
Type of Layer	Output Shape	Other Parameters
Conv1D	(666;128)	Kernel size = 80, Strides = 8, Filters = 128
Batch Normalization	(666;128)	-
Max Pooling 1D	(166;128)	Pool size = 4
Activation	(166;128)	ReLU activation
Conv1D	(163;256)	Kernel size = 4, Filters = 256
Batch Normalization	(163;256)	-
Max Pooling 1D	(40;256)	Pool size = 4
Activation	(40;256)	ReLU activation
Conv1D	(37;256)	Kernel size = 4, Filters = 256
Batch Normalization	(37;256)	-
Max Pooling 1D	(9;256)	Pool size = 4
Activation	(9;256)	ReLU activation
Conv1D	(8;512)	Kernel size = 4, Filters = 512
Batch Normalization	(8;512)	-
Max Pooling 1D	(2;512)	Pool size = 4
Activation	(2;512)	ReLU activation
AveragePooling 1D	(1;512)	Pool size = 2
Flatten	(512)	-
Dropout	(512)	Rate 0.6
Dense	(2)	Regularizer L2 (0.001), Softmax activation

In the output block, the 1D average pooling performed the same operation as the 1D max pooling but took the average window value. After the average pooling, the network had a flatten layer in order to transform multi-dimensional input feature vectors obtained in the previous layer to the appropriate size, as the input of the subsequent layers of the network. The output of the flatten layer is the input of a dense fully connected layer, which uses the Softmax function to predict output classes. Moreover, we used a dropout parameter to prevent overfitting. Dropout is a regularization technique that helps to reduce interdependent learning amongst the neurons. At each training, a set of neurons randomly chosen is dropped out of the net. We used dropout in the dense layer with a fraction of 0.6. With the same aim of preventing overfitting, in the dense layer, we also used a weight regularization approach. We used an L2 regularization penalty (sum of the squared weights) with hyperparameter equal to 0.001 in order to keep small values of weight in the dense layer. The architecture of the proposed 1D-CNN model is shown in Figure 3 and Table 4.

4.4. Validation and Performance Metrics

In order to evaluate the performance of our model, the training set was split in 70% for training and 30% for validation. Then to validate the stability of the model and generalize results, a resampling procedure was performed on the training set. In particular, we implemented k-fold cross-validation with k = 10. Data were split into 10 groups, then each group at a time was used as a validation set and the remaining groups as the training set. Data were split such that no observation could be included both in training and in test sets. The network was fitted on the training set and evaluated on the validation set for 10 times. Results were summarized with mean and standard deviation values of the model performance metrics. Finally, the testing set was used to verify the robustness of the neural network on data not included in the training set.

To evaluate the performance of the neural network, we computed the confusion matrix and the traditional classification metrics. In particular, given TP (true positive) and TN (true negative) the number of events correctly classified, respectively, as successes or failures and FP (false positive) and FN (false negative) the number of events incorrectly classified, respectively, as successes or failures, we calculated

$$\text{Accuracy} = \frac{TP + TN}{TP + TN + FN + FP}, \quad (1)$$

$$\text{Precision} = \frac{TP}{TP + FP}, \quad (2)$$

$$\text{Recall} = \frac{TP}{TP + FN}, \quad (3)$$

$$F1 = \frac{2TP}{2TP + FP + FN}, \quad (4)$$

5. Results and Discussion

We performed the proposed 1D convolution neural network on the MIT-BIH Arrhythmia data processed as segments of 15 s consisting of 5400 samples including 21 different classes of anomalies.

In the first experiment, we split the dataset basing on segments as explained in Section 4.2. The network was trained on 70% of the set and was validated on the remaining 30% for 200 epochs. Results for the validation performed on the training set are shown in Figure 4. The network stabilized in convergence in a training process of 200 epochs. The learning curves of the training and validation loss stabilized below 0.5 and the learning curves of the training and validation accuracy stabilized around 90%, both with a minimal gap between the final values.

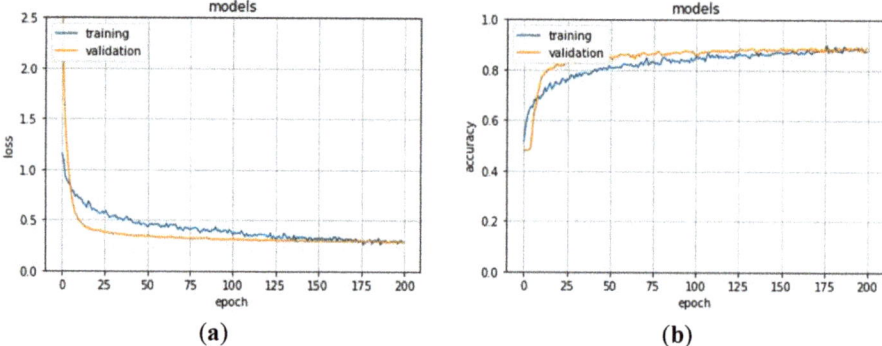

Figure 4. (a) Training and validation loss and (b) training and validation accuracy for the first experimentation. Accuracy metric is defined in Equation (1). Epoch is commonly referred to as the number of a full training pass over the entire dataset.

In order to validate the stability of the proposed method, we used a k-fold cross validation as explained in Section 4.4. The average accuracy of the model was $89.3 \pm 0.26\%$ of standard deviation and the average loss was of $0.28 \pm 0.06\%$ and an average recall $85.6 \pm 0.03\%$.

In order to assess the performance, the network was evaluated on the test set. The confusion matrix and the related metrics were computed (Table 5). The network showed an accuracy of 89.51%, and a recall of 91.09% for normal and 87.79% for anomalous segments, the precision of 91.81% for normal and 86.78% for anomalous segments, and F1-score 91.45% for normal and 87.28% for anomalous segments.

Table 5. Confusion matrix and related performance metrics for the test set in the first experimentation.

		Predicted		Accuracy (%)	Recall (%)	Precision (%)	F1 (%)
		Normal	Anomalous				
True	Normal	583	57	89.51	91.09	91.81	91.45
	Anomalous	52	374		87.79	86.78	87.28

We compared the proposed network with the studies that, at the state of the art, performed the same 1D convolutional neural network using the MIT-BIH Arrhythmia Dataset with the aim to implement an automatic classification of cardiac pathologies based on ECG signals. The results of this comparison are reported in Table 6.

Table 6. Comparison with studies performed using 1D-CNN on the MIT-BIH Arrhythmia Database.

Article	Model	Classes of Anomalies	Accuracy	Recall	F1-Score
[54]	1D-CNN	17 classes	91.3%	83.9%	85.4%
[55]	1D-CNN	5 classes	97.5%	-	-
[56]	1D-CNN	5 classes	92.7%	-	-
[57]	1D-CNN	3 classes	98.33%	98.33%	98.33%
Proposed method	1D-CNN	1 class, including 21 kinds of anomalies	89.51%	87.79%	86.78%

Briefly summarizing, Yıldırım et al. [54] proposed a 1D convolutional neural network model for cardiac arrhythmia (17 classes) detection based on long-duration electrocardiography (ECG) signal analysis. They designed a complete end-to-end structure with neither hand-crafted feature extraction of the signals nor feature selection at any stage using a 16-layer deep network structure including standard CNN layers. The network was tested on MIT-BIH Arrhythmia database considering 10 s ECG signal segments for one lead (MLII) for a total of 1000 ECG signal segments from 45 persons. The network achieved a detection accuracy of 17 cardiac arrhythmia disorders (classes) at a level of 91.33%. Li et al. [55] proposed a 1D-convolutional neural network to classify ECG signals. The network consisted of five layers in addition to the input layer and the output layer, in particular, two convolution layers, two down sampling layers and one full connection layer. The model extracted the effective features from data and classified the features automatically. The wavelet threshold method was used to filter the high frequency noise, while the wavelet transform and reconstruction algorithm to correct the baseline drift, which is a low-frequency noise. Subsequently, the segmentation of ECG signals and the reduction of dimensions were performed by using R peaks that were located by the method of the wavelet transform. The network achieved a detection accuracy of five typical kinds of arrhythmia signals at a level of 97.5%. Zubair et al. [56] proposed an ECG beat classification system based on a 1D-convolutional neural network. The model integrated feature extraction and classification of ECG pattern recognition and consisted of three convolution layers, three pooling layers, a multilayer perceptron and Softmax layer. The classification was performed in three main steps: ECG beat detection, sample extraction, and classification. ECG beat detection stage involves the detection of the individual beat signal from 30 min long ECG recording of each patient, using modified-Lead II signals. Equal numbers of samples (100) on both right and left sides from the Rpeak were extracted and downsampling was performed to represent raw data of each beat by 128 samples. The network classified five different kinds of anomalies with a detection accuracy of 92.7%. Avanzato et al. [57] proposed an automatic heart disease diagnosis system using ECG signals based on the direct application of a 1D-convolutional neural network. The network consisted of three layers in addition to the input layer and the output layer. Unlike the classic CNN, which use fully connected neurons as their output layer, this network performed a single Average pooling layer and then a Softmax followed by a natural logarithm. The structure of the neural network input consisted of 30-s segments where every second of ECG recording was equivalent to 360 samples, for a total of 10,800 samples. The paper evaluated the performance of the network on three classes of anomalies with an accuracy of 98.33%.

Table 6 shows that the proposed method presents remarkable performance compared to the other studies, considering that it is able to detect anomalies in an ECG recording including 21 different classes. In addition, the proposed method is able to classify anomalies even in presence of more than one kind of cardiac pathology in the same ECG segment. It achieves recall and F1-score, respectively of 87.79% and 86.78%, improving results obtained in [54], which considered only 17 classes of anomalies. These results were achieved with a detection accuracy of 89.51%, slightly lower than the accuracy obtained using the method proposed in [54], despite the increase in the number of different kinds of anomalies. The high performance obtained for recall, in spite of a small loss for accuracy, is consistent with the research goal to reduce the number of ECGs sent to the medical specialist for further examination. At the same time, we need to ensure that anomalous ECGs could not escape the medical examination and the prescription of the proper therapy. Although results obtained in [54–56] showed higher performance, in those studies the analysis was carried out including a lower number of anomalies. In particular, [55,56] included in the analysis five classes and obtained an accuracy, respectively, of 97.5% and 92.7%. In [57] the analysis was conducted using three classes with an accuracy of 98.33%. Note that the model in [54] was based on 16 levels architecture (therefore with a large computational complexity to deploy, as an example, on wearable devices) and the models in [55–57], although based on four levels, operate only on a very small number of anomalies.

Analyzing the 52 segments containing anomalies and incorrectly classified as normal (false negative, see Table 5), we observed that, for most of them, at least one of the segments extracted from the same ECG recording was correctly classified as anomalous. Overall, only five ECG recordings from patients affected by cardiac pathologies were not detected at all.

In light of this, we carried out a second experiment, including in the training set only segments extracted from the same ECG recordings, and for the test set, as explained in Section 4.2. Thus, the proposed 1D-CNN was tested on segments extracted from ECG recordings never presented to the network in the training process.

The training set consisted of 3360 segments, 1594 normal, and 1766 anomalous, extracted from 28 ECG recordings, whereas the remaining recordings were included in the test set. In the test set, there were 1800 segments, 435 normal, and 1365 anomalous. To evaluate the performance of the model, the network was trained on 70% of the set and was validated on the remaining 30% for 200 epochs. Figure 5 shows the learning process for training and validation loss and accuracy. The model stabilized in convergence in a training process of 200 epochs. Additionally, in this case, the learning curves of the training and validation loss stabilized around zero and the learning curves of the training and validation accuracy stabilized around 90%.

In order to validate the stability of the proposed method, we used a k-fold cross validation as explained in Section 4.4. The average accuracy of the model was 88.2 ± 0.28% of standard deviation and the average loss was of 0.29 ± 0.07% and an average recall of 87.6 ± 0.03%.

The network was, then, evaluated on the test set. The resulting confusion matrix and the related metrics are shown in Table 7.

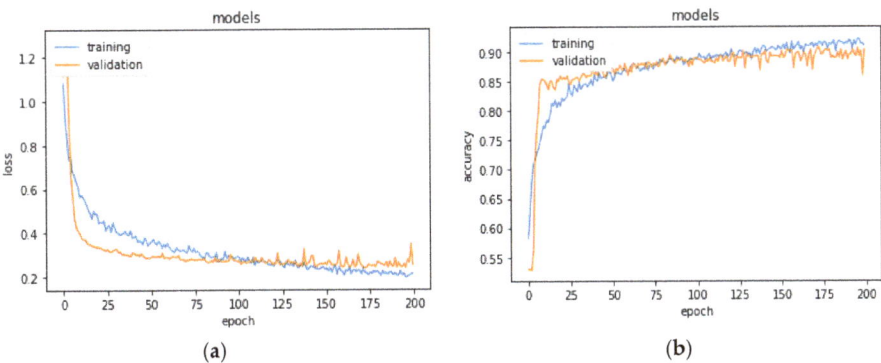

Figure 5. (a) Training and validation loss and (b) training and validation accuracy for the second experimentation.

Table 7. Confusion matrix and related performance metrics for the test set in the second experimentation.

		Predicted		Accuracy	Recall	Precision	F1
		Normal	Anomalous	(%)	(%)	(%)	(%)
True	Normal	241	194	84.94	55.40	75.79	64.01
	Anomalous	77	1288		94.36	86.91	90.48

The network showed an accuracy of 84.94%, and a recall of 55.40% for normal and 94.36% for anomalous segments, the precision of 75.79% for normal and 86.91% for anomalous segments, and F1-score 64.01% for normal and 90.48% for anomalous segments.

The model showed a higher recall for anomalous segments compared to the previous test. Analyzing the 77 segments containing anomalies and incorrectly classified as normal, we observed that, for all of them, at least one of the segments extracted from the same ECG recording was correctly classified as anomalous. This result showed a remarkable improvement in the performance of the proposed method since, thinking in terms of patients rather than segments, the system was able to detect 100% of ECG recordings from patients affected by cardiac pathologies.

Considering this performance, we believe that the unavoidable goal to detect anomalous segments and minimize missed alarms was reached. This claim must be considered in the operative context where the model was deployed, in which the cost of a false alarm was considerably less than a missed one.

Moreover, we want to highlight that these results were achieved with the second experiment whose settings represents a closer scenario in terms of model usage. In the second experiment the model was validated on ECG records of different patients never presented to the model during the training. This experiment design is not common since validation is usually carried out with the usual holdout method, that is, segments from the same ECG recordings could be interleaved between training and test sets. With holdout there are chances that some signal patterns have been already presented to the model in the training phase.

However, it should be noted that the system described here still presents a significant false alarm rate. We are currently investigating different strategies to reduce the required workload due to false alarms. One viable solution is to isolate and collect only anomalous detected segments; when they occur in significant quantities can be sent remotely for the expert verification. Looking only at some of the segments, just those classified as anomalous by our model, can be a very quick job for an expert, certainly less demanding than observing an entire ECG, even more so if referred to a Holter exam.

This operational solution is well suited also for continual and active learning techniques, that is to periodically retrain the model based on new annotations from an expert; in this way, as new examples come into the system a probable gradual decrease in false alarms events is expected, with more balanced performances.

6. Conclusions

The diffusion of personal portable monitoring devices could involve the reporting of millions of ECG recordings every day. Systems able to support the cardiologists' work in the interpretation of ECGs for the diagnosis of cardiac pathologies are required to facilitate health care decision making reducing considerably the expenditure of time and money. In fact, the automated detection of suspicious anomalies in ECG recordings can drastically reduce the number of ECGs that need to be manually examined by the cardiologists, excluding those classified as normal.

In the present paper, we propose a system able to automatically detect the suspect of cardiac pathologies in ECG signals from personal monitoring devices, using a 1D-CNN architecture. The 1D-CNN model overcomes the problems of vanishing gradient and gradient exploding related to recurrent neural networks, making their training difficult. Moreover, the 1D-CNN model allows one to implement real-time and low-cost systems and it is characterized by low computational complexity, feasible implementation on smart devices, and cloud computing. The system was optimized to detect the suspect of anomalies classifying normal and anomalous ECG, regardless of the kind of cardiac pathology. The proposed model was tested on the MIT-BIH ECG Arrhythmia Database, which included 21 different classes of ECG anomalies. Two different experimentations were carried out showing remarkable performance compared to the other studies conducted using the 1D-CNN architecture tested on the MIT-BIH ECG Arrhythmia Database. In particular, the network achieved accuracy and recall, respectively, of 84.94% and 94.36% computed with respect to the ECG signal segments and accuracy and recall of 100% when computed with respect to the patients, therefore considering the detection of anomalies in the entire ECG recordings.

We are now working on a possible personalization of the model, tunable toward a single person. We expect that the performance of this kind of model could be much better than a general one, with an additional cost of model calibration before the actual usage.

In the same study we are also investigating a model trained on "normal" segments of healthy patients and abnormal segments of pathological patients (since it is not possible to obtain abnormal segments from a healthy patient). This will allow us to observe if the model trained on this new dataset presents different characteristics than the model described in this paper. Here, we wanted to compare our study with studies that were as homogeneous as possible, at least in the dataset used, so we did not introduce any further changes regarding the training data.

Author Contributions: Conceptualization, A.N. and G.D.; Data curation, A.N. and M.S.; Formal analysis, P.R.F.; Methodology, F.G., P.R.F. and G.D.; Software, P.R.F. and M.S.; Writing—Original draft, F.G. and G.D. All authors have read and agreed to the published version of the manuscript.

Funding: This research received no external funding.

Institutional Review Board Statement: The used dataset was not recorded by the authors but originated from a 2001 study by Moody et al. [60]. The authors of the database stated that all ethical requirements had been followed. Moreover, the database is available online for an extended period now and has been used extensively in many studies.

Data Availability Statement: The proposed method was tested on the MIT-BIH Arrhythmia Database supplied by PhysioNet, see https://www.physionet.org/content/mitdb/1.0.0/.

Conflicts of Interest: The authors declare no conflict of interest.

References

1. Cai, W.; Hu, D. ECG Interpretation with Deep Learning. In *Feature Engineering and Computational Intelligence in ECG Monitoring*; Liu, C., Li, J., Eds.; Springer: Singapore, 2020; pp. 143–156.
2. Chamley, R.R.; Holdsworth, D.A.; Rajappan, K.; Nicol, E.D. ECG interpretation: Interpretation of the ECG in young, fit, asymptomatic individuals undertaking high-hazard occupations is the topic of the fourth article in the occupational cardiology series. *Eur. Heart J.* **2019**, *40*, 2663–2666. [CrossRef]
3. Dimauro, G.; Caivano, D.; Ciccone, M.M.; Dalena, G.; Girardi, F. Classification of cardiac tones of mechanical and native mitral valves. In *Ambient Assisted Living, Lecture Notes in Electrical Engineering*; Spring: Berlin/Heidelberg, Germany, 2021; Volume 725, ISBN 978-3-030-63107-9.
4. Schläpfer, J.; Wellens, H.J. Computer-Interpreted Electrocardiograms. *J. Am. Coll. Cardiol.* **2017**, *70*, 1183–1192. [CrossRef]
5. Dimauro, G.; de Ruvo, S.; di Terlizzi, F.; Ruggieri, A.; Volpe, V.; Colizzi, L.; Girardi, F. Estimate of Anemia with New Non-Invasive Systems—A Moment of Reflection. *Electronics* **2020**, *9*, 780. [CrossRef]
6. Dimauro, G.; Bevilacqua, V.; Colizzi, L.; di Pierro, D. TestGraphia, a Software System for the Early Diagnosis of Dysgraphia. *IEEE Access* **2020**, *8*, 19564–19575. [CrossRef]
7. Dimauro, G.; Guarini, A.; Caivano, D.; Girardi, F.; Pasciolla, C.; Iacobazzi, A. Detecting Clinical Signs of Anaemia From Digital Images of the Palpebral Conjunctiva. *IEEE Access* **2019**, *7*, 113488–113498. [CrossRef]
8. Kasiviswanathan, S.; Vijayan, T.B.; Simone, L.; Dimauro, G. Semantic Segmentation of Conjunctiva Region for Non-Invasive Anemia Detection Applications. *Electronics* **2020**, *9*, 1309. [CrossRef]
9. Monaco, A.; Cattaneo, R.; Mesin, L.; Fiorucci, E.; Pietropaoli, D. Evaluation of autonomic nervous system in sleep apnea patients using pupillometry under occlusal stress: A pilot study. *Cranio* **2014**, *32*, 139–147. [CrossRef]
10. Castroflorio, T.; Mesin, L.; Tartaglia, G.M.; Sforza, C.; Farina, D. Use of electromyographic and electrocardiographic signals to detect sleep bruxism episodes in a natural environment. *IEEE J. Biomed. Health Inform.* **2013**, *17*, 994–1001. [CrossRef] [PubMed]
11. Bevilacqua, V.; Pietroleonardo, N.; Triggiani, V.; Brunetti, A.; Di Palma, A.M.; Rossini, M.; Gesualdo, L. An innovative neural network framework to classify blood vessels and tubules based on Haralick features evaluated in histological images of kidney biopsy. *Neurocomputing* **2017**, *228*, 143–153. [CrossRef]
12. Buongiorno, D.; Cascarano, G.D.; De Feudis, I.; Brunetti, A.; Carnimeo, L.; Dimauro, G.; Bevilacqua, V. Deep Learning for Processing Electromyographic Signals: A Taxonomy-based Survey. *Neurocomputing* **2020**. [CrossRef]
13. Estes, N.A.M. Computerized Interpretation of ECGs: Supplement Not a Substitute. *Circ. Arrhythm. Electrophysiol.* **2013**, *6*, 2–4. [CrossRef]
14. Kligfield, P.; Gettes, L.S.; Bailey, J.J.; Childers, R.; Deal, B.J.; Hancock, E.W.; van Herpen, G.; Kors, J.A.; Macfarlane, P.; Mirvis, D.M.; et al. Recommendations for the Standardization and Interpretation of the Electrocardiogram: Part II: The Electrocardiogram and Its Technology: A Scientific Statement From the American Heart Association Electrocardiography and Arrhythmias Committee, Council on Clinical Cardiology; the American College of Cardiology Foundation; and the Heart Rhythm Society: Endorsed by the International Society for Computerized Electrocardiology. *Circulation* **2007**, *115*, 1306–1324.
15. Fye, W.B. A History of the origin, evolution, and impact of electrocardiography. *Am. J. Cardiol.* **1994**, *73*, 937–949. [CrossRef]
16. Mesin, L.; Aram, S.; Pasero, E. A neural data-driven algorithm for smart sampling in wireless sensor networks. *J. Wirel. Commun. Netw.* **2014**, *23*, 1–8. [CrossRef]
17. Redlarski, G.; Gradolewski, D.; Palkowski, A. A System for Heart Sounds Classification. *PLoS ONE* **2014**, *9*, e112673. [CrossRef]
18. Liu, W.; Wang, Z.; Liu, X.; Zeng, N.; Liu, Y.; Alsaadi, F.E. A survey of deep neural network architectures and their applications. *Neurocomputing* **2017**, *234*, 11–26. [CrossRef]
19. Zhao, W.; Du, S. Spectral–Spatial Feature Extraction for Hyperspectral Image Classification: A Dimension Reduction and Deep Learning Approach. *IEEE Trans. Geosci. Remote Sens.* **2016**, *54*, 4544–4554. [CrossRef]
20. Dimauro, G.; Deperte, F.; Maglietta, R.; Bove, M.; la Gioia, F.; Renò, V.; Simone, L.; Gelardi, M. A Novel Approach for Biofilm Detection Based on a Convolutional Neural Network. *Electronics* **2020**, *9*, 881. [CrossRef]
21. Renò, V.; Sciancalepore, M.; Dimauro, G.; Maglietta, R.; Cassano, M.; Gelardi, M. A Novel Approach for the Automatic Estimation of the Ciliated Cell Beating Frequency. *Electronics* **2020**, *9*, 1002. [CrossRef]
22. Dimauro, G.; Bevilacqua, V.; Fina, P.; Buongiorno, D.; Brunetti, A.; Latrofa, S.; Cassano, M.; Gelardi, M. Comparative Analysis of Rhino-Cytological Specimens with Image Analysis and Deep Learning Techniques. *Electronics* **2020**, *9*, 952. [CrossRef]
23. Dimauro, G.; Altomare, N.; Scalera, M. PQMET: A digital image quality metric based on human visual system. In Proceedings of the 2014 4th International Conference on Image Processing Theory, Tools and Applications (IPTA), Paris, France, 14–17 October 2014. [CrossRef]
24. Dimauro, G.; Simone, L. Novel Biased Normalized Cuts Approach for the Automatic Segmentation of the Conjunctiva. *Electronics* **2020**, *9*, 997. [CrossRef]
25. Sainath, T.N.; Weiss, R.J.; Wilson, K.W.; Li, B.; Narayanan, A.; Variani, E.; Bacchiani, M.; Shafran, I.; Senior, A.; Chin, K.; et al. Multichannel Signal Processing With Deep Neural Networks for Automatic Speech Recognition. *IEEE/ACM Trans. Audio Speech Lang. Process.* **2017**, *25*, 965–979. [CrossRef]
26. Barletta, V.S.; Caivano, D.; Nannavecchia, A.; Scalera, M. Intrusion Detection for in-Vehicle Communication Networks: An Unsupervised Kohonen SOM Approach. *Future Internet* **2020**, *12*, 119. [CrossRef]

27. Barletta, V.S.; Caivano, D.; Nannavecchia, A.; Scalera, M. A Kohonen SOM Architecture for Intrusion Detection on In-Vehicle Communication Networks. *Appl. Sci.* **2020**, *10*, 5062. [CrossRef]
28. Barletta, V.S.; Caivano, D.; Dimauro, G.; Nannavecchia, A.; Scalera, M. Managing a Smart City Integrated Model through Smart Program Management. *Appl. Sci.* **2020**, *10*, 714. [CrossRef]
29. Renò, V.; Dimauro, G.; Labate, G.; Stella, E.; Fanizza, C.; Cipriano, G.; Carlucci, R.; Maglietta, R. A SIFT-based software system for the photo-identification of the Risso's dolphin. *Ecol. Inform.* **2019**, *50*, 95–101. [CrossRef]
30. Dimauro, G.; Colagrande, P.; Carlucci, R.; Ventura, M.; Bevilacqua, V.; Caivano, D. CRISPRLearner: A Deep Learning-Based System to Predict CRISPR/Cas9 sgRNA On-Target Cleavage Efficiency. *Electronics* **2019**, *8*, 1478. [CrossRef]
31. Ribeiro, A.H.; Ribeiro, M.H.; Paixão, G.M.M.; Oliveira, D.M.; Gomes, P.R.; Canazart, J.A.; Ferreira, M.P.S.; Andersson, C.R.; Macfarlane, P.W.; Meira, W.; et al. Automatic diagnosis of the 12-lead ECG using a deep neural network. *Nat. Commun.* **2020**, *11*, 1760. [CrossRef]
32. Stead, W.W. Clinical Implications and Challenges of Artificial Intelligence and Deep Learning. *JAMA* **2018**, *320*, 1107. [CrossRef]
33. Naylor, C.D. On the Prospects for a (Deep) Learning Health Care System. *JAMA* **2018**, *320*, 1099. [CrossRef] [PubMed]
34. Dimauro, G.; Girardi, F.; Caivano, D.; Colizzi, L. Personal Health E-Record—Toward an Enabling Ambient Assisted Living Technology for Communication and Information Sharing Between Patients and Care Providers. In *Ambient Assisted Living*; Leone, A., Caroppo, A., Rescio, G., Diraco, G., Siciliano, P., Eds.; Springer: Cham, Switzerland, 2019; Volume 544, pp. 487–499. [CrossRef]
35. Ardito, C.; Caivano, D.; Colizzi, L.; Dimauro, G.; Verardi, L. Design and Execution of Integrated Clinical Pathway: A Simplified Meta-Model and Associated Methodology. *Information* **2020**, *11*, 362. [CrossRef]
36. Dimauro, G.; di Pierro, D.; Deperte, F.; Simone, L.; Fina, P.R. A Smartphone-Based Cell Segmentation to Support Nasal Cytology. *Appl. Sci.* **2020**, *10*, 4567. [CrossRef]
37. AliveCor. Available online: https://www.alivecor.com/kardiamobile/ (accessed on 31 August 2020).
38. D-Heart Smartphone ECG Device. Available online: https://www.d-heartcare.com/ (accessed on 31 August 2020).
39. eKuore | Wireless Electronic Stethoscope. Available online: https://www.ekuore.com/ (accessed on 31 August 2020).
40. Wang, H.; Shi, H.; Chen, X.; Zhao, L.; Huang, Y.; Liu, C. An Improved Convolutional Neural Network Based Approach for Automated Heartbeat Classification. *J. Med. Syst.* **2020**, *44*, 1–9. [CrossRef] [PubMed]
41. Duan, L.; Hongxin, Z.; Zhiqing, L.; Juxiang, H.; Tian, W. Deep residual convolutional neural network for recognition of electrocardiogram signal arrhythmias. *J. Biomed. Eng.* **2019**, *36*, 189–198. [CrossRef]
42. Wan, X.; Jin, Z.; Wu, H.; Liu, J.; Zhu, B.; Xie, H. Heartbeat classification algorithm based on one-dimensional convolution neural network. *J. Mech. Med. Biol.* **2020**, *20*, 2050046. [CrossRef]
43. Meintjes, A.; Lowe, A.; Legget, M. Fundamental Heart Sound Classification using the Continuous Wavelet Transform and Convolutional Neural Networks. In Proceedings of the 2018 40th Annual International Conference of the IEEE Engineering in Medicine and Biology Society (EMBC), Honolulu, HI, USA, 18–21 July 2018.
44. Langley, P.; Murray, A. Heart sound classification from unsegmented phonocardiograms. *Physiol. Meas.* **2017**, *38*, 1658–1670. [CrossRef]
45. He, S.; Fataf, N.A.A.; Banerjee, S.; Sun, K. Complexity in the muscular blood vessel model with variable fractional derivative and external disturbances. *Phys. A Stat. Mech. Appl.* **2019**, *526*, 120904. [CrossRef]
46. He, S.; Sun, K.; Wang, H. Complexity Analysis and DSP Implementation of the Fractional-Order Lorenz Hyperchaotic System. *Entropy* **2015**, *17*, 8299–8311. [CrossRef]
47. He, S.; Sun, K.; Banerjee, S. Dynamical properties and complexity in fractional-order diffusionless Lorenz system. *Eur. Phys. J. Plus* **2016**, *131*, 1–12. [CrossRef]
48. Chauhan, S.; Vig, L. Anomaly detection in ECG time signals via deep long short-term memory networks. In Proceedings of the 2015 IEEE International Conference on Data Science and Advanced Analytics (DSAA), Paris, France, 19–21 October 2015.
49. Scalera, M.; Antonella, S. Customer centric strategies for value creation: Academic experimentation. *J. E-Learn. Knowl. Soc.* **2014**, *10*, 65–76.
50. Saadatnejad, S.; Oveisi, M.; Hashemi, M. LSTM-Based ECG Classification for Continuous Monitoring on Personal Wearable Devices. *IEEE J. Biomed. Health Inf.* **2020**, *24*, 515–523. [CrossRef]
51. Thill, M.; Däubener, S.; Konen, W.; Bäck, T. Anomaly Detection in Electrocardiogram Readings with Stacked LSTM. In Proceedings of the ITAT 2019 Information Technologies—Applications and Theory, Donovaly, Slovakia, 20 September 2019.
52. Kiranyaz, S.; Ince, T.; Abdeljaber, O.; Avci, O.; Gabbouj, M. 1-D Convolutional Neural Networks for Signal Processing Applications. In Proceedings of the 2019 IEEE International Conference on Acoustics, Speech and Signal Processing (ICASSP), Brighton, UK, 12–17 May 2019.
53. Kiranyaz, S.; Ince, T.; Abdeljaber, O.; Gabbouj, M. Real-Time Patient-Specific ECG Classification by 1-D Convolutional Neural Networks. *IEEE Trans. Biomed. Eng.* **2016**, *63*, 664–675. [CrossRef]
54. Yıldırım, Ö.; Pławiak, P.; Tan, R.-S.; Acharya, U.R. Arrhythmia detection using deep convolutional neural network with long duration ECG signals. *Comput. Biol. Med.* **2018**, *102*, 411–420. [CrossRef]
55. Li, D.; Zhang, J.; Zhang, Q.; Wei, X. Classification of ECG signals based on 1D convolution neural network. In Proceedings of the 2017 IEEE 19th International Conference on e-Health Networking, Applications and Services (Healthcom), Dalian, China, 12–15 October 2017.

56. Zubair, M.; Kim, J.; Yoon, C. An Automated ECG Beat Classification System Using Convolutional Neural Networks. In Proceedings of the 2016 6th International Conference on IT Convergence and Security (ICITCS), Prague, Czech Republic, 26 September 2016.
57. Avanzato, R.; Beritelli, F. Automatic ECG Diagnosis Using Convolutional Neural Network. *Electronics* **2020**, *9*, 951. [CrossRef]
58. Kamaleswaran, R.; Mahajan, R.; Akbilgic, O. A robust deep convolutional neural network for the classification of abnormal cardiac rhythm using single lead electrocardiograms of variable length. *Physiol. Meas.* **2018**, *39*, 035006. [CrossRef]
59. Hsieh, C.-H.; Li, Y.-S.; Hwang, B.-J.; Hsiao, C.-H. Detection of Atrial Fibrillation Using 1D Convolutional Neural Network. *Sensors* **2020**, *20*, 2136. [CrossRef]
60. Moody, G.B.; Mark, R.G. The impact of the MIT-BIH arrhythmia database. *IEEE Eng. Med. Biol. Mag.* **2001**, *20*, 45–50. [CrossRef] [PubMed]
61. Mondejar, V. Kaggle MIT-BIH Arrhythmia Database. Available online: https://www.kaggle.com/mondejar/mitbih-database (accessed on 31 August 2020).
62. Wang, C.; Xi, Y. *Convolutional Neural Network for Image Classification*; Johns Hopkins University: Baltimore, MD, USA, 1997; Volume 21218.
63. Sivaraks, H.; Ratanamahatana, C.A. Robust and Accurate Anomaly Detection in ECG Artifacts Using Time Series Motif Discovery. *Comput. Math. Methods Med.* **2015**, *2015*, 453214. [CrossRef] [PubMed]

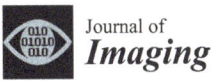

Article

Testing Segmentation Popular Loss and Variations in Three Multiclass Medical Imaging Problems

Pedro Furtado

Dei/FCT/CISUC, University of Coimbra, Polo II, 3030-290 Coimbra, Portugal; pnf@dei.uc.pt

Abstract: Image structures are segmented automatically using deep learning (DL) for analysis and processing. The three most popular base loss functions are cross entropy (crossE), intersect-over-the-union (IoU), and dice. Which should be used, is it useful to consider simple variations, such as modifying formula coefficients? How do characteristics of different image structures influence scores? Taking three different medical image segmentation problems (segmentation of organs in magnetic resonance images (MRI), liver in computer tomography images (CT) and diabetic retinopathy lesions in eye fundus images (EFI)), we quantify loss functions and variations, as well as segmentation scores of different targets. We first describe the limitations of metrics, since loss is a metric, then we describe and test alternatives. Experimentally, we observed that DeeplabV3 outperforms UNet and fully convolutional network (FCN) in all datasets. Dice scored 1 to 6 percentage points (pp) higher than cross entropy over all datasets, IoU improved 0 to 3 pp. Varying formula coefficients improved scores, but the best choices depend on the dataset: compared to crossE, different false positive vs. false negative weights improved MRI by 12 pp, and assigning zero weight to background improved EFI by 6 pp. Multiclass segmentation scored higher than n-uniclass segmentation in MRI by 8 pp. EFI lesions score low compared to more constant structures (e.g., optic disk or even organs), but loss modifications improve those scores significantly 6 to 9 pp. Our conclusions are that dice is best, it is worth assigning 0 weight to class background and to test different weights on false positives and false negatives.

Keywords: computers in medicine; segmentation; machine learning; deep learning; MRI

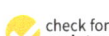

Citation: Furtado, P. Testing Segmentation Popular Loss and Variations in Three Multiclass Medical Imaging Problems. *J. Imaging* **2021**, *7*, 16. https://doi.org/10.3390/jimaging7020016

Academic Editor: Yudong Zhang
Received: 22 December 2020
Accepted: 22 January 2021
Published: 27 January 2021

Publisher's Note: MDPI stays neutral with regard to jurisdictional claims in published maps and institutional affiliations.

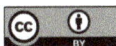

Copyright: © 2021 by the author. Licensee MDPI, Basel, Switzerland. This article is an open access article distributed under the terms and conditions of the Creative Commons Attribution (CC BY) license (https://creativecommons.org/licenses/by/4.0/).

1. Introduction

Various medical imaging modalities are used in different settings to form images of the anatomy and physiological processes of some part of the body. After acquisition, segmentation is an image processing functionality useful for advanced computer-aided analysis, measurements and visualizations related to medical procedures. Deep learning has been applied increasingly in that context to automatically learn how to classify and segment the images. Magnetic resonance imaging (MRI) and computer tomography (CT) are most popular for analysis and diagnosis of multiple affections. Examples of deep learning segmentation on those datasets include acute ischemic lesions [1], brain tumors [2], the striatum [3], organs-at-risks in head and neck [4], polycystic kidneys [5], prostate [6] and spine [7]. References [8,9] review applications in more detail. Analysis of eye-fundus images (EFI) to detect lesions is a very different medical imaging context where precise segmentation can help quantify lesions indicative of diabetic retinopathy [10]. In these, and other medical imaging scenarios, segmentation is a very common operation.

Current state-of-the-art segmentation uses deep convolutional neural networks (DCNN). These systems were first developed to classify images, with some popular architectures being VGG [11] and Resnet [12]. The classification DCNN is made of a sequence of encoder convolution stages (convolutions, activations and pooling) that extract and compress features from the image directly into a feature vector. Next, a fully-connected neural network classifies the image based on the feature vector. The segmentation network is a modified DCNN architecture that classifies each pixel (with a segment label) instead of the image. To achieve this the fully connected layers are replaced by a decoder that successively de-convolves until the full image size is restored. The fully convolutional network (FCN) [13] was one of the first well-structured segmentation network architectures. It uses a DCNN as encoder (e.g., VGG) and replaces the final fully-connected layers by up-sampling interpolation layers. U-Net introduced further innovations [14], with de-convolution stages symmetric to the convolution stages (forming a U-shape) instead of interpolation. DeepLab [15] is another highly accurate segmentation network architecture that introduces important innovations. One such innovation is Atrous spatial pyramid pooling (ASPP), which improves segmentation at multiple scales. Another innovation is the use of conditional random fields (CRF) that applies probabilistic graphical models for improved determination of objects boundaries.

Learning to segment automatically based on training images and groundtruth segments is a crucial step in segmentation DCNNs. In that process, loss is a fundamental measure of the distance between the current quality of segmentation of training images and the groundtruth segmentations that is used as the basis for backpropagation learning. A loss function that fails to reveal deficiencies in segmentation of specific structures will not learn to segment those structures well. Nevertheless, it is difficult to accurately reflect the loss of different target structures, with different characteristics and occurrences, in a single value (the loss). For that reason, it is common in current state-of-the-art to see a final training validation loss of 1% or less at the same time that incorrections in segmentation of some structures are still quite visible. Figure 1 illustrates this problem with a real case segmentation of two MRI test slices (the groundtruth segments are the left images shown on black background). In this example, the final validation loss was very low (less than 1% cross entropy loss), but imperfections are quite visible, especially in the case of (b).

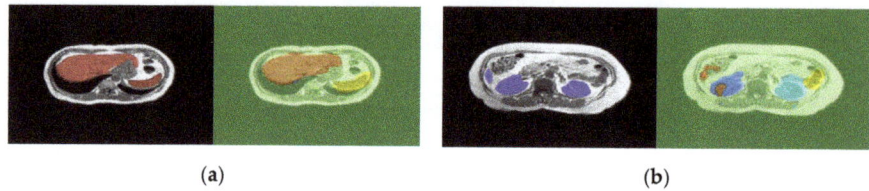

(a) (b)

Figure 1. Example magnetic resonance image (MRI) segmentation of independent test images using DeepLabv3 segmentation network. The left of each image is the groundtruth on a black background, the right is the segmentation: (**a**) is a slice showing the liver and spleen; (**b**) is another slice showing the kidneys and a small extremity of the liver.

The most popular loss functions are cross entropy (crossE), dice and sometimes also IoU (a.k.a Jaccard index). However, given different segmentation contexts in medical imaging, the question arises as to which network, loss function and loss function tuning can optimize the results? In this work, we experiment segmentation in the three imaging contexts (MRI, CT and EFI) to understand which of the three most popular loss functions works better, and to evaluate how changing coefficients weights in the formulas might modify the results. We also evaluate whether it would be preferable to always solve one uniclass segmentation for each target structure or the single multiclass segmentation. In order to reach conclusions we run the following experiments: (1) choose best performing network; (2) compare the three loss functions and variations, such as different weights to false positives and negatives and removal of background class from the formula (zero weighting the background); and (3) evaluate also the alternative of simply replacing multiclass by n uniclass segmentation problems. We observed the following: (1) DeeplabV3 was always better than UNet or FCN; (2) dice is the best in average over the three datasets, followed by IoU and finally crossE; (3) variations were useful in different ways in different datasets: while dice was the best in CT of the liver, IoU with specific weight modifications was the best in the MRI dataset and dice without background was the best alternative in the EFI dataset. From those results, we conclude that: (1) dice is the best scoring alternative in average over all datasets; (2) it is useful to consider different weights variations and to tune for a specific context, because we obtained significant scores improvements; (3) the single multiclass problem was preferable to expressing and solving n uniclass problems.

We also compare segmentation scores of larger and more constant classes, such as the optic disk or organs. In addition, we compare with scores of small and very changing targets, such as small microaneurysms in eye fundus images. We observe that the optic disk (90%) and organs (77 to 86%) score much higher than the smaller, location and conformation changing lesions (18 to 61%). Modifications to loss functions improved scores of the small lesions by 5 to 15%.

Related Work

Deep learning revolutionized segmentation. Prior to the use of deep learning (DL), segmentation of organs in MRI and CT would most frequently be based on multi-atlas approaches (e.g., [16] uses 3D models of the liver and probability maps, [17] is based on histograms and active contours to segment the liver, [18] applies watershed and active contours). Since around 2014, deep learning-based segmentation gradually became the norm. In what concerns recent works on segmentation of MR and CT, Zhou [19] achieved top scores using a fully convolutional networks (FCN) by taking 3-D CT images and applying a majority voting scheme on the output of segmentation of 2D slices taken from different image orientations. Reference [20] applied a similar approach to segmentation of the abdomen from MRI sequences, scoring (dice similarity coefficient = DSC) 0.93, 0.73, 0.78, 0.91, 0.56 for spleen, left and right kidney, liver and stomach respectively. Larsson [21] proposed DeepSeg which segments abdominal organs using multi-atlas, Convolutional Neural Networks (CNN) for pixel binary classification and thresholding to keep only largest connected region (JI: 0.9; 0.87; 0.76; 0.84 for liver, spleen, right and left kidney). Reference [22] proposed multi-slice 2D neural network designed in a way that considers information of subsequent slices, plus augmented data and multiview training. Groza [23] presents an ensemble of DL networks with voting, and [24] tests different architectures (U-Net, deeper U-Net with VGG-19, a cascade of two networks). Loss is considered in [25], where the authors proposed improving deep pancreas segmentation in CT and MRI images via recurrent neural contextual learning and "direct" loss function. They propose a Jaccard Loss (JACLoss): "It empirically works better than the cross-entropy loss or the class-balanced cross-entropy loss when segmenting small objects". Reference [24] also replaced cross-entropy by the dice function to better deal with class imbalance.

Deep learning has also been applied extensively to detection of lesions in eye fundus images. Works include Prentasic et al. [26], Gondal at al. [27], Quellec et al. [28] (exudates, hemorrhages and microaneurysms), Haloi et al. [29], van Grinsven et al. [30], Orlando et al. [31] and Shan et al. [32] (microaneurysms, hemorrhages or both). Some classify small square windows to detect lesions, others extract lesion heat maps from the DCNN and yet others apply segmentation networks directly. In terms of results evaluating segmentation quality, reported sensitivities against one false positive per image (FPI) in some of those works were (HA = hemorrhages, MA = micro-aneurisms, HE = hard exudates, SE = soft exudates): Quellec [28] (HA = 47%; HE = 57%; SE = 70% and MA = 38%), Gondal [27] (HA = 50%; HE = 40%; SE = 64% and MA = 7%) and Orlando [31] (HA:50%, MA: 30%).

The loss function is based on a metric, and the problem of metrics in general is mentioned in [33]: "many scores are artificially high simply because the background is huge and hence the term TN (true negatives) is also huge". In what concerns study of the loss function, the work in [34] compares alternative loss functions for the binary problem only (one class). In a different context, [35] investigated a modified loss function that is useful in our work as well. Ref. [36] investigates the use of prior information, which is the use of information regarding acceptable shapes, conformations, textures or colors to enhance loss function.

Comparing to all the related works we just reviewed, and considering the three different contexts that we have chosen (MRI and CT of organs, and EFI lesions) we ask the question of whether any of the three most popular loss functions has best results along the three contexts, whether different weighting of formula coefficients might be worth and how they compare.

2. Materials and Methods

In this section, we first introduce the MRI, CT and EFI data used in our experimental work, then we describe our investigative methods. We analyze metrics and their limitations, describing the loss function variations and alternatives based on that analysis. Then we describe an experimental setup to evaluate the quality of segmentation with the loss alternatives.

2.1. The Datasets

The three datasets used in this experiment are illustrated briefly in Figure 2. The magnetic resonance imaging (MRI) data used in our experiments are a set of scans available in [37]. The dataset in [37] includes 120 DICOM scans (40 T1-DUAL in phase, 40 T1-DUAL out phase and 40 T2-SPIR), obtained from healthy patients (routine scans, no tumors, lesions or any other diseases). These scans capture abdominal organs (liver, the two kidneys and spleen). In this work, we report our results for 40 in-phase sequences of the T1-DUAL fat suppression protocol. The sequences were acquired by a 1.5T Philips MRI, which produces 12-bit DICOM images with a resolution of 256 × 256. The inter-slice distance ISDs varies between 5.5–9 mm (average 7.84 mm), x-y spacing is between 1.36–1.89 mm (average 1.61 mm) and the number of slices per scan is between 26 and 50 (average 36). Train, test and validation data independent from each other were always obtained by dividing the patients into those subsets. To ensure independent testing, in each run the patients sequences (dataset) were divided into training and testing sequences using a ratio 80%/20%. To obtain multiple runs, the patient sequences were divided randomly into five folds such that each fold has 20% of all patients. In each run, one of the folds was assigned to testing and the remaining folds were used for training. Data augmentation was also added after we verified that it contributes to improved scores, by increasing diversity and size of the dataset. Data augmentation was defined based on random translations of up to 10 pixels, random rotations up to 10 degrees, shearing up to 10 pixels and scaling up to 10%.

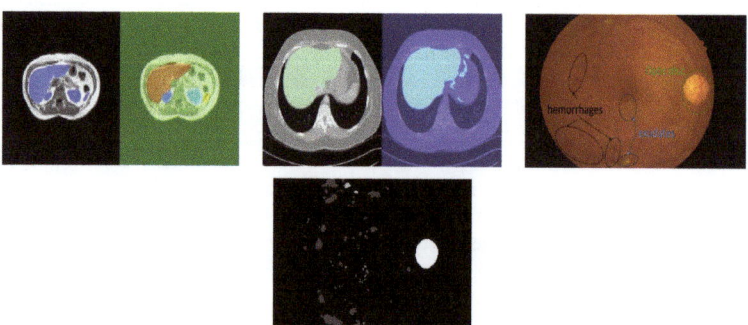

Figure 2. Illustrative examples from the three datasets used. Left: MRI segmentation of liver, spleen, left and right kidneys (groundtruth + segmented); Center: computer tomography (CT) segmentation of liver (groundtruth + segmented); Right: eye fundus image (EFI) with indication of some lesions and example groundtruth.

We also use a computer tomography (CT) dataset composed of upper abdomen sequences from 40 different patients [37]. The images were acquired using equipment—

Philips SecuraCT (Phillips, Amsterdam, Netherlands), 16 detectors, Philips Mx8000, 64 detectors, Toshiba AquilionOne, 320 detectors (equipped with spiral CT). Subjects were all healthy (livers did not exhibit lesions or disease). A contrast agent was used, the abdomen sequences obtained at hepatic phase, i.e., 70–80 s p.i. or 50–60 s after bolus tracking. In this phase, the liver parenchyma enhances through blood supply by the portal vein, resulting in some potential enhancement of the hepatic veins. The resulting 2874 slices have a resolution of 512 × 512, XY spacing 0.7 to 0.8 mm and inter slice distance 3 to 3.2 mm.

The EFI dataset we used is IDRID [10], a dataset that is publicly available for the study of automated detection of diabetic retinopathy and segmentation of characteristic lesions (microaneurysms, hemorrhages, hard exudates, soft exudates), plus the optic disc. It has groundtruth labelled data for each of 83 eye fundus images (EFI), where most images have a large number of instances of each specific lesion, and the groundtruths represent the class that should be assigned to each individual pixel. IDRID contains the pixel groundtruths for micro-aneurisms, hemorrhages, exudates (hard and soft) and the optic disk. The equipment used to acquire the images was a Kowa VX-10 alpha digital fundus camera with 50-degree field of view (FOV), centered near the macula. Image resolution was 4288 × 2848, saved as jpg. Experts validated the quality of the images and their clinical relevance.

2.2. Method

2.2.1. Discussing Metrics and Loss

Both segmentation evaluation metrics and loss function are expected to quantify the difference (error) between the groundtruth (GND), representing a correct segmentation of the image, and the segmentation output (SEG). The loss f(SEG, GND) is a single quantity between 0 and 1, and the quality of segmentation is (quality = 1 − loss). SEG and GND are labelmaps, i.e., each position (pixel) in the labelmap is a class label. In most bibliography, metrics are defined considering a binary classification problem that classifies into two classes: positive (P), with the meaning "is", and negative (N), with the meaning "is not". The quantities TP, TN, FP and FN correspond to the number of pixels that are true positives, true negatives, false positives and false negatives, respectively. Given those quantities, some of the most frequently used metrics are:

$$\text{Accuracy (ac)} = (TP + TN)//TP + TN + FP + FN); \qquad (1)$$

$$\text{Sensitivity (se)} = \text{recall} = \text{True Positive Rate (TPR)} = TP/(TP + FN) \qquad (2)$$

$$\text{Specificity (sp)} = TN/(TN + FP) \qquad (3)$$

$$\text{Precision (p)} = TP/(TP + FP) \qquad (4)$$

$$\text{False Positive Rate (FPR)} = FP/(FP + TN) \qquad (5)$$

$$\text{ROC, a plot of TPR vs. FPR, and AUC, the area under the curve of ROC} \qquad (6)$$

$$\text{IoU} = JI = TP/(TP + FN + FP) \qquad (7)$$

$$\text{Dice (dice)} = DSC = 2TP/(2TP + FP + FN) = 2JI/(JI + 1), \text{ which is highly correlated with JI} \qquad (8)$$

In multiclass problems, we can apply the same formulas, but considering the following quantities instead: a TP pixel is a pixel that belongs to one class c different from background in groundtruth and also in the segmentation; a TN pixel is a pixel that belongs to background in both groundtruth and segmentation; an FP pixel is a pixel that belongs to background in groundtruth but is classified as some other class c in segmentation; an FN pixel is a pixel that belongs to some class c different from background in groundtruth but is then classified as background.

The following three observations are important reasons why the metrics defined in Equations (1)–(8) can fail to evaluate segmentation correctly in many medical imaging contexts:

(1) The number TP is always huge in all metrics, because TP of background pixels is huge. As a consequence, all metrics (1) to (8) report high scores regardless of the actual quality of segmentation of individual classes if evaluated over all pixels;
(2) TN is also huge because it includes a huge number of background pixels that are well classified. It means that specificity (SP), FPR, ROC and AUC do not evaluate the quality of segmentation of individual classes well;
(3) Sensitivity (a.k.a recall or TPR), although useful because it quantifies the fraction of organ pixels classified correctly as such, fails to capture very important possible deficiencies, because it does not include FP (background classified as organ) in the formula, a frequent occurrence.

The problems identified in (a) and (b) are a consequence not only of class imbalance, but most importantly of the fact that background pixels are much easier to segment (score much higher) than pixels of another target class, because they are more constant across most slices and patients (since they include all pixels "framing" the image except the target class itself). The issue identified in (a) means that it is necessary to use metrics that evaluate each class separately instead of computing them over all pixels, requiring modifications to how Equations (1)–(8) were defined above. Additionally, since (b) and (c) discard many metrics that are inappropriate, the metrics that are left for use are jaccard index (JI), and Dice Sorenson Coefficient (DSC) and precision (which should be used together with recall). Given the observations in (a), these need to be evaluated separately for each class. That means each quantity TP, TN, FP and FN must be replaced by TPc, TNc, FPc and FNc respectively, where c is a class, and the metrics should be obtained and reported separately for each class c.

However, while we can report a different value of JI or DSC for each class when evaluating segmentation quality, the loss function needs to output a single value to be used as delta in backpropagation learning. Therefore, the final loss must be averaged over the loss of each class. This solution is still not perfect because the loss of class "background" is in practice always almost zero (due to (a) and (b)), contributing to push the average loss down, even if specific target classes are not very well segmented. Based on these observations, we define the loss functions and variations to consider in the next sub-section.

2.2.2. Defining Metrics and Variations for Use as Loss Function

Based on the previous analysis, we define a set of loss functions besides cross entropy, and a set of variations and alternatives that may contribute to improve the quality of the learning process. We also include the standard cross entropy as one of the options to compare to.

Cross entropy (crossE, the default to compare with): cross-entropy is well-known and the default loss function. Given the set of probabilities p of a single pixel of the segmentation output to be of each possible class, and the real probabilities (one-hot encoding of the class), cross entropy measures dissimilarity between p and q. If t_i and s_i are the groundtruth and the CNN score of each pixel for each class i respectively,

$$crossE = -\sum_i^C t_i \log s_i \qquad (9)$$

By applying a class frequency inverse weight to the value for each pixel, we obtain class-weighted cross-entropy, which is the variant we use and denote as "crossE".

Intersect over the union (IoU): IoU is a convenient measure of the degree of overlap or match between segmentation-obtained regions and the corresponding groundtruth regions. Given the number of true positives (TP), false positives (FP) and false negatives (FN) in the classification of pixels, loss is (1-IoU).

$$IoU(loss) = 1 - IoU = 1 - \frac{TP}{TP + FP + FN} \qquad (10)$$

However, since this *IoU* averages over all pixels and we identified the problem with that measurement, *IoU* averaged over the classes is used instead,

$$IoU(loss) = 1 - \frac{\sum_{I=1}^{C} IoU_i}{C}, IoU_i = 1 - \frac{TP_i}{TP_i + FP_i + FN_i} \quad (11)$$

Dice (dice): The dice or dice similarity coefficient (*DSC*) is a metric that is highly correlated and can be obtained from *IoU* directly. The loss formula for the dice is:

$$dice(loss) = 1 - DSC = 1 - \frac{2TP}{2TP + FP + FN} \quad (12)$$

As with *IoU* we use an average over classes,

$$dice(loss) = 1 - \frac{\sum_{I=1}^{C} dice_i}{C}, dice_i = 1 - \frac{2TP_i}{2TP_i + FP_i + FN_i} \quad (13)$$

Intersect over the union with penalties (*IoUxy*): *IoUxy* is similar to *IoU* but penalizes differently *FP* and *FN* in the denominator of the formula. The resulting formula weighting over classes is:

$$IoU_{xy}(loss) = 1 - \frac{\sum_{I=1}^{C} IoU_{xyi}}{C}, IoU_{xyi} = 1 - \frac{TP_i}{TP_i + \alpha FP_i + \beta FN_i} \quad (14)$$

In these formulas, α and β are such that $\alpha + \beta = 2$, $\alpha, \beta \geq 0$. The question to answer is whether giving different weights to *FN* and *FP* (the two types of unwanted errors) will allow the approach to better segment each organ, and how varying the combination of α and β affects the result. We evaluate this by means of experimentation.

Loss without considering the background (dice noBK): Since the background is easier to segment than the remaining classes and is also huge, dice noBK is an alternative that removes the background from the loss formula (i.e., it averages loss over all classes except the background). The objective is to try to emphasize the need to segment the other classes well. An experimental approach is necessary to evaluate if this alternative improves the outcome.

Uniclass segmentation: instead of a single multi-class problem with a single segmentation network, we can have one specific segmentation network specializing in segmenting each target class. The potential advantage is that we will be replacing a difficult multi-objective optimization problem [38] (minimize loss of segmentation of each organ) by n easier to optimize single objective uniclass problems (each one optimizes segmentation of one organ). Note. however that, on the other hand, in uniclass versions all target classes are marked as background except the one being segmented. An experimental approach is necessary to reach conclusions regarding which alternative scores best, either a single multiclass segmentation network or n uniclass segmentation networks, one for each class.

Summarizing the alternatives, they include the base loss formulas (crossE, IoU, dice), plus versions of dice and IoU that weight false positives and false negatives differently (exemplified here by IoU$_{xy}$), dice or IoU with no background class (exemplified here as dice noBK), and finally the uniclass variation. Additionally, we can specify different combinations of α and β in the IoU$_{xy}$ case. To limit the size of comparisons, we do not test alternatives dice$_{xy}$ and IoU noBK.

2.3. Experimental Setup

The segmentation network architecture is a relevant factor for the quality of segmentation. For this work, we pick well-known segmentation networks, the U-NET [14], FCN [13] and DeepLabV3 [15]. The U-Net uses a 58-layer segmentation network with VGG-16 (7 stages, corresponding to 41 layers) for feature extraction (encoding). The FCN tested here also uses VGG-16 as encoder, and its total network size is smaller than UNet

(51 layers). The decoder stages of U-Net are symmetric to the encoder stages, while FCN uses simple interpolation in the decoder stages. Both networks also include forward connections feeding feature maps from encoder to decoder stages. The two networks (U-Net and FCN) are the most-frequently used ones in segmentation of medical images. The third network, DeepLabV3, is a well-known segmentation network often used in object recognition applications that outperformed most competitors due to some innovations. It is the deepest network tested in this work, with 100 layers and uses Resnet-18 as feature extractor (8 stages, totaling 71 layers). DeepLabV3 incorporates two important segmentation quality enhancing improvements, the Atrous spatial pyramid pooling (ASPP) (improving segmentation of objects at multiple scales) and fully connected conditional random fields (CRF) for improved localization of object boundaries using mechanisms from probabilistic graphical models. All segmentation networks were pre-trained versions based on object recognition data.

The experiments reported in this work were preceded by a set of iterations tuning configurations to the best possible results. The final network training parameters after tuning, to be used in our experimental work, were: learning function stochastic gradient descent with momentum (SGDM), with an initial learning rate = 0.005, piecewise learning rate with drop period of 20 and learn rate drop factor of 0.9 (i.e., the learn rate would decrease to 90% every 20 epochs). Training iterations were 500 epochs; minibatch sz = 32; momentum = 0.9. The factor that most improved performance in our initial tuning prior to experiments was data augmentation, which we described before. A machine with a GPU NVIDIA G Force GTX1070 was used for the experiments.

Class balancing was applied in the pixel classification layer. Class balancing is a common operation in machine learning for datasets where classes have very different numbers of representatives (class imbalance). In medical images, class imbalance biases the result of the iterative backpropagation learning process to favor background over the target structures or organs. To illustrate the class imbalance problem, a classifier that classifies every pixel as background will guess correctly 95% of times if the background represents 95% of all pixels, yet it does not segment any structures or organs correctly. To solve this problem, class balancing multiplies the contribution of each pixel or class in the computation of the loss function by the inverse of its frequency in the whole dataset. Those class weights are added to the last layer, the pixel classification layer.

The experiments were divided into two phases. The first phase chose the best performing segmentation network among the three candidates, using the default cross entropy loss function. Using the best performing chosen network (DeepLabV3), we then tested the various loss functions. The loss functions used are cross entropy (crossE), IoU (IoU11) and IoUxy with different configurations of x and y, dice and dice without considering the background (dice noBK). In the case of IoUxy, we first test the following options: IoU11 = IoUxy with $\alpha = 1$, $\beta = 1$, IoU1505 = IoUxy with $\alpha = 1.5$, $\beta = 0.5$, IoU0515 = IoUxy with $\alpha = 0.5$, $\beta = 1.5$. Afterwards, we run a sensitivity experiment testing all combinations of α and β with steps 0.25. Finally, we compare multiclass versus n-uniclass segmentations. In what concerns metrics used to evaluate the quality of the resulting segmentations, we focused mostly our analysis on per-class IoU (JI), since it allows us to assess the quality of segmentation of each organ/lesion separately, and mean IoU over all classes.

3. Results

3.1. Choose Best-Performing Network

All experiments ran on independent test datasets after training and are the average over 5 cross-validation runs. For MRI and CT data, patient sequences were divided randomly into 5 folds such that each fold has 20% of all patients. This allowed us to run 5 experiments, each one considering one fold as containing the testing sequences and the remaining folds as training sequences (80% training/20% testing). Table 1 shows the IoU (JI) of UNet, FCN and DeeplabV3 (with cross-entropy crossE loss) for the MRI, CT and EFI datasets (Table 4 details example cross-validation runs for the MRI dataset).

Table 1. Intersect-over-the-union (IoU) of segmentation networks with base crossE loss (MRI, CT and EFI).

MRI Data	DeepLabV3	FCN	UNET	CT Data	DeepLabV3	FCN	UNET	EFI Data	DeepLabV3	FCN	UNET
Background	0.99	0.99	0.98					Background	0.97	0.89	0.75
Liver	0.86	0.86	0.74	Liver	0.86	0.77	0.75	Microaneurysms	0.13	0.02	0.01
Spleen	0.82	0.74	0.73					Hemorrhages	0.24	0.23	0.10
Rt Kidney	0.77	0.78	0.75					Hard Exudates	0.52	0.20	0.08
Lt Kidney	0.81	0.77	0.78					Soft Exudates	0.41	0.29	0.08
								Optic Disc	0.90	0.83	0.26
Avg IoU	0.85	0.83	0.80						0.53	0.31	0.21

Table 2 shows the results of different loss variations for MRI and EFI data, and Table 3 shows the corresponding results for CT data. The base loss functions tested were crossE, IoU and dice. Variants tested were no background (dice noBK) and different combinations of weights in IoU (different weights α and β applied to false negatives and false positives). Table 4 details cross-validation runs for the MRI dataset, to show that the difference of scores is statistically relevant. We report the mean IoU of each fold, average mean (IoU) over the 5 folds, the standard deviation, the 90% CI interval limits and the p-value (the p-value evaluates the null hypothesis that the differences observed between each of the loss functions and that of iou0515 might be purely by chance).

Table 2. IoU of segmentation network DeepLabV3 with diff. loss functions, two datasets (MRI, EFI).

MRI	CrossE	IoU	IoU	Iou	Dice	Dice noBK	EFI	CrossE	IoU	Dice	Dice noBK
α	-	1	1.5	0.5							
β	-	1	0.5	1.5							
BackGround	0.99	0.99	0.99	1.00	0.99	0.99	Background	0.97	0.98	0.98	0.98
liver	0.86	0.84	0.69	0.88	0.87	0.84	Microaneurysm.	0.13	0.17	0.16	0.18
spleen	0.82	0.84	0.80	0.87	0.80	0.81	Hemorrhages	0.24	0.1	0.28	0.32
Rt kidney	0.77	0.82	0.77	0.88	0.81	0.82	Hard Exudates	0.52	0.61	0.61	0.61
Lt kidney	0.81	0.74	0.73	0.85	0.76	0.79	Soft Exudates	0.41	0.49	0.51	0.56
							Optic Disc	0.90	0.91	0.91	0.90
avg	0.84	0.86	0.82	0.90	0.85	0.85	avg	0.53	0.53	0.57	0.59

Table 3. IoU of segmentation network DeepLabV3 on CT data.

	CrossE	Iou11	Iou0515	Dice	Dice noBK
BackGround	0.98	0.96	0.98	0.99	0.98
liver	0.75	0.82	0.76	0.84	0.79
avg	0.86	0.89	0.87	0.91	0.89

Table 4. IoU of segmentation network DeepLabV3 for diff folds (CVi = cross validation fold) on MRI.

Mean (IoU)	CV1	CV2	CV3	CV4	CV5	Avg	stdev	Avg – CI	Avg + CI	p-Value
CrossE	0.843	0.834	0.829	0.833	0.836	0.835	0.006	0.831	0.842	0.000007
dice	0.848	0.851	0.864	0.849	0.852	0.853	0.007	0.845	0.859	0.00015
iou11	0.836	0.875	0.855	0.876	0.857	0.860	0.019	0.838	0.876	0.007
iou0515	0.879	0.901	0.903	0.895	0.881	0.892	0.011	0.871	0.892	-

3.2. Loss Formula Weights: Sensitivity Run Using IoU_{xy} Loss Function

Since variations of weights were useful for MRI data, in this experiment we vary the alpha and beta coefficients of the denominator of IoU loss function ($\alpha FP_i + \beta FN_i$) using a step of 0.25 for the MRI dataset. Table 5 shows the evolution of the mean IoU for different values of alpha in one run.

Table 5. IoU of segmentation network DeepLabV3 for different values of alpha in MRI.

Alpha	0	0.25	0.5	0.75	1	1.25	1.5	1.75	2
MeanIoU	0.63	0.82	0.89	0.88	0.87	0.84	0.83	0.79	0.16

3.3. Would It Be Worth Running by n-Uniclass Problems Instead of One Multiclass Problem?

Table 6 compares the scores of the multiclass problem with those obtained for n uniclass problems considering the MRI dataset (n = 4, one for each organ), and for the EFI dataset (n = 5, one for each lesion). The objective is to evaluate whether running n-uniclass segmentations, one for each organ/lesion, would improve or degrade scores. To compare the two options, the next experiment reports results of two runs: (1) multiclass segmentation (all organs/lesions in a single network); (2) uniclass segmentation for each organ/lesion separately. For the MRI dataset, multiclass scores were higher for any loss function: crossE, dice and IoU improved from (0.77, 0.73, 0.79) to (0.84, 0.86, 0.85) using multiclass. Looking at the details per organ, only the liver scores the same (crossE, dice) or better (IoU11) using the uniclass alternative. In the case of EFI, uniclass scores were also similar or lower than multiclass scores in most cases, and the average IoU scores are higher for the multiclass alternative as well.

Table 6. IoU achieved with multiclass vs. uniclass on MRI and EFI.

MRI	Multiclass			Uniclass			EFI	Multiclass		Uniclass	
	CrossE	IoU	Dice	CrossE	IoU	Dice		CrossE	Dice	CrossE	Dice
BackGround	0.99	0.99	0.99	-	-	-	Background	0.97	0.98	-	-
liver	0.86	0.84	0.87	0.86	0.89	0.87	Microaneurysm.	0.13	0.16	0.16	0.12
spleen	0.82	0.84	0.80	0.58	0.62	0.52	Hemorrhages	0.24	0.28	0.31	0.25
Rt kidney	0.77	0.82	0.81	0.72	0.50	0.79	Hard Exudates	0.52	0.61	0.43	0.60
Lt kidney	0.81	0.74	0.76	0.70	0.67	0.79	Soft Exudates	0.41	0.51	0.45	0.36
							Optic Disc	0.9	0.91	0.87	0.91
avg	0.84	0.86	0.85	0.77	0.73	0.79	avg	0.53	0.57	0.45	0.45

4. Discussion

According to the results shown in Table 1, the best-performing network was DeepLabV3. Since UNet is a popular network for medical imaging, this result was surprising. As part of our future work, we are currently studying the details that contribute to this difference. The use of Resnet residue-based encoder network, ASPP and CRF should be important factors when compared with UNets' VGG-16. In the same table, we can also see that MRI organ scores are much better than EFI lesions scores. In EFI, the background and optic disk score high (90% to 97%), but lesions score much lower (13 to 52% using crossE). Most of the background is fairly constant, and the optic disk also has relatively constant location and shape. In MRI, organs score reasonably high (77% to 86%). Organs in MRI are also located in similar places and have similar conformations, although their shape varies between different slices. Eye fundus lesions, on the other hand, are much smaller and/or have varying conformations and sometimes also lack adequate contrast. In general, there are also more errors near region borders in MRI and EFI, so that small/thin regions have higher error rates relative to their area. By modifying the loss function, Table 2 shows that scores of lesions in EFI improved from (13% to 52% using crossE) to (18% to 61% using dice noBK).

From Table 2 (comparison of scores of loss alternatives for MRI and EFI data), and Table 3 (same for CT data), we conclude that the best performing loss function differed slightly depending on the dataset, but there were some common patterns. Dice was the best for the liver CT dataset (91% versus 86% of crossE); IoU0515 (i.e., IoU with modified FP and FN weights) was the best performing loss variant for the MRI dataset (90% versus 84% of crossE); Finally, dice with no background was the top performing alternative for EFI data

(59% versus 53% of crossE). Evaluating only the base loss functions (no variations) over the three datasets, dice scores best (85% MRI, 57% EFI, 91% CT), followed by IoU (86% MRI, 53% EFI and 89% CT) and finally crossE (84% MRI, 53% EFI, 86% CT). This means that dice loss improved scores by an average of one percentage point (pp), 4pp and 5pp for MRI, EFI and CT datasets, respectively, when comparing with crossE. Considering weight variations (different weights to false positives and negatives, zero weight on background = noBK) the score improvement is larger. Tuning α and β weights of false positives vs. false negatives improved scores further in MRI by 6 pp for a total of 12 pp, while assigning zero weight to class background improved scores in EFI dataset by 4 pp for a total of 6 pp. The top improvement per class considering the best variations were 11% for the right kidney in MRI, 15% for soft exudates in EFI and 9% for the liver in the CT dataset.

Tables 4 and 5 show additional details. Table 4 details cross validation runs for the MRI dataset, showing that the differences observed between for instance IoU$_{xy}$ and cross entropy are statistically significant. Table 5 shows how scores varied in MRI as α and β weights on false positives versus false negatives are modified in steps of 0.25. It shows that values of α between 0.5 and 0.75 scored highest for the MRI dataset.

The last experiment (Table 6) concerned evaluating whether replacing the multiclass problem by a set of n-uniclass problems, one for each non-background class, would improve or worsen the results, using the MRI dataset and the EFI dataset as well. Multiclass scores were better for any loss function: in the case of MRI, crossE, dice and IoU improved from (0.77, 0.73, 0.79) to (0.84, 0.86, 0.85) using multiclass. Looking at the details per organ, only the liver scores the same (crossE, dice) or better (IoU11) using the uniclass alternative. For the EFI dataset, taking the example of dice loss, we have multiclass (0.16, 0.28, 0.61, 0.51, 0.91) and uniclass (0.12, 0.25, 0.60, 0.36, 0.91). The conclusion is that the multiclass problem scored higher in general. The potential advantage of considering the uniclass problem would be that loss would only have to optimize for one class. However, organs/lesions that are not the target in each independent run can be more easily confounded with other organs/lesions that are now part of the background in that run (e.g., in the case of MRI, left and right kidney, or spleen with left kidney). The conclusion is that multiclass segmentation was better.

The final conclusions from the previous experiments are: (1) dice is the best in average over the three datasets when considering base loss functions without modifications, but IoU has scores similar. Cross entropy (crossE) was worse than both; and variations were useful in different ways in different datasets. While dice was the best in CT of the liver, IoU with specific weight modification was the best in the MRI dataset and dice without background was the best alternative in the EFI dataset. From those results, we conclude that dice should be used, but also that it is useful to consider different variations (dice$_{xy}$ and dice noBK), tuning for a specific context. Another important conclusion from our experiments is that the single multiclass problem is preferable to expressing and solving n uniclass problems.

In what concerns generalization of our conclusions, we were careful to run multiple datasets and independent experiments, therefore, the results should be generalizable to other multiclass medical imaging problems in general.

5. Comparison with Related Work on MRI

For completion, in this section we review briefly results obtained by other authors segmenting MRI and CT scans (results for lesions segmentation on EFI images were reviewed briefly in related work section). Tables 7 and 8 show the IoU reported by related MRI and CT segmentation approaches by other authors. Table 8 compares our scores with those of a few other approaches running on the same MRI dataset as ours (therefore, directly comparable), where we can see that our best performing approach was superior to those compared. Table 8 shows a broader picture of scores reported in other works, which implemented enhanced networks with architectural modifications added to improve segmentation quality of CT and MRI scans of abdominal organs. These works use different datasets from ours, and many of them segment CT instead of MRI, therefore they are not directly comparable to our results, however it is interesting to analyze their scores. In those results [39,40], achieved highest scores in segmentation of MRI images, and Hu et al. [41,42] obtained the best scores for CT. The results we obtained in this work, in spite of using only a general-purpose segmentation network and not testing other architectural modifications that were proposed in each of the works referenced in Table 8, are still "competitive". Most importantly, they can be experimented with in future work with any of those works. Note also that, in general, in Table 8 segmentation of CT scans achieved better top scores than segmentation of MRI scans.

Table 7. Comparing to IoU of related approaches (CHAOS dataset).

MRI JI = IoU	Liver	Spleen	R Kidney	L Kidney
teamPK [24]				
U-Net	0.73	0.76	0.79	0.83
V19UNet	0.76	0.79	0.84	0.85
V19pUNet	0.85	0.83	0.85	0.86
V19pUnet1-1	0.86	0.83	0.86	0.87
deeplabV3 iou 0.5/1.5	0.88	0.87	0.88	0.85

Table 8. IoU as reported in some related approaches (MRI and CT).

MRI JI = IoU	Liver	Spleen	R Kidney	L Kidney
[20]	0.84	0.87	0.64	0.57
[40]	0.90(LiverNet)	-	-	-
[39]	0.91	-	0.87	0.87
CT JI = IoU	Liver	Spleen	R Kidney	L Kidney
[43]	0.938	0.945		
[44]	0.85	-		
[19]	0.88	0.77		
[41]	0.92	0.89		
[42]	0.96	0.94	0.96	0.94
[45]	0.9	-	0.84	0.80
[23]				
F-net	0.86	0.79	0.79	0.80
BRIEF	0.74	0.60	0.60	0.60
U-Net	0.89	0.80	0.77	0.78
[21]	0.90	0.87	0.76	0.84

6. Conclusions and Future Work

The loss function is an important part of optimization in deep learning-based segmentation of medical images. It is important to analyze the effects of loss alternatives and whether they differ depending on datasets. In this paper, we investigate how the most popular loss functions (cross entropy, IoU and dice) and variations based on differently weighting factors compare in three different datasets. The objective was to find common patterns and to investigate if the variations that can be introduced in the base formulas can contribute to improve segmentation scores.

We have discussed metrics, loss functions and variations. Taking three different medical image segmentation problems we quantified the quality of loss, evaluating how the three popular loss functions compare in different settings, and how a set of variations affect the result. Experimentally, we firstly needed to choose the top-scoring network, considering UNet, FCN and DeepLabV3. We have concluded that DeeplabV3 outperformed the other two. Then we ran a set of experiments to explore how loss functions and their variations influence scores. Dice was the best in average over the three datasets, but we also concluded that variations were very useful in different ways in different datasets. In particular, we found that differently weighting of false positives and false negatives improved scores significantly for the MRI data, while removing class background from the loss formula improved scores significantly for the EFI dataset. However, these improvements were dependent on the dataset, hence we conclude that it is worth tuning the loss function taking into consideration these variations to adapt to the medical imaging context. We also analyzed how characteristics of different structures influence scores and how loss modifications can help overcome difficulties related to those characteristics. Finally, we compared single multiclass problem versus n uniclass problems in the MRI data.

There are a number of open challenges for future work that result from this work: one challenge is to determine why, based on architectural features, Deeplab3 outperforms UNet and FCN. This involves understanding the contribution of using a residue-based encoder (Resnet in DeepLabV3) versus VGG-16 (tested in UNet and FCN), as well as the contribution of other architectural features (e.g., ASPP and CRF of DeepLabV3). Another challenge is to understand what factors influence different scores of different variations in different medical imaging contexts. A direct extension of the work presented in this paper is to apply differentiated weights to other loss functions, and to extend the study to other advanced loss functions. However, the most important future challenge is how to improve quality of segmentation of the most difficult small and varying conformance targets, such as lesions in eye fundus images.

Funding: This research received no external funding.

Institutional Review Board Statement: Not Applicable.

Informed Consent Statement: Not Applicable.

Data Availability Statement: Data is contained within the article itself, code used for coding loss is in https://github.com/pedronunofurtado/codingLOSS.

Acknowledgments: We used publicly available MRI, CT and IDRID datasets for our experiments. The references for the datasets are [10,37]. We acknowledge the organizers for allowing researchers to use this data.

Conflicts of Interest: The authors declare no conflict of interest.

References

1. Chen, L.; Bentley, P.; Rueckert, D. Fully automatic acute ischemic lesionsegmentation in DWI using convolutional neural networks. *NeuroImage Clin.* **2017**, *15*, 633–643. [CrossRef]
2. Havaei, M.; Davy, A.; Warde-Farley, D.; Biard, A.; Courville, A.; Bengio, Y.; Pal, C.; Jodoin, P.M.; Larochelle, H. Brain tumor segmentation with deep neural networks. *Med. Image Anal.* **2017**, *35*, 18–31. [CrossRef]
3. Choi, H.; Jin, K.H. Fast and robust segmentation of the striatumusing deep convolutional neural networks. *J. Neurosci. Methods* **2016**, *274*, 146–153. [CrossRef] [PubMed]
4. Ibragimov, B.; Xing, L. Segmentation of organs-at-risks in head andneck CT images using convolutional neural networks. *Med. Phys.* **2017**, *44*, 547–557. [CrossRef] [PubMed]
5. Kline, T.L.; Korfiatis, P.; Edwards, M.E.; Blais, J.D.; Czerwiec, F.S.; Harris, P.C.; King, B.F.; Torres, V.E.; Erickson, B.J. Performance of an artificial multi-observer deep neural net-work for fully automated segmentation of polycystic kidneys. *J. Digit. Imaging* **2017**, *30*, 442–448. [CrossRef]
6. Guo, Y.; Gao, Y.; Shen, D. Deformable MR prostate segmentation viadeep feature learning and sparse patch matching. *IEEE Trans. MedImaging* **2016**, *35*, 1077–1089.
7. Li, X.; Dou, Q.; Chen, H.; Fu, C.W.; Qi, X.; Belavý, D.L.; Armbrecht, G.; Felsenberg, D.; Zheng, G.; Heng, P.A. 3D multi-scaleFCN with random modality voxel dropout learning for intervertebraldisc localization and segmentation from multi-modality MR images. *Med. Image Anal.* **2018**, *45*, 41–54. [CrossRef] [PubMed]
8. Litjens, G.; Kooi, T.; Bejnordi, B.E.; Setio, A.A.; Ciompi, F.; Ghafoorian, M.; Van Der Laak, J.A.; Van Ginneken, B.; Sánchez, C.I. A survey on deep learning in medical image analysis. *Med. Image Anal.* **2017**, *42*, 60–88. [CrossRef] [PubMed]
9. Ching, T.; Himmelstein, D.S.; Beaulieu-Jones, B.K.; Kalinin, A.A.; Do, B.T.; Way, G.P.; Ferrero, E.; Agapow, P.M.; Zietz, M.; Hoffman, M.M.; et al. Opportunities and obstacles for deep learning in biology andmedicine. *J. R. Soc. Interface* **2018**, *15*, 20170387. [CrossRef] [PubMed]
10. Porwal, P.; Pachade, S.; Kamble, R.; Kokare, M.; Deshmukh, G.; Sahasrabuddhe, V.; Meriaudeau, F. Indian Diabetic Retinopathy Image Dataset (IDRiD): A Database for Diabetic Retinopathy Screening Research. *Data* **2018**, *3*, 25. [CrossRef]
11. Simonyan, K.; Zisserman, A. Very deep convolutional networks for large-scale image recognition. *arXiv* **2014**, arXiv:1409.1556.

12. He, K.; Zhang, X.; Ren, S.; Sun, J. Deep residual learning for image recognition. In Proceedings of the IEEE Conference on Computer Vision and Pattern Recognition, Las Vegas, NV, USA, 27–30 June 2016; pp. 770–778.
13. Long, J.; Shelhamer, E.; Darrell, T. Fully convolutional networks for semantic segmentation. In Proceedings of the IEEE Conference on Computer Vision and Pattern Recognition, Boston, MA, USA, 7–12 June 2015; pp. 3431–3440.
14. Ronneberger, O.; Fischer, P.; Brox, T. U-net: Convolutional networks for biomedical image segmentation. In Proceedings of the International Conference on Medical Image Computing and Computer-Assisted Intervention, Munich, Germany, 5–9 October 2015; pp. 234–241.
15. Chen, L.C.; Papandreou, G.; Kokkinos, I.; Murphy, K.; Yuille, A.L. Deeplab: Semantic image segmentation with deep convolutional nets, atrous convolution, and fully connected crfs. *IEEE Trans. Pattern Anal. Mach. Intell.* **2017**, *40*, 834–848. [CrossRef]
16. Bereciartua, A.; Picon, A.; Galdran, A.; Iriondo, P. Automatic 3D model-based method for liver segmentation in MRI based on active contours and total variation minimization. *Biomed. Sign. Process. Control.* **2015**, *20*, 71–77. [CrossRef]
17. Le, N.; Bao, P.; Huynh, H. Fully automatic scheme for measuring liver volume in 3D MR images. *Bio-Med. Mater. Eng.* **2015**, *26*, 1361–1369. [CrossRef] [PubMed]
18. Huynh, H.; Le, N.; Bao, P.; Oto, A.; Suzuki, K. Fully automated MR liver volumetry using watershed segmentation coupled with active contouring. *Int. J. Comput. Assist. Radiol. Surg.* **2018**, *12*, 235–243. [CrossRef]
19. Zhou, X.; Takayama, R.; Wang, S.; Zhou, X.; Hara, T.; Fujita, H. Automated segmentation of 3D anatomical structures on CT images by using a deep convolutional network based on end-to-end learning approach. In Proceedings of the Medical Imaging 2017: Image Processing, Orlando, FL, USA, 11–16 February 2017; Volume 10133, p. 1013324.
20. Bobo, M.; Bao, S.; Huo, Y.; Yao, Y.; Virostko, J.; Plassard, A.; Landman, B. Fully convolutional neural networks improve abdominal organ segmentation. In Proceedings of the Medical Imaging 2018: Image Processing, Houston, TX, USA, 10–15 February 2018; Volume 10574, p. 105742V.
21. Larsson, M.; Zhang, Y.; Kahl, F. Deepseg: Abdominal organ segmentation using deep convolutional neural networks. In Proceedings of the Swedish Symposium on Image Analysis 2016, Göteborg, Sweden, 14–16 March 2016.
22. Chen, Y.; Ruan, D.; Xiao, J.; Wang, L.; Sun, B.; Saouaf, R.; Yang, W.; Li, D.; Fan, Z. Fully Automated Multi-Organ Segmentation in Abdominal Magnetic Resonance Imaging with Deep Neural Networks. *arXiv* **2019**, arXiv:1912.11000.
23. Groza, V.; Brosch, T.; Eschweiler, D.; Schulz, H.; Renisch, S.; Nickisch, H. Comparison of deep learning-based techniques for organ segmentation in abdominal CT images. In Proceedings of the 1st Conference on Medical Imaging with Deep Learning (MIDL 2018), Amsterdam, The Netherlands, 4–6 July 2018; pp. 1–3, 15, 16.
24. Conze, P.; Kavur, A.; Gall, E.; Gezer, N.; Meur, Y.; Selver, M.; Rousseau, F. Abdominal multi-organ segmentation with cascaded convolutional and adversarial deep networks. *arXiv* **2020**, arXiv:2001.09521.
25. Cai, J.; Lu, L.; Zhang, Z.; Xing, F.; Yang, L.; Yin, Q. Pancreas segmentation in MRI using graph-based decision fusion on convolutional neural networks. In Proceedings of the MICCAI 2016, LNCS, Athens, Greece, 17–21 October 2016; Ourselin, S., Joskowicz, L., Sabuncu, M.R., Unal, G., Wells, W., Eds.; Springer Nature: Cham, Switzerland, 2016; Volume 9901, pp. 442–450.
26. Prentašić, P.; Lončarić, S. Detection of exudates in fundus photographs using convolutional neural networks. In Proceedings of the 2015 9th International Symposium on Image and Signal Processing and Analysis (ISPA), Edinburgh, UK, 6–8 September 2015; pp. 188–192.
27. Gondal, W.M.; Köhler, J.M.; Grzesick, R.; Fink, G.A.; Hirsch, M. Weakly-supervised localization of diabetic retinopathy lesions in retinal fundus images. In Proceedings of the 2017 IEEE International Conference on Image Processing (ICIP), Beijing, China, 17–20 September 2017; pp. 2069–2073.
28. Quellec, G.; Charrière, K.; Boudi, Y.; Cochener, B.; Lamard, M. Deep image mining for diabetic retinopathy screening. *Med. Image Anal.* **2017**, *39*, 178–193. [CrossRef]
29. Haloi, M. Improved microaneurysm detection using deep neural networks. *arXiv* **2015**, arXiv:1505.04424.
30. Van Grinsven, M.J.; van Ginneken, B.; Hoyng, C.B.; Theelen, T.; Sánchez, C.I. Fast convolutional neural network training using selective data sampling: Application to hemorrhage detection in color fundus images. *IEEE Trans. Med. Imaging* **2016**, *35*, 1273–1284. [CrossRef]
31. Orlando, J.I.; Prokofyeva, E.; del Fresno, M.; Blaschko, M.B. An ensemble deep learning based approach for red lesion detection in fundus images. *Comput. Methods Progr. Biomed.* **2018**, *153*, 115–127. [CrossRef] [PubMed]
32. Shan, J.; Li, L. A deep learning method for microaneurysm detection in fundus images. In Proceedings of the 2016 IEEE First International Conference on Connected Health: Applications, Systems and Engineering Technologies (CHASE), Washington, DC, USA, 27–29 June 2016; pp. 357–358.
33. Zhang, X.; Thibault, G.; Decencière, E.; Marcotegui, B.; Laÿ, B.; Danno, R.; Cazuguel, G.; Quellec, G.; Lamard, M.; Massin, P.; et al. Exudate detection in color retinal images for mass screening of diabetic retinopathy. *Med. Image Anal.* **2014**, *18*, 1026–1043. [CrossRef] [PubMed]
34. Jadon, S. A survey of loss functions for semantic segmentation. *arXiv* **2020**, arXiv:2006.14822.
35. Salehi, S.S.; Erdogmus, D.; Gholipour, A. Tversky loss function for image segmentation using 3D fully convolutional deep networks. In *International Workshop on Machine Learning in Medical Imaging*; Springer: Cham, Switzerland, 2017.
36. Jurdia, R.E.; Petitjean, C.; Honeine, P.; Cheplygina, V.; Abdallah, F. High-level Prior-based Loss Functions for Medical Image Segmentation: A Survey. *arXiv* **2020**, arXiv:2011.08018.

37. Kavur, A.; Sinem, N.; Barış, M.; Conze, P.; Groza, V.; Pham, D.; Chatterjee, S.; Ernst, P.; Ozkan, S.; Baydar, B.; et al. CHAOS Challenge—Combined (CT-MR) Healthy Abdominal Organ Segmentation. *arXiv* **2020**, arXiv:2001.06535. [CrossRef]
38. Deb, K. Multi-objective optimization. In *Search Methodologies*; Springer: Boston, MA, USA, 2014; pp. 403–449.
39. Fu, Y.; Mazur, T.; Wu, X.; Liu, S.; Chang, X.; Lu, Y.; Harold, H.; Kim, H.; Roach, M.; Henke, L.; et al. A novel MRI segmentation method using CNN-based correction network for MRI-guided adaptive radiotherapy. *Med. Phys.* **2018**, *45*, 5129–5137. [CrossRef]
40. Chlebus, G.; Meine, H.; Thoduka, S.; Abolmaali, N.; van Ginneken, B.; Hahn, H.; Schenk, A. Reducing inter-observer variability and interaction time of MR liver volumetry by combining automatic CNN-based liver segmentation and manual corrections. *PLoS ONE* **2019**, *14*, e0217228. [CrossRef]
41. Hu, P.; Wu, F.; Peng, J.; Bao, Y.; Chen, F.; Kong, D. Automatic abdominal multi-organ segmentation using deep convolutional neural network and time-implicit level sets. *Int. J. Comput. Assist. Radiol. Surg.* **2017**, *12*, 399–411. [CrossRef]
42. Wang, Y.; Zhou, Y.; Shen, W.; Park, S.; Fishman, E.; Yuille, A. Abdominal multi-organ segmentation with organ-attention networks and statistical fusion. *Med. Image Anal.* **2019**, *55*, 88–102. [CrossRef]
43. Roth, R.; Shen, C.; Oda, H.; Sugino, T.; Oda, M.; Hayashi, H.; Misawa, K.; Mori, K. A multi-scale pyramid of 3D fully convolutional networks for abdominal multi-organ segmentation. In Proceedings of the International Conference on Medical Image Computing and Computer-Assisted Intervention, Granada, Spain, 16–20 September 2018; pp. 417–425.
44. Gibson, E.; Giganti, F.; Hu, Y.; Bonmati, E.; Bandula, S.; Gurusamy, K.; Davidson, B.; Pereira, S.; Clarkson, M.; Barratt, D. Towards image-guided pancreas and biliary endoscopy: Automatic multi-organ segmentation on abdominal ct with dense dilated networks. In Proceedings of the MICCAI, Quebec City, QC, Canada, 11–13 September 2017; Springer Nature: Cham, Switzerland, 2017; pp. 728–736.
45. Kim, J.; Lee, J. Deep-learning-based fast and fully automated segmentation on abdominal multiple organs from CT. In Proceedings of the International Forum on Medical Imaging in Asia 2019, Singapore, 7–9 January 2019; Volume 11050, p. 110500K.

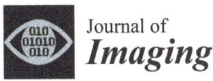

Article

Hand Motion-Aware Surgical Tool Localization and Classification from an Egocentric Camera

Tomohiro Shimizu [1,*], Ryo Hachiuma [1], Hiroki Kajita [2], Yoshifumi Takatsume [2] and Hideo Saito [1]

1. Faculty of Science and Technology, Keio University, Yokohama, Kanagawa 223-8852, Japan; ryo-hachiuma@keio.jp (R.H.); hs@keio.jp (H.S.)
2. Keio University School of Medicine, Shinjuku-ku 160-8582, Tokyo, Japan; jmrbx767@keio.jp (H.K.); tsume@keio.jp (Y.T.)
* Correspondence: tomy1201@keio.jp

Abstract: Detecting surgical tools is an essential task for the analysis and evaluation of surgical videos. However, in open surgery such as plastic surgery, it is difficult to detect them because there are surgical tools with similar shapes, such as scissors and needle holders. Unlike endoscopic surgery, the tips of the tools are often hidden in the operating field and are not captured clearly due to low camera resolution, whereas the movements of the tools and hands can be captured. As a result that the different uses of each tool require different hand movements, it is possible to use hand movement data to classify the two types of tools. We combined three modules for localization, selection, and classification, for the detection of the two tools. In the localization module, we employed the Faster R-CNN to detect surgical tools and target hands, and in the classification module, we extracted hand movement information by combining ResNet-18 and LSTM to classify two tools. We created a dataset in which seven different types of open surgery were recorded, and we provided the annotation of surgical tool detection. Our experiments show that our approach successfully detected the two different tools and outperformed the two baseline methods.

Keywords: object detection; surgical tools; open surgery; egocentric camera

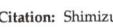

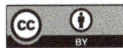

1. Introduction

Recording plastic surgeries in operating rooms with cameras has been indispensable for a variety of purposes, such as education, sharing surgery technologies and techniques, performing case studies of diseases, and evaluating medical treatments [1,2]. Due to the development of mobile hardware, egocentric cameras such as GoPro [3] or Tobii [4] have been introduced to many fields [5] to analyze activities from a first-person perspective while not disturbing the action of the recorder [6].

From the recorded video of the surgery, many tasks have been proposed to analyze surgery, such as workflow analysis [7], phase recognition [8], video segmentation [9], skill assessment [10], and video summarization [11]. The presence and positions of surgical tools are essential information for analyzing surgical procedures [7,8,10,12,13].

Predicting the objects' rough positions, sizes, and classifications is known as the object detection task. In the computer vision field, the task of object detection is well studied [14,15]. However, these approaches have only been tested with common object detection datasets, such as MS-COCO [16] or Pascal VOC [17], which include the images captured in the daily-life for detecting variety of objects. As a result that there is a huge domain gap between images from everyday life and those associated with plastic surgery, the detection models which are trained on these datasets [16,17] have difficulty detecting the detailed surgical tools with the category information. In the medical vision field, object detection in endoscopic surgery is well studied. Endoscopic surgery is the surgery where the surgeon sees the images through the endoscope camera. An example image of the endoscopic surgery is shown in Figure 1 (left). It can be seen that the surgical tools are clearly seen in the image.

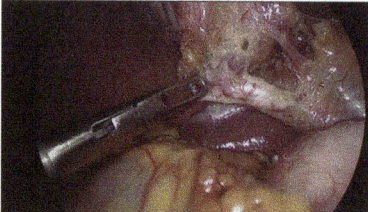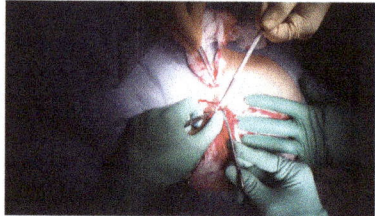

Figure 1. The comparison figure between the images of endoscopic surgery [18] **(left)** and open surgery **(right)**.

However, in the case of open surgery video captured with the egocentric camera, there are several difficulties in detecting the surgical tools. The example image of open surgery recorded with the egocentric camera is shown in Figure 1 (right). First, the surgical tools are severely occluded by the surgeon's hand or the other surgical tools. Second, even though there is no occlusion of the tools, it is difficult to classify the tools because their shapes and textures are similar. For example, the overall shapes of the scissors and needle holders (Figure 2) are very similar. Only the tip of them and the grasping part are different, but these parts are mostly occluded by hands or the surgical field.

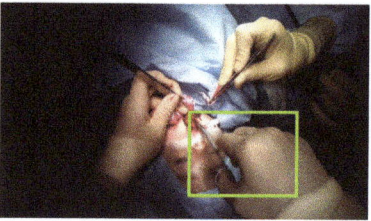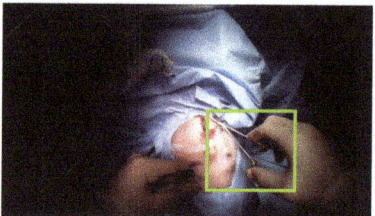

Figure 2. The comparison figure between the scissors **(left)** and the needle holders **(right)**.

This paper tackles the detection and classification task of surgical tools from egocentric images for open surgery analysis. A naive approach for detecting the objects is applying a recently proposed deep learning based model, such as Faster R-CNN [15], SSD [19] or YOLO [14]. These methods simultaneously detect and classify the objects from RGB images using their shape and texture information. However, as the textures of the tools are metallic and shiny and shapes are similar among the surgical tools, it might be easy to detect but difficult to classify.

Even though the shapes of the surgical tools are similar, the tools are used for completely different purposes. For example of the scissors and the needle holders, the function of the scissors is to cut the object, but the function of the needle holders is to suture by holding suture materials. However, it is difficult to predict the function of the tools from the images so we assume that the hand motions of the surgeons are different when using different surgical tools. We focus on the motion of the surgeon's hand to classify surgical tools instead of the textures and shapes of the tools. Figure 3 shows an example of the hand motions associated with the scissors (a) and the needle holders (b). It can be seen that the motion is completely different among tools according to their usage.

We present a framework for detecting and classifying similarly shaped surgical tools, such as scissors and needle holders, from an egocentric video. In the first stage, we detect surgical tools and hands in the image using Faster R-CNN [15]. In this stage, the surgical tools are detected, but are classified as tools but not classified by tool type. In the second stage, as multiple hands such as those belonging to assistants or that do not play a role in the procedure are seen in the image, we select the surgeon's hand using the maximum overlap ratio between the tools and hands. At the last stage, the sequentially selected hand regions are classified into different tool categories using convolutional neural network (CNN) and long short-term memory (LSTM) module [20].

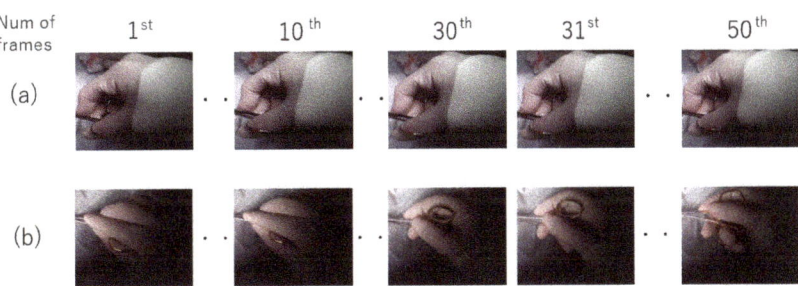

Figure 3. The comparison of the hands' motion between the surgical tools: (**a**) scissors, (**b**) needle holder.

As there is no dataset available to the public containing open surgery videos via egocentric camera, we recorded our own dataset. The actual plastic surgeries were recorded at our university's school of medicine. We recorded seven different types of surgery with Tobii cameras [4] attached to the surgeon's head. We validate our proposed model with this dataset, and we quantitatively evaluate our approach against two baseline methods to verify the effectiveness of our approach. The experiments show that our approach can detect the two surgical instruments separately.

In summary, our contributions are as follows: (1) To the best of our knowledge, this is the first approach to improve the accuracy of surgical tool detection (localization and classification) with similar shape in open surgical videos. (2) We employed hand motion information for classifying surgical tools, instead of tool shape. (3) We created a dataset of a variety of open surgeries recorded with egocentric cameras, we manually annotate detection labels of surgical tools, scissors and needle holders. We conducted extensive experimentation from qualitative and quantitative perspectives to verify the effectiveness of the proposed method.

2. Related Work

2.1. Object Detection Using Hand Appearance

Many studies have been conducted to improve the accuracy of object detection using information other than that of the target object. For example, Cue et al. [21] developed object detection by estimating the location of target objects from hand segmentation results. They detected hands, and cropped the area where the target object was estimated to be located by using detected hands area. From the resulting cropped image, they classified the target object by using CNN. That is, their method consisted of two modules: the part that estimates the location of the target object and the part that classifies the target object. Ren et al. [22] used optical flow to separate the background from the hand-held objects to improve the accuracy of detection. Since the target videos were first person videos, the calculation of optical flow was greatly influenced by the motion of the body and head. Therefore, they normalized the optical flow by using background motion in the video.

Cue and Ren used hand information to estimate the location of the object, but not to classify or label it. Our study differs from those studies because we used hand motion information to classify tools rather than estimate the position of the target object. In addition, although motion information can be obtained by using optical flow, for firstperson video it is necessary to normalize the optical flow as in Ren et al. [22]. However, in our study, hand motion is used in the classification part of object detection, so it is not appropriate to normalize or otherwise alter the raw data. Therefore, the motion information is not obtained by using optical flow; instead, CNN and LSTM [20] are used to extract features from images.

2.2. Surgery Video Analysis and Surgical Tool Detection

Studies of surgical tool detection have been mainly focused on procedures in which the surgeon sees the surgical field not directly but through a camera, such as cataract and endoscopic surgery. There are some datasets for the surgical tool detection, such as Cholec80 [23], ITEC [24], M2CAI2016 [18], CATARACT2017 [25] dataset. These datasets cannot be applied to our task as the domain of the surgery in these datasets is different from the domain of the open surgery.

Using these datasets, many methods have been proposed for detecting the surgical tools of the cataract and endoscopic surgery [26–29] and generating the realistic surgery images [30]. For example, Colleoni et al. [26] proposed a method for detecting the surgical tools and estimating the articulation of the tools for the laparoscopic surgery analysis. Du et al. [27] presented a fully-convolutional network-based articulated 2D pose estimation of the surgical tools for microsurgery video analysis.

In addition, although there are studies about surgical tool detection using the edge and texture information of surgical tools [31,32], many studies have used features obtained by fine-tuning existing CNN algorithms that have been trained with the Imagenet dataset [33]. For example, Twinada et al. [23] fine-tuned Alexnet [34], Roychowdhury et al. [35] fine-tuned Inception-v4 [36], ResNet-50 [37], and NASNet [38], and Raju et al. [39] fine-tuned GoogleNet [40], VGG-16 [41], and Inception-v3. In addition, in the study by Cadene et al. [42], the detection accuracy was improved by inputting the 15-frame presence probability of each tool, obtained by fine-tuning ResNet-200 and Inception-v3, into a hidden Markov process. Thus, there are many studies that take into account temporal information in surgical tool detection. The reason for this is that information about which tools have been used in previous frames helps in identifying which surgical tools are in the current frame. Mishra et al. [43] used LSTM [20] for making it possible to classify tools with multiple labels. In addition, Ai et al. [25] studied surgical tool detection while simultaneously training the CNN and recurrent neural network (RNN) for cataract surgery. In this case, the problem was that as they were simultaneously trained, the loss of the RNN across each frame was not propagated back to the CNN. Therefore, by using the boosting algorithm, they made it possible to train the CNN while and after training the RNN.

In summary, these studies focused on surgeries in which surgeons observed the surgical field through a camera, such as cataract surgery or endoscopic surgery. The relevant work is the work presented by Zhang et al. [44]. They applied RetinaNet [45], which is trained with annotated Youtube open surgery videos, and Simple Online and Realtime Tracking (SORT) algorithm to detect and track the hand during the open surgery. They did not aim to localize and classify the surgical tools.

As this is the first study which aims to detect the surgical tools for open surgery video analysis, we localize and classify the tools which have the similar shapes, scissors, and forceps as seen in Figure 2. As the shapes and textures are similar between two surgical tools, it is difficult to classify these tools using the conventional object detection methods such as Faster R-CNN [15]. In our study, hand appearance features are extracted with ResNet-18 for each frame. Hand motion information is then extracted with LSTM for surgical tool detection labeling.

3. Proposed Framework for Surgical Tools Localization and Classification

Our task was to detect the surgical tools that have similar shapes and textures, such as needle holders and scissors. The overview of our surgical tool detection and classification framework is visualized in Figure 4, and the abstract of it is visualized in Figure 5. Our proposed framework consists of three phases: surgical tool and hand localization, selection of the target hand, and surgical tool classification from the motion of the target hand. First, we employ Faster R-CNN to jointly detect the hands and the surgical tools. Note that surgical tools are detected as tools and the specific tool category is not labeled at this stage. Second, as multiple hands can be seen in the image that are irrelevant to the surgical tool classification, we use the overlap ratio between the bounding boxes of the hand operating the tool and the tool itself, respectively, to select the appropriate single hand. Finally, the surgical tool is classified from the sequentially selected target hand frames. We employ ResNet-18 [37] to extract the visual context features for each frame. These features are inputted to LSTM to aggregate the sequential features from which the surgical tool label is predicted. The following explains the details of the proposed framework.

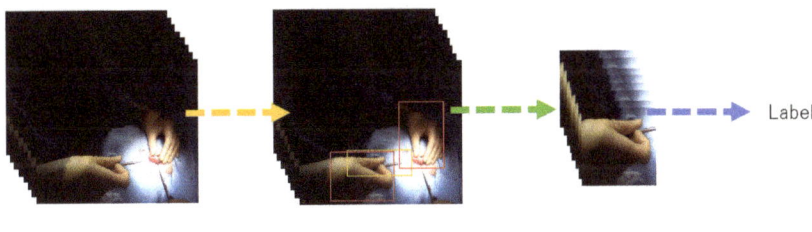

(1) Localization   (2) Hand selection   (3) Classification

Figure 4. The overview of the proposed surgical tool detection and classification.

3.1. Surgical Tool and Hand Localization

First, we apply Faster R-CNN [15] to detect the surgical tools and hands in the image. Faster R-CNN is one of the major two-staged object detectors. It predicts the object proposal regions using a region proposal network from the image feature encoded with CNN. Then, the refined bounding box and its category are predicted for each object proposal region. Note that all of the surgical tools are detected as tools and each tool category is not predicted in this stage.

3.2. Target Hand Selection

Second, we select the single hand which operates the surgical tool in the image. During open surgery, multiple hands from multiple surgeons can be seen in the egocentric image. To classify the category of the surgical tool, the hand which operates the target tool should be selected among multiple detected hand bounding boxes. From the i-th hand multiple bounding box b_i^{hand}, we calculate the overlap ratio r_{ik} with the k-th target surgical tool bounding box b_k^{tool} as follows:

$$r_{ik}(b_i^{hand}, b_k^{tool}) = \frac{b_i^{hand} \cap b_k^{tool}}{b_i^{hand} \cup b_k^{tool}}. \quad (1)$$

To select the single hand bounding box i^* which operates surgical tool k, the hand bounding box with the maximum ratio is selected:

$$i^* = \arg\max_{i \in \mathcal{V}} \{r_{ik}(b_i^{hand}, b_k^{tool})\}, \quad (2)$$

where $\mathcal{V}$ denotes the set of bounding boxes labeled as the hand. We use the bounding box i^* to classify the surgical tool k.

3.3. Surgical Tool Classification from Hand Motion

To obtain the motion of the hand, we crop hand image $I_t(0 \leq t \leq T)$ which is selected at the previous step. T denotes the number of frames for inputting into the LSTM for surgical tool classification. That is, only when the target hand is detected for T consecutive frames, it is used as input data for classification.

3.3.1. Network Architecture

First, from the hand-cropped images I_t, a visual feature is extracted from each cropped image. In this paper, ResNet-18 [37] is employed as a visual feature extractor, and the cropped image I_t is resized to 252 × 252 (pixels) to make the image size of ResNet-18 input consistent. We extract the visual feature $\psi_t \in \mathbb{R}^{128}$ from each image I_t.

After extraction, the visual features of the hands are used as input for LSTM to obtain hand motion information. Then, we aggregate the context features over time, $\hat{\psi}_1 \ldots \hat{\psi}_t \ldots \hat{\psi}_T = \mathbb{B}(\psi_1, \ldots \psi_t \ldots \psi_T)$, where $\mathbb{B}$ is a sequential feature aggregation module that computes the sequential feature $\hat{\psi}_t$. In our experiments, we employ an LSTM recurrent neural network with one hidden layer for $\mathbb{B}$.

The output feature $\hat{\psi}_1, \ldots, \hat{\psi}_T$ is then fed to a multilayer perceptron (MLP) with one hidden layer and rectified linear units (ReLU) activation function [46] to predict the label probability $p_1, \ldots, p_T$. The sigmoid activation function is applied to the output layer.

3.3.2. Loss Function

We formulate the task of surgical tool detection as the surgical tool and hand detection, and surgical tool classification using the cropped hand images. At this stage, we employ weighted cross-entropy loss for classifying the sequential hand images into the surgical tools for considering the imbalance of images for surgical tool category in the training dataset.

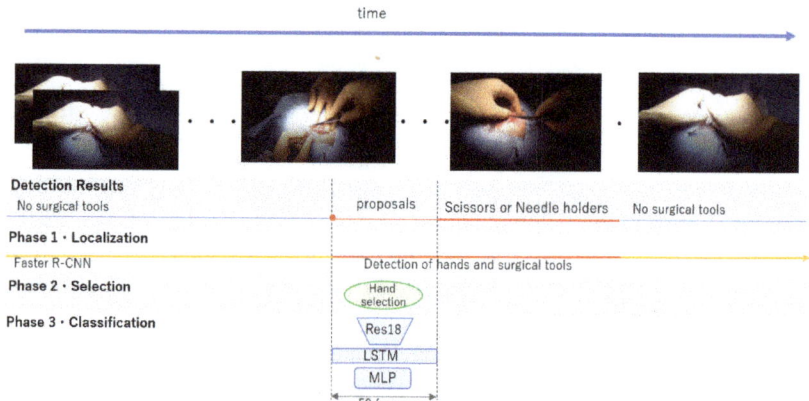

Figure 5. The abstract of the proposed method.

4. Experiment

4.1. Dataset

As there is no dataset available that contains open surgery recordings, we use Tobii cameras to create our dataset. The surgeries are recorded at Keio University School of Medicine. Video recording of the patients is approved by the Keio University School of Medicine Ethics Committee, and written informed consent is obtained from all patients or their parents. We record seven different types of surgery with Tobii cameras attached to the surgeon's head. Among the surgical videos, three glove colors, including green, skin-colored, and white, were used, and three surgeons performed the surgery. Five videos were for training and two were for testing. Patient diagnoses included Stahl's ear, open fracture, lipoma, skin tumor, nevus cell nevus, cryptotia, and cleft palate. Images from each surgery video are shown in Figure 6. Each surgery video is about 20 min long, and was recorded at 25 frames per second (FPS). The frame size of each video is 1920 × 1080 (pixels).

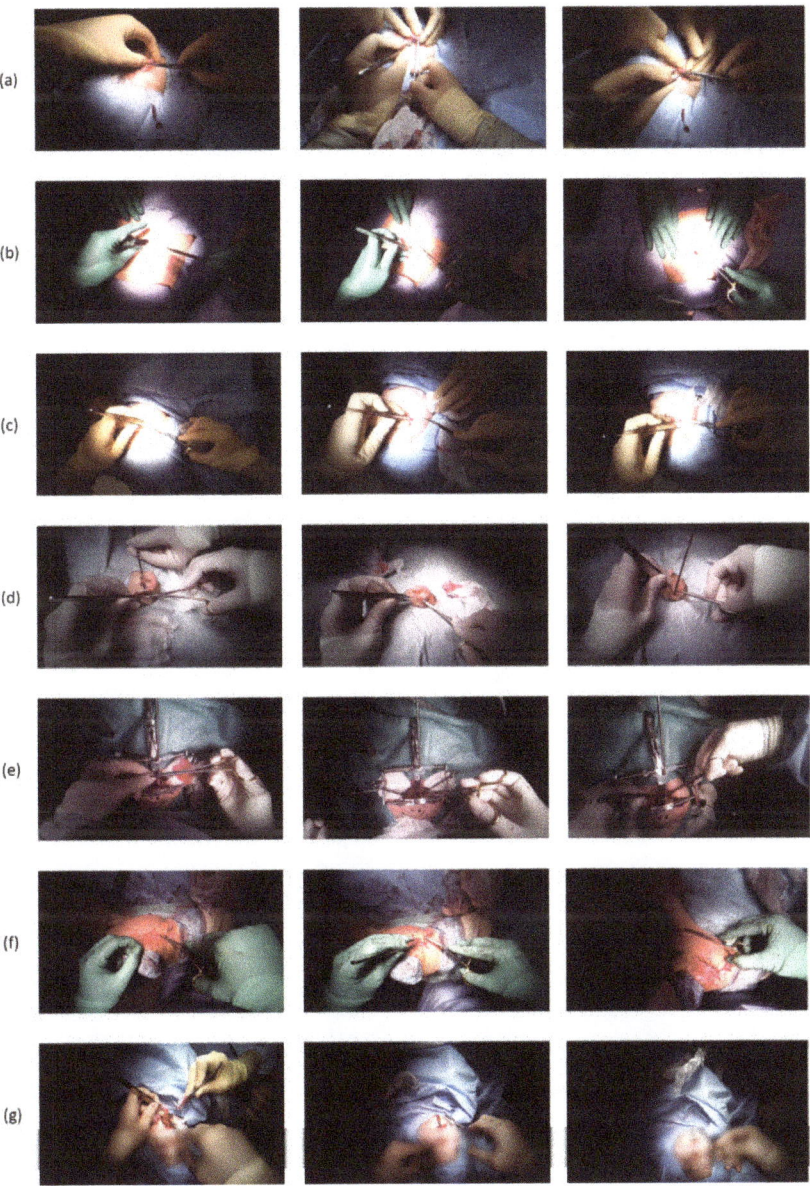

Figure 6. Images of videos we used for the experiment: (**a**) Stahl's ear, (**b**) lipoma, (**c**) skin tumor, (**d**) cryptotia, (**e**) cleft palate, (**f**) open fracture, and (**g**) nevus cell nevus.

4.2. Faster R-CNN Training

In Phase 1, it is necessary to train the system to detect surgical tools and hands using Faster R-CNN. Therefore, we randomly sampled 2000 images from five surgical videos for training and annotated them with two labels: hand and tool, which did not distinguish between needle holders and scissors, to create a dataset. Using this dataset, we performed tool and hand localization by training in Faster R-CNN. We employ VGG-16 [41] as the backbone of Faster R-CNN, and VGG-16 was pre-trained by using the Imagenet dataset.

4.3. Network Training

For Phase 2, we employ an Adam optimizer [47] with a learning rate of 1.0×10^{-3}. When training the model, we randomly sample a data fragment of $T = 50$ frames. The model converged after 15 epochs, which takes about 48 hours on a GeForce RTX 2080. We apply dropout with probability 0.5 during training. We used Keras library (https://github.com/fchollet/keras) to implement the models. The weights of ResNet-18 are initialized with the pretrained ImageNet dataset [33]. The number of frames for inputting into the LSTM was set to 50 because the movie is at 25 fps and 50 frames is equivalent to 2 s. Basic procedures, such as making incisions or suturing, are recognized by humans within 2 s, so 50 frames was appropriate. The number of dimensions of the output of LSTM is 128, and an activation function we employed is the hyperbolic tangent function. We train the model with batch size 5.

4.4. Baseline

As a result that there is no other study that has attempted detection of similarly shaped tools in open surgical videos, we defined two baselines by ourselves and performed a comparison experiment.

The first is Faster R-CNN. That is, we compare a method for surgical tool detection that distinguishes two tools with only Faster R-CNN. In the experiment, the same dataset as the proposed method was annotated with scissors and needle holders as separate tools and trained from five surgical videos, and two surgical videos that were not used for training were used for comparison. The detection result is based on whether or not the intersection over union (IOU), with the threshold set to 0.5, is above the threshold. In comparison to this baseline, we validate the effectiveness of using motion information for tool classification.

Second, we distinguish two tools from the single hand-cropped image only. That is, in Phase 3, we verify whether we can distinguish between needle holders and scissors using visual features of the hands without time series information. ResNet-18 was fine-tuned and compared with those pre-trained by the ImageNet dataset. In the experiments, the same data set as the proposed method was annotated with scissors and needle holders as separate tools and trained from five surgical videos, and two surgical videos that were not used for training were used for comparison. Compared to this baseline, we verify that not hand appearance but hand motion (but not appearance) is effective for classification.

4.5. Procedure Lengths

In this experiment, we verify the effectiveness of the proposed method by changing the number of frames T. That is, we verify how many frames are appropriate as input data. The comparison is made with 25 frames, 50 frames, 100 frames.

5. Results and Discussion

5.1. Localization and Selection Results

As mentioned earlier, our method is divided into three modules, localization, selection, and classification. Therefore, the lower the accuracy of localization and selection, the lower the accuracy of the proposed method. Using 300 test images from two videos, the test results are shown in Tables 1 and 2. The correctness of the localization result is measured by whether the IOU, whose threshold is set to 0.5, is above the threshold or not, and the results of the target hand are whether the target hand is selected from detected hands. As shown in Table 1, there are a few cases in which the tools are miss-classified, but the probability of miss-classification over 50 consecutive frames is considered to be very low, which indicates that the recognition of tools (scissors or needle holders) is accurate. As shown in Table 2, the selection of target hand areas is also found to be accurate. As a result that our localization and selection methods have been demonstrated to be accurate, we expect a similar level of accuracy from our proposed classification method.

Table 1. Results of localization.

	AP
tools	0.925
hands	0.713

Table 2. Results of selection.

Method	Accuracy	Recall	Precision	F-Measure
target hand	0.943	0.996	0.946	0.971

5.2. Proposed Method

The proposed method and the baseline method were trained on five videos and tested on two videos that were not used for training. The number of sequences of scissors were 756, and that of needle holders were 2894. The results are shown in Table 3 and Figure 7. ROC curve and learning curve of the proposed method are shown in Figures 8 and 9.

Table 3. Results of the proposed method.

Method	Accuracy	Recall	Precision	F-Measure
proposed method	0.895	0.810	0.981	0.888
only Faster R-CNN	0.663	0.811	0.970	0.883
only hand	0.524	0.559	0.230	0.326

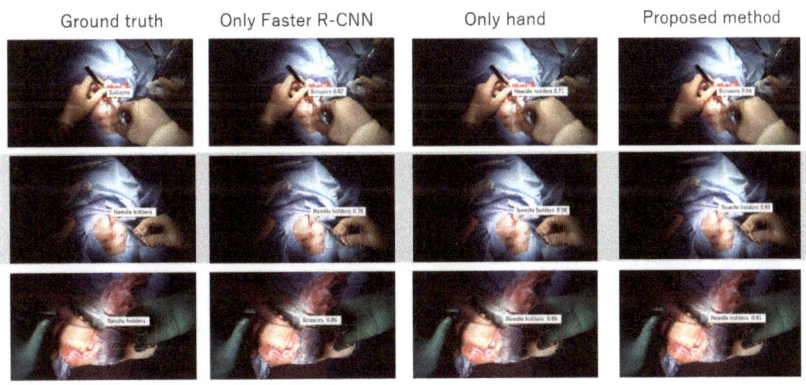

Figure 7. Examples of results.

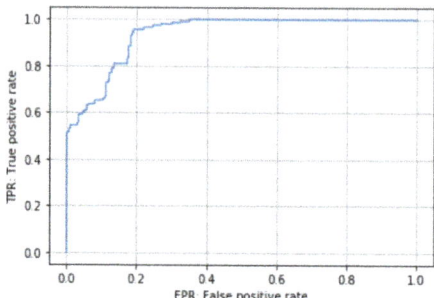

Figure 8. ROC curve.

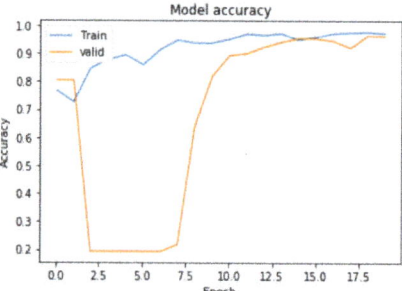

Figure 9. Learning curve.

As show in Table 3, the proposed method is more accurate in detection than the baseline method. Our task is a binary classification, so the chance rate is 0.5. Therefore, the result of only hand means that it is difficult to detect two tools by only hand appearance. Faster R-CNN alone can also make detection with greater accuracy than chance rate, but the value is lower than the proposed method. That is, the proposed method effectively detects scissors and needle holders.

5.3. Procedure Length

In this experiment, we verify the effectiveness of the proposed method by changing the number of frames T. The comparison is made with 25 frames, 50 frames, and 100 frames. The results are shown in Table 4.

Table 4. Results using varying frame numbers in the input data.

Num of Frames	Accuracy	Recall	Precision	F-Measure
25	0.728	0.956	0.703	0.810
50	0.895	0.810	0.981	0.888
100	0.563	0.903	0.500	0.644

As shown in Table 4, the result of 50 frames has the highest accuracy. In the case of 25 frames, the accuracy is lower than that of 50 frames. The reason for this may be that the surgeon sometimes does not finish suturing the thread with the forceps in one second, and the hand rotation, which is a characteristic movement, may not occur. On the other hand, in the case of 100 frames, the accuracy is close to a chance rate. The reason for this may be that there were too much input data and the learning process was not successful. Moreover, it is also possible that hand movements other than holding the scissors, such as rotational movements, were used by the surgeon for cutting multiple parts of the body with the scissors.

6. Conclusions

In this paper, we proposed a method for object detection of similarly shaped tools using hand motion information. The proposed method is divided into three modules, localization, selection, and classification. Faster R-CNN is used for localization and ResNet-18 and LSTM are used for classification. In the experiment, the two tools were detected separately in open surgery videos with an accuracy of 89.5%. In this paper, we detect only two tools by hand motion information. Therefore we would like to develop our method to detect other tools, such as tweezers and forceps, in the future work.

Author Contributions: Conceptualization, T.S.; data curation, T.S. and Y.T.; formal analysis, T.S.; funding acquisition, H.K. and H.S.; investigation, T.S.; methodology, T.S.; project administration, H.K. and H.S.; resources, Y.T.; supervision, H.S.; validation, T.S.; visualization, T.S.; writing—original draft, T.S.; writing—review and editing, R.H. and H.S. All authors have read and agreed to the published version of the manuscript.

Funding: This research was funded by JST-Mirai Program Grant Number JPMJMI19B2, ROIS NII Open Collaborative Research 2020-20S0404, the MIC/SCOPE #201603003, and MHLW Program Grant Number JPMH20AC1004.

Institutional Review Board Statement: The study was conducted according to the guidelines of the Declaration of Helsinki, and approved by the Ethics Committee of Keio University School of Medicine (protocol code 20180111 and date of approval: 2 August 2018).

Informed Consent Statement: Not applicable

Data Availability Statement: The data presented in this study are available on request from the corresponding author. The data are not publicly available due to privacy protection.

Conflicts of Interest: The authors declare no conflict of interest.

References

1. Matsumoto, S.; Sekine, K.; Yamazaki, M.; Funabiki, T.; Orita, T.; Shimizu, M.; Kitano, M. Digital video recording in trauma surgery using commercially available equipment. *Scand. J. Trauma Resusc. Emerg. Med.* **2013**, *21*, 27. [CrossRef] [PubMed]
2. Sadri, A.; Hunt, D.; Rhobaye, S.; Juma, A. Video recording of surgery to improve training in plastic surgery. *J. Plast. Reconstr. Aesthetic Surg.* **2013**, *66*, 122–123. [CrossRef]
3. Graves, S.N.; Shenaq, D.S.; Langerman, A.J.; Song, D.H. Video capture of plastic surgery procedures using the GoPro HERO 3+. *Plast. Reconstr. Surg. Glob. Open* **2015**, *3*, e312. [CrossRef] [PubMed]
4. Olsen, A. *The Tobii I-VT Fixation Filter*; Tobii Technology: Danderyd, Sweden, 2012; pp. 1–21.
5. Li, Y.; Ye, Z.; Rehg, J.M. Delving Into Egocentric Actions. In Proceedings of the IEEE Conference on Computer Vision and Pattern Recognition, Boston, MA, USA, 7–12 June 2015.
6. Damen, D.; Doughty, H.; Farinella, G.M.; Fidler, S.; Furnari, A.; Kazakos, E.; Moltisanti, D.; Munro, J.; Perrett, T.; Price, W.; et al. The EPIC-KITCHENS Dataset: Collection, Challenges and Baselines. *arXiv* **2020**, arXiv:2005.00343.
7. Primus, M.J.; Putzgruber-Adamitsch, D.; Taschwer, M.; Münzer, B.; El-Shabrawi, Y.; Böszörmenyi, L.; Schoeffmann, K. Frame-based classification of operation phases in cataract surgery videos. In Proceedings of the International Conference on Multimedia Modeling, Bangkok, Thailand, 5–7 February 2018; pp. 241–253.
8. Zisimopoulos, O.; Flouty, E.; Luengo, I.; Giataganas, P.; Nehme, J.; Chow, A.; Stoyanov, D. Deepphase: surgical phase recognition in cataracts videos. In Proceedings of the International Conference on Medical Image Computing and Computer-Assisted Intervention, Granada, Spain, 16–20 September 2018; pp. 265–272.
9. Volkov, M.; Hashimoto, D.A.; Rosman, G.; Meireles, O.R.; Rus, D. Machine learning and coresets for automated real-time video segmentation of laparoscopic and robot-assisted surgery. In Proceedings of the IEEE International Conference on Robotics and Automation, Singapore, 29 May–3 June 2017; pp. 754–759. [CrossRef]
10. Jin, A.; Yeung, S.; Jopling, J.; Krause, J.; Azagury, D.; Milstein, A.; Fei-Fei, L. Tool detection and operative skill assessment in surgical videos using region-based convolutional neural networks. In Proceedings of the IEEE Winter Conference on Applications of Computer Vision, Lake Tahoe, NV, USA, 12–15 March 2018; pp. 691–699.

11. Liu, T.; Meng, Q.; Vlontzos, A.; Tan, J.; Rueckert, D.; Kainz, B. Ultrasound Video Summarization Using Deep Reinforcement Learning. In *Medical Image Computing and Computer Assisted Intervention*; Martel, A.L., Abolmaesumi, P., Stoyanov, D., Mateus, D., Zuluaga, M.A., Zhou, S.K., Racoceanu, D., Joskowicz, L., Eds.; Springer International Publishing: Cham, Switzerland, 2020; pp. 483–492.
12. DiPietro, R.; Lea, C.; Malpani, A.; Ahmidi, N.; Vedula, S.S.; Lee, G.I.; Lee, M.R.; Hager, G.D. Recognizing Surgical Activities with Recurrent Neural Networks. *arXiv* **2016**, arXiv:1606.06329.
13. Lea, C.; Hager, G.D.; Vidal, R. An Improved Model for Segmentation and Recognition of Fine-Grained Activities with Application to Surgical Training Tasks. In Proceedings of the IEEE Winter Conference on Applications of Computer Vision, Waikoloa, HI, USA, 6–9 January 2015; pp. 1123–1129. [CrossRef]
14. Redmon, J.; Divvala, S.; Girshick, R.; Farhadi, A. You only look once: Unified, real-time object detection. In Proceedings of the IEEE Conference on Computer Vision and Pattern Recognition, Las Vegas, USA, 27–30 June 2016; pp. 779–788.
15. Ren, S.; He, K.; Girshick, R.; Sun, J. Faster r-cnn: Towards real-time object detection with region proposal networks. In Proceedings of the Advances in Neural Information Processing Systems, Montreal, QC, Canada, 7–12 December 2015; pp. 91–99.
16. Lin, T.Y.; Maire, M.; Belongie, S.; Hays, J.; Perona, P.; Ramanan, D.; Dollár, P.; Zitnick, C.L. Microsoft coco: Common objects in context. In Proceedings of the European Conference on Computer Vision, Zurich, Switzerland, 6–12 September 2014; pp. 740–755.
17. Everingham, M.; Van Gool, L.; Williams, C.K.; Winn, J.; Zisserman, A. The pascal visual object classes (voc) challenge. *Int. J. Comput. Vis.* **2010**, *88*, 303–338. [CrossRef]
18. Stauder, R.; Ostler, D.; Kranzfelder, M.; Koller, S.; Feußner, H.; Navab, N. The TUM LapChole dataset for the M2CAI 2016 workflow challenge. *arXiv* **2017**, arXiv:1610.09278.
19. Liu, W.; Anguelov, D.; Erhan, D.; Szegedy, C.; Reed, S.; Fu, C.Y.; Berg, A.C. Ssd: Single shot multibox detector. In Proceedings of the European Conference on Computer Vision, Amsterdam, The Netherlands, 11–14 October 2016; pp. 21–37.
20. Hochreiter, S.; Schmidhuber, J. Long short-term memory. *Neural Comput.* **1997**, *9*, 1735–1780. [CrossRef]
21. Lee, K.; Kacorri, H. Hands holding clues for object recognition in teachable machines. In Proceedings of the Conference on Human Factors in Computing Systems, Scotland, UK, 4–9 May 2019; pp. 1–12.
22. Ren, X.; Gu, C. Figure-ground segmentation improves handled object recognition in egocentric video. In Proceedings of the IEEE Computer Society Conference on Computer Vision and Pattern Recognition, San Francisco, CA, USA, 13–18 June 2010; pp. 3137–3144. [CrossRef]
23. Twinanda, A.P.; Shehata, S.; Mutter, D.; Marescaux, J.; De Mathelin, M.; Padoy, N. Endonet: A deep architecture for recognition tasks on laparoscopic videos. *IEEE Trans. Med. Imaging* **2016**, *36*, 86–97. [CrossRef]
24. Schoeffmann, K.; Husslein, H.; Kletz, S.; Petscharnig, S.; Muenzer, B.; Beecks, C. Video retrieval in laparoscopic video recordings with dynamic content descriptors. *Multimed. Tools Appl.* **2018**, *77*, 16813–16832. [CrossRef]
25. Al Hajj, H.; Lamard, M.; Conze, P.H.; Cochener, B.; Quellec, G. Monitoring tool usage in surgery videos using boosted convolutional and recurrent neural networks. *Med. Image Anal.* **2018**, *47*, 203–218. [CrossRef] [PubMed]
26. Colleoni, E.; Moccia, S.; Du, X.; De Momi, E.; Stoyanov, D. Deep learning based robotic tool detection and articulation estimation with spatio-temporal layers. *IEEE Robot. Autom. Lett.* **2019**, *4*, 2714–2721. [CrossRef]
27. Du, X.; Kurmann, T.; Chang, P.L.; Allan, M.; Ourselin, S.; Sznitman, R.; Kelly, J.D.; Stoyanov, D. Articulated multi-instrument 2-D pose estimation using fully convolutional networks. *IEEE Trans. Med. Imaging* **2018**, *37*, 1276–1287. [CrossRef]
28. Sarikaya, D.; Corso, J.J.; Guru, K.A. Detection and Localization of Robotic Tools in Robot-Assisted Surgery Videos Using Deep Neural Networks for Region Proposal and Detection. *IEEE Trans. Med. Imaging* **2017**, *36*, 1542–1549. [CrossRef]
29. Wang, S.; Xu, Z.; Yan, C.; Huang, J. Graph Convolutional Nets for Tool Presence Detection in Surgical Videos. In *Information Processing in Medical Imaging*; Chung, A.C.S., Gee, J.C., Yushkevich, P.A., Bao, S., Eds.; Springer International Publishing: Cham, Switzerland, 2019; pp. 467–478.
30. Marzullo, A.; Moccia, S.; Catellani, M.; Calimeri, F.; De Momi, E. Towards realistic laparoscopic image generation using image-domain translation. *Comput. Methods Programs Biomed.* **2020**, 105834. [CrossRef]
31. Bouget, D.; Benenson, R.; Omran, M.; Riffaud, L.; Schiele, B.; Jannin, P. Detecting Surgical Tools by Modelling Local Appearance and Global Shape. *IEEE Trans. Med. Imaging* **2015**, *34*, 2603–2617. [CrossRef] [PubMed]
32. Voros, S.; Orvain, E.; Cinquin, P.; Long, J. Automatic detection of instruments in laparoscopic images: A first step towards high level command of robotized endoscopic holders. In Proceedings of the First IEEE/RAS-EMBS International Conference on Biomedical Robotics and Biomechatronics, Pisa, Italy, 20–22 February 2006; pp. 1107–1112. [CrossRef]
33. Russakovsky, O.; Deng, J.; Su, H.; Krause, J.; Satheesh, S.; Ma, S.; Huang, Z.; Karpathy, A.; Khosla, A.; Bernstein, M.; Berg, A.C.; Fei-Fei, L. ImageNet Large Scale Visual Recognition Challenge. *Int. J. Comput. Vis.* **2015**, *115*, 211–252. [CrossRef]
34. Krizhevsky, A.; Sutskever, I.; Hinton, G.E. Imagenet classification with deep convolutional neural networks. *Commun. Assoc. Comput. Mach.* **2017**, *60*, 84–90. [CrossRef]
35. Roychowdhury, S.; Bian, Z.; Vahdat, A.; Macready, W.G. *Identification of Surgical Tools Using Deep Neural Networks*; Technical Report; D-Wave Systems Inc.: Burnaby, BC, Canada, 2017.
36. Szegedy, C.; Ioffe, S.; Vanhoucke, V.; Alemi, A. Inception-v4, inception-resnet and the impact of residual connections on learning. *arXiv* **2016**, arXiv:1602.07261.
37. He, K.; Zhang, X.; Ren, S.; Sun, J. Deep residual learning for image recognition. In Proceedings of the IEEE Conference on Computer Vision and Pattern Recognition, Las Vegas, USA, 27–30 June 2016; pp. 770–778.

38. Zoph, B.; Vasudevan, V.; Shlens, J.; Le, Q.V. Learning transferable architectures for scalable image recognition. In Proceedings of the IEEE Conference on Computer Vision and Pattern Recognition, Salt Lake City, UT, USA, 18–22 June 2018; pp. 8697–8710.
39. Raju, A.; Wang, S.; Huang, J. M2CAI surgical tool detection challenge report. In Proceedings of the Workshop and Challenges on Modeling and Monitoring of Computer Assisted Intervention (M2CAI), Athens, Greece, 21 October 2016.
40. Szegedy, C.; Liu, W.; Jia, Y.; Sermanet, P.; Reed, S.; Anguelov, D.; Erhan, D.; Vanhoucke, V.; Rabinovich, A. Going deeper with convolutions. In Proceedings of the IEEE Conference on Computer Vision and Pattern Recognition, Boston, MA, USA, 7–12 June 2015; pp. 1–9.
41. Simonyan, K.; Zisserman, A. Very deep convolutional networks for large-scale image recognition. *arXiv* **2014**, arXiv:1409.1556.
42. Cadene, R.; Robert, T.; Thome, N.; Cord, M. M2CAI workflow challenge: Convolutional neural networks with time smoothing and hidden markov model for video frames classification. *arXiv* **2016**, arXiv:1610.05541.
43. Mishra, K.; Sathish, R.; Sheet, D. Learning latent temporal connectionism of deep residual visual abstractions for identifying surgical tools in laparoscopy procedures. In Proceedings of the IEEE Conference on Computer Vision and Pattern Recognition Workshops, Honolulu, HI, USA, 21–26 July 2017; pp. 58–65.
44. Zhang, M.; Cheng, X.; Copeland, D.; Desai, A.; Guan, M.Y.; Brat, G.A.; Yeung, S. Using Computer Vision to Automate Hand Detection and Tracking of Surgeon Movements in Videos of Open Surgery. *arXiv* **2020**, arXiv:2012.06948.
45. Lin, T.; Goyal, P.; Girshick, R.; He, K.; Dollár, P. Focal Loss for Dense Object Detection. In Proceedings of the 2017 IEEE International Conference on Computer Vision (ICCV), Venice, Italy, 22–29 October 2017; pp. 2999–3007. [CrossRef]
46. Xu, B.; Wang, N.; Chen, T.; Li, M. Empirical Evaluation of Rectified Activations in Convolutional Network. *arXiv* **2015**, arXiv:1505.00853.
47. Kingma, D.P.; Ba, J. Adam: A Method for Stochastic Optimization. In Proceedings of the International Conference on Learning Representations, San Diego, CA, USA, 7–9 May 2015.

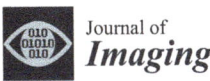

Article

Bayesian Learning of Shifted-Scaled Dirichlet Mixture Models and Its Application to Early COVID-19 Detection in Chest X-ray Images

Sami Bourouis [1,*], Abdullah Alharbi [1] and Nizar Bouguila [2]

1 Department of Information Technology, College of Computers and Information Technology, Taif University, Taif, P.O. Box 11099, Taif 21944, Saudi Arabia; amharbi@tu.edu.sa
2 The Concordia Institute for Information Systems Engineering (CIISE), Concordia University, Montreal, QC H3G 1T7, Canada; nizar.bouguila@concordia.ca
* Correspondence: s.bourouis@tu.edu.sa

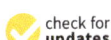

Citation: Bourouis, S.; Alharbi, A.; Bouguila, N. Bayesian Learning of Shifted-Scaled Dirichlet Mixture Models and Its Application to Early COVID-19 Detection in Chest X-ray Images. *J. Imaging* **2021**, *7*, 7. https://doi.org/10.3390/jimaging7010007

Received: 11 November 2020
Accepted: 7 January 2021
Published: 10 January 2021

Publisher's Note: MDPI stays neutral with regard to jurisdictional claims in published maps and institutional affiliations.

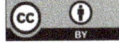

Copyright: © 2021 by the authors. Licensee MDPI, Basel, Switzerland. This article is an open access article distributed under the terms and conditions of the Creative Commons Attribution (CC BY) license (https://creativecommons.org/licenses/by/4.0/).

Abstract: Early diagnosis and assessment of fatal diseases and acute infections on chest X-ray (CXR) imaging may have important therapeutic implications and reduce mortality. In fact, many respiratory diseases have a serious impact on the health and lives of people. However, certain types of infections may include high variations in terms of contrast, size and shape which impose a real challenge on classification process. This paper introduces a new statistical framework to discriminate patients who are either negative or positive for certain kinds of virus and pneumonia. We tackle the current problem via a fully Bayesian approach based on a flexible statistical model named shifted-scaled Dirichlet mixture models (SSDMM). This mixture model is encouraged by its effectiveness and robustness recently obtained in various image processing applications. Unlike frequentist learning methods, our developed Bayesian framework has the advantage of taking into account the uncertainty to accurately estimate the model parameters as well as the ability to solve the problem of overfitting. We investigate here a Markov Chain Monte Carlo (MCMC) estimator, which is a computer-driven sampling method, for learning the developed model. The current work shows excellent results when dealing with the challenging problem of biomedical image classification. Indeed, extensive experiments have been carried out on real datasets and the results prove the merits of our Bayesian framework.

Keywords: infection detection; COVID-19; X-ray images; image classification; bayesian inference; shifted-scaled dirichlet distribution; MCMC; gibbs sampling

1. Introduction and Related Works

Pneumonia is a severe disease issue resulting in inflammation of the lungs where a large number of people lose their lives every day. The causes of this infectious disease could be attributed to viruses or bacteria. Today, the SARS-CoV-2 virus named COVID-19 pneumonia is causing a significant outbreak around the world, having a serious impact on the health and life of several people. In particular, it causes pneumonia in humans and carries severe infections between people. Patients with COVID-19 can have acute symptoms and some may die of major organ failure. One of the critical steps in the fight against this disease is the possibility to quickly detect and track contaminated persons and place them under particular care. Early inspection of confirmed cases is of great urgency because of its infectious nature. One of the many ways of detecting the disease is by a chest radiographs of the patient. Recently, some studies have shown that studying COVID-19 from Chest X-ray images may be considered as the quickest solution to diagnose patients [1]. It is noteworthy that chest X-ray radiography is one of the interesting imaging to diagnose several related chest diseases such as pneumonia, lung cancer, emphysema and pulmonary edema [2,3]. However, sometimes this medical imaging can be subject to error for inexperienced radiologists, while being tedious for experienced ones. Visual examination of these radiographs is generally restricted due to low infectious disease specificity. In addition, the presence of noise, the contrast which is often insufficient between the soft tissues and the overlap in appearance properties are often sources of error for an accurate diagnosis [1,4]. These inconsistencies can result in important biased decisions for clinicians.

To deal with these drawbacks and to detect infected patients, it is necessary to develop effective and automated computerized support tools able to offer radiologists desirable measures about the disease severity. These tools should also allow rapid detection and prediction of any possible infection, in particular COVID-19. Nevertheless, performing a precise analysis of big biomedical data is too difficult and time consuming because these images contain various patterns and symptoms at different stages (early, middle, advanced) [4,5]. For instance at the early stage, it is not easy at all to discover COVID-19 symptoms having acute respiratory distress syndrome in chest X-ray (CXR) scans because these symptoms can look similar to other viral infections like RSV pneumonia. Consequently, it is important to consider such assumption and to take into account robust features extraction techniques when implementing new systems.

Several promising algorithms have been implemented in the past decades to deal especially with infection detection. Some traditional machine learning-based methods are applied to support pneumonia diagnosis in children by classifying chest radiographs into normal or pneumonia cases [6]. Haar wavelet transform is also investigated as an effective feature extraction technique. Some classifiers such as FCM, DWT and WFT [2] and K-nearest neighbor (k-NN) [3] were exploited in this context to detect pneumonia infection. Nevertheless, these conventional methods fail to identify properly lung with lesions. It is true that traditional methods helped the specialists in their diagnosis, but the resulting accuracy was poor. Thus, other image processing-based systems have been proposed to address the problems of infection localization and detecting malicious lesions using, for example, SVM, Neural Networks (NN) and Deep NN (DNN) [5,7–9].

The Fully CN (FCN) method is also applied for segmenting lung in CXR [10]. Another work which is conducted using deep learning method is proposed in [11] to classify CT scan and chest X-ray into three classes: influenza-A viral pneumonia, COVID-19, and normal. The obtained accuracy is 89.3%. As a result, the accuracy is 89.3% and the training process takes a long time. After studing the related work, it is obvious that the success of supervised CNN and deep learning methods to classify CXR images and detect COVID-19 relies mainly on the size of training data. For smaller data set, these techniques are not suitable since this size is responsible for poor performances and in many cases, it becomes too difficult to generate more training data. Thus, it is important to look for other alternatives. Features extraction methods are also exploited in conjuction with some classifiers in order to extrcat ans select relevant visual features. For instance, the ResNet50 feature extractor is used with SVM and CNN for detecting and classifying lung nodule disease in chest CT- images [12]. Other approaches such as registration and active shape models [13,14] are exploited with pixel-based statistical classification methods in order find the boundary/region targets. For example, the lung region is determined through a non-rigid registration step between the chest radiograph of the image patient and a reference model [13].

The good results obtained from applying artificial intelligence and machine learning models to some previous epidemics are motivating researchers to provide new perspective for addressing this novel coronavirus outbreak. In particular, classifying non-Gaussian data in an unsupervised way can be of great interest for automated medical applications. Among the main existing methods to tackle this problem, statistical mixture models have recently gained considerable interest from both the theoretical and practical points of view [15–20]. This approach has led to the design of new more efficient tools. Our work is mainly based on recent research findings that have shown modeling visual data (such as images) effectively is very important for further applications such as image classification. In particular, the taking into account of the distribution of Dirichlet is very interesting to deal with non-Gaussian data modelling [21]. Other derived models such as the scaled Dirichlet mixture (a generalization of the Dirichlet) [16] have also been shown to be effective for data grouping and classification. Further works have show that it is possible to improve these last two models by introducing an additional parameter which leads to a more flexible model. The resulting statistical mixture is called shifted-scaled Dirichlet mixture (SSDMM) and is assumed to be a generalization of the scaled model (here the Shifted term mean a perturbation in the simplex). This new model has been applied successfully for a variety of applications [22].

2. Motivations

The work developed in [22] is based on a shifted-scaled Dirichlet mixture model (SSDMM) and evaluated for data clustering and writer identification. Two important issues arise when deploying mixture models which are calculating the parameters of the mixture and determining the exact number of components that best describes the data set. These issues have been tackled recently by learning the SSDMM via deterministic Maximum Likelihood Estimator (MLE) [22]. Nevertheless, it is known that MLE has major shortcomings linked to its sensitivity at the initialization step. Therefore, a better solution especially for our case (i.e., when dealing with complex medical noisy data including COVID-19 infection) is to develop a more robust alternative based on fully Bayesian inference approach. We recall that Bayesian estimation has attracted a lot of attention for many applications [23–33]. It is also known that the Bayesian approach may be more practical due to the existance of powerful simulation techniques like MCMC [29]. Moreover, the model complexity can be easily solved using for example the marginal likelihood-based technique. Thus, our focus in this paper is to implement an effective Bayesian learning method for SSDMM in order to take into account the complexity of medical data and to overcome the drawbacks of frequentist (deterministic) approaches [34,35]. To the best of our knowledge, such an approach has never been tackled before, especially for the problem of chest x-ray images classification.

The rest of this paper is organized as follows. In next section, the finite shifted-scaled Dirichlet mixture model and the Bayesian approach are exposed. Experimental results and the merits of our approach are introduced in Section 4. Finally, we end this work and provide some possible extensions to be treated in the future.

3. Bayesian Framework for the Shifted-Scaled Dirichlet Mixture Model

We start this section by revising both the Dirichlet and scaled Dirichlet distributions, and then introduce a new generalization of these distributions named shifted-scaled Dirichlet distribution (SSDD). The finite shifted-scaled Dirichlet mixture model is also presented. Then, we develop a fully Bayesian framework for learning the parameters of this finite mixture model.

3.1. Dirichlet and Scaled-Dirichlet Distributions

Definition 1 (Dirichlet distribution). *Let us consider a random vector $Y = (y_1, \ldots, y_D) \in S^D$ (sample space), where $\sum_{d=1}^{D} y_d = 1$. We say that Y has a D-variate Dirichlet distribution with parameter $\vec{\alpha} = (\alpha_1, \ldots, \alpha_D) \in \mathbb{R}_+^D$ if its density function is:*

$$Y \sim Dir^D(\vec{\alpha})$$

$$f(\vec{Y}) = p(\vec{Y}|\theta) = \frac{\Gamma(\alpha_+)}{\prod_{i=1}^{D} \Gamma(\alpha_i)} \prod_{i=1}^{D} y_i^{\alpha_i - 1} \qquad (1)$$

where $\vec{\alpha}$ denotes a shape parameter, $\alpha_+ = \sum_{i=1}^{D} \alpha_i$ and Γ indicates the Euler gamma function.

It is noted that the Dirichlet distribution with D parameters ($Y \sim Dir^D(\vec{\alpha})$) is still popular, especially when it comes to analyzing composition data, and this popularity is due to its its conjugate property with the multinomial likelihood.

Definition 2 (Scaled Dirichlet distribution). *If Y follows a scaled Dirichlet distribution, then its density function is given as:*

$$Y \sim SDir^D(\vec{\alpha}, \vec{\beta})$$

$$f(\vec{Y}) = p(\vec{Y}|\theta) = \frac{\Gamma(\alpha_+)}{\prod_{i=1}^{D} \Gamma(\alpha_i)} \frac{\prod_{i=1}^{D} \beta_i^{\alpha_i} y_i^{\alpha_i - 1}}{(\sum_{i=1}^{D} \beta_i y_i)^{\alpha_+}} \quad (2)$$

$\vec{\alpha} = (\alpha_1, \ldots, \alpha_D)$ and $\vec{\beta} = (\beta_1, \ldots, \beta_D) \in \mathbb{R}_+^D$ are the parameters of this distribution. β is a scale parameter.

The scaled Dirichlet distribution has $2D$ parameters and in this case we have $Y \sim SDir^D(\vec{\alpha}, \vec{\beta})$. If the parameter β is fixed, then we obtain a Dirichlet model.

3.2. Finite Shifted-Scaled Dirichlet Mixture Model

Definition 3 (Shifted-Scaled Dirichlet distribution). *Suppose that Y follows a shifted scaled Dirichlet distribution with parameters* $\vec{\alpha} = (\alpha_1, \ldots, \alpha_D) \in \mathbb{R}_+^D$, $\vec{\lambda} = (\lambda_1, \ldots, \lambda_D) \in S^D$ *and* $a \in \mathbb{R}_+$. *Then, the density probability of this distribution is given as:*

$$Y \sim pSDir^D(\vec{\alpha}, \vec{\lambda}, a)$$

$$f(\vec{Y}) = p(\vec{Y}|\theta) = \frac{\Gamma(\alpha_+)}{\prod_{i=1}^{D} \Gamma(\alpha_i)} \frac{1}{a^{D-1}} \frac{\prod_{i=1}^{D} \lambda_i^{-(\alpha_i/a)} y_i^{(\alpha_i/a)-1}}{(\sum_{i=1}^{D} (y_i/\lambda_i)^{(1/a)})^{\alpha_+}} \quad (3)$$

where $\vec{\lambda}$ denotes a location parameter.

The shifted-scaled Dirichlet distribution has $2D$ parameters and in this case we have $Y \sim pSDir^D(\vec{\alpha}, \vec{\lambda}, a)$. If the parameter $a = 1$, then we obtain a scaled Dirichlet model.

Now, suppose that we have a set of vectors $\mathcal{Y} = \{\vec{Y}_1, \vec{Y}_2, \ldots, \vec{Y}_N\}$, where each vector $\vec{Y}_n = (y_{n1}, \ldots, y_{nD})$ follows a mixture of SSD, then the corresponding likelihood is defined as:

$$p(\mathcal{Y}|\Theta) = \prod_{n=1}^{N} \sum_{k=1}^{K} \pi_k p(\vec{Y}_n|\theta_k) \quad (4)$$

where the model's parameters are defined by $\Theta = (\vec{\pi}, \theta)$ and $\{\pi_k\}$ are positive mixing parameters ($\sum_k \pi_k = 1$). Each vector is supposed coming from one component as $\vec{Y}_n \sim pSDir^D(\vec{\alpha}, \vec{\lambda}, a)$. The shape parameter has the role to describe the form of the shifted SDMM. The scale (a) checks how the plotting of the density is distributed and $\vec{\lambda}$ follows the location of the data densities. In the next section, we will develop our Bayesian approach based on the presented mixture of SSDD.

3.3. Fully Bayesian Learning Algotithm

In many cases, the deterministic approach (named also maximum likelihood-based technique) via the well known EM algorithm [36] is used to estimate the parameters of finite mixture models due to its simplicity. Deterministic approach assumes that $\mathcal{Z} = (\vec{Z}_1, \ldots, \vec{Z}_N)$, is a missing data. Thus, if $\vec{Y}_n \in j$ then $Z_{ij} = 1$, else $Z_{nj} = 0$. Because the likelihood-technique depends on initial values and is sensitive to local minima, we propose here to overcome these limitations by developing an efficient way based on Bayesian inference to better learn the Shifted-Scaled Dirichlet mixture model. More precisely, we propose to investigate one of the effective simulation techniques called Markov Chain Monte Carlo (MCMC) via Gibbs sampler [37,38]. Thus, the complete likelihood is defined as:

$$p(\mathcal{Y}, \mathcal{Z}|\Theta) = \prod_{n=1}^{N} \prod_{k=1}^{K} (\pi_k p(\vec{Y}_n|\theta_k))^{Z_{nk}} \quad (5)$$

Using Bayes formula, the likelihood and the priors will be expressed together to define the posterior distribution like this:

$$p(\Theta|\mathcal{Y}, \mathcal{Z}) \propto p(\mathcal{Y}, \mathcal{Z}|\Theta)p(\Theta) \tag{6}$$

The proposed Bayesian algorithm for SSDMM parameters' learning is based on the following steps:

1. Initialization
2. Step t: For t = 1,...

   (a) Generate $\vec{Z}_i^{(t)} \sim \mathcal{M}(1; \hat{Z}_{i1}^{(t-1)}, \ldots, \hat{Z}_{iM}^{(t-1)})$
   (b) Generate $\vec{\pi}^{(t)}$ from $p(\pi|\mathcal{Z}^{(t)})$
   (c) Generate $(\theta)^{(t)}$ from $p(\theta|\mathcal{Z}^{(t)}, \mathcal{Y})$

where $\mathcal{M}(1; \hat{Z}_{i1}^{(t-1)}, \ldots, \hat{Z}_{iM}^{(t-1)})$ is a multinomial distribution of order one with parameters $(p(1|\vec{Y}_i)^{(t-1)}, \ldots, p(M|\vec{Y}_i)^{(t-1)})$. Based on this algorithm, we have to evaluate $p(\pi|\mathcal{Z})$ and $p(\theta|\mathcal{Z}, \mathcal{Y})$.

3.3.1. Priors and Posteriors

The choice of priors is one of the most crucial steps in Bayesian modeling. These priors reflect our belief about the the model's parameters and are updated and enhanced according to the observed data (see for example details in [39]). In the following, the choice of the priors is addressed as well as the determining of the resulting posteriors for our fully Bayesian approach.

Estimating the posterior will lead to have our parameters $\Theta \sim p(\Theta|\mathcal{Y}, \mathcal{Z})$. In order to perform this step, we proceed with an elegant sampling technique called Gibbs sampler. This method allows the use of conditional posterior distribution in order to update each parameter.

Since no convenient conjugate prior exist for $\vec{\alpha}_k$ and a_k, we adopt a common choice for them which is the Gamma distribution $\mathcal{G}(.)$:

$$p(\alpha_{kd}) = \mathcal{G}(\alpha_{kd}|u_{kd}, v_{kd}) \tag{7}$$

$$p(a_k) = \mathcal{G}(a_k|g_k, h_k) \tag{8}$$

Then, we determine the posterior distributions according to these priors and by considering the following:

$$p(\vec{\alpha}_k|\mathcal{Z}, \mathcal{Y}) \propto p(\vec{\alpha}_k) \prod_{Z_{ik}=1} p(\vec{Y}_i|\theta_k) \propto \prod_{d=1}^{D} p(\alpha_{kd}) \prod_{Z_{ik}=1} p(\vec{Y}_i|\theta_k) \tag{9}$$

$$p(a_k|\mathcal{Z}, \mathcal{Y}) \propto p(a_k) \prod_{Z_{ik}=1} p(\vec{Y}_i|\theta_k) \tag{10}$$

Regarding the parameter $\vec{\lambda}_k$, since it is defined in a simplex, therefore, it is a common and classic choice in Bayesian inference to choose the Dirichlet distribution as prior with parameters $\eta_k = (\eta_{k1}, \ldots, \eta_{kD})$. So, it is expressed as:

$$p(\vec{\lambda}_k|\eta_k) = \frac{\Gamma(\sum_{j=1}^{D} \eta_{kj})}{\prod_{j=1}^{D} \Gamma(\eta_{kj})} \prod_{j=1}^{D} p_{kj}^{\eta_{kj}-1} \tag{11}$$

Knowing this prior, we can estimate the posterior distribution using the following equation:

$$p(\vec{\lambda}_k|\mathcal{Z}, \mathcal{Y}) \propto p(\vec{\lambda}_k|\eta_k) \prod_{Z_{ik}=1} p(\vec{Y}_i|\theta_k) \tag{12}$$

For the prior of mixing weight $\vec{\pi}$, the common choice is the Dirichlet distribution since $\sum_{j=1}^{K} \pi_j = 1$. So, the mixing weight prior is expressed as:

$$p(\vec{\pi}|K, \delta) = \frac{\Gamma(\sum_{j=1}^{K} \delta_j)}{\prod_{j=1}^{K} \Gamma(\delta_j)} \prod_{j=1}^{K} \pi_j^{\delta_j - 1} \quad (13)$$

The selected prior of $\mathcal{Z}$ (membership variable) is defined as :

$$p(\mathcal{Z}|\vec{\pi}, K) = \prod_{j=1}^{K} \pi_j^{n_j} \quad (14)$$

where n_j is the tiotal vectors in cluster j. Given the former equations Equations (13) and (14) we have

$$p(\vec{\pi}|\ldots) \propto p(\mathcal{Z}|\vec{\pi}, K) p(\vec{\pi}|K, \delta)$$

$$\propto \prod_{j=1}^{K} \pi_j^{n_j} \frac{\Gamma(\sum_{j=1}^{K} \delta_j)}{\prod_{j=1}^{K} \Gamma(\delta_j)} \prod_{j=1}^{K} \pi_j^{\delta_j - 1} \propto \frac{\Gamma(\sum_{j=1}^{K} \delta_j)}{\prod_{j=1}^{K} \Gamma(\delta_j)} \prod_{j=1}^{K} \pi_j^{n_j + \delta_j - 1} \quad (15)$$

This posterior is proportional to the Dirichlet distribution $(\delta_1 + n_1, \ldots, \delta_K + n_K)$. In addition, the posterior of the membership $\mathcal{Z}$ may be deduced as:

$$p(Z_i = j|\ldots) \propto \pi_j p(\vec{Y}_n|\theta_j) \quad (16)$$

Finally, we choose the uniform distribution as an appropriate prior for K. This value can vary between 1 and K_{max} (K_{max} is a predefined value). We summarize the proposed model in the following graphical representation Figure 1.

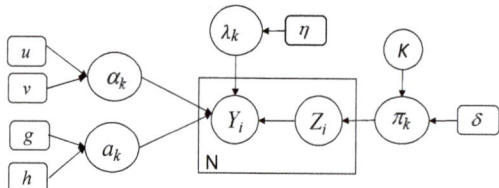

Figure 1. Graphical representation of our developed Bayesian finite shifted-scaled Dirichlet mixture model. Fixed hyperparameters are indicated by rounded boxes and random variables by circles. Y is the observed variable, Z represents the latent variable, the large box indicates repeated process, and the arcs show the dependencies between variables.

3.3.2. Complete Bayesian Estimation-Algorithm

The Gibbs sampling technique is mainly based on alternating conditional distributions for several steps. Indeed, for each iteration t, the resulted estimate Θ^t is sampled from its previous approximate Θ^{t-1}. Having all these posterior probabilities in hand, the complete MCMC-based Bayesian algorithm to learn the parameters of our finite mixture model and especially the steps of our Gibbs sampler are as follows:

1. Initialization
2. Step t: For t = 1,...
   (a) Generate $Z_i^{(t)} \sim \mathcal{M}(1; \hat{Z}_{i1}^{(t-1)}, \ldots, \hat{Z}_{iK}^{(t-1)})$
   (b) Compute $n_k^{(t)} = \sum_{i=1}^{N} \mathbb{I}_{Z_{ik}^{(t)} = j}$
   (c) Generate $\vec{\pi}^{(t)}$ from Equation (15)
   (d) Generate $\vec{\alpha}_k^{(t)}$, $a_k^{(t)}$, and $\vec{\lambda}_k^{(t)}$ ($k = 1, \ldots, K$) from Equations (9), (10) and (12), respectively, using random-walk Metropolis-Hastings (M-H) algorithm [40,41].

where $\mathcal{M}(1; \hat{Z}_{i1}^{(t-1)}, \ldots, \hat{Z}_{iM}^{(t-1)})$ is a multinomial distribution of order one with parameters $(p(1|\vec{Y}_i)^{(t-1)}, \ldots, p(M|\vec{Y}_i)^{(t-1)})$.

4. Experimental Results

The goal of this section is to evaluate and validate the developed statistical model with the different inference techniques. We have considered several real data sets of images including COVID-19 and different pneumonia types.

4.1. Data Sets

The first main COVID-19dataset (https://github.com/ieee8023/covid-chestxray-dataset) for our experiments is the one developed by Cohen et al. [42]. It contains 542 Chest X-ray (CXR) images. A subset of 434 CXR images represent patients positive to COVID-19 and the rest are COVID-19 negative. The image dimension is 4248 × 3480 pixels. Main statistics of this dataset are given in Table 1. An illustrative sample of confirmed Coronavirus Disease 2019 (COVID-19) is given in Figure 2. This image is from a 53-year-old female who had a fever and cough for 5 days. Indeed, Multifocal patchy opacities can be seen in both lungs (arrows) [43].

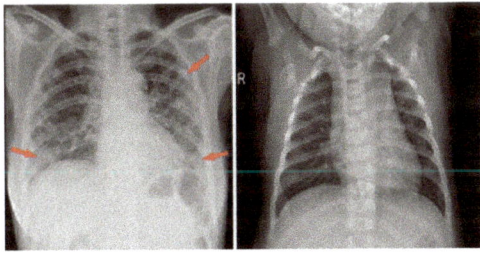

COVID-19 image   Healthy image

Figure 2. Illustrative sample of Chest X-Rays image with COVID-19 [43].

Table 1. Data description.

Dataset	Class	Train	Validation	Test	Total
CXR-COVID	Non-COVID-19	70	20	18	108
	COVID-19	328	80	26	434
CXR-Augmented-COVID	Non-COVID-19	512	100	300	912
	COVID-19	512	100	300	912
CXR-Pneumonia	Normal	1341	8	234	1583
	Pneumonia	3875	8	390	4273

We run also our implemented framework on another available dataset named Augmented COVID-19 Dataset (https://data.mendeley.com/datasets/2fxz4px6d8/4). It is collected from the previous dataset and the Kaggle one (kaggle.com/paultimothymooney/chest-xray-pneumonia). It is made up of augmented radiographics with and without COVID-19. Here, the number of images is larger than the previous dataset. Our aim is to study the performance of our model when the size of the data increases. This dataset contains 912 COVID-19 images and 912 non COVID-19 images. The augmentation process takes into account some geometric transformations and other ones such as translation, rotation, scaling, flipping, noising, bluring, etc. Some illustrative augmented images are given in Figure 3.

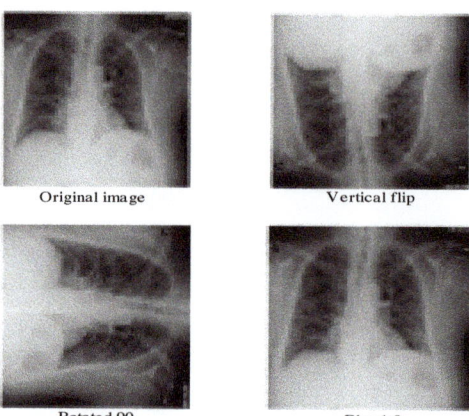

Figure 3. Illustrative examples of augmented Chest X-Rays with COVID-19 from the dataset [44].

Finally, we use the chest-xray-pneumonia to evaluate the performance. Thus, we rum our algorithm on big dataset (viral, bacterial infection, and normal) Kaggle (https://www.kaggle.com/paultimothymooney/chest-xray-pneumonia). It contains 5856 CXR images where 1583 are normal and 4273 are infected with pneumonia. The image dimension is 1024 × 1024 pixels. This dataset is structured into three folders: train, test and val. Some samples are given in Figure 4. Statistics about this dataset are shown in Table 1.

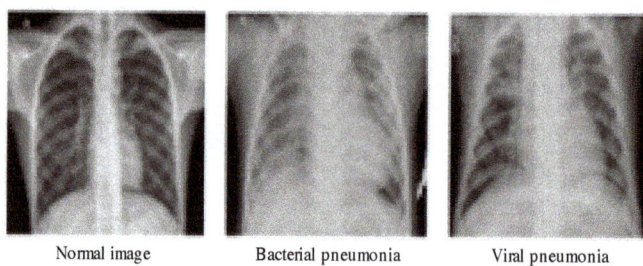

Figure 4. Illustrative samples of chest-xray-pneumonia from the dataset in [45].

4.2. Methodology

The developed model is applied to classify several images from different datasets as normal or COVID-19 affected patients using CXR images. To deal with this objective, we proceed with some preprocessing steps. After a pre-segmentation step of the lung region, we extracted some relevant features based on texture analysis. Indeed, several recently published works have shown that the lung is the basic organ which is affected by the corona COVID-19 virus. The classification is performed into two classes: normal and abnormal. Each image is modelled with a mixture of SSDDMM, then we apply the MCMC algorithm to estimate the parameters of each component. Here, the classification problem is presented in terms of assigning each image to the appropriate class using the Bayes rules. In other word, each image is affected to the class that has the greatest posterior probability. The pipeline of the proposed method is given in Figure 5.

It is noted that, in many cases, medical images such as chest x-rays are not easy to interpret; thus, it is mandatory to identify important patterns to interpret better and improve the decision. Feature extraction problem is the process of acquiring relevant information such as texture. The step of feature extraction has the role to improve the performance and accelerate the processing time. In particular, texture's structures (e.g., fine, smooth, coarse or grained) characterize effectively visual patterns in the image. In the state of the art, many texture extraction methods have been proposed such as statistical ones which are based on different statistics order of the gray-level value. For complex images like medical ones, the use of single feature value cannot lead to satisfactory results; thus, it is important to consider more features to increase the expected performance [46]. In this work, we focus on investigating the so-called Gray Level Co-occurrence Matrix (GLCM)-based features, which has been shown to be efficient and offer interesting results in term of classification accuracy. GLCM matrix provides a co-occurrence matrix of joint probability density of the gray levels of two pixels. In this work, the second-order statistics are investigated to compute some features in order to well-discriminate lung abnormalities. In particular, the following features [47] are calculated for each image: contrast (large differences between neighboring pixels), correlation, energy, entropy, difference variance, difference entropy, inverse difference normalized, information measure of correlation, information measure of correlation. In our analysis, we focused on extracting the lungs area using image thresholding and segmentation processing which leads to identify the left and right lungs from CXR images. In order to remove noise, we applied the Gaussian filter. In Figure 6, we illustrate the obtained segmented lung using the above method. After isolating the lungs, we proceed with feature extraction step and then with classification using the proposed statistical model. The required time for feature extraction for each image is a few seconds and the model fitting taken between 20 to 30 min for the different data sets.

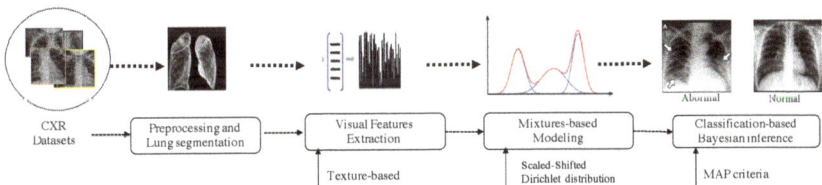

Figure 5. The pipeline of the proposed method. First, the lungs are segmented, then robust visual features are extracted. Features are modelled using the proposed mixture model (SSDDMM) and a Bayesian framework is applied to estimate the parameters of the model. Finally, images are classified on the basis of Bayes rule.

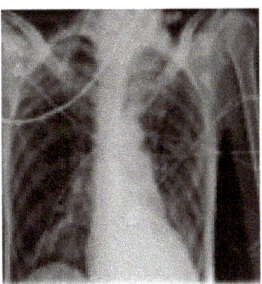 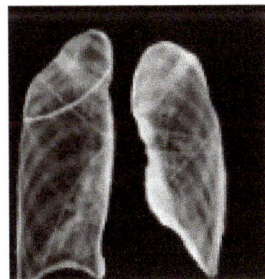

Figure 6. Process of lungs regions extraction applied on image sample from [42].

4.3. Results Analysis

In this section, we investigate our approach for COVID-19 detection. The ultimate first goal is to prove the potential of our Bayesian learning algorithm as compared to other learning method named maximum likelihood (ML) estimation. The second goal is to compare the performance of the proposed shifted-scaled Dirichlet mixture model with other methods which are Gaussian mixture-based, Gamma mixture-based, Dirichlet mixture-based and scaled Dirichlet mixture-based method. For performance investigation, we evaluate the performance of our Bayesian learning method and the rest of methods in terms of overall accuracy (ACC), detection rate (DR), and false-positive rate (FPR).

Tables 2–4, show the classification accuracies for the Test sets of each dataset when applying different generative approaches namely: Gaussian mixture model with maximum likelihood (**GMM-ML**), with Bayesian inference (**GMM-B**), Gamma mixture model with maximum likelihood (**ΓMM-ML**), Dirichlet mixture with maximum likelihood (**DMM-ML**), with Bayesian inference (**DMM-B**), scaled Dirichlet mixture with maximum likelihood (**SDMM-ML**), with Bayesian inference (**SDMM-B**), shifted scaled Dirichlet mixture with maximum likelihood (**SSDMM-ML**), and our proposed method named as shifted scaled Dirichlet mixture with Bayesian inference (**SSDMM-B**).

According to these tables, we can see clearly that, in general, all mixture models provide encouraging results taking into account the difficulty of the unsupervised learning problem. It is clear that our proposed Bayesian method for the shifted scaled Dirichlet mixture outperforms, according to the used metrics, the rest of methods. Indeed, our work has better accuracy as well as lowest false positive rate than both Dirichlet and Gaussian mixtures. We can also see that Bayesian learning provides better results than the ML approach for all models. As we can see, for CXR-COVID dataset, the SSDMM-B outperforms other models with accuracy of 89.57% compared to 88.08% for SDMM-B, 88.04% for DMM and 82.44% for GMM. Our Bayesian model is slightly better than SSDMM-MML [22]. Likewise, we came to the same conclusion for the other datasets and we reach the highest accuracy of 93.03% with our model **SSDMM-B** for the CXR-Pneumonia dataset. According to this last result, it is clear that the precision increases (and the false positive decreases) as the dataset size increases. This is can be viewed for CXR-Augmented-COVID and CXR-Pneumonia datasets which contain more images than CXR-COVID. On the basis of the overall accuracy (ACC) for three datasets (CXR-COVID, CXR-Pneumonia, and CXR-Augmented-COVID), it is obviously clear that the difference between the highest and lowest accuracy is between 5.2% and 7.46% for each dataset. The difference between some methods is about 2.26% which is also considered significant according to t-student test. The obtain results confirm the merits of the fully Bayesian formalism for shifted-scaled Dirichlet mixture which is more flexible (since it has more degrees of freedom) than the Dirichlet and the scaled Dirichlet mixtures. Its flexibility also makes it possible to easily integrate more knowledge and especially features selection mechanism into the proposed framework. On the other hand, even a small improvement is worthwhile taking into account the difficulty of the problem especially with the availability of strong machines to do the processing and simulations. Concerning the modeling uncertainty quantification, this is something that distinguishes our approach from deep learning models (black boxes). We are currently working with clinicians to be able to quantify the uncertainty and extract interpretations, as well as explanations from our models which is possible thanks to the generative nature of the deployed model.

Table 2. Overall accuracy for chest x-ray (CXR)-COVID Dataset.

Approach/Metrics	ACC(%)	DR(%)	FPR(%)
GMM-ML [48]	82.11	81.02	0.18
GMM-B [49]	83.44	82.14	0.17
ΓMM-ML [50]	85.22	83.76	0.16
DMM-ML [51]	87.99	87.88	0.14
DMM-B [52]	88.04	87.78	0.13
SDMM-ML [16]	88.08	87.84	0.13
SDMM-B [31]	88.22	88.07	0.13
SSDMM-ML [22]	89.13	88.24	0.12
SSDMM-B (our method)	**89.57**	**88.61**	**0.12**

Table 3. Overall accuracy for CXR-Pneumonia Dataset.

Approach/Metrics	ACC(%)	DR(%)	FPR(%)
GMM-ML [48]	87.66	85.80	0.13
GMM-B [49]	88.90	86.98	0.11
ΓMM-ML [50]	90.54	88.54	0.10
DMM-ML [51]	91.81	91.03	0.09
DMM-B [52]	92.01	91.33	0.09
SDMM-ML [16]	92.43	91.32	0.09
SDMM-B [31]	92.81	91.77	0.09
SSDMM-ML [22]	92.85	92.01	0.08
SSDMM-B (our method)	93.03	92.90	0.08

Table 4. Overall accuracy for CXR-Augmented COVID-19 Dataset.

Approach/Metrics	ACC(%)	DR(%)	FPR(%)
GMM-ML [48]	85.13	83.99	0.14
GMM-B [49]	86.77	84.08	0.13
ΓMM-ML [50]	90.24	89.14	0.10
DMM-ML [51]	88.01	87.57	0.12
DMM-B [52]	88.44	87.96	0.12
SDMM-ML [16]	89.01	88.12	0.11
SDMM-B [31]	89.88	89.12	0.10
SSDMM-ML [22]	90.10	89.01	0.09
SSDMM-B (our method)	90.33	89.12	0.09

It is also noted that the lung segmentation step is difficult particularly when it includes acute respiratory distress syndrome. This difficulty is due to the little contrast at the boundary of the lung. Moreover, when the number of images in this dataset is too small, the obtained results are lower than the case of big datasets. We can conclude that the obtained results are considered very encouraging given that we approach the classification problem in an unsupervised manner. In fact, the flexibility of the shifted-scaled mixture model and the robustness of texture-based features lead to more stable results. For COVID-19 identification through CXR images, the proposed fully Bayesian learning approach for SSDMM has confirmed that it is capable to discriminate images according to texture properties. In order to further improve these results, perhaps other descriptors are needed, especially the consideration of a robust feature selection mechanism to filter out unreliable features and keep only the most relevant ones. Please note that various studies have been proposed in the state of the art [53] which show that textures are very promising for many medical applications [54]. Here, the comparison between different feature-based techniques is beyond the scope of this article. Instead, we investigated in this work one robust texture-based descriptor to have interesting results for the classification of chest x-ray (CXR) images and corona virus convid-19 detection.

5. Conclusions

In this paper, we have addressed the problems of modeling and classification of multidimensional non-Gaussian data via a purely Bayesian learning approach based on a shifted scaled Dirichlet mixture model. We have especially tackled the problems of chest x-ray (CXR) images classification and COVID-19 detection. The flexibility and capability of the proposed statistical framework is evaluated through three public datasets related to COVID-19 and Pneumonia diseases. Unlike other statistical methods, which assume the heavy assumption that input data are Gaussian, which is not always ture especially for real medical applications, the treated data in our work are modelled via non-Gaussian model and using finite mixtures of shifted scaled Dirichlet distributions that offer reasonable explanations. Our framework has provided promising results and outperforms other methods. In particular, the Bayesian inference results are more interesting thanks to the consideration of the joint posterior distribution. In this work we have investigated an effective MCMC-based approximation technique given that exact inference in fully Bayesian methods is not easy to compute. Our implemented approach has also the advantage of being more general and extensible enough to be applied for large scale data presenting various infection's type. Future works could be devoted to extending the proposed framework via nonparametric approaches. Other promising future works include the integration of feature selection mechanism into the statistical model to improve the generalization capabilities. We hope also that many other real-world problems, including medical ones, will be addressed within the proposed framework.

Author Contributions: Conceptualization, S.B. and A.A.; methodology, N.B.; software, N.B.; validation, S.B. and A.A. and N.B.; formal analysis, S.B.; investigation, S.B. and A.A.; resources, N.B.; data curation, N.B.; writing—original draft preparation, S.B. and A.A.; writing—review and editing, N.B.; visualization, A.A.; supervision, N.B.; project administration, S.B.; funding acquisition, S.B. All authors have read and agreed to the published version of the manuscript.

Funding: This work was supported by the Research Groups Program funded by Deanship of Scientific Research, Taif University, Ministry of Education, Saudi Arabia, under grant number 1-441-50.

Institutional Review Board Statement: Not applicable.

Informed Consent Statement: Not applicable.

Data Availability Statement: https://github.com/ieee8023/covid-chestxray-dataset; https://www.kaggle.com/paultimothymooney/chest-xray-pneumonia; https://data.mendeley.com/datasets/2fxz4px6d8/4

Acknowledgments: Authors would like to thank the Deanship of Scientific Research, Taif University, Kingdom of Saudi Arabia, for their funding support under grant number 1-441-50.

Conflicts of Interest: The authors declare no conflict of interest.

References

1. Jacobi, A.; Chung, M.; Bernheim, A.; Eber, C. Portable chest X-ray in coronavirus disease-19 (COVID-19): A pictorial review. *Clin. Imaging* **2020**, *64*, 35–42. [CrossRef] [PubMed]
2. Parveen, N.; Sathik, M.M. Detection of pneumonia in chest X-ray images. *J. X-ray Sci. Technol.* **2011**, *19*, 423–428. [CrossRef] [PubMed]
3. Ginneken, B.V.; Stegmann, M.B.; Loog, M. Segmentation of anatomical structures in chest radiographs using supervised methods: A comparative study on a public database. *Med. Image Anal.* **2006**, *10*, 19–40. [CrossRef] [PubMed]
4. Minaee, S.; Kafieh, R.; Sonka, M.; Yazdani, S.; Soufi, G.J. Deep-COVID: Predicting COVID-19 from chest X-ray images using deep transfer learning. *Med. Image Anal.* **2020**, *65*, 101794. [CrossRef] [PubMed]
5. Gordienko, Y.; Gang, P.; Hui, J.; Zeng, W.; Kochura, Y.; Alienin, O.; Rokovyi, O.; Stirenko, S. Deep learning with lung segmentation and bone shadow exclusion techniques for chest x-ray analysis of lung cancer. In *International Conference on Computer Science, Engineering and Education Applications*; Springer: Berlin/Heidelberg, Germany, 2018; pp. 638–647.
6. Oliveira, L.L.G.; e Silva, S.A.; Ribeiro, L.H.V.; de Oliveira, R.M.; Coelho, C.J.; Andrade, A.L.S.S. Computer-aided diagnosis in chest radiography for detection of childhood pneumonia. *Int. J. Med. Inform.* **2008**, *77*, 555–564. [CrossRef]
7. Litjens, G.; Kooi, T.; Bejnordi, B.E.; Setio, A.A.A.; Ciompi, F.; Ghafoorian, M.; van der Laak, J.A.W.M.; van Ginneken, B.; Sánchez, C.I. A survey on deep learning in medical image analysis. *Med. Image Anal.* **2017**, *42*, 60–88. [CrossRef]
8. Greenspan, H.; van Ginneken, B.; Summers, R.M. Guest Editorial Deep Learning in Medical Imaging: Overview and Future Promise of an Exciting New Technique. *IEEE Trans. Med. Imaging* **2016**, *35*, 1153–1159. [CrossRef]
9. Zhao, B.; Feng, J.; Wu, X.; Yan, S. A survey on deep learning-based fine-grained object classification and semantic segmentation. *Int. J. Autom. Comput.* **2017**, *14*, 119–135. [CrossRef]
10. Novikov, A.A.; Lenis, D.; Major, D.; Hladůvka, J.; Wimmer, M.; Bühler, K. Fully convolutional architectures for multiclass segmentation in chest radiographs. *IEEE Trans. Med Imaging* **2018**, *37*, 1865–1876. [CrossRef]
11. Xu, X.; Jiang, X.; Ma, C.; Du, P.; Li, X.; Lv, S.; Yu, L.; Chen, Y.; Su, J.; Lang, G.; et al. Deep Learning System to Screen Coronavirus Disease 2019 Pneumonia. *Engineering* **2020**, *6*, 1122–1129. [CrossRef]
12. da Nóbrega, R.V.M.; Filho, P.P.R.; Rodrigues, M.B.; da Silva, S.P.P.; Júnior, C.M.J.M.D.; de Albuquerque, V.H.C. Lung nodule malignancy classification in chest computed tomography images using transfer learning and convolutional neural networks. *Neural Comput. Appl.* **2020**, *32*, 11065–11082. [CrossRef]

13. Candemir, S.; Jaeger, S.; Palaniappan, K.; Musco, J.P.; Singh, R.K.; Xue, Z.; Karargyris, A.; Antani, S.; Thoma, G.; McDonald, C.J. Lung Segmentation in Chest Radiographs Using Anatomical Atlases With Nonrigid Registration. *IEEE Trans. Med. Imaging* **2014**, *33*, 577–590. [CrossRef] [PubMed]
14. Xu, T.; Mandal, M.K.; Long, R.; Cheng, I.; Basu, A. An edge-region force guided active shape approach for automatic lung field detection in chest radiographs. *Comput. Med. Imaging Graph.* **2012**, *36*, 452–463. [CrossRef] [PubMed]
15. Mashrgy, M.A.; Bdiri, T.; Bouguila, N. Robust simultaneous positive data clustering and unsupervised feature selection using generalized inverted Dirichlet mixture models. *Knowl. Based Syst.* **2014**, *59*, 182–195. [CrossRef]
16. Oboh, B.S.; Bouguila, N. Unsupervised learning of finite mixtures using scaled dirichlet distribution and its application to software modules categorization. In Proceedings of the 2017 IEEE International Conference on Industrial Technology (ICIT), Toronto, ON, Canada, 22–25 March 2017; pp. 1085–1090.
17. Channoufi, I.; Bourouis, S.; Bouguila, N.; Hamrouni, K. Image and video denoising by combining unsupervised bounded generalized gaussian mixture modeling and spatial information. *Multimed. Tools Appl.* **2018**, *77*, 25591–25606. [CrossRef]
18. Fan, W.; Bouguila, N. Spherical data clustering and feature selection through nonparametric Bayesian mixture models with von Mises distributions. *Eng. Appl. Artif. Intell.* **2020**, *94*, 103781. [CrossRef]
19. Najar, F.; Bourouis, S.; Bouguila, N.; Belghith, S. Unsupervised learning of finite full covariance multivariate generalized Gaussian mixture models for human activity recognition. *Multimed. Tools Appl.* **2019**, *78*, 18669–18691. [CrossRef]
20. Najar, F.; Bourouis, S.; Zaguia, A.; Bouguila, N.; Belghith, S. Unsupervised Human Action Categorization Using a Riemannian Averaged Fixed-Point Learning of Multivariate GGMM. In Proceedings of the Image Analysis and Recognition-15th International Conference, ICIAR, Póvoa de Varzim, Portugal, 27–29 June 2018; pp. 408–415.
21. Bourouis, S.; Mashrgy, M.A.; Bouguila, N. Bayesian learning of finite generalized inverted Dirichlet mixtures: Application to object classification and forgery detection. *Expert Syst. Appl.* **2014**, *41*, 2329–2336. [CrossRef]
22. Alsuroji, R.; Zamzami, N.; Bouguila, N. Model Selection and Estimation of a Finite Shifted-Scaled Dirichlet Mixture Model. In Proceedings of the 17th IEEE International Conference on Machine Learning and Applications, ICMLA, Orlando, FL, USA, 17–20 December 2018; pp. 707–713.
23. Alroobaea, R.; Rubaiee, S.; Bourouis, S.; Bouguila, N.; Alsufyani, A. Bayesian inference framework for bounded generalized Gaussian-based mixture model and its application to biomedical images classification. *Int. J. Imaging Syst. Technol.* **2020**, *30*, 18–30. [CrossRef]
24. Kayabol, K.; Kutluk, S. Bayesian classification of hyperspectral images using spatially-varying Gaussian mixture model. *Digit. Signal Process.* **2016**, *59*, 106–114. [CrossRef]
25. Li, Z.; Xia, Y.; Ji, Z.; Zhang, Y. Brain voxel classification in magnetic resonance images using niche differential evolution based Bayesian inference of variational mixture of Gaussians. *Neurocomputing* **2017**, *269*, 47–57. [CrossRef]
26. Li, F.; Perona, P. A Bayesian Hierarchical Model for Learning Natural Scene Categories. In Proceedings of the 2005 IEEE Computer Society Conference on Computer Vision and Pattern Recognition (CVPR 2005), San Diego, CA, USA, 20–26 June 2005; pp. 524–531.
27. Bourouis, S.; Al-Osaimi, F.R.; Bouguila, N.; Sallay, H.; Aldosari, F.M.; Mashrgy, M.A. Bayesian inference by reversible jump MCMC for clustering based on finite generalized inverted Dirichlet mixtures. *Soft Comput.* **2019**, *23*, 5799–5813. [CrossRef]
28. Robert, C. *The Bayesian Choice: From Decision-Theoretic Foundations to Computational Implementation*; Springer Science & Business Media: New York, NY, USA, 2007.
29. Marin, J.M.; Robert, C. *Bayesian Core: A Practical Approach to Computational Bayesian Statistics*; Springer Science & Business Media: New York, NY, USA, 2007.
30. Chen, P.; Nelson, J.D.B.; Tourneret, J. Toward a Sparse Bayesian Markov Random Field Approach to Hyperspectral Unmixing and Classification. *IEEE Trans. Image Process.* **2017**, *26*, 426–438. [CrossRef] [PubMed]
31. Bourouis, S.; Laalaoui, Y.; Bouguila, N. Bayesian frameworks for traffic scenes monitoring via view-based 3D cars models recognition. *Multimed. Tools Appl.* **2019**, *78*, 18813–18833. [CrossRef]
32. Barber, D.; Williams, C.K.I. Gaussian Processes for Bayesian Classification via Hybrid Monte Carlo. In Proceedings of the Advances in Neural Information Processing Systems 9, NIPS, Denver, CO, USA, 2–5 December 1996; Mozer, M., Jordan, M.I., Petsche, T., Eds.; MIT Press: Cambridge, MA, USA, 1996; pp. 340–346.
33. Bourouis, S.; Al-Osaimi, F.R.; Bouguila, N.; Sallay, H.; Aldosari, F.M.; Mashrgy, M.A. Video Forgery Detection Using a Bayesian RJMCMC-Based Approach. In Proceedings of the 14th IEEE/ACS International Conference on Computer Systems and Applications, AICCSA 2017, Hammamet, Tunisia, 30 October–3 November 2017; pp. 71–75.
34. Fan, W.; Bouguila, N.; Bourouis, S.; Laalaoui, Y. Entropy-based variational Bayes learning framework for data clustering. *IET Image Process.* **2018**, *12*, 1762–1772. [CrossRef]
35. Bourouis, S.; Zaguia, A.; Bouguila, N. Hybrid Statistical Framework for Diabetic Retinopathy Detection. In *Image Analysis and Recognition, Proceedings of the 15th International Conference, ICIAR 2018, Póvoa de Varzim, Portugal, 27–29 June 2018*; Lecture Notes in Computer Science; Campilho, A., Karray, F., ter Haar Romeny, B.M., Eds. Springer: Cham, Switzerland, 2018; Volume 10882, pp. 687–694.
36. Dempster, A.P.; Laird, N.M.; Rubin, D.B. Maximum likelihood from incomplete data via the EM algorithm. *J. R. Stat. Soc. Ser. B* **1977**, *39*, 1–38.

37. Bouguila, N. Bayesian hybrid generative discriminative learning based on finite Liouville mixture models. *Pattern Recognit.* **2011**, *44*, 1183–1200. [CrossRef]
38. Gelman, A.; Carlin, J.B.; Stern, H.S.; Rubin, D.B. *Bayesian Data Analysis*, 3rd ed.; Chapman and Hall/CRC: New York, NY, USA, 2013.
39. Geiger, D.; Heckerman, D. Parameter priors for directed acyclic graphical models and the characterization of several probability distributions. In Proceedings of the Fifteenth Conference on Uncertainty in Artificial Intelligence, Stockholm, Sweden, 30 July–1 August 1999; pp. 216–225.
40. Congdon, P. *Applied Bayesian Modelling*; John Wiley and Sons: Hoboken, NJ, USA, 2003.
41. Chib, S.; Greenberg, E. Understanding the Metropolis-Hastings Algorithm. *Am. Stat.* **1995**, *49*, 327–335.
42. Cohen, J.P.; Morrison, P.; Dao, L.; Roth, K.; Duong, T.Q.; Ghassemi, M. COVID-19 Image Data Collection: Prospective Predictions Are the Future. *arXiv* **2020**, arXiv:2006.11988.
43. Zu, Z.Y.; Jiang, M.D.; Xu, P.P.; Chen, W.; Ni, Q.Q.; Lu, G.M.; Zhang, L.J. Coronavirus disease 2019 (COVID-19): A perspective from China. *Radiology* **2020**, *296*, 200490. [CrossRef]
44. Alqudah, A.; Qazan, S. Augmented COVID-19 X-ray images dataset. *Mendeley Data* **2020**, *4*. [CrossRef]
45. Mooney, P. Chest X-ray Images (Pneumonia). 2020. Available online: https://www.kaggle.com/paultimothymooney/chest-xray-pneumonia (access on November 2020).
46. Xie, J.; Jiang, Y.; Tsui, H. Segmentation of kidney from ultrasound images based on texture and shape priors. *IEEE Trans. Med. Imaging* **2005**, *24*, 45–57. [PubMed]
47. Pourghassem, H.; Ghassemian, H. Content-based medical image classification using a new hierarchical merging scheme. *Comput. Med. Imaging Graph.* **2008**, *32*, 651–661. [CrossRef] [PubMed]
48. Fernando, B.; Fromont, É.; Muselet, D.; Sebban, M. Supervised learning of Gaussian mixture models for visual vocabulary generation. *Pattern Recognit.* **2012**, *45*, 897–907. [CrossRef]
49. Figueiredo, M.A.T.; Jain, A.K. Unsupervised Learning of Finite Mixture Models. *IEEE Trans. Pattern Anal. Mach. Intell.* **2002**, *24*, 381–396. [CrossRef]
50. Sallay, H.; Bourouis, S.; Bouguila, N. Online Learning of Finite and Infinite Gamma Mixture Models for COVID-19 Detection in Medical Images. *Computers* **2021**, *10*, 6. [CrossRef]
51. Bouguila, N.; Ziou, D. Using unsupervised learning of a finite Dirichlet mixture model to improve pattern recognition applications. *Pattern Recognit. Lett.* **2005**, *26*, 1916–1925. [CrossRef]
52. Ma, Z.; Rana, P.K.; Taghia, J.; Flierl, M.; Leijon, A. Bayesian estimation of Dirichlet mixture model with variational inference. *Pattern Recognit.* **2014**, *47*, 3143–3157. [CrossRef]
53. Smith, G.; Burns, I. Measuring texture classification algorithms. *Pattern Recognit. Lett.* **1997**, *18*, 1495–1501. [CrossRef]
54. Melendez, J.; van Ginneken, B.; Maduskar, P.; Philipsen, R.H.H.M.; Reither, K.; Breuninger, M.; Adetifa, I.M.O.; Maane, R.; Ayles, H.; Sánchez, C.I. A Novel Multiple-Instance Learning-Based Approach to Computer-Aided Detection of Tuberculosis on Chest X-Rays. *IEEE Trans. Med. Imaging* **2015**, *34*, 179–192. [CrossRef]

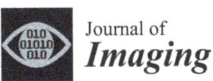

Article

Data Augmentation Using Adversarial Image-to-Image Translation for the Segmentation of Mobile-Acquired Dermatological Images

Catarina Andrade [1,*], Luís F. Teixeira [2,3], Maria João M. Vasconcelos [1] and Luís Rosado [1]

1. Fraunhofer Portugal AICOS, Rua Alfredo Allen, 4200-135 Porto, Portugal; maria.vasconcelos@fraunhofer.pt (M.J.M.V.); luis.rosado@fraunhofer.pt (L.R.)
2. Faculty of Engineering, University of Porto, Rua Dr. Roberto Frias, 4200-465 Porto, Portugal; luisft@fe.up.pt
3. INESC TEC, Rua Dr. Roberto Frias, 4200-465 Porto, Portugal
* Correspondence: catarina.andrade@fraunhofer.pt

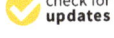

Citation: Andrade, C.; Teixeira, L.F.; Vasconcelos, M.J.; Rosado, L. Data Augmentation Using Adversarial Image-to-Image Translation for the Segmentation of Mobile-Acquired Dermatological Images. *J. Imaging* **2021**, *7*, 2. https://dx.doi.org/10.3390/jimaging7010002

Received: 9 November 2020
Accepted: 16 December 2020
Published: 24 December 2020

Publisher's Note: MDPI stays neutral with regard to jurisdictional claims in published maps and institutional affiliations.

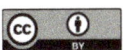

Copyright: © 2020 by the authors. Licensee MDPI, Basel, Switzerland. This article is an open access article distributed under the terms and conditions of the Creative Commons Attribution (CC BY) license (https://creativecommons.org/licenses/by/4.0/).

Abstract: Dermoscopic images allow the detailed examination of subsurface characteristics of the skin, which led to creating several substantial databases of diverse skin lesions. However, the dermoscope is not an easily accessible tool in some regions. A less expensive alternative could be acquiring medium resolution clinical macroscopic images of skin lesions. However, the limited volume of macroscopic images available, especially mobile-acquired, hinders developing a clinical mobile-based deep learning approach. In this work, we present a technique to efficiently utilize the sizable number of dermoscopic images to improve the segmentation capacity of macroscopic skin lesion images. A Cycle-Consistent Adversarial Network is used to translate the image between the two distinct domains created by the different image acquisition devices. A visual inspection was performed on several databases for qualitative evaluation of the results, based on the disappearance and appearance of intrinsic dermoscopic and macroscopic features. Moreover, the Fréchet Inception Distance was used as a quantitative metric. The quantitative segmentation results are demonstrated on the available macroscopic segmentation databases, SMARTSKINS and Dermofit Image Library, yielding test set thresholded Jaccard Index of 85.13% and 74.30%. These results establish a new state-of-the-art performance in the SMARTSKINS database.

Keywords: convolutional neural network; CycleGAN; data augmentation; dermoscopic images; domain transfer; macroscopic images; skin lesion segmentation

---

1. Introduction

Skin cancer is one of the most prevalent malignancy worldwide and has a reported yearly growing incidence with no signs of plateauing. In 2018, almost three-hundred thousand malignant melanoma (MM) were diagnosed worldwide and over a million non-melanoma skin cancers (NMSC) [1]. However, this number excludes basal cell carcinoma, the most frequent skin cancer, since most go unreported [2]. The majority of NMSC and MM are highly curable if diagnosed in the early stages. The estimated 5-year survival rate for MM drops from over 98% to 23% if detected when the metastases are distant from the origin point [1]. Moreover, the effective diagnosis is compromised by the almost identical clinical presentation of benign and malignant skin lesions. Therefore, timely and accurate diagnosis is a paramount measure in controlling this pre-eminent global public health problem.

The growing usage of smartphones added to the robustness of deep learning models makes a mobile-based deep learning approach a well-suited possibility for the automatic cutaneous cancer triage [3,4]. Notwithstanding, the limited volume of mobile acquired images, such as macroscopic or close-up images, proves to be an obstacle in the development of a robust model specific to the macroscopic image type. Dermoscopy is the standard procedure for skin cancer preliminary diagnosis, it allows the visualization of inner layers of the skin which are not visible to the naked eye. This visualization method added to the procedural algorithms, allowed an expert diagnostic accuracy of 75% to 84% [5–7], which compelled the generation of several sizeable databases of this type of images. Yet, the direct inference between the two domains, macroscopic and dermoscopic, is not advisable and may even prove to be a detriment for the robustness of the model [8,9]. These image acquisition formats generate images with very different characteristics and challenges [10] and even for the clinical diagnosis, there are rules and methods specific for each domain [11].

This work aims to evaluate the possibility of designing a deep learning algorithm for the precise segmentation of lesion in macroscopic images capable to fully operate in the mobile environment. To assemble such a model, we explore the capitalization of the sizable dermoscopic databases by using a Cycle-Consistent Adversarial Network (CycleGAN) [12] for the translation between the two domains, macroscopic and dermoscopic.

2. Related Work

One of the fundamental challenges of the medical imaging computer vision analysis is to achieve satisfactory results with limited labelled datasets. Even in the era of Big data, there are still some challenges for which the amount of available data is still severely lacking. This is the case for the macroscopic segmentation challenge.

The lack of macroscopic images may be the reason for the few efforts into developing segmentation algorithms [10,13–18]. Examples of segmentation techniques used are—thresholding [14,16,17], unsupervised dictionary learning methods [13] and support vector machines [15]. Rosado et al. [16] used an adaptive thresholding technique with strong pre and post-processing techniques. The usage of deep learning methods has also been reported [10,18]. In Fernandes et al. [18], a convolution neural network (CNN), with gossip blocks, combined with a backpropagation technique was used to improve the segmentation masks by maximizing the expected quality. In the previous work [10] several architectural modifications of two widely used segmentation CNNs, U-Net and DeepLab, were tested to infer the best macroscopic segmentation CNNs. Here, two methodologies were tested to attempt to mitigate the small size of the macroscopic databases: heavy classical augmentation and transfer learning. The highest reported segmentation performance obtained, in a macroscopic database, was in Reference [10] with an 82.64% Jaccard index.

One of the techniques used to lessen the small datasets is data augmentation through basic image manipulation such as flipping, rotating and addition of noise [10,18]. However, with very small datasets extensive classical data augmentation may promote overfitting [19]. Another strategy used for data augmentation is the creation of artificial instances through generative adversarial networks. This type of framework samples from simple distributions and learn to transform it into the complex high dimensional distributions. For this purpose, two networks are used: one generating network which creates real-looking images, and a discriminator network which tries to distinguish between the real and fake images. Several techniques have been attempted for the skin lesion generation [20–23] however most are used for data augmentation applied to classification task, or to generate skin lesions from random noise without little to no prior knowledge of the complexity of the lesion.

More recently, Gu et al. [9] used a CycleGAN to perform cross-domain skin diseases classification between different disease databases. The CycleGAN algorithm performs image-to-image translation without the need for paired training samples, where the referred work proved the suitability of this approach to reduce the domain shift between different datasets. Thus, in this paper, we propose the CycleGAN to transform the dermatoscopic images into macroscopic. This transformation would allow the use of the vast amount of available dermatological images to increase the robustness of approaches in the macroscopic domain, while maintaining structural information of the lesions and some of their characteristics.

3. Materials and Methods

3.1. Databases

The growing interest in computer-aided diagnosis systems for automated detection and classification of skin lesions led to the creation of several databases. Most of these have been used by researchers to develop algorithms for automated segmentation of lesion borders.

3.1.1. Segmentation Databases

Macroscopic Segmentation Databases Although many databases provide matching binary segmentation masks of cutaneous lesions only the Dermofit image Library [24] and the SMARTSKINS database [25] are of the macroscopic domain. The Dermofit digital image database consists of 1300 high-quality colour skin lesions images taken with standard cameras–with matching binary segmentation masks and class labels, the lesions belong to 10 different diseases with 819 benign and 481 carcinogenic images, annotated by individual disease classes. The SMARTSKINS database was obtained at the Skin Clinic of the Portuguese Institute of Oncology of Porto [25]. This database was acquired with mobile devices and it comprises several subsets captured in different years. One of the subset consists of 80 melanocytic lesions together with the corresponding segmentation masks, as well as medical annotations regarding ABCD score and overall risk.

Dermoscopic Segmentation Databases In terms of dermoscopic databases, we used the three publicly available International Skin Imaging Collaboration (ISIC) challenges datasets (2016 [26], 2017 [27] and 2018 [28,29]), as well as the PH2 database [30]. The ISIC database is a collection of multiple databases used in a recurrent challenge, which aims to improve melanoma detection in dermoscopic images. The ISIC Challenge is broken into 3 tasks—lesion segmentation, lesion attribute detection and disease classification. The PH2 database was obtained at the Dermatology Service of Hospital Pedro Hispano. Each case contains a dermoscopic image, the segmentation of the lesion provided by a doctor, as well as clinical and histological diagnosis and the assessment of several dermoscopic criteria.

The splitting process performed on these databases is summarized in Table 1, which is the same used in Reference [10]. Essentially, the Dermofit and PH2 databases suffer an 80/20 split, between the train and test subsets, and the SMARTSKINS a 50/50 split due to its relative small size. For the three ISIC challenges, the images were merged and the ISIC 2017 test instances were reserved for the test subset. Figure 1 shows illustrative examples of the macroscopic and dermoscopic segmentation databases in pairs A and B.

Table 1. Overview of available segmentation macroscopic and dermoscopic databases and separation into train/validation and test subsets.

Set	Database	No. Images (Type)	No. Train/Val.	No. Test
set M	Dermofit	1300 (MD)	1036	264
	SMARTSKINS	80 (MP)	39	41
set D	ISIC	2594 (De)	1994	600
	PH2	200 (De)	160	40

set M—set of macroscopic images; set D—set of dermoscopic images; No-Number of images, De-Dermoscopic images, MD-Macroscopic images acquired with a digital camera, MP-Macroscopic images acquired with a mobile phone.

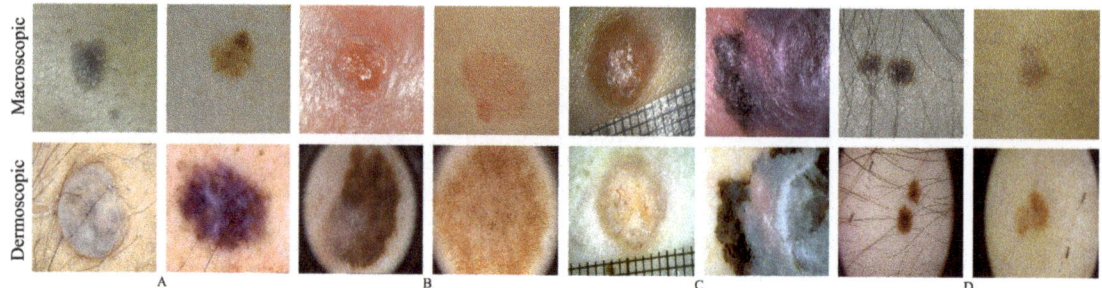

Figure 1. Illustrative examples of macroscopic (row above) and dermoscopic (below) skin lesions. (**A**) above: SMARTSKINS (Set M); below: ISIC (set D); (**B**) above: Dermofit (Set M); below: PH2 (set D); (**C**) EDRA ; (**D**) SMARTSKINS 2014/2015.

3.1.2. Macroscopic and Dermoscopic Databases

The particular characteristic of these databases is that for each skin lesion it has both macroscopic and dermoscopic image. Two databases were found that enter this category—the EDRA database [31] and a subset of the SMARTSKINS database [25]. Figure 1 shows illustrative examples of the two aforementioned databases in pairs C and D, each column has above the macroscopic images and below the dermoscopic counterpart. The EDRA database comprises over 1000 cases of skin lesions. Each clinical case is properly annotated with the clinical data, histopathological results, diagnosis, level of difficulty and the macroscopic and dermoscopic image of the lesion. The subset SMARTSKINS database (SMARTSKINS 2014/2015) was acquired with two smartphones and classified by the overall risk of the lesions. This subset contained over 170 cases of lesions, each of them had one dermoscopic image and two macroscopic.

These databases were used to form the macroscopic and dermoscopic dataset. The division of these databases, into train and test subsets, was performed in a stratified manner in accordance with the classification. Subsequently, it was added to the train subset the ISIC macroscopic images [32] and the training and validation subsets of Set D and Set M. The final configuration of the dermoscopic and macroscopic datasets can be seen in Table 2.

Table 2. Formation of dermoscopic and macroscopic datasets and separation into train and test subsets.

Database	Train		Test	
	MD\MP	De	MD\MP	De
EDRA	802	802	209	209
SMARTSKINS 2014/2015	295	148	56	28
PH2 (Set D)	-	160	-	40
ISIC (Set D)	-	1994	-	600
Dermofit (Set M)	1036	-	-	-
SMARTSKINS (Set M)	39	-	-	-
ISIC Archive	104	-	-	-
Total	2158	3057	242	869

De-Dermoscopic images, MD-Macroscopic images acquired with a digital camera, MP-Macroscopic images acquired with a mobile phone.

3.2. Methodology

3.2.1. Generation of Macroscopic Images

CycleGAN was introduced in 2017 by Zhu et al. [12], this framework is a technique used for the adversarial "unsupervised" training of image translation between two different domains. The most notable capacity is the ability to transform within two domains without using paired data. This lack of pixel-to-pixel correspondence happens in the macroscopic and dermoscopic images, even if images correspond to the same lesion as each acquisition implies different illumination, resolution and distance to the lesion. The framework consists of two mapping functions $G: X-> Y$ and $F: Y-> X$ in conjunction with the respective adversarial discriminators, Dx and Dy, that distinguishes x from F(y) and y from G(x), respectively. These duos are trained with an adversarial loss (L_{GAN}) in association with a cycle consistency loss (L_{cyc}).

In this work, the objective function used in the computation of the L_{GAN} was a combination of the sigmoid cross-entropy between the generated images and an array of ones, and the L1 loss interpolated from the generated image and the target image. Nevertheless, the L_{GAN} alone is not enough to produce images of quality, since it imposes the generated output to be in the desired domain, but does not promote the recognizability between the source and target domain. To enable this mode of learning, Zhu et al. [12] proposed L_{cyc}. This mechanism, which can be seen in Figure 2, relies on the expectation that if an image is converted to another domain and back again it will be comparable to the original image. This generates two cycle-consistency losses: the forward cycle and the backward cycle.

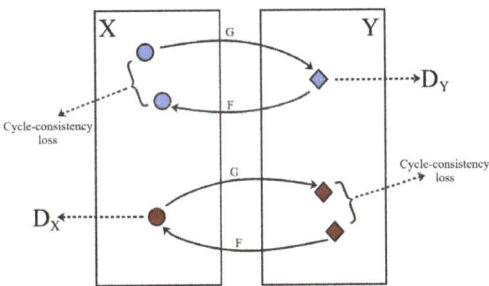

Figure 2. CycleGAN framework and training strategy. Blue—Forward cycle-consistency loss; Red — Backwards cycle-consistency loss.

The full loss is a weighted sum of the adversarial loss of both mapping functions ($L_{GAN}(F, D_X, Y, X)$) and $L_{GAN}(G, D_Y, X, Y)$) and the cycle consistent loss ($L_{cyc}(G, F)$), where the $L_{cyc}(G, F)$ was favoured by a $\lambda = 10$ as shown in (1).

$$L(G, F, D_X, D_Y) = L_{GAN}(F, D_X, Y, X) + L_{GAN}(G, D_Y, X, Y) + \lambda L_{cyc}(G, F). \quad (1)$$

Generator Architecture The architecture adopted is based on the approach described by Johnson et al. [33] in 2016, which was used for neural style transfer and superresolution. This network can be divided into three sections: the encoder, the transformer and the decoder. The encoder is comprised of three sets of padding and convolutional layers followed by instance normalization and the ReLU activation function. The first convolutional layer has a 7×7 kernel and stride 1, and the last two have 3×3 kernels and stride 2. Afterwards, more representative features are produced with the transformer, which encompasses a series of twelve residual blocks of 3×3 kernels and stride 1, instead of the nine residual blocks used in the Johnson et al. [33]. Lastly, the feature maps are expanded by the decoder, which is comprised of two transposed convolutions, with 3×3 filters and stride 2, and one output convolutional layer with 7×7 kernels and stride 1. This last layer has the typical *tanh* activation function to produce the final image in RGB.

Discriminator Architecture For the discriminator, the PatchGAN [34] was used. This CNN looks at a "patch" of the input image and ascertains the probability of being real. This fully connected network is comprised of five convolutional layers with 4×4 kernels and stride 2. Each layer is followed by an instance normalization and the Leaky

ReLU activation function. The output layer uses a sigmoid function to perform the binary classification between real and fake images.

Implementation Details The implementation of the CycleGAN was made with Tensorflow API r1.15 in Python 3.7.3 on an NVIDIA Tesla V100 PCIe 32GB GPU. As training protocol, the one proposed on the original paper [12] was followed. In short, we employ a learning rate of 0.0002 with the weights initialized from a Gaussian distribution ranging from 0 to 0.02. The stopping criteria took into consideration the stabilization of the loss values of the generators, as well as the immutability of the TransMacro and TransDermo images, which were visually analysed during training. In the limiting case in which none of the criteria were satisfied, the CycleGAN model had the final criteria of 1000 epochs. The dataset used in the training and testing of this network is described in Table 2.

3.2.2. Segmentation Network

The segmentation network employed was the optimized encoder-decoder network selected in Reference [10], which used a modified DeepLabV3+ [35]. Initially, the encoder was replaced by a MobileNetV2 [36] reduced with a width multiplier, which allows the manipulation of the input width of a layer, of $\alpha = 0.35$. Additionally, the last convolutional layer was adjusted to a 1×1 convolutional layer with a sigmoid activation function, which is more appropriate for a binary segmentation.

Before the training procedure, the images were scaled and resized to 512×512 pixels. The following classic data augmentation procedure was applied: the images were randomly flipped vertically and horizontally, randomly transposed, randomly modify brightness, saturation, contrast and hue, and randomly add Gaussian noise. To optimize the network, we followed the procedure from the previous work [10]: the stochastic optimization of the model was performed with the soft Dice Loss ($1 - $ Dice), with a batch size of 4, a 90/10 partition for the training/validation subsets and the Adam optimizer associated with a cyclic learning rate [37].

3.2.3. Evaluation

Although the evaluation the generated images is still an active frontier of research [38], they may be analysed by visual inspection, metrics of similarity and the impact of using them in segmentation can also be calculated.

CycleGAN evaluation metrics The visual inspection was based on domain-specific knowledge of intrinsic dermoscopic features, such as pigmented networks and diffused pigmentation, the appearance of macroscopic artefacts, for instance, the surface glare and reflections, and, lastly, the generation of the outward aspect of depth and the modification of the background skin tonality.

To quantitatively evaluate the similarity between the generated and the real images, the Fréchet Inception Distance (FID) [39] was used. This metric measures the distance between the features spaces of specific CNN layer, typically the last pooling layer of InceptionV3 [40], for the real and real and generated images. Since it is based on a distance metric, a lower FID score means that the two analysed distributions are similar. FID is considered a discriminative, robust metric, and evidence shows that it is consistent with human judgement [39,41].

Segmentation evaluation metrics For the evaluation of the segmentation results, the six metrics used in the ISIC challenge of 2018 [28] were adopted, namely: threshold Jaccard coefficient (TJA), Jaccard coefficient (JA), dice coefficient (DI), accuracy (AC), sensitivity (SE) and specificity (SP). The TJA is a metric created specifically for the skin lesion segmentation, which introduces the measure of incorrectness. If the value of JA, on each image, is below 65% threshold then JA is considered 0.

4. Results and Discussion

4.1. Evaluation of the Generated Images

4.1.1. Visual Inspection

A visual assessment was performed to evaluate the outputs' realism, by identifying the loss or preservation of some dermoscopic structures. The datasets that had both dermoscopic and macroscopic for the same skin lesion were used, namely the EDRA and SMARTSKINS 2014/2015. The same analysis was carried out with images from the ISIC and PH2 test subsets; these images were not used during the training phase of the CycleGAN.

EDRA Figure 3a shows the results obtained from the trained CycleGAN in the test subset of the EDRA dataset—It is possible to compare the macroscopic image to the dermoscopic image translated into the macroscopic domain (TransMacro) and the macroscopic image translated into the dermoscopic domain (TransDermo). In the case of the dermoscopic to macroscopic translation, we can observe that the model was able to generate plausible macroscopic images from dermoscopic images. In particular, several successful transformations unique to the macroscopic domain were obtained, such as: (i) The generation of depth in the TransMacro images, that is, lesion images with nodular aspect from flat dermoscopic images, shown in Figure 3a (row 1); (ii) The expected appearance of surface glare and change of skin tonality due to the absence of polarized light in macroscopic images, which can be seen in Figure 3a (rows 1, 2, and 3); and (iii) The loss of dermoscopic characteristics such as specific pigmentations or diffuse borders, as illustrated in Figure 3a (rows 1 and 2). It should be noted that failure cases occur when there is the presence of gel or ruler markings and round black borders. These three characteristics never appear in macroscopic images, so, understandably, the model could not learn how to address these artefacts. Where there is gel in the lesion, the model only performed slight modifications to the input, as shown in Figure 3a row 4.

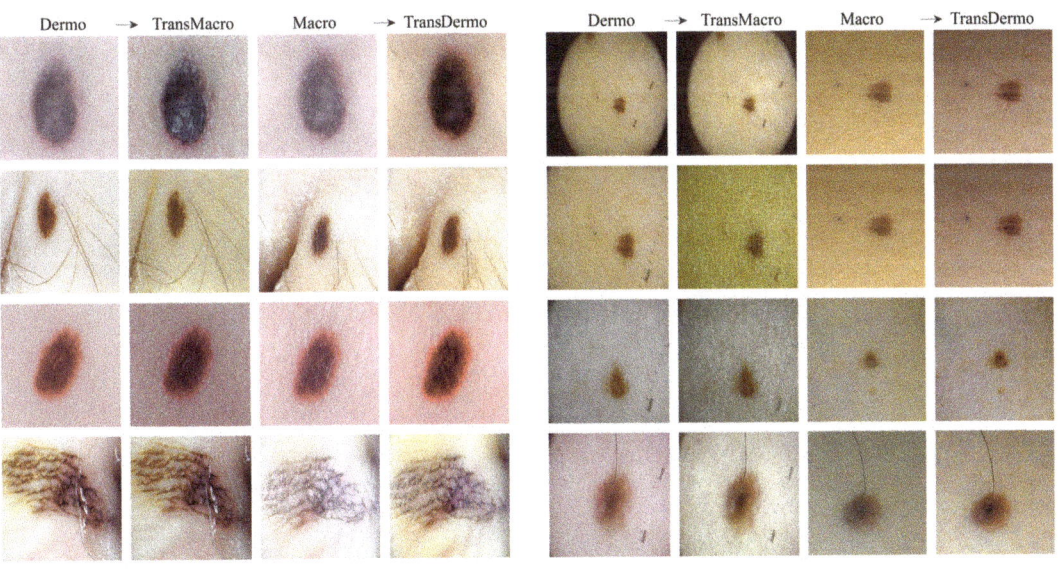

(a) EDRA (b) SMARTSKINS 2014/2015

Figure 3. Examples of the translation between domains in EDRA (**a**) and SMARTSKINS 2014/2015 (**b**) tests subsets. For each subfigure, from left to right: pair Dermo→TransMacro and pair Macro→TransDermo.

However, the inverse transformation seems to lead to unsatisfactory results. One possible explanation is the incapacity of the model of extrapolating the greater details of the dermoscopic images. Considering all the specific details normally obtained in the dermoscopic image, the model was not able to capture sufficient features to solve this task.

SMARTSKINS 2014/2015 This dataset proved quite challenging for the model due to the dark corners in all dermoscopic images. Figure 3b (row 1) shows this failure case, which usually results in minimal to no changes in the TransMacro result. Since we suspected that the cause of failure was the fact that macroscopic images never have these dark borders, and consequently the generator does not learn how to deal with the characteristic, the dark corners were removed, by cropping the image. This pre-processing step led to a considerable improvement in the results. Figure 3b (row 2), shows the translation of the same dermoscopic image, this time cropped. Here, the model was able to generate an appearance of reflection and modify the skin tonality, which can be seen in Figure 3b (rows 2, 3, and 4). In this dataset, the generation of depth skin lesion can also be seen in Figure 3b (row 4), however not as evidently as in the previous dataset.

In this dataset, an interesting result was obtained in the macroscopic to dermoscopic translation. Figure 3b (row 4) shows the generation of a region with red colouration in the left inferior area of the lesion of the TransDermo image. This colouration, which was not present in the original macroscopic image, is also present in the original dermoscopic image. Another transformation detected, in this image was the accentuation in the contrast of the two brown tonalities of the lesion.

ISIC Figure 4 shows the results obtained from the trained CycleGAN in the ISIC test subset. As expected, the best transformations occured in this subset, as the ISIC images represented a large portion of the training dataset. For the most part, the conversions in this dataset can be categorised into four main ones which are shown in Figure 4 in the top row: (i) the appearance of surface glare and reflections; (ii) generation of depth; (iii) loss of dermoscopic structures; and (iv) generation of squamous appearance. Regarding the generation of surrounding skin with colourization and surface glared, typical of the macroscopic domain (Figure 4, pair A, top row), this modification is usually accompanied by the loss on any structure typical of the dermoscopic domain. This loss can be from the diffuse borders, regression structure or pigmented networks (Figure 4, pairs A, B and C, top row). Another frequent modification is the generation of squamous like plaque or nodular appearance (Figure 4 pair D of the top row). The generation of an appearance of depth in the image is also very prevalent (Figure 4, pairs A, B and C, top row).

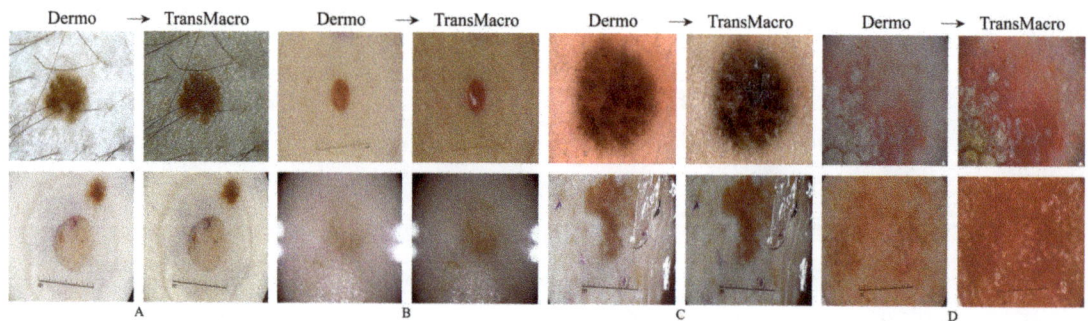

Figure 4. Examples of successful (**top row**) and failure cases (**bottom row**) of translation from the dermoscopic domain to the macroscopic domain in ISIC test subset. The letters A, B, C and D represent pairs of Dermo→TransMacro.

In the translation of dermoscopic to the macroscopic domain, there are several noticeable limitations, as shown in Figure 4 (bottom row). The appearance of artefacts such as black frames, dark corners, gel substances, intensive illuminations spots, ink marks and air bubbles can lead to translations with no noticeable modifications (Figure 4, pairs A, B and C, bottom row). Another main concern is the transformation to an uncharacteristic lesion which does not resemble any specific domain. Normally these translated images have a reddish tone or complete loss of definition (Figure 4, pair D, bottom row).

PH2 Figure 5 shows the results obtained from the trained CycleGAN in the PH2 test subset. In order to obtain reasonable results, it was necessary to crop the image to remove the dark corners just as it was done in the SMARTSKINS 2014/2015 dataset. After this pre-processing step, the most successful transformations were the change in the tonality of the surrounding skin, the addition of reflections, the darkening of the lesion and some elevation of the lesions. However, it should be noted that the results were not as satisfactory as in the previous test subsets.

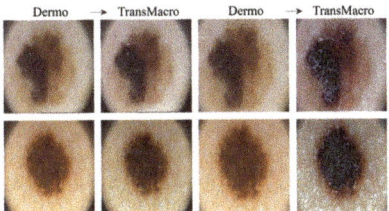

Figure 5. Examples of successful (column 1 and 2) and failure cases (column 3 and 4) of translation from the dermoscopic domain to the macroscopic domain in the PH2 test subset. From Left to right: pair Dermo→TransMacro, cropped pair Dermo→TransMacro.

4.1.2. Fréchet Inception Distance Results

The FID metric was used to ascertain the feasibility of using the CycleGAN to translate between the macroscopic and dermoscopic domains. For this purpose, the distance between three pairs of domains was analysed: (i) Macro/Dermo, between the macroscopic and dermoscopic original images; (ii) Macro/TransMacro, between the original macroscopic image and the dermoscopic image translated into the macroscopic domain; (iii) Dermo/TransDermo, between the original dermoscopic image and the macroscopic image translated into the dermoscopic domain. Since the first pair, Macro/Dermo, compares original images, it can be considered our reference value. If the FID value of the other pairs is lower than the reference value, it means that the translation led to an approximation of the translated images to the target domain, implying a transfer of characteristics between domains.

This change can also be directly compared using the variation ratio (VR), VR = $\frac{ReferenceValue - Value}{ReferenceValue}$, which will directly compare the change of similarity between the original domains (reference value) and the translated domains. Table 3 presents the computed FID scores, using the official implementation in TensorFlow [39], on the test subsets of EDRA, SMARTSKINS 2014/2015, PH2 (set D) and ISIC (set D). Since PH2 (set D) and ISIC (set D) do not have a macroscopic image for each dermoscopic image, they were compared with the macroscopic images of the train subset of Dermofit (set M) and SMARTSKINS (set M).

Table 3. Fréchet Inception Distance (FID) and Variation Ratio (VR) results in the test subsets of EDRA, SMARTSKINS 2014/2015, PH2 and ISIC.

Domains	EDRA		SMARTSKINS 2014/2015				ISIC (Set D)		PH2 (Set D)	
			Uncropped		Cropped				Cropped	
	FID	VR	FID	VR	FID	VR	FID	VR	FID	VR
Macro/Dermo (reference value)	167.9		331.7		294.2		180.9		292.9	
Macro/TransMacro	160.2	0.05	285.1	0.15	177.5	0.40	123.7	0.31	285.7	0.02
Dermo/TransDermo	186.4	−0.11	285.6	0.14	263.6	0.10	-		-	

When analysing the FID results, it is possible to confirm several findings reached in the visual inspection. In the EDRA test subset, the FID score of 160.2 between the domains Macro/TransMacro is lower than the value 167.9 between the Macro/Dermo. This shows that the translations of the dermoscopic images to macroscopic was successful and implies that the images gain specific macroscopic characteristic. In contrast, the value between Dermo/TransDermo is much higher, reaching 186.4. When comparing to the reference value, it leads to a negative VR, which indicates that translating the macroscopic images into dermoscopic made the domains more dissimilar. This further corroborates the conclusion of the visual analysis that the macroscopic to dermoscopic translation was not successful.

In the SMARTSKINS 2014/2015 test subset, the macroscopic images were compared with the uncropped and cropped dermoscopic images, as in the visual analysis. Considering that the decay between the reference FID score with the cropped dermoscopic (Macro/TransMacro) is much higher than decay between the reference value using the uncropped dermoscopic images, it can be stated that this preprocessing step improves the results. In fact, the VR of the Macro/TransMacro with cropped dermoscopic is the highest among test subsets. When analysing the other translation (Dermo/TransDermo), the absolute value of the FID score with the cropped dermoscopic (263.6) is lower than with the uncropped dermoscopic (285.6). However, the VR is also lower, which means that the preprocessing did not improve as much the results.

In the ISIC (Set D) test subset, the dermoscopic images were compared with the train images of Set M. Upon translation, the absolute FID score is the lowest of the test subsets (123.7), validating the assessment made in the visual inspection—the best results were obtained in this dataset.

The PH2 test subset was also compared with the train images of Set M. Here, the FID value obtained was the highest absolute value with the lowest percentage of variation, which is consistent with the small changes observed in the visual inspection.

Lastly, the CycleGAN was used to translate the training/validation images from Set D to the macroscopic domain. This led to the creation of the Set $M_{artificial}$ to augment the macroscopic images. Table 4 shows the results of the FID between the segmentation training datasets set M and Set D and the new generated Set $M_{artificial}$. The FID score between Set M/set $M_{artificial}$ (102.4) is much lower than the reference value between Set M/Set D (181.1). This drop leads to the most significant change in the variation ratio between the reference value and the Macro/TransMacro domains. Considering also the low absolute value of the FID score (102.4), it is possible to conclude that the images of Set $M_{artificial}$ obtain several key features of the macroscopic domain.

Table 4. Fréchet Inception Distance (FID) and Variation Ratio (VR) results between set M, set D and set $M_{artificial}$.

Domains	Segmentation Sets	FID	VR
Macro/Dermo (reference value)	Set M/Set D	181.1	
Macro/TransMacro	Set M/set $M_{artificial}$	102.4	0.43

4.2. Segmentation Results

The final objective of translating the images to the macroscopic domain was improving the model's segmentation capacity for macroscopic images. Thus, the reduced Mobile DeepLab model was trained with two different datasets, first with the merging of Set M and Set D and, after, with the combined Set M and Set $M_{artificial}$. The first dataset (Set M + Set D) serves to check if the performance improvement is due to more samples or the addition of the translated images. The datasets had a total of 3230 samples: being Set D + Set M composed of 2/3 of dermoscopic images, while the Set M + Set $M_{artificial}$ is composed of 2/3 of macroscopic images artificially generated with the CycleGAN.

Table 5 compares the methods described in the related work [10,16,18], which exploit the SMARTSKINS database, with the two aforementioned models. The addition of the translated macroscopic images, Set M + Set $M_{artificial}$ (Table 5, row 6), outperforms the other methods by a considerable margin. This augmentation technique leads to an improvement even when compared to the classical augmentation methods (Table 5, row 3), to the transfer learning technique (Table 5, row 4) and to the addition of the original dermoscopic images (Table 5, row 5). With an 85.13% TJA and 86.69% JA, our method, that includes the translated macroscopic images, sets a new state-of-the-art performance in the SMARTSKINS database.

Table 5. Comparison between the proposed methods and related studies using the SMARTSKINS database. The best result, for each of the metrics in the present table, is identified in boldface.

Method	TJA	JA	DI	AC	SE	SP
Adaptive Thresholding [16]	-	81.58	-	97.38	-	-
Gossip Network [18]	-	-	83.36	-	-	-
Reduce Mobile DeepLab (Macroscopic) [10]	78.51	82.64	90.14	98.96	95.40	99.15
Reduce Mobile DeepLab (Transfer Learning) [10]	78.04	82.21	89.89	98.90	96.05	99.09
Our Method (Set M + Set D)	78.27	82.58	90.22	98.88	98.39	98.89
Our Method (Set M + Set $M_{artificial}$)	**85.13**	**86.69**	**92.74**	**99.18**	96.36	**99.32**

For the Dermofit database, there was only one record of the use of this database for segmentation [10], which is compared with our methods in Table 6. In the Dermofit test subset, the addition of artificial macroscopic images (Table 6, row 4) has similar results to the model trained with Set M + Set D (Table 6, row 3). In fact, both models, while outperforming the classical data augmentation (Table 6, row 1), seem to underperform when compared with the transfer learning method (Table 6, row 2) used in Reference [10]. However, it is only possible to make a distinction with the TJA metric, which features a 1.16% decrease. This underperformance means that only four more images were below the 65% threshold in the model trained with the artificial macroscopic images (Table 6, row 4) than with the transfer learning method (Table 6, row 2).

Table 6. Comparison between the proposed methods and related studies using the Dermofit Image Library database. The best result, for each of the metrics in the present table, is identified in boldface.

Method	TJA	JA	DI	AC	SE	SP
Reduce Mobile DeepLab (Macroscopic) [10]	72.97	80.26	88.26	93.51	87.56	**96.86**
Reduce Mobile DeepLab (Transfer Learning) [10]	**75.46**	**81.03**	**88.79**	**93.78**	89.68	96.13
Our Method (Set M + Set D)	74.42	80.88	88.75	93.53	**90.74**	95.14
Our Method (Set M + Set $M_{artificial}$)	74.30	80.90	88.62	93.54	88.91	95.84

The fundamental reason behind this discrepancy in the results between the two databases can be the melanocytic bias present in most of the databases. Since the past research focused on the distinction between melanocytic lesions [29], almost all databases are heavily biased towards this type of lesions. Nowadays, there has been an attempt to solve this issue, however, this is mainly in dermoscopic datasets [28,29]. Since SMARTSKINS database has this biased distribution of lesions it leads to a significant improvement. However, Dermofit Image Library has a high non-melanocytic percentage of images. Due to this disparity with all other available databases the improvement is not as substantial.

It is of note that in Dermofit questionable ground truth segmentation masks were found as depicted in Figure 6. Both these labels appear to be the result of a segmentation method which over-segmented the lesion due to the hair artefacts present in the images, which is a common occurrence when the removal of the hairs is ineffective [42].

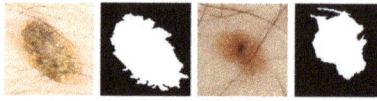

Figure 6. Examples of questionable segmentation labels of the Dermofit Database.

Figure 7a,b show various examples of the predicted segmentation mask of the model trained with the addition of the artificial images, Set M + Set $M_{artificial}$, compared with the ground truth label. The juxtaposition of the predicted segmentation mask with the ground truth originated a plot which makes it possible to ascertain the viability of the segmentation by colour code. Fundamentally, the yellow represents where both masks overlap (true positives), the red the over-segmented areas (false positives) and the green the under-segmented areas (false negatives). Over the entire test subset, the normalized value of false positive pixels is of 0.12 for the Dermofit and 0.032 for the SMARTSKINS dataset and the normalized value of false negatives is of 0.04 and 0.007, respectively.

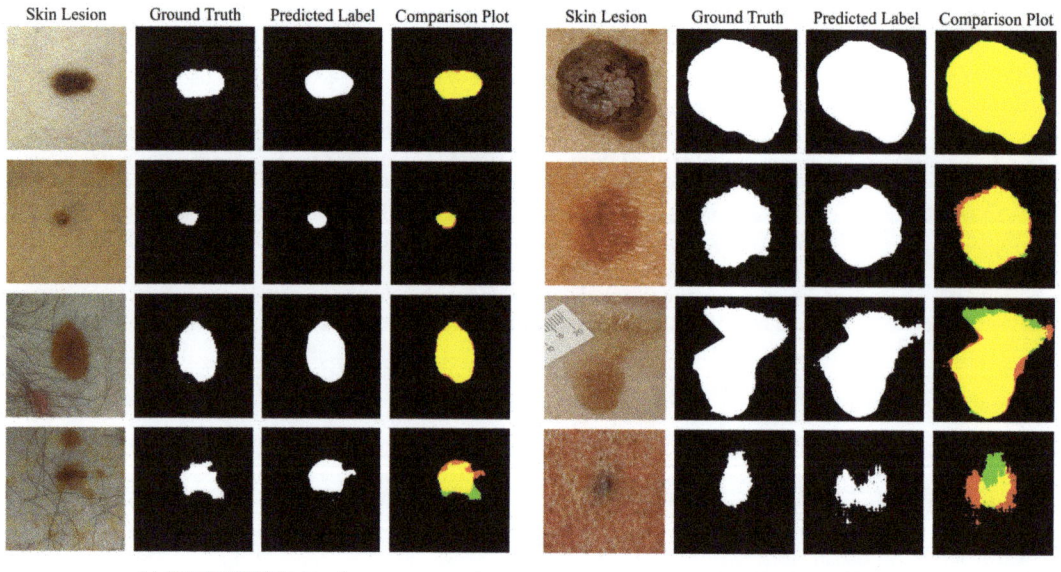

(a) SMARTSKINS test subset. (b) Dermofit test subset.

Figure 7. Segmentation results of the Set M + Set $M_{artificial}$ from the tests subsets. In the comparison images: yellow —true positives; red —false positives; green —false negatives; black—true negatives.

When analysing the results in detail when using the model that includes generated macroscopic images from each of the test subsets, it is possible to observe that all segmentation results are almost identical in shape to the ground truth when dealing with melanocytic lesions with high contrast with the surrounding skin and no artefacts present (Figure 7a,b row 1). This high performance is maintained with lesions with low contrast and uneven pigmentation (Figure 7a,b row 2). Furthermore, if we observe Figure 7a,b row 3, it is possible to see that the model is able to correctly segment in the proximity of regions with the red colouration, with hairs and superimposed artefacts. However, the model seems to underperform when the lesion presents a dysplastic form, with the hair artefact, and with heavily porous skin and low contrast (Figure 7a,b row 4).

5. Conclusions

Nowadays, with skin cancer's ever-growing incidence, developing a robust system capable of assisting physicians in cancer screening is of paramount importance. The ubiquitous spread of smartphones combined with deep learning models' robustness makes mobile teledermatology a possible tipping point for the early diagnosis of skin lesions. However, this has been hindered by the small size of macroscopic datasets available.

In this paper, we tackle the challenge of improving the macroscopic skin lesion segmentation performance by effectively taking advantage of the large dermoscopic datasets available. Using a CycleGAN, it was possible to translate between the two domains and generate natural-looking artificial macroscopic skin lesions. Furthermore, we demonstrate the quality of the generated images quantitatively using the FID score. This analysis confirmed most of the visual inspection conclusions and demonstrated the artificial macroscopic images' fidelity.

Regarding the use of macroscopic artificial images to improve the segmentation capacity, it was demonstrated the overall effectiveness of this method. In both available databases, there was an improvement when comparing with classical data augmentation method. As future work, we should consider to examine the segmentation masks of the Dermofit Image Library, in order to correct them, however it should be noted that this segmentation should be done preferable by experts.

Undeniably, the assessment of the images by an expert dermatologist would be interesting to further evaluate the relevance of the generated medical data. However, this is not critical since the final objective is to improve the segmentation model's performance.

Further work is needed to overcome the melanocytic bias of the databases. This could begin with the collection of new non-melanocytic macroscopic images. However, when taking into consideration the arduousness of collecting healthcare data, the applications of differentiated augmentation techniques should be studied. This can include the analysis of loss functions that represent more faithfully our design goals, such as condition-specific losses or texture-focused losses as in Reference [22]. Other improvements can also be made to the generator architecture of the CycleGAN framework since its goal is the translation of style, and it has limited translation capacity in form transfiguration.

Author Contributions: Conceptualization, C.A., L.F.T., M.J.M.V. and L.R.; Data curation, C.A.; Formal analysis, C.A.; Funding acquisition, M.J.M.V.; Investigation, C.A.; Methodology, C.A., L.F.T. and L.R.; Project administration, M.J.M.V.; Resources, M.J.M.V.; Software, C.A.; Supervision, L.F.T., M.J.M.V. and L.R.; Validation, C.A., L.F.T., M.J.M.V. and L.R.; Visualization, C.A.; Writing—original draft, C.A.; Writing—review & editing, L.F.T., M.J.M.V. and L.R. All authors have read and agreed to the published version of the manuscript.

Funding: This work was done under the scope of project "DERM.AI: Usage of Artificial Intelligence to Power Teledermatological Screening" and supported by national funds through 'FCT—Foundation for Science and Technology, I.P.', with reference DSAIPA/AI/0031/2018.

Institutional Review Board Statement: Not applicable.

Informed Consent Statement: Not applicable.

Data Availability Statement: International Skin Imaging Collaboration (ISIC) challenges datasets: Publicly available dataset was analyzed in this study. This data can be found here: https://challenge.isic-archive.com/data. PH2 dataset: Publicly available dataset was analyzed in this study. This data can be found here: https://www.fc.up.pt/addi/ph2%20database.html. SMARTSKINS segmentation and 2014/2015: The data presented in this study are available on request from the corresponding author. The data are not publicly available due to privacy reasons. Dermofit image Library: Restrictions apply to the availability of these data. Data was obtained from The University of Edinburgh and are available at https://licensing.edinburgh-innovations.ed.ac.uk/i/software/dermofit-image-library.html with the permission of The University of Edinburgh. EDRA: Restrictions apply to the availability of these data. Data was obtained from DS Medica srl and are available at http://www.dermoscopy.org/atlas/order_cd.asp with the permission of DS Medica srl based in

Milan in Viale Monza 133 - CF. and VAT number 12676030153.

Conflicts of Interest: The authors declare no conflict of interest.

References

1. Society, A.C. Cancer Facts and Figures 2019. 2019. Available online: https://www.cancer.org/content/dam/cancer-org/research/cancer-facts-and-statistics/annual-cancer-facts-and-figures/2019/cancer-facts-and-figures-2019.pdf (accessed on 17 June 2019).
2. Perera, E.; Gnaneswaran, N.; Staines, C.; Win, A.K.; Sinclair, R. Incidence and prevalence of non-melanoma skin cancer in Australia: A systematic review. *Australas. J. Dermatol.* **2015**, *56*, 258–267. [CrossRef]
3. de Carvalho, T.M.; Noels, E.; Wakkee, M.; Udrea, A.; Nijsten, T. Development of smartphone apps for skin cancer risk assessment: progress and promise. *JMIR Dermatol.* **2019**, *2*, e13376. [CrossRef]
4. Xiong, M.; Pfau, J.; Young, A.T.; Wei, M.L. Artificial Intelligence in Teledermatology. *Curr. Dermatol. Rep.* **2019**, *8*, 85–90. [CrossRef]
5. Kittler, H.; Pehamberger, H.; Wolff, K.; Binder, M. Diagnostic accuracy of dermoscopy. *Lancet Oncol.* **2002**, *3*, 159–165. [CrossRef]
6. Carli, P.; Quercioli, E.; Sestini, S.; Stante, M.; Ricci, L.; Brunasso, G.; De Giorgi, V. Pattern analysis, not simplified algorithms, is the most reliable method for teaching dermoscopy for melanoma diagnosis to residents in dermatology. *Br. J. Dermatol.* **2003**, *148*, 981–984. [CrossRef] [PubMed]
7. Vestergaard, M.; Macaskill, P.; Holt, P.; Menzies, S. Dermoscopy compared with naked eye examination for the diagnosis of primary melanoma: a meta-analysis of studies performed in a clinical setting. *Br. J. Dermatol.* **2008**, *159*, 669–676. [CrossRef]
8. Litjens, G.; Kooi, T.; Bejnordi, B.E.; Setio, A.A.A.; Ciompi, F.; Ghafoorian, M.; Van Der Laak, J.A.; Van Ginneken, B.; Sánchez, C.I. A survey on deep learning in medical image analysis. *Med. Image Anal.* **2017**, *42*, 60–88. [CrossRef]
9. Gu, Y.; Ge, Z.; Bonnington, C.P.; Zhou, J. Progressive Transfer Learning and Adversarial Domain Adaptation for Cross-Domain Skin Disease Classification. *IEEE J. Biomed. Health Inform.* **2019**, *24*, 1379–1393. [CrossRef]
10. Andrade, C.; Teixeira, L.F.; Vasconcelos, M.J.M.; Rosado, L. Deep Learning Models for Segmentation of Mobile-Acquired Dermatological Images. In *International Conference on Image Analysis and Recognition*; Springer: Póvoa de Varzim, Portugal, 2020; pp. 228–237.
11. Korotkov, K.; Garcia, R. Computerized analysis of pigmented skin lesions: A review. *Artif. Intell. Med.* **2012**, *56*, 69–90. [CrossRef]
12. Zhu, J.Y.; Park, T.; Isola, P.; Efros, A.A. Unpaired image-to-image translation using cycle-consistent adversarial networks. In Proceedings of the IEEE International Conference on Computer Vision, Venice, Italy, 22–29 October 2017; pp. 2223–2232.
13. Flores, E.; Scharcanski, J. Segmentation of melanocytic skin lesions using feature learning and dictionaries. *Expert Syst. Appl.* **2016**, *56*, 300–309. [CrossRef]
14. Cavalcanti, P.G.; Scharcanski, J. A coarse-to-fine approach for segmenting melanocytic skin lesions in standard camera images. *Comput. Methods Programs Biomed.* **2013**, *112*, 684–693. [CrossRef] [PubMed]
15. Oliveira, R.B.; Marranghello, N.; Pereira, A.S.; Tavares, J.M.R. A computational approach for detecting pigmented skin lesions in macroscopic images. *Expert Syst. Appl.* **2016**, *61*, 53–63. [CrossRef]
16. Rosado, L.; Vasconcelos, M. Automatic segmentation methodology for dermatological images acquired via mobile devices. In Proceedings of 8th International Conference on Health Informatics, Lisbon, Portugal, 12–15 January 2015; pp. 246–251.
17. Cavalcanti, P.G.; Yari, Y.; Scharcanski, J. Pigmented skin lesion segmentation on macroscopic images. In Proceedings of the 2010 25th International Conference of Image and Vision Computing, Queenstown, New Zealan, 8–9 November 2010; pp. 1–7.
18. Fernandes, K.; Cruz, R.; Cardoso, J.S. Deep image segmentation by quality inference. In Proceedings of the 2018 International Joint Conference on Neural Networks (IJCNN), Rio de Janeiro, Brazil, 8–13 July 2018; pp. 1–8.
19. Shorten, C.; Khoshgoftaar, T.M. A survey on image data augmentation for deep learning. *J. Big Data* **2019**, *6*, 60. [CrossRef]
20. Mikołajczyk, A.; Grochowski, M. Data augmentation for improving deep learning in image classification problem. In Proceedings of the 2018 International Interdisciplinary PhD Workshop (IIPhDW), Swinoujscie, Poland, 9–12 May 2018; pp. 117–122.
21. Baur, C.; Albarqouni, S.; Navab, N. Generating highly realistic images of skin lesions with GANs. In *OR 2.0 Context-Aware Operating Theaters, Computer Assisted Robotic Endoscopy, Clinical Image-Based Procedures, and Skin Image Analysis*; Springer: Granada, Spain, 2018; pp. 260–267.
22. Ghorbani, A.; Natarajan, V.; Coz, D.; Liu, Y. DermGAN: Synthetic Generation of Clinical Skin Images with Pathology. *arXiv* **2019**, arXiv:1911.08716.
23. Ali, I.S.; Mohamed, M.F.; Mahdy, Y.B. Data Augmentation for Skin Lesion using Self-Attention based Progressive Generative Adversarial Network. *arXiv* **2019**, arXiv:1910.11960.
24. Ltd, E.I. Dermofit Image Library—Edinburgh Innovations. 2019. Available online: https://licensing.eri.ed.ac.uk/i/software/dermofit-image-library.html (accessed on 11 June 2019).
25. Vasconcelos, M.J.M.; Rosado, L.; Ferreira, M. Principal axes-based asymmetry assessment methodology for skin lesion image analysis. In *International Symposium on Visual Computing*; Springer: Las Vegas, NV, USA,2014; pp. 21–31.
26. Gutman, D.; Codella, N.C.F.; Celebi, E.; Helba, B.; Marchetti, M.; Mishra, N.; Halpern, A. Skin Lesion Analysis toward Melanoma Detection: A Challenge at the International Symposium on Biomedical Imaging (ISBI) 2016, hosted by the International Skin Imaging Collaboration (ISIC). *arXiv* **2016**, arXiv:1605.01397.

27. Codella, N.C.F.; Gutman, D.; Celebi, M.E.; Helba, B.; Marchetti, M.A.; Dusza, S.W.; Kalloo, A.; Liopyris, K.; Mishra, N.; Kittler, H.; et al. Skin lesion analysis toward melanoma detection: A challenge at the 2017 International symposium on biomedical imaging (ISBI), hosted by the international skin imaging collaboration (ISIC). In Proceedings of the 2018 IEEE 15th International Symposium on Biomedical Imaging (ISBI 2018), Washington, DC, USA, 4–7 April 2018; [CrossRef]
28. Codella, N.; Rotemberg, V.; Tschandl, P.; Celebi, M.E.; Dusza, S.; Gutman, D.; Helba, B.; Kalloo, A.; Liopyris, K.; Marchetti, M.; et al. Skin Lesion Analysis Toward Melanoma Detection 2018: A Challenge Hosted by the International Skin Imaging Collaboration (ISIC). *arXiv* **2019**, arXiv:1902.03368.
29. Tschandl, P.; Rosendahl, C.; Kittler, H. The HAM10000 dataset, a large collection of multi-source dermatoscopic images of common pigmented skin lesions. *Sci. Data* **2018**, *5*, 180161. [CrossRef]
30. Mendonça, T.; Ferreira, P.M.; Marques, J.S.; Marcal, A.R.; Rozeira, J. PH 2-A dermoscopic image database for research and benchmarking. In Proceedings of the 2013 35th Annual International Conference of the IEEE Engineering in Medicine and Biology Society (EMBC), Osaka, Japan, 3–7 July 2013; pp. 5437–5440.
31. Argenziano, G.; Soyer, H.; De Giorgi, V.; Piccolo, D.; Carli, P.; Delfino, M. *Interactive Atlas of Dermoscopy (Book and CD-ROM)*; Edra Medical Publishing & New Media: Milan, Italy, 2000.
32. ISIC Archive. 2019. Available online: https://www.isic-archive.com/#!/topWithHeader/onlyHeaderTop/gallery (accessed on 11 June 2019).
33. Johnson, J.; Alahi, A.; Fei-Fei, L. Perceptual losses for real-time style transfer and super-resolution. In *European Conference on Computer Vision*; Springer: Amsterdam, The Netherlands 2016; pp. 694–711.
34. Isola, P.; Zhu, J.Y.; Zhou, T.; Efros, A.A. Image-to-image translation with conditional adversarial networks. In Proceedings of the IEEE Conference on Computer Vision and Pattern Recognition, Honolulu, HI, USA, 21–26 July 2017; pp. 1125–1134.
35. Chen, L.C.; Zhu, Y.; Papandreou, G.; Schroff, F.; Adam, H. Encoder-decoder with atrous separable convolution for semantic image segmentation. In Proceedings of the European Conference on Computer Vision (ECCV), Munich, Germany, 8–14 September 2018; pp. 801–818.
36. Sandler, M.; Howard, A.; Zhu, M.; Zhmoginov, A.; Chen, L.C. MobileNetV2: Inverted Residuals and Linear Bottlenecks. In Proceedings of the 2018 IEEE/CVF Conference on Computer Vision and Pattern Recognition, Salt Lake City, UT, USA, 18–23 June 2018; [CrossRef]
37. Smith, L.N. Cyclical learning rates for training neural networks. In Proceedings of the 2017 IEEE Winter Conference on Applications of Computer Vision (WACV), Santa Rosa, CA, USA, 24–31 March 2017; pp. 464–472.
38. Goodfellow, I. NIPS 2016 Tutorial: Generative Adversarial Networks. *arXiv* **2016**, arXiv:1701.00160.
39. Heusel, M.; Ramsauer, H.; Unterthiner, T.; Nessler, B.; Klambauer, G.; Hochreiter, S. GANs Trained by a Two Time-Scale Update Rule Converge to a Nash Equilibrium. *arXiv* **2017**, arXiv:1706.08500.
40. Szegedy, C.; Vanhoucke, V.; Ioffe, S.; Shlens, J.; Wojna, Z. Rethinking the Inception Architecture for Computer Vision. In Proceedings of the 2016 IEEE Conference on Computer Vision and Pattern Recognition (CVPR), Las Vegas, NV, USA, 27–30 June 2016; [CrossRef]
41. Xu, Q.; Huang, G.; Yuan, Y.; Guo, C.; Sun, Y.; Wu, F.; Weinberger, K. An empirical study on evaluation metrics of generative adversarial networks. *arXiv* **2018**, arXiv:1806.07755.
42. Abbas, Q.; Celebi, M.E.; García, I.F. Hair removal methods: A comparative study for dermoscopy images. *Biomed. Signal Process. Control* **2011**, *6*, 395–404. [CrossRef]

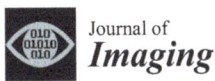

Article

Musculoskeletal Images Classification for Detection of Fractures Using Transfer Learning

Ibrahem Kandel [1,*], Mauro Castelli [1] and Aleš Popovič [1,2]

[1] Nova Information Management School (NOVA IMS), Universidade Nova de Lisboa, Campus de Campolide, 1070-312 Lisboa, Portugal; mcastelli@novaims.unl.pt (M.C.); ales.popovic@ef.uni-lj.si (A.P.)
[2] School of Economics and Business, University of Ljubljana, Kardeljeva Ploščad 17, 1000 Ljubljana, Slovenia
* Correspondence: D20181143@novaims.unl.pt

Received: 20 August 2020; Accepted: 20 November 2020; Published: 23 November 2020

Abstract: The classification of the musculoskeletal images can be very challenging, mostly when it is being done in the emergency room, where a decision must be made rapidly. The computer vision domain has gained increasing attention in recent years, due to its achievements in image classification. The convolutional neural network (CNN) is one of the latest computer vision algorithms that achieved state-of-the-art results. A CNN requires an enormous number of images to be adequately trained, and these are always scarce in the medical field. Transfer learning is a technique that is being used to train the CNN by using fewer images. In this paper, we study the appropriate method to classify musculoskeletal images by transfer learning and by training from scratch. We applied six state-of-the-art architectures and compared their performance with transfer learning and with a network trained from scratch. From our results, transfer learning did increase the model performance significantly, and, additionally, it made the model less prone to overfitting.

Keywords: transfer learning; computer vision; convolutional neural networks; image classification; musculoskeletal images; deep learning; medical images

1. Introduction

Bone fractures are among the most common conditions that are treated in emergency rooms [1]. Bone fractures represent a severe condition that could result from an accident or a disease like osteoporosis. The fractures can lead to permanent damage or even death in severe cases. The most common way of detecting bone fractures is by investigating an X-ray image of the suspected organ. Reading an X-ray is a complex task, especially in emergency rooms, where the patient is usually in severe pain, and the fractures are not always visible to doctors. Musculoskeletal images are a subspecialty of radiology, which includes several techniques like X-ray, Computed Tomography (CT), and Magnetic Resonance Imaging (MRI), among others. For detecting fractures, the most commonly used method is the musculoskeletal X-ray image [2]. This process involves the radiologists, who are the doctors responsible for classifying the musculoskeletal images, and the emergency physicians, who are the doctors present in the emergency room where any patient with a sudden injury is admitted once arrived at the hospital. Emergency physicians are not very experienced in reading X-ray images like the radiologists, and they are prone to errors and misclassifications [3,4]. Image-classification software can help emergency physicians to accurately and rapidly diagnose a fracture [5], especially in emergency rooms, where a second opinion is much needed and, usually, is not available.

Deep learning is a recent breakthrough in the field of artificial intelligence, and it has demonstrated its potential in learning and prioritizing essential features of a given dataset without being explicitly programmed to do so. The autonomous behavior of deep learning makes it particularly suitable in the field of computer vision. The area of computer vision includes several tasks, like image segmentation, image detection, and image classification. Deep learning was successfully applied in many computer vision tasks, like in retinal image segmentation [6], histopathology image classification [7], and MRI image classification [8], among others.

Focusing on image classification, in 2012, Krizhevsky et al. [9] proposed a convolutional neural network CNN-based model, and they won a very popular image classification challenge called ILSVRC. Afterward, CNNs gained popularity in the area of computer vision, and it is nowadays considered the state-of-the-art technique for image classification. The process of training a classifier is time-consuming and requires large datasets to be correctly trained. In the medical field, there is always a scarcity of images that can be used to train a classifier, mainly due to the regulations implemented in the medical field. Transfer learning is a technique that is usually used to train CNNs, when there are not enough images available or when obtaining new images is particularly difficult. Transfer learning is about training a CNN to classify large non-medical datasets and then use the weights of such a CNN as a starting point for classifying other target images, in our case, X-ray images.

Several studies addressed the classification of musculoskeletal images using deep learning techniques. Rajpurkar et al. [10] introduced a novel dataset called MURA dataset that contains 40,005 musculoskeletal images. The authors used DenseNet169 CNN to compare the performance of the CNN against three radiologists. The model achieved an acceptable performance compared to the predictions of the radiologists. Chada [11] investigated the performance of three state-of-the-art CNNs, namely DenseNet169, DenseNet201, and InceptionResNetV2, on the MURA dataset. The author fine-tuned the three architectures using Adam optimizer with a learning rate of 0.0001. Fifty epochs were used with a batch size of eight images to train the model. The author reported that DenseNet201 achieved the best performance for the humerus images, with a Kappa score of 0.764, and InceptionResNetV2 achieved the best performance for the finger images, with a Kappa score of 0.555.

To demonstrate the importance of deep learning in the emergency room for fracture detections, Lindsey et al. [5] investigated the usage of CNNs to detect wrist fractures. Subsequently, they measured the radiologists' performance of detecting fractures with and without the help of CNN. The authors reported that, by using a CNN, the performance of the radiologists increased significantly. Kitamura et al. [12] studied the possibility of detecting ankle fractures with CNNs, using InceptionV3, ResNet, and Xception networks for their experiments. The authors trained a CNN from scratch without any transfer learning, and they used a private dataset and an ensemble of the three architectures and reported an accuracy of 81%.

In this paper, we are extending the work of Rajpurkar et al. [10] and Chada [11] by investigating the usage of transfer learning of a CNN to classify X-ray images to detect bone fractures. To do so, we used six state-of-the-art CNN architectures that were previously trained on the ImageNet dataset (an extensive non-medical dataset). To the best of our knowledge, this is the first paper that performs a rigorous investigation on the use of transfer learning in the context of musculoskeletal image classification. More in detail, we investigate the following:

1. The effect of transfer learning on image classification performance. To do that, we compare the performance of six CNN architectures that were trained on ImageNet to classify fractures images. Then, we train the same datasets with the same networks, but without the ImageNet weights.
2. The best classifier that achieves the best results on the musculoskeletal images.
3. The effect of the fully connected layers on the performance of the network. To do that, two fully connected layers were added after each network, and then we recorded their performance. Subsequently, the layers are removed, and the performance of the networks is recorded as well.

The paper is organized as follows: In Section 2, we present the methodology used. In Section 3, we present the results achieved by training the MURA dataset on the considered CNNs. In Section 4, we present a discussion about the results obtained, and we compare them to other state-of-the-art results. In Section 5, we conclude the paper by summarizing the main findings of this work.

2. Methodology

In this section, we briefly describe the main methods used in this paper.

2.1. Convolutional Neural Networks and Transfer Learning

A convolutional neural network is a feed-forward neural network with at least one convolution layer. A convolution layer is a hidden neural network layer that has a convolution operation, where the convolution operation is a mathematical operation that is used to make use of the spatial information presented in images. Training a CNN requires a significant amount of images, and this is one of the most severe limitations in deep learning. In particular, deep learning has a very strong dependence on massive training data compared to traditional machine learning methods because it needs a large amount of data to understand the latent patterns of data. Unfortunately, there are problems in which insufficient training data are an inescapable issue. This may happen in domains in which obtaining new observations are either expensive, time-consuming, or impossible. In these situations, transfer learning provides a suitable way for training a CNN. More in detail, transfer learning is a technique used in the deep learning field to make use of knowledge that can be shared by different domains. According to Pan and Yang [13], transfer learning can be defined as improving the predictive function, $f_T(.)$ by using the knowledge acquired from the source domain, D_S, into the target domain, D_T. Transfer learning relaxes the hypothesis that the training data must be independent and identically distributed with the test data. This allows us to use transfer learning for training CNNs in a given domain and to use them to subsequently address a problem in which data scarcity is a significant limitation. For more details on transfer learning, the interested reader is referred to Pan and Yang [13].

2.2. State-of-the-Art Architectures

Many CNNs were introduced to participate in the ILSVRC challenge. In this section, we present different CNNs that are considered in this study.

2.2.1. VGG

Simonyan et al. [14] introduced the VGG network in 2014. The VGG was implemented in many variations like VGG16 and VGG19, which only differ in the number of convolution layers used in each. In this paper, we use VGG19 because it is the largest one, and it usually produces better performance than VGG16. VGG19 consists of 19 convolution layers and one dense layer with 4096 neurons to classify the ImageNet images. For more information, the reader is referred to the corresponding paper [14].

2.2.2. Xception

Chollet [15] introduced a novel architecture called Xception (extreme inception), where the author replaced the conventional convolutional layers with depthwise separable convolutional layers. These modified layers decreased the network parameters without decreasing its capacity, which yielded a robust network with fewer parameters and so less computational resources needed for training. For more information, the reader is referred to the corresponding paper [15].

2.2.3. ResNet

ResNet architecture was introduced by He et al. [16] in 2015. ResNet was developed by exploiting the concept of residual connections. The authors introduced the concept of a residual connection to minimize the effect of the vanishing gradient. The ResNet architecture comes in many variants. In this paper, we use the ResNet50 network, which contains 50 layers. For more information, the reader is referred to the corresponding paper [16].

2.2.4. GoogLeNet

GoogLeNet architecture was introduced by Szegedy et al. [17] in 2014. The authors proposed a novel idea called the inception module, which takes the aspect ratio of each image into account. There are many variants for GoogLeNet architecture, and we use the InceptionV3 network. For more information, the reader is referred to the corresponding paper [17].

2.2.5. InceptionResNet

Längkvist et al. [18] created a novel architecture called InceptionResNet, where the authors combined the inception module idea from GoogLeNet architecture [17] with the residual idea from ResNet architecture [16]. InceptionResNet is more computationally efficient than both ResNet and Inception architectures and achieved higher results than both on the ImageNet dataset. For more information, the reader is referred to the corresponding paper [18].

2.2.6. DenseNet

Huang et al. [19] introduced a novel architecture called DenseNet. In this architecture, the convolution blocks are densely connected to each other, and the convolution blocks are concatenated to each other instead of being added like in the ResNet network. For more information, the reader is referred to the corresponding paper [19].

2.3. Evaluation Metrics

Two evaluation metrics are being used to assess the performance of each network. Accuracy and Kappa. Below, we briefly summarize each metric:

2.3.1. Accuracy

This metric quantifies how accurate the classifier is. It is calculated as the number of correctly classified data points divided by the total number of the data points. The formula is shown in Equation (1).

$$\text{Accuracy} = \frac{TN + TP}{TP + TN + FP + FN} \quad (1)$$

where TP stands for true positive, TN stands for true negative, FP stands for false positive, and FN stands for false negative. In the context of this study, images without fractures belong to the negative class, whereas images with a bone fracture belong to the positive class.

2.3.2. Kappa

This is an evaluation metric that is usually used to take into account the probability of selecting by chance, especially in cases of unbalanced datasets, and it was introduced by Cohen [20]. The upper limit of the Kappa metric is 1, which means that the classifier classified everything correctly. At the same time, the lower bound can go below zero, which indicates the classifier is just classifying by luck. The Kappa formula is presented in Equation (2).

$$\text{Kappa} = \frac{\text{Agreement}_{Observed} - \text{Agreement}_{Expected}}{1 - \text{Agreement}_{Expected}} \quad (2)$$

2.4. Statistical Analysis

A statistical analysis was performed to assess the statistical significance of the results. We considered a confidence interval with a 95% error rate (95% CI) and a hypothesis test. Two hypothesis tests can be used: ANOVA or Kruskal–Wallis test. The choice of the test mainly depends on the normality of the data under observation. The ANOVA test is a parametric test that assumes that the data have a normal distribution. The null hypothesis of the ANOVA test is that the considered samples have the same mean, and the alternative hypothesis is that the samples have a different mean.

The non-parametric test is the Kruskal–Wallis hypothesis test [21]. This test does not make any assumption on the normality of the data, and it compares the medians of different samples. The null and alternative hypotheses tested are the following:

Hypothesis 0 (H0). *The populations medians are all equal.*

Hypothesis 1 (H1). *The populations medians are not all equal.*

In this paper, we first tested the normality assumption by using the Shapiro–Wilk test. Considering that the test does not allow to reject the alternative hypothesis (i.e., data not normally distributed), the Kruskal–Wallis test was used to test the significance of the results obtained. To make the hypothesis test and to report means and significance errors, each setting was repeated 30 times using different seeds and different validation split. In this way, each approach's stability can be assessed by also mitigating the effect of lucky seeds [22].

2.5. Dataset

The dataset used in this paper is the publicly available MURA dataset [10]. The dataset consists of seven different skeletal bones: elbow, finger, forearm, hand, humerus, shoulder, and wrist. Each category has a binary label, indicating if the image presents a broken bone or not. The dataset contains a total of 40,005 images. The authors of the dataset split it into training and test sets. The train set included 21,935 images without fractures (54.83% of the dataset) and 14,873 images with fractures (37.17% of the dataset), and the test set contained 1667 images without fractures (4.16% of the dataset) and 1530 images with fractures (3.84% of the dataset).

All in all, 92% of the dataset is used for training, and 8% of the dataset is used for testing the results. The summary of the dataset is presented in Table 1. A sample of the MURA dataset is presented in Figure 1.

Table 1. MURA dataset summary.

Category	Training Dataset		Test Dataset	
	Normal	Fractured	Normal	Fractured
Elbow	2925	2006	235	230
Finger	3138	1968	214	247
Hand	4059	1484	271	189
Humerus	673	599	148	140
Forearm	1164	661	150	151
Shoulder	4211	4168	285	278
Wrist	5765	3987	364	295
Total	21,935	14,873	1667	1530

Broken Forearm

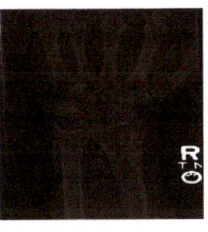
Normal Forearm

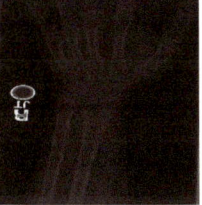
Broken Wrist

Normal Wrist

Figure 1. A sample of the MURA dataset.

3. Results

Throughout the experiments, all the hyperparameters were fixed. All the networks were either fine-tuned completely or trained from scratch. Adam optimizer [21] was used in all the experiments. As noted by studies [22,23], the learning rate should be low to avoid dramatically changing the original weights, so we set the learning rate to be 0.0001. All the images were resized to 96 × 96 pixels. Binary cross-entropy was used as the loss function because the images are binary classified. An early stopping criterion of 50 epochs would be used to stop the algorithms if no updates happened to the validation score. The batch size was selected to be 64, and the training dataset was split into 80% to train and 20% to validate the results during training. Four image augmentation techniques were used to increase the training dataset's size and make the network more robust against overfitting; the augmentation techniques used are horizontal and vertical flips, 180 rotations, and zooming.

Additionally, image augmentation is performed to balancing the number of images in the two target classes, thus achieving 50% of images without fractures and 50% of images with fractures in the training set. After the training, each network's performance was tested using the dataset that was supplied by the owner and creator of the dataset. The test dataset was not used during the training phase, but only in the final testing phase. The hyperparameters used are presented in Table 2. In the following sections, Kappa is the metric considered for comparing the performance of the different architectures.

Table 2. The hyperparameters were used for all the experiments.

Framework	Keras with Python
Optimizer	Adam
Learning Rate	0.0001
Loss Function	Binary Cross-entropy
Early Stopping	50 epochs
Batch Size	64
Validation Split	20%
Image Augmentation	Horizontal flips Vertical flips 180 rotations Zooming

3.1. Wrist Images Classification Results

Two main sets of experiments were performed: the first consists of adding two fully connected layers after each architecture to act as a classifier block. The second consists of adding only a sigmoid layer after the network. Both the results of the first set and the second set are presented in Table 3.

In the first set of experiments, the fine-tuned VGG19 network had a Kappa score of 0.5989, while the network that was trained from scratch had a score of 0.5476. For the Xception network, the transfer learning score was higher than the one trained from scratch by a large margin. The ResNet50 network performance improved significantly by using transfer learning rather than training it from scratch. This indicates that transfer learning is fundamental for this network, that it could not learn the features of the images from scratch. Both the fine-tuned InceptionV3, InceptionResNetV2, and DenseNet121 networks have a higher score than training them from scratch. Overall, fine-tuning the networks did yield better results than training the networks from scratch. The best performance for the first set of experiments was achieved by fine-tuning the DenseNet121 network.

In the second set of experiments, all the networks' performance increased by fine-tuning than by training from scratch. The ResNet network was the network with the highest difference between fine-tuning and training from scratch. Overall, the best performance for the second set of experiments was achieved by fine-tuning the Xception network. Comparing the first set of experiments to the second set, we see that the best performance for classifying wrist images was the fine-tuned DenseNet121 network with fully connected layers. The presence of fully connected layers did not have any noticeable increase in performance; however, it is worth noting that the ResNet network with fully connected layers did not converge when trained from scratch.

Table 3. Accuracy and Kappa scores of classifying wrist images with and without fully connected layers (±95% CI).

Network	Method	With FC		Without FC	
		Mean Accuracy	Mean Kappa	Mean Accuracy	Mean Kappa
VGG19	TL	80.45% ± 1.26%	0.5989 ± 2.39%	80.63% ± 1.64%	0.6035 ± 3.33%
	Scratch	78.07% ± 0.94%	0.5476 ± 2.11%	79.89% ± 1.84%	0.5846 ± 3.74%
InceptionV3	TL	79.92% ± 2.07%	0.5886 ± 3.61%	79.94% ± 1.46%	0.5876 ± 2.77%
	Scratch	77.01% ± 2.98%	0.5241 ± 6.49%	77.59% ± 1.51%	0.5389 ± 3.03%
ResNet	TL	78.76% ± 0.88%	0.5647 ± 2.04%	80.85% ± 1.70%	0.6046 ± 3.63%
	Scratch	58.65% ± 8.70%	0.0836 ± 21.31%	70.99% ± 4.20%	0.4018 ± 8.27%
Xception	TL	80.93% ± 0.88%	0.6098 ± 1.69%	81.18% ± 0.47%	0.6133 ± 0.94%
	Scratch	77.44% ± 1.99%	0.5333 ± 4.41%	77.14% ± 1.86%	0.5318 ± 3.32%
DenseNet	TL	81.71% ± 0.94%	0.6245 ± 1.98%	78.76% ± 2.27%	0.5663 ± 4.29%
	Scratch	76.40% ± 2.30%	0.5083 ± 5.17%	76.68% ± 3.62%	0.5214 ± 7.25%
InceptionResNet	TL	80.1% ± 1.66%	0.5917 ± 3.32%	80.55% ± 1.06%	0.6010 ± 2.25%
	Scratch	77.77% ± 1.59%	0.5450 ± 2.85%	78.55% ± 1.70%	0.5580 ± 3.48%

3.2. Hand Images Classification Results

As done with the wrist images, two sets of experiments were performed. Both the results of the first set and the second set are presented in Table 4.

In the first set of experiments, for the VGG19 and the ResNet networks, fine-tuning the networks resulted in significantly higher performance than training the networks from scratch. The networks trained from scratch did not converge to an acceptable result. This fact highlights that the importance of transfer learning for these networks, that are not able to learn the images' features from scratch. For the remaining networks, fine-tuning achieved significantly better performance than by training the networks from scratch. Overall, all the fine-tuned networks achieved better results than by training from scratch. The best performance of the first set of experiments was obtained with the fine-tuned Xception network.

Table 4. Accuracy and Kappa scores of classifying hand images with and without fully connected layers (±95% CI).

Network	Method	With FC		Without FC	
		Mean Accuracy	Mean Kappa	Mean Accuracy	Mean Kappa
VGG19	TL	70.11% ± 9.23%	0.3089 ± 25.42%	73.04% ± 1.27%	0.3960 ± 3.23%
	Scratch	58.91% ± 0%	0 ± 0%	63.22% ± 5.90%	0.1312 ± 15.90%
InceptionV3	TL	70.25% ± 1.34%	0.3261 ± 3.57%	72.10% ± 0.79%	0.3829 ± 2.15%
	Scratch	66.38% ± 3.80%	0.2382 ± 9.76%	66.56% ± 2.48%	0.2361 ± 6.07%
ResNet	TL	72.25% ± 1.25%	0.3754 ± 3.55%	71.12% ± 1.94%	0.3503 ± 5.44%
	Scratch	59.28% ± 0.93%	0.0103 ± 2.65%	62.10% ± 1.21%	0.0971 ± 3.26%
Xception	TL	75.36% ± 2.56%	0.4621 ± 6.27%	72.50% ± 2.0%	0.3778 ± 5.41%
	Scratch	66.74% ± 2.58%	0.2277 ± 7.20%	66.81% ± 3.60%	0.2334 ± 10.05%
DenseNet	TL	72.21% ± 1.69%	0.3746 ± 4.33%	70.22% ± 3.28%	0.3243 ± 9.03%
	Scratch	63.33% ± 1.16%	0.1308 ± 3.47%	62.79% ± 1.50%	0.1231 ± 4.39%
InceptionResNet	TL	71.96% ± 1.80%	0.3709 ± 4.33%	71.81% ± 1.91%	0.3670 ± 4.65%
	Scratch	68.48% ± 1.53%	0.2788 ± 4.36%	69.09% ± 1.04%	0.3071 ± 2.43%

In the second set of experiments, the performance of all the networks increased by fine-tuning than by training from scratch. The ResNet network was the network with the highest difference between fine-tuning and training from scratch. Overall, the best network was the VGG19 network. Comparing the first set of experiments to the second set, we see that the best performance for classifying hand images was the fine-tuned Xception network with fully connected layers. The presence of fully connected layers did not significantly increase the performance; however, it is important to point out that the VGG19 network with fully connected layers did not converge when it was trained from scratch.

3.3. Humerus Images Classification Results

For the humerus images, the results of both the first and second sets of experiments are presented in Table 5. In the first set of experiments, fine-tuning VGG19 architecture did not converge to any acceptable results, while training the VGG19 from scratch did yield higher performance. For the rest of the networks, fine-tuning did achieve better results than training the networks from scratch. The highest difference was between fine-tuning the ResNet network and training it from scratch. Overall, the best network in the first sets of experiments was the fine-tuned DenseNet network, with a Kappa score of 0.6260.

In the second set of experiments, fine-tuning did achieve better results for all the networks than training the networks from scratch. The best-achieved network was the VGG19 network, with a Kappa score of 0.6333. Comparing the first set of experiments to the second set, we see that the best performance for classifying humerus images was the fine-tuned VGG19 network without fully connected layers. Just as in the previous experiments, the fully connected layers' presence did not provide any significant performance improvement; however, fine-tuning the VGG19 with fully connected layers did not converge compared to fine-tuning the same network without any fully connected layers.

Table 5. Accuracy and Kappa scores of classifying humerus images with and without fully connected layers (±95% CI).

Network	Method	With FC		Without FC	
		Mean Accuracy	Mean Kappa	Mean Accuracy	Mean Kappa
VGG19	TL	51.39% ± 0%	0 ± 0%	81.66% ± 2.74%	0.6333 ± 5.43%
	Scratch	62.04% ± 3.67%	0.239 ± 8.01%	69.44% ± 8.28%	0.3893 ± 16.77%
InceptionV3	TL	80.32% ± 2.74%	0.6070 ± 5.51%	80.56% ± 1.48%	0.6114 ± 2.94%
	Scratch	67.77% ± 3.12%	0.3603 ± 6.08%	64.06% ± 3.51%	0.2879 ± 6.81%
ResNet	TL	80.38% ± 2.55%	0.6084 ± 5.03%	78.18% ± 2.20%	0.5647 ± 4.31%
	Scratch	54.28% ± 7.46%	0.0849 ± 14.97%	65.63% ± 5.19%	0.3171 ± 10.26%
Xception	TL	80.03% ± 1.92%	0.6010 ± 3.81%	79.75% ± 1.67%	0.5942 ± 3.40%
	Scratch	66.55% ± 2.84%	0.3386 ± 5.46%	66.32% ± 4.72%	0.3334 ± 9.11%
DenseNet	TL	81.31% ± 1.88%	0.6260 ± 3.81%	77.84% ± 1.52%	0.5563 ± 3.16%
	Scratch	70.54% ± 5.85%	0.4134 ± 11.37%	71.93% ± 2.74%	0.4406 ± 5.35%
InceptionResNet	TL	78.41% ± 1.84%	0.5697 ± 3.61%	78.76% ± 2.56%	0.5761 ± 5.07%
	Scratch	65.34% ± 3.89%	0.3135 ± 7.61%	65.34% ± 4.37%	0.3139 ± 8.47%

3.4. Elbow Images Classification Results

For the elbow images, we performed the same two sets of experiments performed with the previously analyzed datasets. Both the results of the first set and the second set are presented in Table 6. In the first set of experiments, the fine-tuned VGG19 score was less than training the same network from scratch. For the rest of the networks, fine-tuning did achieve higher performance than training the networks from scratch. The ResNet network achieved the highest difference between fine-tuning and training from scratch. Overall, the best network was the fine-tuned DenseNet121, with a Kappa score of 0.6510.

In the second set of experiments, no fully connected layers were added. For all the networks, fine-tuning did achieve higher results than training from scratch. Overall, the best network was the fine-tuned Xception network, with a Kappa score of 0.6711. Comparing the first set of experiments to the second set, we see that the best performance for classifying elbow images was the fine-tuned Xception network without fully connected layers.

Table 6. Accuracy and Kappa scores of classifying elbow images with and without fully connected layers (±95% CI).

Network	Method	With FC		Without FC	
		Mean Accuracy	Mean Kappa	Mean Accuracy	Mean Kappa
VGG19	TL	71.36% ± 16.95%	0.4232 ± 13.01%	81.61% ± 1.56%	0.6316 ± 3.12%
	Scratch	75.81% ± 34.45%	0.5136 ± 26.45%	76.52% ± 13.45%	0.5279 ± 27.33%
InceptionV3	TL	81.72% ± 0.91%	0.6339 ± 1.84%	80.93% ± 2.3%	0.6180 ± 4.6%
	Scratch	77.96% ± 2.92%	0.5583 ± 5.84%	76.09% ± 4.29%	0.5208 ± 8.6%
ResNet	TL	81.79% ± 3.28%	0.6351 ± 6.61%	81.9% ± 2.22%	0.6374 ± 4.44%
	Scratch	56.20% ± 9.60%	0.1161 ± 19.68%	71.04% ± 4.02%	0.4191 ± 8.09%
Xception	TL	82.15% ± 1.21%	0.6425 ± 2.42%	83.58% ± 1.64%	0.6711 ± 3.31%
	Scratch	78.21% ± 2.83%	0.5631 ± 5.70%	78.49% ± 1.88%	0.5690 ± 3.75%
DenseNet	TL	82.58% ± 1.97%	0.6510 ± 3.92%	81.08% ± 2.23%	0.6208 ± 4.47%
	Scratch	75.38% ± 3.36%	0.5060 ± 6.82%	73.84% ± 4.70%	0.4754 ± 9.49%
InceptionResNet	TL	80.82% ± 0.61%	0.6159 ± 1.21%	80.47% ± 1.68%	0.6087 ± 3.37%
	Scratch	79.82% ± 1.45%	0.5955 ± 2.91%	78.49% ± 1.28%	0.5694 ± 2.58%

3.5. Finger Images Classification Results

As with the previous datasets, two main sets of experiments were performed. Both the results of the first set and the second set are presented in Table 7. In the first set of experiments, fine-tuning achieved better results than training the networks from scratch for all the networks. The best-achieved network was the fine-tuned VGG19, with a Kappa score of 0.4379. In the second set of experiments, fine-tuning produced better results than training from scratch for all the six networks. The best network was the fine-tuned InceptionResNet network, with a Kappa score of 0.4455. Comparing the first set of experiments to the second set, we see that the best performance for classifying finger images was the fine-tuned InceptionResNet network without fully connected layers. Moreover, in this case, the presence of the fully connected layers did not provide any significant advantage in terms of performance.

Table 7. Accuracy and Kappa scores of classifying finger images with and without fully connected layers (±95% CI).

Network	Method	With FC		Without FC	
		Mean Accuracy	Mean Kappa	Mean Accuracy	Mean Kappa
VGG19	TL	71.4% ± 1.84%	0.4379 ± 3.59%	68.44% ± 2.76%	0.3847 ± 5.10%
	Scratch	66.78% ± 2.83%	0.3505 ± 5.22%	66.16% ± 3.10%	0.3413 ± 5.26%
InceptionV3	TL	67.68% ± 2.15%	0.3686 ± 3.87%	68.55% ± 3.19%	0.3834 ± 5.97%
	Scratch	63.52% ± 2.66%	0.2911 ± 4.82%	63.88% ± 2.15%	0.2916 ± 4.09%
ResNet	TL	70.17% ± 1.16%	0.4129 ± 2.17%	69.02% ± 2.52%	0.3900 ± 4.44%
	Scratch	60.34% ± 8.07%	0.2341 ± 13.90%	66.41% ± 2.98%	0.3431 ± 5.68%
Xception	TL	71.37% ± 2.43%	0.4369 ± 4.42%	70.64% ± 2.27%	0.4234 ± 4.28%
	Scratch	64.75% ± 2.79%	0.3109 ± 5.33%	64.57% ± 2.72%	0.3055 ± 5.31%
DenseNet	TL	66.78% ± 2.64%	0.3552 ± 4.66%	66.81% ± 1.92%	0.3512 ± 3.61%
	Scratch	62.18% ± 2.10%	0.2692 ± 3.60%	64.32% ± 3.16%	0.3051 ± 5.64%
InceptionResNet	TL	70.97% ± 2.05%	0.4294 ± 3.80%	71.8% ± 1.49%	0.4455 ± 2.88%
	Scratch	64.64% ± 3.07%	0.3112 ± 5.70%	65.29% ± 3.09%	0.3204 ± 5.72%

3.6. Forearm Images Classification Results

As with the previous datasets, two sets of experiments were performed on the forearm images dataset. Both the results of the first set and the second set are presented in Table 8. In the first set of experiments, fine-tuning all the networks produced better results than training from scratch. Training of ResNet network from scratch did not yield any satisfactory results, which can imply that fine-tuning this network was crucial for obtaining a good result. The best network was the DenseNet121 network, with a Kappa score of 0.5851. Moreover, in the second set of experiments, fine-tuning achieved better results than training from scratch. The best network was the fine-tuned ResNet network, with a Kappa score of 0.5673. Comparing the first set of experiments to the second set, we see that the best performance for classifying forearm images was the fine-tuned DenseNet network with fully connected layers. As observed in other datasets, the presence of the fully connected layers did not have any significant advantage in terms of performance.

Table 8. Accuracy and Kappa scores of classifying forearm images with and without fully connected layers (±95% CI).

Network	Method	With FC		Without FC	
		Mean Accuracy	Mean Kappa	Mean Accuracy	Mean Kappa
VGG19	TL	77.02% ± 1.27%	0.5408 ± 2.54%	76.3% ± 2.16%	0.5264 ± 4.31%
	Scratch	64.29% ± 9.50%	0.2870 ± 18.91%	71.15% ± 6.41%	0.4237 ± 12.75%
InceptionV3	TL	76.52% ± 1.46%	0.5308 ± 2.91%	77.46% ± 1%	0.5496 ± 1.99%
	Scratch	64.84% ± 5.50%	0.2973 ± 11.01%	65.84% ± 4.95%	0.3171 ± 9.89%
ResNet	TL	74.7% ± 1.20%	0.4943 ± 2.38%	78.35% ± 3.46%	0.5673 ± 6.92%
	Scratch	50.11% ± 0.56%	0.0055 ± 1.11%	63.79% ± 3.58%	0.2764 ± 7.12%
Xception	TL	75.08% ± 1.84%	0.5022 ± 3.69%	76.08% ± 1.66%	0.5222 ± 3.32%
	Scratch	66.00% ± 2.54%	0.3204 ± 5.08%	65.73% ± 5.31%	0.3148 ± 10.64%
DenseNet	TL	79.24% ± 0.53%	0.5851 ± 1.05%	76.14% ± 2.32%	0.5232 ± 4.63%
	Scratch	68.77% ± 3.75%	0.3755 ± 7.51%	69.66% ± 3.12%	0.3935 ± 6.25%
InceptionResNet	TL	74.7% ± 2.64%	0.4945 ± 5.27%	74.86% ± 1.98%	0.4977 ± 3.95%
	Scratch	65.45% ± 3.36%	0.3096 ± 6.69%	69.1% ± 6.07%	0.3824 ± 12.12%

3.7. Shoulder Images Classification Results

In the first set of experiments, the VGG19 network did not converge to an acceptable result by using both methods. For the rest of the networks, fine-tuning the networks achieved better results than training the networks from scratch. The best network was the fine-tuned Xception network, with a Kappa score of 0.4543. Both the results of the first set and the second set are presented in Table 9. In the second set of experiments, training the ResNet network from scratch achieved slightly better results than fine-tuning. For the rest of the networks, fine-tuning achieved better results. The best network was the fine-tuned VGG19, with a Kappa score of 0.4502. Comparing the first set of experiments to the second set, we see that the best performance for classifying shoulder images was the fine-tuned Xception network with fully connected layers. The presence of the fully connected layers did not show any significant advantage in terms of performance. Anyhow, the VGG19 network with fully connected layers did not converge to any satisfactory result compared to the same network without any fully connected layers.

3.8. Kruskal–Wallis Results

We applied the Kruskal–Wallis test to assess the statistical significance of different settings. The Kruskal–Wallis test yielded a p-value < 0.05 for all the results, which indicates to reject the null hypothesis that the settings have the same median and to accept the alternative hypothesis that there is a statistically significant difference between different settings (transfer learning "with and without fully connected layers" vs. training from scratch "with and without fully connected layers").

Table 9. Accuracy and Kappa scores of classifying shoulder images with and without fully connected layers (±95% CI).

Network	Method	With FC		Without FC	
		Mean Accuracy	Mean Kappa	Mean Accuracy	Mean Kappa
VGG19	TL	77.02% ± 1.27%	0.5408 ± 2.54%	76.3% ± 2.16%	0.5264 ± 4.31%
	Scratch	64.29% ± 9.50%	0.2870 ± 18.91%	71.15% ± 6.41%	0.4237 ± 12.75%
InceptionV3	TL	76.52% ± 1.46%	0.5308 ± 2.91%	77.46% ± 1%	0.5496 ± 1.99%
	Scratch	64.84% ± 5.50%	0.2973 ± 11.01%	65.84% ± 4.95%	0.3171 ± 9.89%
ResNet	TL	74.7% ± 1.20%	0.4943 ± 2.38%	78.35% ± 3.46%	0.5673 ± 6.92%
	Scratch	50.11% ± 0.56%	0.0055 ± 1.11%	63.79% ± 3.58%	0.2764 ± 7.12%
Xception	TL	75.08% ± 1.84%	0.5022 ± 3.69%	76.08% ± 1.66%	0.5222 ± 3.32%
	Scratch	66.00% ± 2.54%	0.3204 ± 5.08%	65.73% ± 5.31%	0.3148 ± 10.64%
DenseNet	TL	79.24% ± 0.53%	0.5851 ± 1.05%	76.14% ± 2.32%	0.5232 ± 4.63%
	Scratch	68.77% ± 3.75%	0.3755 ± 7.51%	69.66% ± 3.12%	0.3935 ± 6.25%
InceptionResNet	TL	74.7% ± 2.64%	0.4945 ± 5.27%	74.86% ± 1.98%	0.4977 ± 3.95%
	Scratch	65.45% ± 3.36%	0.3096 ± 6.69%	69.1% ± 6.07%	0.3824 ± 12.12%

4. Discussion

In this paper, we compared the performance of fine-tuning on six state-of-the-art CNNs to classify musculoskeletal images. Training a CNN network from scratch can be very challenging, especially in the case of data scarcity. Transfer learning can help solve this problem by initiating the weights with values learned from a large dataset instead of initializing the weights from scratch. Musculoskeletal images play a fundamental role in classifying fractures. However, these images are always challenging to be analyzed, and a second opinion is often required, which will not always be available, especially in the emergency room. As pointed out by Lindsey et al. [5], the presence of an image classifier in the emergency room can significantly increase physicians' performance in classifying fractures.

For the first research question, about the effect of transfer learning, we noted that transfer learning produced better results than training the networks from scratch. For our second research question, the classifier that achieved the best result for wrist images was the fine-tuned DenseNet121 with fully connected layers; the classifier that achieved the best performance for elbow images was the fine-tuned Xception network without fully connected layers; for finger images, the best classifier was the fine-tuned InceptionResNetV2 network without fully connected layers; for forearm images, the best classifier was the fine-tuned DenseNet network with fully connected layers; for hand images, the best classifier was a fine-tuned Xception network with fully connected layers; the best classifier for humerus images was the fine-tuned VGG19 network without fully connected layers; finally, the best classifier for classifying the shoulder images was the fine-tuned Xception network with fully connected layers. A summary of the best CNNs is presented in Table 10. Concerning the third research question, the fully connected layers had a negative effect on the performance of the considered CNNs. In particular, in many cases, it decreased the performance of the network. Further research is needed to study, in more detail, the impact of fully connected layers, especially in the case of transfer learning.

The authors of the MURA dataset [10] assessed the performance of three radiologists on the dataset and compared their performance against the one of a CNN. In Table 11, we present their results, along with our best scores.

For classifying elbow images, the first radiologist achieved the best score, and our score was comparable to other radiologists [10]. For finger images, our score was higher than the three radiologists. For forearm images, our score was lower than the radiologists. For hand images, our score was the lowest. For humerus images, shoulder images, and wrist images, our score was lower than the radiologists. We still believe that the scores achieved in this paper are promising, keeping in mind that these scores came from off-the-shelf models that were not designed for medical images in the first place and that the images were resized to be 96 × 96 pixels due to hardware limitations. Nevertheless, additional efforts are needed to outperform the performance of experienced radiologists.

Table 10. The best convolutional neural network (CNN) for each image category.

Fracture	CNN
Wrist	DenseNet
Elbow	Xception
Finger	InceptionResNetV2
Forearm	DenseNet121
Hand	Xception
Humerus	VGG19
Shoulder	Xception

Table 11. Kappa scores of three radiologists reported in Reference [10] compared to our results.

Fracture	1st Radiologist	2nd Radiologist	3rd Radiologist	Our Score
Elbow	0.850	0.710	0.719	0.671
Finger	0.304	0.403	0.410	0.445
Forearm	0.796	0.802	0.798	0.585
Hand	0.661	0.927	0.789	0.462
Humerus	0.867	0.733	0.933	0.633
Shoulder	0.864	0.791	0.864	0.454
Wrist	0.791	0.931	0.931	0.625

On the other side of the spectrum, there is the study of Raghu et al. [24], where the authors argued that transfer learning is not good enough for medical images and will be less accurate compared to training from scratch or compared to novel networks explicitly designed for the problem at hand. The authors studied the effect of transfer learning on two medical datasets, namely, retina images and chest X-ray images. The authors stated that designing a lightweight CNN can be more accurate than using transfer learning. In our study, we did not consider "small" CNNs trained from scratch. Thus, it is not possible to directly compare the results obtained to the ones presented in Raghu et al. [24]. Anyway, more studies are needed to better understand the effect of transfer learning on medical-image classification.

5. Conclusions

In this paper, we investigated the effect of transfer learning on classifying musculoskeletal images. We find that, out of the 168 results obtained that were performed by using six different CNN architectures and seven different bone types, transfer learning achieved better results than training a CNN from scratch. Only in 3 out of the 168 results did training from scratch achieve slightly better results than transfer learning. The weaker performance of the training-from-scratch approach could be related to the number of images in the considered dataset, as well as to the choice of the hyperparameters. In particular, the CNNs taken into account are characterized by the presence of a large number of trainable parameters (i.e., weights), and the number of images used to train these networks is too small to build a robust model. Concerning the hyperparameters, we highlight the importance of the learning rate. While we used a small value of the learning rate in the fine-tuning approach, to avoid changing the architectures' original weights dramatically, the training-from-scratch approach could require a higher value of the learning rate. A complete study on the hyperparameters' effect will be considered in future work, aiming to fully understand the best approach to be used when dealing with fracture images. Focusing on this study's results, it is possible to state that transfer learning is recommended in the context of fracture images. In our future work, we plan to introduce a novel CNN to classify musculoskeletal images, aiming at outperforming fine-tuned CNNs. This would be the first step towards the design of a CNN-based system, which classifies the image and provides the probable position of the fracture if the fracture is present in the image.

Author Contributions: Conceptualization, I.K. and M.C.; methodology, I.K.; software, I.K.; validation, I.K., M.C. and A.P.; writing—original draft preparation, I.K.; writing—review and editing, M.C. and A.P.; supervision, M.C.; project administration, A.P.; funding acquisition, M.C. and A.P. All authors have read and agreed to the published version of the manuscript.

Funding: This work was supported by national funds through FCT (Fundação para a Ciência e a Tecnologia) by the project GADgET (DSAIPA/DS/0022/2018). Mauro Castelli and Aleš Popovič acknowledge the financial support from the Slovenian Research Agency (research core funding No. P5-0410).

Conflicts of Interest: The authors declare no conflict of interest.

References

1. CDC. *National Hospital Ambulatory Medical Care Survey: 2017 Emergency Department Summary Tables*; CDC: Atlanta, GA, USA, 2017.
2. Tanzi, L.; Vezzetti, E.; Moreno, R.; Moos, S. X-Ray Bone Fracture Classification Using Deep Learning: A Baseline for Designing a Reliable Approach. *Appl. Sci.* **2020**, *10*, 1507.
3. Hallas, P.; Ellingsen, T. Errors in fracture diagnoses in the emergency deparment—Characteristics of patients and diurnal variation. *BMC Emerg. Med.* **2006**, *6*, 4.
4. Moonen, P.-J.; Mercelina, L.; Boer, W.; Fret, T. Diagnostic error in the Emergency Department: Follow up of patients with minor trauma in the outpatient clinic. *Scand. J. Trauma. Resusc. Emerg. Med.* **2017**, *25*, 13. [PubMed]
5. Lindsey, R.; Daluiski, A.; Chopra, S.; Lachapelle, A.; Mozer, M.; Sicular, S.; Hanel, D.; Gardner, M.; Gupta, A.; Hotchkiss, R.; et al. Deep neural network improves fracture detection by clinicians. *Proc. Natl. Acad. Sci. USA* **2018**, *115*, 11591–11596. [PubMed]
6. Almubarak, H.; Bazi, Y.; Alajlan, N. Two-Stage Mask-RCNN Approach for Detecting and Segmenting the Optic Nerve Head, Optic Disc, and Optic Cup in Fundus Images. *Appl. Sci.* **2020**, *10*, 3833.
7. Kandel, I.; Castelli, M. A novel architecture to classify histopathology images using convolutional neural networks. *Appl. Sci.* **2020**, *10*, 2929.
8. Farooq, A.; Anwar, S.; Awais, M.; Rehman, S. A deep CNN based multi-class classification of Alzheimer's disease using MRI. In Proceedings of the 2017 IEEE International Conference on Imaging Systems and Techniques (IST), Beijing, China, 18–20 October 2017; pp. 1–6.
9. Krizhevsky, A.; Sutskever, I.; Hinton, G.E. ImageNet Classification with Deep Convolutional Neural Networks. In Proceedings of the Neural Information Processing Systems, Lake Tahoe, NV, USA, 3–6 December 2012; Volume 25.
10. Rajpurkar, P.; Irvin, J.; Bagul, A.; Ding, D.Y.; Duan, T.; Mehta, H.; Yang, B.J.; Zhu, K.; Laird, D.; Ball, R.L.; et al. MURA: Large Dataset for Abnormality Detection in Musculoskeletal Radiographs. *arXiv* **2017**, arXiv:1712.06957.
11. Chada, G. Machine Learning Models for Abnormality Detection in Musculoskeletal Radiographs. *Reports* **2019**, *2*, 26.
12. Kitamura, G.; Chung, C.Y.; Moore, B.E. Ankle Fracture Detection Utilizing a Convolutional Neural Network Ensemble Implemented with a Small Sample, De Novo Training, and Multiview Incorporation. *J. Digit. Imaging* **2019**, *32*, 672–677. [PubMed]
13. Pan, S.; Yang, Q. A Survey on Transfer Learning. *IEEE Trans. Knowl. Data Eng. Knowl. Data Eng.* **2010**, *22*, 1345–1359.
14. Simonyan, K.; Zisserman, A. Very Deep Convolutional Networks for Large-Scale Image Recognition. *arXiv* **2014**, arXiv:1409.1556.
15. Chollet, F. Xception: Deep Learning with Depthwise Separable Convolutions. In Proceedings of the IEEE Conference on Computer Vision and Pattern Recognition (CVPR), Honolulu, HI, USA, 21–26 July 2017.
16. He, K.; Zhang, X.; Ren, S.; Sun, J. Deep Residual Learning for Image Recognition. In Proceedings of the 2016 IEEE Conference on Computer Vision and Pattern Recognition (CVPR), Las Vegas, NV, USA, 27–30 June 2016; pp. 770–778.

17. Szegedy, C.; Liu, W.; Jia, Y.; Sermanet, P.; Reed, S.; Anguelov, D.; Erhan, D.; Vanhoucke, V.; Rabinovich, A. Going deeper with convolutions. In Proceedings of the 2015 IEEE Conference on Computer Vision and Pattern Recognition (CVPR), Boston, MA, USA, 7–12 June 2015; pp. 1–9.
18. Längkvist, M.; Karlsson, L.; Loutfi, A. Inception-v4, Inception-ResNet and the Impact of Residual Connections on Learning. *Pattern Recognit. Lett.* **2014**, *42*, 11–24.
19. Huang, G.; Liu, Z.; Van der Maaten, L.; Weinberger, K.Q. Densely Connected Convolutional Networks. In Proceedings of the 2017 IEEE Conference on Computer Vision and Pattern Recognition (CVPR), Honolulu, HI, USA, 21–26 July 2017; pp. 2261–2269.
20. Cohen, J. A Coefficient of Agreement for Nominal Scales. *Educ. Psychol. Meas.* **1960**, *20*, 37–46.
21. Kruskal, W.H.; Wallis, W.A. Use of Ranks in One-Criterion Variance Analysis. *J. Am. Stat. Assoc.* **1952**, *47*, 583–621.
22. Schmidt, R.; Schneider, F.; Hennig, P. Descending through a Crowded Valley—Benchmarking Deep Learning Optimizers. *arXiv* **2020**, arXiv:2007.01547.
23. Kingma, D.; Ba, J. Adam: A Method for Stochastic Optimization. In Proceedings of the International Conference on Learning Representations (ICLR), Banff, AB, Canada, 14–16 April 2014.
24. Raghu, M.; Zhang, C.; Kleinberg, J.; Bengio, S. Transfusion: Understanding Transfer Learning with Applications to Medical Imaging. *arXiv* **2019**, arXiv:1902.07208.

Publisher's Note: MDPI stays neutral with regard to jurisdictional claims in published maps and institutional affiliations.

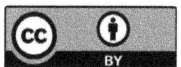

© 2020 by the authors. Licensee MDPI, Basel, Switzerland. This article is an open access article distributed under the terms and conditions of the Creative Commons Attribution (CC BY) license (http://creativecommons.org/licenses/by/4.0/).

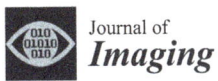

Article

Fully 3D Active Surface with Machine Learning for PET Image Segmentation

Albert Comelli

Ri.MED Foundation, 90133 Palermo, Italy; acomelli@fondazionerimed.com; Tel.: +39-3333967105

Received: 26 August 2020; Accepted: 20 October 2020; Published: 23 October 2020

Abstract: In order to tackle three-dimensional tumor volume reconstruction from Positron Emission Tomography (PET) images, most of the existing algorithms rely on the segmentation of independent PET slices. To exploit cross-slice information, typically overlooked in these 2D implementations, I present an algorithm capable of achieving the volume reconstruction directly in 3D, by leveraging an active surface algorithm. The evolution of such surface performs the segmentation of the whole stack of slices simultaneously and can handle changes in topology. Furthermore, no artificial stop condition is required, as the active surface will naturally converge to a stable topology. In addition, I include a machine learning component to enhance the accuracy of the segmentation process. The latter consists of a forcing term based on classification results from a discriminant analysis algorithm, which is included directly in the mathematical formulation of the energy function driving surface evolution. It is worth noting that the training of such a component requires minimal data compared to more involved deep learning methods. Only eight patients (i.e., two lung, four head and neck, and two brain cancers) were used for training and testing the machine learning component, while fifty patients (i.e., 10 lung, 25 head and neck, and 15 brain cancers) were used to test the full 3D reconstruction algorithm. Performance evaluation is based on the same dataset of patients discussed in my previous work, where the segmentation was performed using the 2D active contour. The results confirm that the active surface algorithm is superior to the active contour algorithm, outperforming the earlier approach on all the investigated anatomical districts with a dice similarity coefficient of 90.47 ± 2.36% for lung cancer, 88.30 ± 2.89% for head and neck cancer, and 90.29 ± 2.52% for brain cancer. Based on the reported results, it can be claimed that the migration into a 3D system yielded a practical benefit justifying the effort to rewrite an existing 2D system for PET imaging segmentation.

Keywords: 3D segmentation; machine learning; active surface; discriminant analysis; PET imaging

1. Introduction

In oncological studies, the main motivation to image segmentation is to recognize the portions of ill tissues so that treatment can be better directed (e.g., radio-therapy, [1–3]) and chances of survival improved [4–7]. Furthermore, segmentation is a pre-requisite to advanced studies such as radiomics feature extraction [8–10]. The present study discusses the segmentation of Positron Emission Tomography images leveraging a fully 3D hybrid algorithm which combines traditional segmentation (e.g., active surface) with machine learning (ML). Unlike several algorithms based on the segmentation of independent Positron Emission Tomography (PET) slices, the present algorithm is capable of segmenting all the slices in a PET data set simultaneously with the immediate advantage of exploiting valuable cross-slice information which would be ignored otherwise (e.g., [11–13]). In addition, in order to improve the accuracy of the final result, I included a machine learning component. A term based on information from a classifier (i.e., discriminant analysis) is included in the formulation of the energy function driving the surface evolution. The main advantage brought by artificial intelligence is that these approaches are designed to "learn" a non-obvious input–output relation directly from data. In the clinical context, artificial intelligence is used to obtain the morphology of organs or for the delineation of pathological tissue. Examples include the identification of cancer within the head and the neck using deep learning [14,15], classification using a kernel support vector machine [16], thyroid volume computation in 3D ultrasound imaging using random forest and convolutional neural network (CNN) [17], etc. It could be observed that deep learning techniques are more efficient than classical statistical approaches and, consequently, they are applied in many biomedical image segmentation tasks [18]. Nevertheless, while such methods are commonly used in magnetic resonance or computerized tomography imaging, their application on PET is still rather scarce and not much is found in the literature [19]. The reason is that in order to be successful, deep learning approaches require datasets containing hundreds of labelled examples, which is rarely the case in nuclear medicine. Vice versa, deep learning is largely used to classify patients in terms of outcome based on quantitative features extracted from previously delineated tumors for radiomics analyses of PET images [20]. Furthermore, to date, artificial intelligence algorithms are often employed as a stand-alone tool. Conversely, such a class of algorithms can be leveraged to improve the performance of more traditional approaches as well. For example, in [11], the k-means clustering technique was used to support a random walk segmentation algorithm, while, in [21], a convolutional neural network was used to obtain an initial delineation, successively refined by threshold segmentation and morphological methods. Moreover, an enhanced active contour (AC) algorithm has been proposed to delineate tumor in PET datasets in a semi-automatic way [22]. In detail, Comelli et al. [22] developed a 2D algorithm based on an AC enhanced by the inclusion of tissue classification information [23–25]. In these studies, authors reconstructed the 3D tumor shape by separately segmenting 2D PET slices because the main goal was to obtain a delineation method capable of being efficient, repeatable and real time. The core of such volume reconstruction was an active contour segmentation of PET images (i.e., 2D), performed marching through the PET slices and where the converged segmentation of one slice was used to initialize segmentation on the next. Nevertheless, the distance between consecutive PET slices is typically much greater than their voxel size. This feature introduces a sort of preferential direction in the data which may influence the reconstructed volume. In addition, the 2D contour evolution on one PET slice does not retain memory of what actually happened in the previous slice, nor does it takes into account what is the information in the slice that will come next.

Based on these considerations, the present study proposes a fully 3D active surface (AS) driven by a 3D machine learning component (i.e., 3D tissue classification). Starting from a region placed around the target, the AS deforms and moves to fit the target minimizing an "energy", defined as a multi-parameter function. In addition, the ML component, trained trough examples generated by expert human operators, learns to classify the PET data (i.e., the voxels in the slices) and introduces insight into the AS on which tissue portions are to be considered tumor or healthy. Therefore, to some extent, the algorithm learns to "mimic" how a human would perform this complex task and to avoid false positives. Although several classifiers were considered in previous publications (k-nearest neighbors, Naive Bayes, and Discriminant Analysis [23–25]), it is worth noting that the discriminant analysis provided consistently better performances [24]. As such, since a quite large comparative work was performed in [23–25], and since a full investigation on which classification approach would perform best within the new 3D framework is beyond the scope of the present study, the discriminant analysis is the algorithm of choice for this publication as well.

Summarizing, the key aspect of the proposed study is the evolution of a 3D surface embedded in the data volume, henceforth referred to as active surface, the evolution of which is driven by the minimization of a cost function specifically built to take into account information contained in the data and from 3D tissue classification. To evaluate the performance of the algorithm, fifty-eight patient studies are considered. In detail, eight studies are used for training and testing of the artificial intelligence component and fifty to test the full 3D reconstruction algorithm.

2. Materials and Methods

2.1. Overview of the 3D as Proposed Method and Differences with the Previous 2D AC Method

This study proposes a re-engineering of the algorithm from my previous work and focuses on the development of a 3D AS for the volume delineation augmented with the inclusion of a discriminant analysis (DA) component for 3D tissue classification. Figure 1 compares the 2D DA system proposed in [24] and the new 3D DA implementation discussed here to highlight differences and improvements.

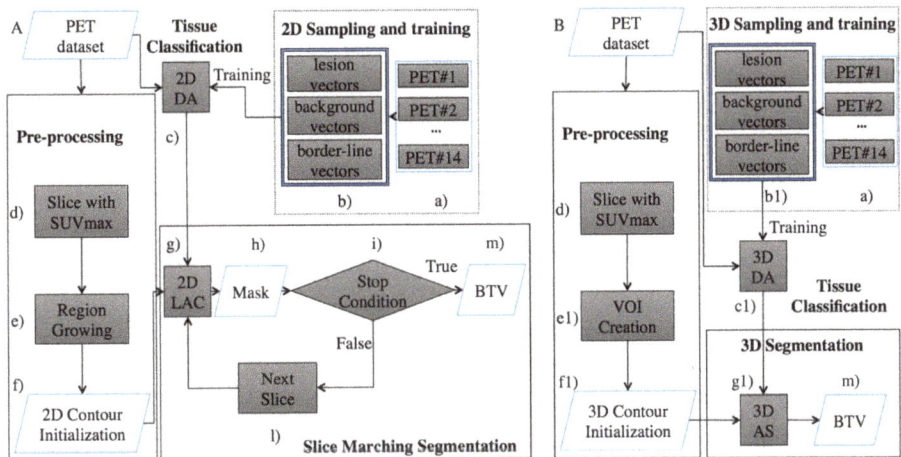

Figure 1. Comparison of the Positron Emission Tomography (PET) system proposed in the previous work (**A**) [24], and the implementation set out here (**B**). The proposed implementation substitutes the 'Slice Marching Segmentation' block (**A**) with the fully "3D Segmentation" block (**B**). Therefore, cross-slice information previously ignored is now being completely exploited. Moreover, the artificial stopping condition (step i) is no longer necessary. Additionally, (steps b, c, f, and g) were modified in order to provide a 3D sampling and training (step b1), a 3D tissue classification (step c1), 3D contour initialization (step f1), and 3D AS (step g1).

Figure 1A describes the system from my previous work [24]. Here, the "Pre-processing" block consisted of a pre-segmentation where the user draws, on a single PET slice, a contour roughly encircling the cancer area. This input is required to minimize the risk of incurring in false positives. Such an input was used to generate a user-independent mask which could be located on a different slice from the one chosen by the operator. By construction, this mask belonged to the same anatomical anomaly and included the radio-tracer maximum absorption area. After this step, the initial mask was fed to the next block of the workflow ("Slice Marching Segmentation" step), where the segmentation was obtained using a local region-based AC in which the contour evolved while minimizing its energy function. Information from the "2D Sampling and training" block consisted of labels associated to the PET image's pixels which identified each pixel as "lesion", "background", or "border-line" tissue. The different tissues in the PET slices were automatically identified using a 2D floating window (3 × 3 voxels). Finally, this algorithm used a slice-by-slice marching strategy to obtain an accurate segmentation, which began at the slice containing the user-independent mask and propagated upward and downward. Every time a slice segmentation was completed, the contour was propagated to the nearest adjacent slice until the stop condition was finally met. The final 3D shape consisted of the union of all contours obtained on each slice.

The algorithm presented here (Figure 1B) inherits the same pre-segmentation workflow of [24], although a 3D shape is required as the output of the pre-segmentation step. Specifically, to initialize the AS (step "g1" in Figure 1B), the pre-segmentation step (step "f1" in Figure 1B) must output a 3D shape transforming the user independent mask (step "f" in Figure 1A) in an ellipsoid (the 3D shape needed to start the 3D AS method). It is worth noting that the only requirement for the ellipsoid is that it envelops a portion of the tumor, including the voxel with the maximum intensity value (requirement already satisfied in [24] and naturally inherited from the ellipsoid). The energy function being minimized depends on the shape of the curves generated by the intersection of the AS with the planes containing the PET slices. Consequently, the ellipsoid around the tumor changes shape and moves towards the tumor borders with the aim of minimizing the energy function. Information from the 3D classifier is now included in the energy function in terms of labelled voxels combining, during the classification process, information involving multiple slices. As in the previous 2D classifier [24], the proposed 3D classifier labels the tissue as "lesion", "background" or "border-line" and drives the 3D AS algorithm ("3D Sampling and training" block), although the classification occurs now in terms of voxels and not pixels. This task comprises the training and validation steps of the DA classifier. Different tissues (i.e., lesion, background, or border-line tissue) are automatically identified in the PET data volume using a 3D floating window (i.e., $3 \times 3 \times 3$ voxels). The highlighted values are then arranged for every window into 27-element vectors describing the volume sample being investigated. The "training and testing" step needs to be performed only once. When completed, the classifier is capable of labelling new tissue and, subsequently, this information will be used to guide the segmentation process. A thorough explanation of this aspect will be provided in Section 2.1.1. The main advantage of leveraging a AS is that it is free to intersect the whole volume of PET images (i.e., all slices) and therefore segments them all at once, using cross-slice information, both in terms of data volume and tissue labels, that could not be leveraged before (i.e., in the system of Figure 1A). Details of this part will be given in Section 2.1.2. Finally, an operator-independent biological tumor volume (BTV) is obtained (step "m" in Figure 1B).

The following subsections will provide detailed discussion of the various components of system 1-A.

2.1.1. The 3D Discriminant Analysis

The DA was used to classify PET tissues into three clusters: background, lesion, and border-line tissues. The training needs to be done only once, after which DA is able to classify newly encountered tissues and can be re-used at any time.

Three clinicians with different expertise segmented 58 patients [24] (see Section 2.2 for more details). The STAPLE tool [26] was used to combine the three manual segmentations and to define a consolidated reference to be used as gold standard. Only eight patients (considering multiple PET slices for each study) were used for the training and testing of the 3D tissue classification algorithm. These comprised 2 with brain metastases, 4 with head and neck cancers, and 2 with lung cancers, respectively. The sampling process produced 13,762,560 vectors divided into 28,152 lesion vectors, 16,107 border-line vectors, and 13,718,301 background vectors. Specifically, in order to extract such samples, each PET slice was processed using a 3D floating window (i.e., $3 \times 3 \times 3$ voxels). The values in every window were arranged into 27-element vectors. Such a sample size was empirically determined to provide the best results on the current data set.

Of the generated samples, 80% were used for the training step, while the remaining 20% were used for the testing step (as stated by the Pareto principle, also known as the 80/20 rule). The K-Fold cross-validation was used to obtain a robust classification and to eliminate over-fitting. Accordingly, the dataset was split into K equal folds, and the holdout method repeated K times. Every time one of the K folds was used as a validation set, and the remaining K-1 subsets were assembled to form a training set. The variance of the resulting estimate decreased as K increased. Samples with no more than 17 lesion voxels or totally outside the gold standard were labelled as "border-line" and "background" tissue, respectively. In all other instances, the label "lesion" was assigned. Once the training process was completed, a validation stage to test the efficiency of the classification followed.

2.1.2. The Active Surface Algorithm

Starting from the model proposed by Lankton et al. [27], which benefits purely local edge-based active contours and more global region-based active contours, I propose a more efficient segmentation technique that segments all slices simultaneously by developing a single surface inside the corresponding 3D PET volume [28], and a new mathematical formulation of the active surface energy including the 3D classifier information.

Summarizing, the obtained algorithm possesses the following novelty and improvements:

- A new active surface volumetric energy formulation.
- A full 3D development so leveraging cross-slice information.
- Inclusion of 3D tissue information.

These aspects are further detailed below.

First, a new formulation of the energy driving the AS by the inclusion of information from the 3D classifier is introduced.

In view of the fact that the tumor and the background regions are not easily split into two distinct regions, the energy was modified to include a new energy term based on tissue classes generated by the 3D classifier:

$$\chi_{lesion}(x) = \begin{cases} 1 & \text{when } 3D\ DA(x) = lesion; \\ 0 & \text{otherwise}; \end{cases} \quad (1)$$

$$\chi_{border-line}(x) = \begin{cases} 1 & \text{when } 3D\ DA(x) = borderline; \\ 0 & \text{otherwise}; \end{cases} \quad (2)$$

$$\chi_{background}(x) = \begin{cases} 1 & \text{when } 3D\ DA(x) = background; \\ 0 & \text{otherwise}; \end{cases} \quad (3)$$

where the characteristic functions $\chi_{lesion}(x)$, $\chi_{border-line}(x)$ and $\chi_{background}(x)$ represent the 3D tissue's classification for lesion, border-line, and background, respectively.

In Functional Energy Equation (4), the first term is basically a prior term penalizing the overlap between regions which are classified in a conflicting way by the 3D AS and the 3D classifier (in regions classified as "border-line" no penalty is applied).

To integrate the standardized uptake value (SUV) and to insert this new prior term in the mathematical model and formulate it in a fully 3D setup, the active surface energy to be minimized for PET image segmentation is defined as:

$$E = \int_S \lambda \left(\int_{R_{in}} \chi_l(x,s) \overline{Pout}_l(x)\ dx + \int_{R_{out}} \chi_l(x,s) \overline{Pin}_l(x)\ dx \right) + \\ (1-\lambda) \left(\int_{R_{in}} \chi_l(x,s)(SUV(x) - u_l(s))^2 dx + \int_{R_{out}} \chi_l(x,s)(SUV(x) - v_l(s))^2 dx \right) dS \quad (4)$$

- $\lambda \in R^+$ was chosen equal to 0.01, because such value proved to yield the best result;
- $\overline{Pin}_l(x)$ and $\overline{Pout}_l(x)$ indicate the 3D local mean DA classification within the portions of the local neighborhood $\chi_l(x)$ inside and outside the surface, respectively (within Ω);
- S is the 3D AS and dS is the surface area measure;
- s is the 3D surface parameter;
- x is a point within the 3D volume and dx the volume measure;
- R_{in} and R_{out} are the corresponding 3D regions inside and outside the surface;
- $\chi_l(x,s)$ is the indicator function around the surface point $S(s)$ of a local neighborhood.

Such neighborhoods are spheres of radius l centered around each point of the surface S. It was equal to 3 as proposed in [19].

$$\overline{P\text{in}}_l(x) = \frac{\int_\Omega \chi_l(x)\chi_{lesion}(x)\,dx}{\int_\Omega \chi_l(x)\,dx}, \quad \overline{P\text{out}}_l(x) = \frac{\int_\Omega \chi_l(x)\chi_{background}(x)\,dx}{\int_\Omega \chi_l(x)\,dx} \tag{5}$$

In practice, the 3D surface obtained after pre-segmentation is used as initialization to the AS and evolved to minimize the energy E until it finally fits the tumor silhouette.

2.2. The Clinical Dataset

In order to compare the performance of this new algorithm to its 2D predecessor, I considered the same dataset discussed in [24], which comprises 12 lung, 29 head and neck, and 17 brain cancers for a total of 58 PET studies. Eight PET datasets (2 with brain metastases, 4 with head and neck cancers, 2 with lung cancers) were used to train and test the 3D DA classifier while the remaining fifty PET datasets (i.e., 10 lung, 25 head and neck, and 15 brain cancers) were used to evaluate the performance of the proposed segmentation method.

Segmentations were done off-line and the findings did not affect either the treatment plan or the care of the patient. No personal information on patients has been released. Concerning the use of dataset, written consent was released by patients.

The PET investigation protocol was approved by the institutional Hospital Medical Ethics Review Board. Acquisitions were performed on a Discovery 690 PET/CT scanner with time of flight (General Electric Medical Systems, Milwaukee, WI, USA) and produced PET images with resolution of 256 × 256 voxels with grid spacing of 2.73 mm^3, thickness of 3.27 mm^3 and voxel size 2.73 × 2.73 × 3.27 mm^3.

2.3. Framework for Performance Evaluation

The following parameters are used here for performance evaluation:

$$Sensitivity = \frac{True\ Positive}{True\ Positive + False\ Negative} \tag{6}$$

$$Specificity = \frac{True\ Negative}{True\ Negative + False\ Positive} \tag{7}$$

$$positive\ predictive\ value\ (PPV) = \frac{True\ Positive}{True\ Positive + False\ Positive} \tag{8}$$

$$Accuracy(ACC) = \frac{True\ Positive + True\ Negative}{True\ Positive + False\ Positive + False\ Negative + True\ Negative} \tag{9}$$

$$Dice\ similarity\ coefficient\ (DSC) = \frac{2 \times True\ Positive}{2 \times True\ Positive + False\ Positive + False\ Negative} \tag{10}$$

$$Hausdorff\ distance\ (HD) = \max\{d(A,B), d(B,A)\} \tag{11}$$

$$Pearson\ correlation\ coefficient\ (PCC) = \frac{COV(X,Y)}{\sigma X \sigma Y} \tag{12}$$

The PCC can take a value between +1 and −1, where +1 and −1 show total correlation (no difference between two segmentations), while 0 means no correlation (totally difference between two segmentations).

The proposed fully 3D DA segmentation method was implemented in Matlab R2019a and run on MacBook Pro computer with a 2.5 GHz Intel Core i7 processor, 16 GB 1600 MHz DDR3 memory, and OS X Sierra.

3. Results

Segmentation Results

To train and test the classifier, tumor, background and border-line tissues were automatically identified on PET images using the strategy described in Section 2.1.1. Starting from eight patient cases, the sampling process produced 13,762,560 vectors divided into 28,152 lesion vectors, 16,107 border-line vectors, and 13,718,301 background vectors. In total, 80% of the samples were used for training, while the remaining 20% were used for testing. Concerning the K-Fold cross-validation, the optimal k value was determined through the trial-and-error method (k ranged: 5–15, step size of 5), k = 5 corresponded to the highest classification accuracy. The capability of the 3D DA classifier in discerning different tissues achieved excellent result with a sensitivity of 99.09%, a specificity of 90.58%, a precision of 98.53%, and an accuracy of 96.46%. Figure 2 shows the receiver operating characteristic (ROC) analysis performed to assess the efficiency of 3D DA classification after the training phase. The area under the curve (AUC) is 0.99538. The maximum AUC is 1, which corresponds to the perfect classifier. After this training, the classifier is able to label new tissues and is ready to be integrated in the segmentation process (as described in Section 2.1.2).

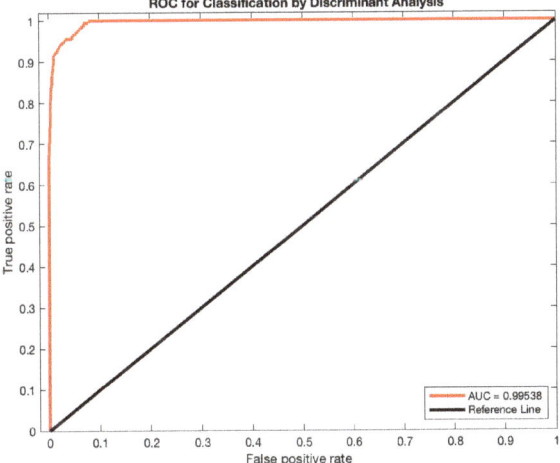

Figure 2. Classification performance of the 3D DA classifier was evaluated by calculating the area under the receiver operating characteristic (ROC) curve (AUC) using the ROC analysis.

To assess the performance of the segmentation method, ten patient studies with lung cancer (^{18}F-fluorodeoxyglucose PET), 25 with head and neck cancer (^{18}F-fluorodeoxyglucose PET), and 15 with brain cancer (^{11}C-methionine PET) were considered. Table 1 summarizes the results of the three previous anatomical districts including the results from the previous study [24]. Since the 2D slice-by-slice approach worked better than several other state-of-the-art approaches [24], I felt judged comparison with additional approaches to be unnecessary.

Table 1. Sensitivities, PPVs, DSCs and HDs for cancer studies using the 3D and 2D algorithms.

	3D Active Surface with 3D Discriminant Analysis		
	Lung	Head and Neck	Brain
	Mean ± std	Mean ± std	Mean ± std
Sensitivity	90.09 ± 6.50%	86.05 ± 5.70%	89.61 ± 4.29%
PPV	91.36 ± 3.89%	91.19 ± 5.30%	91.27 ± 4.52%
DSC	90.47 ± 2.36%	88.30 ± 2.89%	90.29 ± 2.52%
HD	1.40 ± 0.72	1.33 ± 0.57	1.04 ± 0.49
	2D Active Contour with 2D Discriminant Analysis		
	Lung	Head and Neck	Brain
	Mean ± std	Mean ± std	Mean ± std
Sensitivity	88.00 ± 5.41%	89.28 ± 5.70%	89.58 ± 3.40%
PPV	88.19 ± 4.73%	85.53 ± 5.13%	89.76 ± 3.31%
DSC	88.01 ± 4.23%	87.15 ± 3.23%	89.58 ± 2.37%
HD	1.53 ± 0.54	1.18 ± 0.39	1.07 ± 0.61

As confirmed by the analysis of variance (ANOVA) (see Table 2), the proposed 3D AS DA algorithm generated better results than the previous 2D algorithm. This was further demonstrated by the statistical difference (ANOVA p-value < 0.047) in the DSC comparison. In addition, Pearson correlation coefficient (PCC) analysis has been performed to evaluate the similarity of the proposed segmentation with the previous method [24], across all the fifty cases. The fully 3D AS DA approach, with a mean DSC of 89.69 ± 1.21%, not only performed overall better than the old method (DSC = 87.24 ± 4.59%), but with PCC~0.53 provided significantly different results as well (p-value = 0.000044).

Table 2. ANOVA and PCC on the DSC showed statistical differences between 2D and 3D segmentation methods.

Active Surface with Discriminant Analysis	ANOVA p-Value	Mean DSC Difference	PCC	PCC p-Value
2D vs. 3D	0.046	2.45%	0.53	0.000044

Figure 3 shows the qualitative comparison between the proposed method and the algorithm proposed in [24].

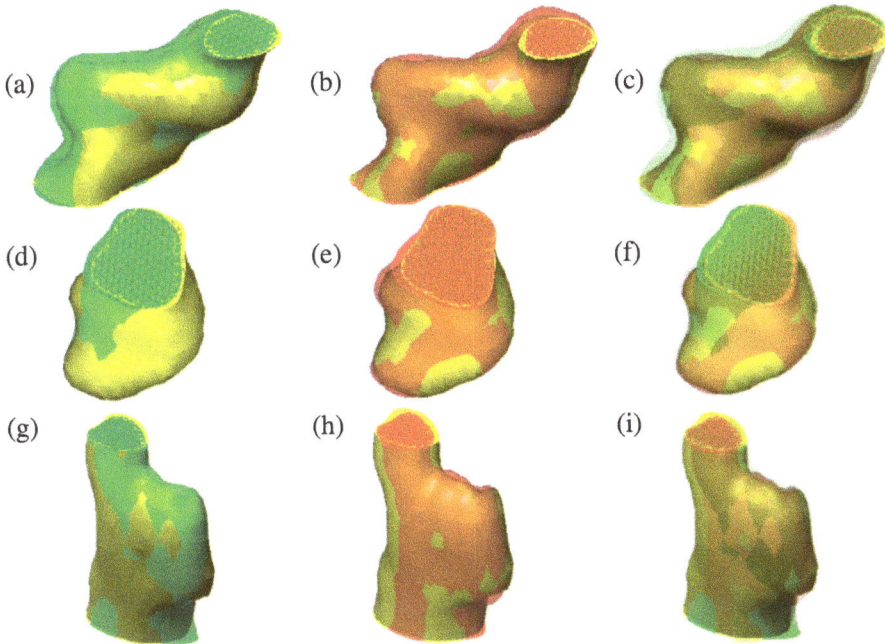

Figure 3. Three different tumors reported in the figure show the difference between 2D active contours (**a,d,g**) [24] and 3D active surface (**b,e,h**) segmentations guided by the 3D classifier. The reconstructed surfaces (green and red) and the gold standards (in yellow) are rendered partially transparent for better comparison. In the last column, the overlap of both methods and the gold standard is shown (**c,f,i**). Specifically, an over-segmentation of the 2D approach compared to 3D can be observed. (Color images can be found on the electronic version of this article).

4. Discussion

In this study, I discuss the inclusion of 3D tissue labelling with in the energy to be minimized during the 3D segmentation based on AS. The key improvement over the previous work [24] is a new segmentation algorithm obtained by evolving a 3D active surface, not only according to the PET data itself, but also leveraging information conveyed by a purposely-trained 3D DA classifier. Such information is included directly in the energy formulation. Previously [24], the 3D shape reconstruction challenge was addressed by using a reconstruction strategy based on a 2D approach, where the tumor segmentation was performed on each slice independently, and marching from one slice to the next until a stop condition is satisfied. While this represented an important step toward 3D delineation, it introduced a preferential direction (the direction of the marching) in the algorithm. In addition, the presence of a preferential direction is an embedded feature of PET data itself, being the distance between pet slices much greater than their planar resolution. While this particular aspect did not seem to influence the outcome of [24], it is nevertheless possible to conceive tumor topologies for which the marching 2D algorithm could actually ignore part of the tumor. To remove such a risk, I wanted to perform the shape reconstruction using an algorithm capable of handling any topology and where no preferential direction is present, either implicitly or explicitly. For this reason, the BTV delineation in this work is obtained through the evolution of a fully 3D surface. While some key features of the present system remained unchanged with respect to the previous version [24], such as (i) input is minimal and consist of just one manual delineation on one pet slice (see Section 2.1.), (ii) conversion of PET images into SUV images (see Section 2.1.2), and (iii) an optimal mask is retrieved during the pre-segmentation step, the core approach to segmentation, the initialization strategy and the DA labelling underwent consistent changes. In particular, initialization is now provided in form of a 3D shape and the DA has been re implemented to handle voxels, as opposed to pixels.

Finally, for better comparison, I used the same PET dataset as in Comelli et al. [24] where I demonstrated that the 2D approach already performed better than many commonly employed delineation methods. My results clearly show that both the migration from assembled 2D to full 3D, and the inclusion of tissue classification contributed to improve performance regardless of the anatomical district considered. In particular, in terms of DSC the improvement can be summarized as follows: 90.47 ± 2.36% versus 88.01 ± 4.23% for lung cancer, 88.30 ± 2.89% versus 87.15 ± 3.23% for head and neck cancer, and 90.29 ± 2.52% versus 89.58 ± 2.37% for brain cancer. Moreover, it is worth noting that, with the active surface, no stopping condition is needed and any preferential direction is removed. The converged active surface delivers a final, fully operator-independent 3D segmentation. In addition, I included the tissue classification, which was implemented in 3D as well. In this way, both the evolving shape and the tissue classification included in the energy, and consequently in the shape evolution, exploit cross-slice information that has never been exploited before. Despite (from a surficial search of the literature) the impression that the combination of ML with the active surface approach has been investigated by many authors, most studies have instead kept active surface and ML as independent entities. In contrast, I integrated ML directly in the energy of the active surface approach.

5. Conclusions

In this study, I discussed the inclusion of 3D tissue classification into fully 3D segmentation based on the evolution of an active surface. The obtained algorithm outperforms my previous formulation in which the tumor delineation was achieved using a 2D active contour approach. As an immediate advantage, the active surface is capable of segmenting all volume at once. Additionally, I enriched such an algorithm with the inclusion of a machine learning component, which consists of a 3D tissue classification based on discriminant analysis and compared the results with previous work. Noteworthy, both shape evolution and tissue classification can now leverage cross-slice information that was not available before. Based on the reported results, I can claim that migrating the system into 3D yielded a practical benefit justifying the effort to rewrite an existing 2D system for PET imaging segmentation.

Funding: This research received no external funding.

Acknowledgments: I would like to thank Alessandro Stefano, Samuel Bignardi, Anthony Yezzi, Giorgio Russo, Maria Gabriella Sabini, and Massimo Ippolito, who provided crucial suggestions and high-quality observations during the preparation of this study. Additionally, I would like to acknowledge my family, for their continuous support and encouragement.

Conflicts of Interest: The author declares no conflict of interest.

References

1. Niyazi, M.; Landrock, S.; Elsner, A.; Manapov, F.; Hacker, M.; Belka, C.; Ganswindt, U. Automated biological target volume delineation for radiotherapy treatment planning using FDG-PET/CT. *Radiat. Oncol.* **2013**, *8*, 180. [CrossRef]
2. Borasi, G.; Russo, G.; Alongi, F.; Nahum, A.; Candiano, G.C.; Stefano, A.; Gilardi, M.C.; Messa, C. High-intensity focused ultrasound plus concomitant radiotherapy: A new weapon in oncology? *J. Ther. Ultrasound* **2013**, *1*, 6. [CrossRef] [PubMed]
3. Guo, Z.; Guo, N.; Gong, K.; Zhong, S.; Li, Q. Gross tumor volume segmentation for head and neck cancer radiotherapy using deep dense multi-modality network. *Phys. Med. Biol.* **2019**, *64*, 205015. [CrossRef] [PubMed]
4. Wahl, R.L.; Jacene, H.; Kasamon, Y.; Lodge, M.A. From RECIST to PERCIST: Evolving Considerations for PET response criteria in solid tumors. *J. Nucl. Med.* **2009**, *50*, 122S. [CrossRef] [PubMed]
5. Cegla, P.; Kazmierska, J.; Gwozdz, S.; Czepczynski, R.; Malicki, J.; Cholewinski, W. Assessment of biological parameters in head and neck cancer based on in vivo distribution of 18F-FDG-FLT-FMISO-PET/CT images. *Tumori* **2019**, *106*, 33–38. [CrossRef] [PubMed]

6. Banna, G.L.; Anile, G.; Russo, G.; Vigneri, P.; Castaing, M.; Nicolosi, M.; Strano, S.; Gieri, S.; Spina, R.; Patanè, D.; et al. Predictive and Prognostic Value of Early Disease Progression by PET Evaluation in Advanced Non-Small Cell Lung Cancer. *Oncology* **2017**, *92*, 39–47. [CrossRef]
7. Stefano, A.; Porcino, N.; Banna, G.; Russoa, G.; Mocciaro, V.; Anile, G.; Gieri, S.; Cosentino, S.; Murè, G.; Baldari, S.; et al. Metabolic response assessment in non-small cell lung cancer patients after platinum-based therapy: A preliminary analysis. *Curr. Med. Imaging Rev.* **2015**, *11*, 218–227. [CrossRef]
8. Gillies, R.J.; Kinahan, P.E.; Hricak, H. Radiomics: Images Are More than Pictures, They Are Data. *Radiology* **2016**, *278*, 563–577. [CrossRef]
9. Stefano, A.; Gioè, M.; Russo, G.; Palmucci, S.; Torrisi, S.E.; Bignardi, S.; Basile, A.; Comelli, A.; Benfante, V.; Sambataro, G.; et al. Performance of Radiomics Features in the Quantification of Idiopathic Pulmonary Fibrosis from HRCT. *Diagnostics* **2020**, *10*, 306. [CrossRef]
10. Comelli, A.; Stefano, A.; Coronnello, C.; Russo, G.; Vernuccio, F.; Cannella, R.; Salvaggio, G.; Lagalla, R.; Barone, S. Radiomics: A New Biomedical Workflow to Create a Predictive Model. In *Annual Conference on Medical Image Understanding and Analysis*; Springer: Cham, Switzerland, 2020; pp. 280–293.
11. Stefano, A.; Vitabile, S.; Russo, G.; Ippolito, M.; Sabini, M.G.; Sardina, D.; Gambino, O.; Pirrone, R.; Ardizzone, E.; Gilardi, M.C. An enhanced random walk algorithm for delineation of head and neck cancers in PET studies. *Med. Biol. Eng. Comput.* **2017**, *55*, 897–908. [CrossRef]
12. Abdoli, M.; Dierckx, R.A.J.O.; Zaidi, H. Contourlet-based active contour model for PET image segmentation. *Med. Phys.* **2013**, *40*, 082507. [CrossRef]
13. Foster, B.; Bagci, U.; Mansoor, A.; Xu, Z.; Mollura, D.J. A review on segmentation of positron emission tomography images. *Comput. Biol. Med.* **2014**, *50*, 76–96. [CrossRef] [PubMed]
14. Guo, Z.; Guo, N.; Li, Q.; Gong, K. Automatic multi-modality segmentation of gross tumor volume for head and neck cancer radiotherapy using 3D U-Net. In *Medical Imaging 2019: Computer-Aided Diagnosis*; San Diego, CA, USA, 16–21 February 2019; International Society for Optics and Photonics: Bellingham, WA, USA, 2009.
15. Huang, B.; Chen, Z.; Wu, P.M.; Ye, Y.; Feng, S.T.; Wong, C.Y.O.; Zheng, L.; Liu, Y.; Wang, T.; Li, Q.; et al. Fully Automated Delineation of Gross Tumor Volume for Head and Neck Cancer on PET-CT Using Deep Learning: A Dual-Center Study. *Contrast Media Mol. Imaging* **2018**, *2018*. [CrossRef] [PubMed]
16. Comelli, A.; Terranova, M.C.; Scopelliti, L.; Salerno, S.; Midiri, F.; Lo Re, G.; Petrucci, G.; Vitabile, S. A Kernel Support Vector Machine Based Technique for Crohn's Disease Classification in Human Patients. In *Conference on Complex, Intelligent, and Software Intensive Systems*; Springer: Cham, Switzerland, 2018; pp. 262–273.
17. Poudel, P.; Illanes, A.; Sheet, D.; Friebe, M. Evaluation of Commonly Used Algorithms for Thyroid Ultrasound Images Segmentation and Improvement Using Machine Learning Approaches. *J. Healthc. Eng.* **2018**, *2018*. [CrossRef]
18. Çiçek, Ö.; Abdulkadir, A.; Lienkamp, S.S.; Brox, T.; Ronneberger, O. 3D U-net: Learning dense volumetric segmentation from sparse annotation. In Proceedings of the Lecture Notes in Computer Science (including subseries Lecture Notes in Artificial Intelligence and Lecture Notes in Bioinformatics), 25 January 2016; Springer: Cham, Switzerland, 2016; Volume 9901, pp. 424–432.
19. Hatt, M.; Lee, J.A.; Schmidtlein, C.R.; El Naqa, I.; Caldwell, C.; De Bernardi, E.; Lu, W.; Das, S.; Geets, X.; Gregoire, V.; et al. Classification and evaluation strategies of auto-segmentation approaches for PET: Report of AAPM task group No. 211. *Med. Phys.* **2017**, *44*, e1–e42. [CrossRef]
20. Avanzo, M.; Wei, L.; Stancanello, J.; Vallières, M.; Rao, A.; Morin, O.; Mattonen, S.A.; El Naqa, I. Machine and deep learning methods for radiomics. *Med. Phys.* **2020**, *47*, e185–e202. [CrossRef] [PubMed]
21. Feng-Ping, A.; Zhi-Wen, L. Medical image segmentation algorithm based on feedback mechanism convolutional neural network. *Biomed. Signal Process. Control* **2019**, *53*, 101589. [CrossRef]
22. Comelli, A.; Stefano, A.; Russo, G.; Sabini, M.G.; Ippolito, M.; Bignardi, S.; Petrucci, G.; Yezzi, A. A smart and operator independent system to delineate tumours in Positron Emission Tomography scans. *Comput. Biol. Med.* **2018**, *102*, 1–15. [CrossRef] [PubMed]
23. Comelli, A.; Stefano, A.; Russo, G.; Bignardi, S.; Sabini, M.G.; Petrucci, G.; Ippolito, M.; Yezzi, A. K-nearest neighbor driving active contours to delineate biological tumor volumes. *Eng. Appl. Artif. Intell.* **2019**, *81*, 133–144. [CrossRef]
24. Comelli, A.; Stefano, A.; Bignardi, S.; Russo, G.; Sabini, M.G.; Ippolito, M.; Barone, S.; Yezzi, A. Active contour algorithm with discriminant analysis for delineating tumors in positron emission tomography. *Artif. Intell. Med.* **2019**, *94*, 67–78. [CrossRef]

25. Comelli, A.; Stefano, A.; Bignardi, S.; Coronnello, C.; Russo, G.; Sabini, M.G.; Ippolito, M.; Yezzi, A. Tissue Classification to Support Local Active Delineation of Brain Tumors. In *Proceedings of the Communications in Computer and Information Science*; Springer: Cham, Switzerland, 2020; Volume 1065, pp. 3–14.
26. Warfield, S.K.; Zou, K.H.; Wells, W.M. Simultaneous truth and performance level estimation (STAPLE): An algorithm for the validation of image segmentation. *IEEE Trans. Med. Imaging* **2004**, *23*, 903–921. [CrossRef] [PubMed]
27. Lankton, S.; Nain, D.; Yezzi, A.; Tannenbaum, A. Hybrid geodesic region-based curve evolutions for image segmentation. In *Proceedings of the Medical Imaging 2007: Physics of Medical Imaging*; Hsieh, J., Flynn, M.J., Eds.; International Society for Optics and Photonics: Bellingham, WA, USA, 2007; Volume 6510, p. 65104U.
28. Comelli, A.; Bignardi, S.; Stefano, A.; Russo, G.; Sabini, M.G.; Ippolito, M.; Yezzi, A. Development of a new fully three-dimensional methodology for tumours delineation in functional images. *Comput. Biol. Med.* **2020**, *120*, 103701. [CrossRef] [PubMed]

Publisher's Note: MDPI stays neutral with regard to jurisdictional claims in published maps and institutional affiliations.

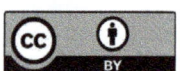

© 2020 by the author. Licensee MDPI, Basel, Switzerland. This article is an open access article distributed under the terms and conditions of the Creative Commons Attribution (CC BY) license (http://creativecommons.org/licenses/by/4.0/).

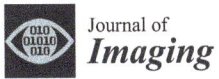

Article

Morphological Estimation of Cellularity on Neo-Adjuvant Treated Breast Cancer Histological Images

Mauricio Alberto Ortega-Ruiz [1,2,*], Cefa Karabağ [2], Victor García Garduño [3] and Constantino Carlos Reyes-Aldasoro [4,*]

1. Universidad del Valle de México, Departamento de Ingeniería, Campus Coyoacán, Ciudad de México 04910, Mexico
2. Department of Electrical & Electronic Engineering, School of Mathematics, Computer Science and Engineering, City, University of London, London EC1V 0HB, UK; cefa.karabag.1@city.ac.uk
3. Departamento de Ingeniería en Telecomunicaciones, Facultad de Ingeniería, Universidad Nacional Autónoma de México, Av. Universidad 3000, Ciudad Universitaria, Coyoacán, Ciudad de México 04510, Mexico; france@marconi.fi-b.unam.mx
4. giCentre, Department of Computer Science, School of Mathematics, Computer Science and Engineering, City, University of London, London EC1V 0HB, UK
* Correspondence: mauricio.ortega@city.ac.uk (M.A.O.-R.); reyes@city.ac.uk (C.C.R.-A.)

Received: 31 July 2020; Accepted: 21 September 2020; Published: 27 September 2020

Abstract: This paper describes a methodology that extracts key morphological features from histological breast cancer images in order to automatically assess Tumour Cellularity (TC) in Neo-Adjuvant treatment (NAT) patients. The response to NAT gives information on therapy efficacy and it is measured by the residual cancer burden index, which is composed of two metrics: TC and the assessment of lymph nodes. The data consist of whole slide images (WSIs) of breast tissue stained with Hematoxylin and Eosin (H&E) released in the 2019 SPIE Breast Challenge. The methodology proposed is based on traditional computer vision methods (K-means, watershed segmentation, Otsu's binarisation, and morphological operations), implementing colour separation, segmentation, and feature extraction. Correlation between morphological features and the residual TC after a NAT treatment was examined. Linear regression and statistical methods were used and twenty-two key morphological parameters from the nuclei, epithelial region, and the full image were extracted. Subsequently, an automated TC assessment that was based on Machine Learning (ML) algorithms was implemented and trained with only selected key parameters. The methodology was validated with the score assigned by two pathologists through the intra-class correlation coefficient (ICC). The selection of key morphological parameters improved the results reported over other ML methodologies and it was very close to deep learning methodologies. These results are encouraging, as a traditionally-trained ML algorithm can be useful when limited training data are available preventing the use of deep learning approaches.

Keywords: neo-adjuvant treatment; digital pathology; tumour cellularity; machine learning

1. Introduction

Digital pathology has recently become a major player in Cancer research, disease detection, classification, and even in outcome prognosis [1–4]. Perhaps the most common imaging technique is Hematoxylin and Eosin (H&E), where H stains nuclei blue and E stains cytoplasm pink [5]. Additionally, other immunohistochemistry methods (IHC) that use antibodies to stain antigens or proteins in the tissue are more specific and they can complement H&E [6]. For instance, the cluster of differentiation 31 (CD31), which is commonly found on endothelial cells, is used as an indication of the growth of blood vessels in tumours, or angiogenesis [7–9]. CD34 is found on hematopoietic cells, mesenchymal stem cells, and it is required in certain processes, like infiltration of eosinophils into the colon [10], or the dendritic cell trafficking and pathology in pneumonitis [11], Ki67 is normally associated with cell proliferation and it can be used as a prognostic factor for gliomas [12], breast cancer [13], and colorectal adenocarcinomas [14]. Computer-assisted diagnosis (CAD) [2] is based on the quantitative analysis to grade the level of the disease, but, recently, other clinical-pathological relationships with the data have been explored [15,16]. For example, a better understanding of mechanisms of the disease evolution process [1] and even prognosis information [3].

Breast Cancer is a common disease both in terms of incidence and deaths, with approximately 252,710 new cases and 40,610 deaths in 2017 in the United States alone [17]. In 2018, 30% of new cases Cancer among females cases in the US were breast cancer, which placed it the second place in mortality [18]. Numerous imaging analysis methods are employed in order to study these cancers [19]. Common treatments for breast cancer are surgery, radiation, chemotherapy, or targeted therapy. Breast cancer neo-adjuvant treatment (NAT) is a therapy for advanced cases that provides useful information for breast-conserving surgery [20]. NAT provides prognostic and survival information [21] as well as a rate of local recurrence [22]. The efficacy of NAT is determined by means of the pathological complete response (pCR) and this can be assessed by the Residual Cancer Burden (RCB) [23]. RCB is supported by two metrics: residual Tumour Cellularity (TC) within the Tumour Bed (TB) and the assessment of lymph nodes. RCB is scored in a continuous value, but it is further categorised in four classes RCB-0 to RCB-III. Subsequently, TC, which is defined as the fraction of malignant cells within the image patch, is a key parameter for RCB computation [24,25]. Currently, TC is manually assessed by an eye-balling routine estimating the proportion of TB and this procedure is time-consuming and requires an experienced pathologist.

Neo-adjuvant treatment (NAT) chemotherapy refers to a treatment that is administered before Cancer surgery [26–28]. The first successful results of NAT chemotherapy were demonstrated in the 1980s [29,30]. Some of the benefits of NAT are: tumour size reduction, better prognostics, and, even in some cases, surgery can be avoided [31]. In addition, patients with large tumours could be eligible for breast-conserving or a less tumour size surgery extraction.

TC assessment problem was first addressed by a hand engineering approach based on nuclei segmentation and feature extraction. In the first step, nuclei segmentation needs to be implemented [1]. This is a challenging task and some common techniques are based on active contours [32], watersheds [33], or graph cuts [34], which are either designed for nuclei [33] or lymphocytes segmentation. [32] Based on the segmentation application, speed, accuracy, or automation level might be required [34]. In the present study, automated segmentation is performed and, as it has been reported in some tissue classification studies, accuracy nuclei segmentation does not guarantee better outcome assessment between benign and malignant tissue [2]. When processing a high number of image files, speed constraint is preferable. After segmentation, many features can be extracted, for instance, cell shape, size, and texture [33–35], and also, features from regional and the global image can provide valuable information [36]. These parameters can be used for diagnostic purposes to classify tissue malignancy [36–39] and also for grade disease level assignment. Ref. [33] For instance, a study conducted by Dong and co-authors [40] categorised intraductal lesions in breast cancer by an adequate feature extraction and machine learning (ML) classification.

ML algorithms are trained to learn from the parameters extracted [15]. Some supervised algorithms are Support Vector Machines [41], Boosted Trees [42], and K-Nearest Neighbours [43]. Besides diagnosis, different new clinicopathological relationships with features have been discovered, for example, [16] revealed the relation between stroma morphology and prognosis of breast cancer patients and [44] studied quantification and distribution of tumour-infiltrating lymphocytes (TILs) as prognostic and predictive biomarker.These type of digital pathology methodologies can also useful for TC assessment. A full hand-engineering method for this task was proposed by Peikari [45]. This methodology was based on the extraction of a vector with 125 parameters [45].

Separate to traditional ML techniques, another approach to estimate TC is by Deep Learning (DL) techniques. In the last decade, there has been increased interest in DL methods. One of the main architectures or models is based on the use of neural networks, and a particular case is a Convolutional Neural Network (CNN) [46]. The main advantage of DL techniques is that they do not require the extraction of features manually or by training, as the network learns a series of parameters and weights by itself. However, to achieve this, the network requires a relatively large number of training images with labels, and the number of training data can impact on the performance. In many histopathology applications, labelled training data are still limited as compared to other imaging applications, such as everyday images, like cats and dogs. With the spread use of whole slide digital scanners [47], numerous histopathology images have become available for research purposes. Some have been released to the research community in general in the form of challenges (e.g., https://grand-challenge.org/challenges/) in order to encourage research groups globally to work together, gather annotations, provide training, and testing data sets and benchmark algorithms. The present work follows the 2019 SPIE-AAPM-NCI BreastPathQ: Cancer Cellularity Challenge with the specific objective of "development of quantitative biomarkers for the determination of cancer cellularity from whole slide images (WSI) of breast cancer hematoxylin and eosin (H&E) stained pathological slides" (https://breastpathq.grand-challenge.org/) and addresses the development of quantitative biomarkers for the challenge.

CNNs have been used for different Histopathology tasks, like segmentation [48,49], detection of a specific image properties [50] , and image grade classification [38,51]. Breast cancer tumour cellularity has also been addressed by deep techniques. For instance, Ziang Pei [52] implemented a direct method based on deep and transfer learning approach with the advantage of avoiding cell segmentation. Akbar [20] presented a traditional hand-engineering approach and a deep neural network.

The methodology in this study is based on a hand-engineering approach similar to the one that was described by [45] based on a 125 parameter vector size, but we selected 22 parameters after a correlation analysis of extracted features with TC. Additionally, the methodology described here is similar to Dong et al. parameters from nuclei; we also include parameters from the neighbourhood of the nuclei and from the full image patch. The study by Fondon [36] also analysed regions around the nuclei; however, our study includes morphology parameters from whole breast ducts region. Thus, the main contributions of this paper in the methodology are the segmentation algorithm that is based on the enhancement of the nuclei region, and an algorithm for breast ducts detection and the parameter derivation and selection and its correlation to tumour cellularity. In the results, the correlation analysis of the morphological parameters with cellularity revealed that stroma concentration has the strongest correlation with TC, which is in agreement with the results that were presented by [16]. Finally, the results were validated with the ICC and compared with similar studies [20,45] indicating an increase in ICC. The methodology described only requires a reduced set of training parameters. Therefore, the methodology described in this paper improves previous results and it may be useful in cases when large training data sets, which are normally required for deep learning approaches, are not available.

2. Materials and Methods

2.1. Materials

The data set used in this work consists of 2579 patches of tissue stained with H&E, which were extracted from 64 different patients under Neo-adjuvant Treatment. The size of each patch is 512 × 512 pixels. As a reference, a breast tissue is formed of a connective tissue, named stroma, as seen in pink. Lymphocytes can be seen as dark blue round objects and fat zones as white areas. It also contains ducts,which are responsible for carrying milk, and sometimes arteries, which can be seen as regular clusters of darker blue nuclei grouped into the region (Figure 1).

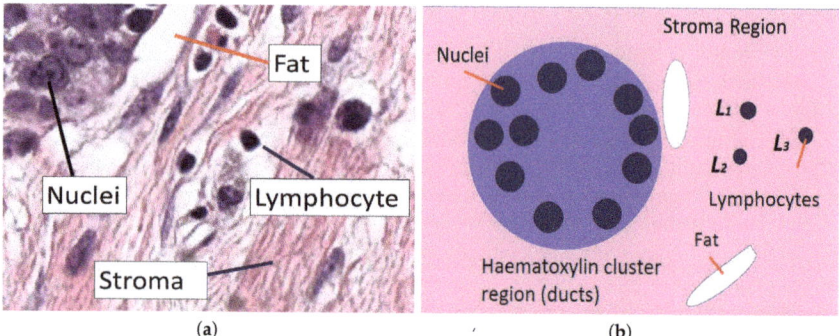

Figure 1. (**a**) Stroma region which shows several clusters, regions of fat as well as some lymphocytes. (**b**) Graphical description of the elements that are analysed in this work. Within a stroma, the connective tissue shown in pink region, ducts appear as clusters stained with haematoxylin and contain several nuclei. Outside these ducts, regions of fat appear white and lymphocytes appear purple.

The residual cellularity of each patch was evaluated by 2 pathologists and this assessment was considered to be the ground truth (GT) for this study. The data was released as part of the challenge 2019 and it was collected at the Sunnybrook Health Sciences Centre, Toronto. It comprises a set of whole slide images (WSIs) that have been stained with H&E [45] from 64 patients with residual invasive breast cancer on re-section specimens following NAT therapy. The specimens were handled according to routine clinical protocols and WSIs were scanned at 20× magnification (0.5 μm/pixel).

The images were divided into a training and validation set of images. The cellularity value distribution for the whole data-set is uneven, i.e., most of the patches correspond to cellularity zero and fewer patches were available for higher cellularity. The training images were selected uniformly distributed from cellularity zero to one in order to have an even amount of benign and malignant nuclei. First, 212 images with selected cellularity values from 0 to 1 were processed and 4533 nuclei cells from those selected images were extracted and its corresponding features computed and used as a training set. The remaining 2367 patches were used for validation. Figure 2 shows the selected patches with different levels of cellularity. A third set of test data of 1119 images was available for the challenge contest. These three sets were used in this work.

2.2. Methodology

The proposed methodology consists of a sequence of traditional image processing routines, computer vision, and machine learning algorithms that automatically process the full validation set. A large amount of morphological parameters can be extracted and stored orderly in an output table file. A master control routine is responsible for selecting one by one the corresponding image patch to be processed. There are two operational modes. A manualmode useful to train machine learning algorithms. In this mode, nuclei from the selected image with a known classification assignment are fed to the algorithm and output features are saved in an output data file. Subsequently, an automated mode processes the full validation set and gives a TC estimation. This mode is able to process thousands of patch images. Figure 3 presents this process in a diagram.

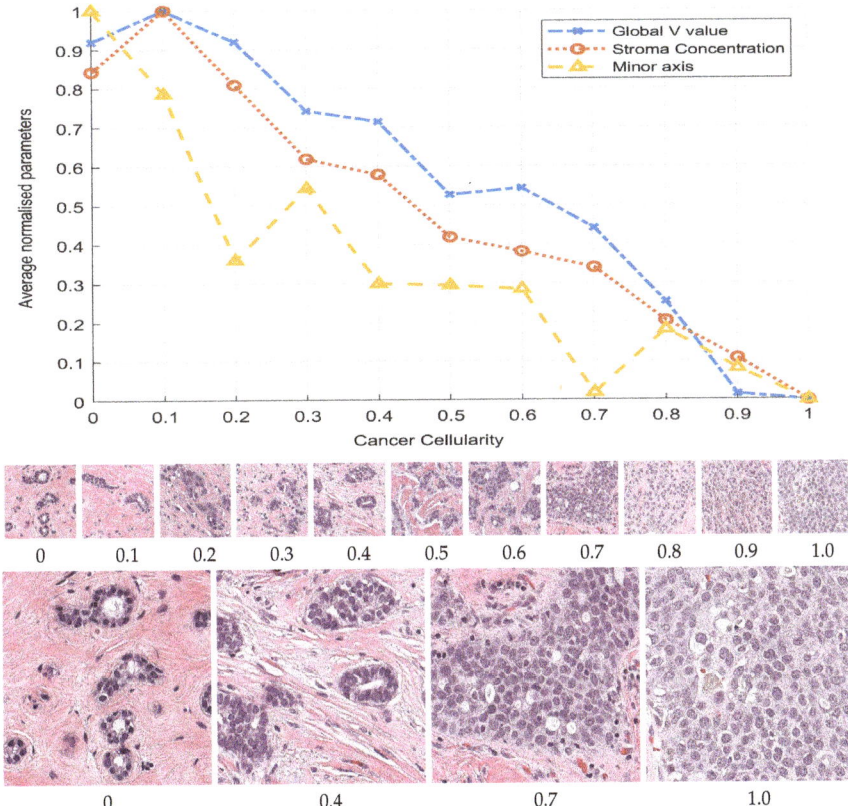

Figure 2. Graphical display of three selected morphological parameters against the cellularity: Global stroma filtered region (o), minor axis (△) and Value concentration in region (x). Cellularity was manually ranked by a pathologist and the parameters automatically extracted. The plots represent average parameter value normalised with maximum value to be compared in the same graph. The graph indicates an inverse relationship between respective parameter and cellularity. Thumbnails show images with cellularity values from zero to one and magnified versions of cases with values 0, 0.4, 0.7, and 1, where the prevalence of cancerous cells can be clearly observed.

The methodology was implemented in Matlab® (The Mathworks™, Natick, MA, USA) 2019b version, with functions from the digital image processing, statistical, and machine learning toolboxes. Additionally, QuPath [53], an open source software for digital pathology image analysis, was used to validate the segmentation results obtained by the methodology. Three regions of interest were selected from each image patch, and more than 150 morphological parameters were extracted at inner segmented cell region, neighbourhood around segmented cell, and the full image patch.

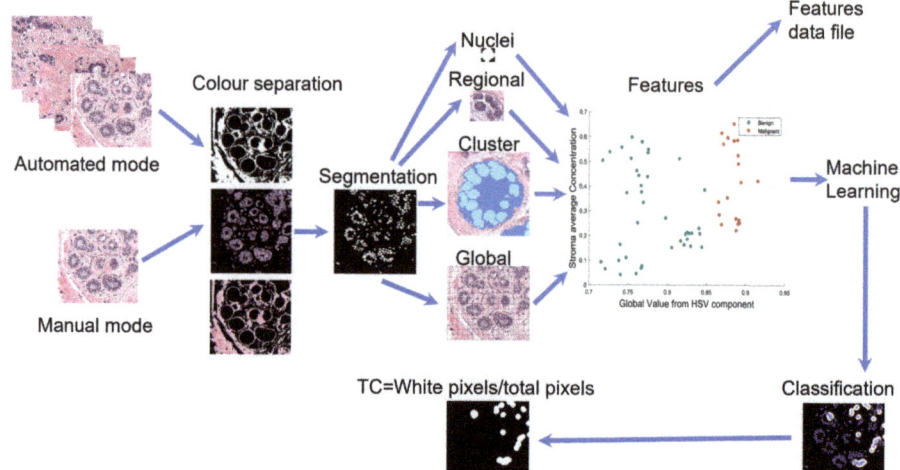

Figure 3. Graphical illustration of the pipeline of the methodology. Under two operational modes images are processed to extract features at nuclei, regional, cluster, and global image regions either to classify and assign Cellularity or to extract same features in order to an archive output.

2.3. Segmentation of Nuclei

At the nuclei region, cells from the image patch are segmented by colour separation and binarisation. The image is converted to HSV colour space and, by K-means clustering [54], three main colour images are extracted, say Ip for pink, Ib for blue, and Iba for the remaining background component image. A special procedure enhances Ib and weakens background region is calculated as:

$$In = K_1(Io. * Im) + K_2 Io + \gamma(Im, 0.1) \tag{1}$$

where Io is the RGB image converted to gray levels and Im is gray image after a median filter of size 3×3 was applied. γ is the gamma correction Im of parameter 0.1 represented as $\gamma(Im, 0.1)$. This value was selected as low to start from a lighter background. K_1 and K_2 are constants that control enhancement of nuclei and weaken background intensity, respectively, and they were experimentally adjusted. First, both of the constants were fixed to 0.5 and, as K_1 is increased and K_2 is reduced, the nuclei region is enhanced. The enhanced image In is binarised by Otsu's algorithm [55] combined with watershed [56] separation of touching nuclei. This segmentation procedure is seen in Figure 4 for three TC cases. A validation analysis of this procedure was done by means of Jaccard Index [57], as shown in (e). The reference images were obtained by a manual segmentation while using the QuPath platform. The results indicate an average Jaccard index of 0.73 after comparing cases of low, medium, and high TC. Although this result might be improved, Peikari and co-authors [45] suggest that cell segmentation accuracy does not have a significant effect in TC assessment.

2.4. Extraction of Morphological Parameters

Using the binary image, a set of morphological parameters has been obtained: area, perimeter, roundness, eccentricity, centroid X, centroid Y, major axis, minor axis, and orientation angle. Additionally, a sub region inside the segmented cell body was determined in order to compute the texture and mean HSV values of the nuclei cell body.

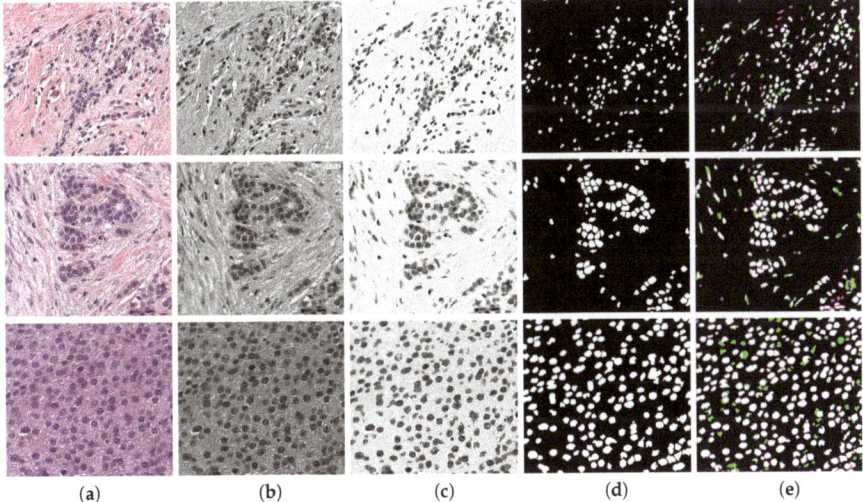

Figure 4. Enhancement of nuclei area. First row corresponds to a Tumour Cellularity (TC) value of zero, second row is an example of TC= 0.5 and third row is TC= 1. Images in column (**a**) are the original image, (**b**) gray level images, (**c**) enhanced images, notice that the nuclei region is darker whilst background becomes lighter, (**d**) Binary image obtained with an adaptive threshold value estimated directly from strongest correlated parameter, and (**e**) validation of nuclei segmentation by Jaccard index. Reference image was manually segmented by using QuPath Platform.

The parameters were extracted from different window sizes surrounding the segmented cell: 30×30, 60×60, 90×90, and 120×120 pixels. The statistical analysis indicated that the best correlation was obtained from the smallest window size. The parameters estimated are the four bins histogram from HSV image and also the regional concentration R of Ip, Iba, and Ib from its binary image, determined by the ratio of total white pixels T_W by total pixels T_P inside window neighbourhood region, $R = T_W/T_P$. Figure 5 shows a sample patch image, with its corresponding pink, blue, binary, and concentration image components. Brown areas indicate low concentration and white and yellow areas are high concentration. Breast normal tissue images present ducts and sometimes arteries, which are clearly seen as regular clusters of darker blue nuclei grouped into the region, see Figure 6. These are detected based on set theory: let U be the full image, D be the cluster or duct, $D \subseteq U \neq \emptyset$. Subsequently, D regions are obtained by subtracting background image Iba from original image U. The following morphological parameters can be extracted from these regions: total cluster area, roundness, number of cells inside cluster, and distance from cells centroid to cluster centroid.

Concentration parameters from the complete full image patch were computed using original RGB image and transformed to HSV. Additionally, a pink colour filter was implemented by means of the Matlab® colour thresholder, which extracts stroma region from the image and computes its mean value. A summary of the full set of features extracted is presented in Table 1; notice that regional parameters are computed at the different window sizes.

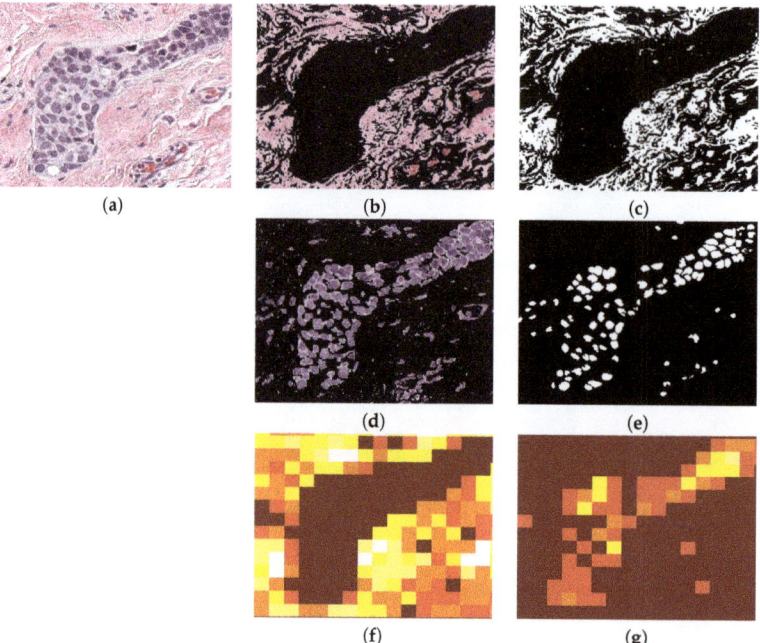

Figure 5. Regional analysis of the data. (**a**) Original image. (**b**) Ip, stroma region image obtained from colour separation. (**c**) Binarised Ip image. (**d**) Ib nuclei image obtained from colour separation. (**e**) Binarised Ib image. (**f**) Regional image concentration of Ip in which brown colour indicates the lowest and white is the highest region concentration. (**g**) Regional density concentration of Ib. This example was processed at 30×30 pixels window.

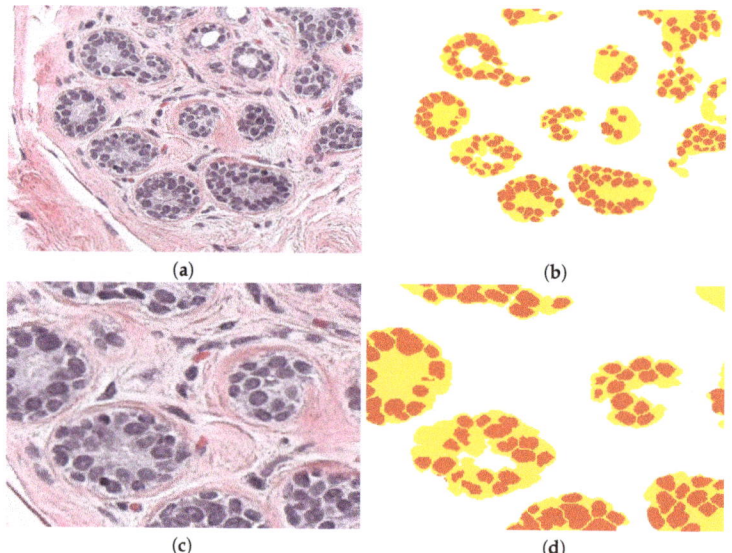

Figure 6. (**a**) The original patch with clear breast ducts. (**b**) Clusters detected by the methodology, every duct or cluster is in yellow and cells inside are in red. Background is labelled in white. (**c**,**d**) Magnified regions of (**a**,**b**).

Table 1. Summary of extracted features. Features at regional level are computed at four different window sizes. Features from the full image represent average values.

Nuclei	Area	Eccentricity	Roundness	Centroid x, y
	Perimeter	Orientation	Major Axis	Minor Axis
	Mean Texture Contrast 1	Mean Texture Contrast 2	Mean Texture Homogenity 1	Mean Texture Homogenity 2
	Mean H value inside nuclei	Mean V value inside nuclei	Mean S value inside nuclei	
Regional Concentrations	Stroma Ip	Background Iba	Nuclei Ib	Epithelial tissue from Ib
	Mean H in window	Mean S in window 2	Mean V in window	
	Mean intensity Histogram H 1	Mean intensity Histogram H 2	Mean intensity Histogram H 3	Mean intensity Histogram H 4
	Mean intensity Histogram S 1	Mean intensity Histogram S 2	Mean intensity Histogram S 3	Mean intensity Histogram S 4
	Mean intensity Histogram V 1	Mean intensity Histogram V 2	Mean intensity Histogram V 3	Mean intensity Histogram V 4
Clusters (ducts)	Cluster area	Cluster roundness	Cells inside cluster	Distance to centroid
Global Image Concentrations	Stroma Ip	Background Iba	Nuclei Ib	
	H value	V Value	S Value	

2.5. Correlation Analysis of Morphological Parameters to TC

The full training set was processed to determine all of the morphological parameters at the three region of interest and those corresponding to Cellularity values equal to (0, 0.1, 0.2, ..., 1.0) were selected, and their mean, standard deviation, maximum, and minimum values were computed. Subsequently, a linear regression and lasso analysis were determined from both analyses. Parameters of coefficient above 0.80 from linear regression and in concordance with lasso selected parameters after redundant removal yield 22 parameters that have the strongest correlation with TC. The plot in in Figure 2 illustrates three parameters with the strongest correlation with TC.

First, the morphological parameters related to segmented nuclei are: eccentricity, roundness, major axis, minor axis, and perimeter. Subsequently, parameters computed at neighbourhood region are: nuclei density concentration, Hue, Value, and Saturation histograms of the regional HSV colour map image. Finally, parameters that are computed from the full image are: HSV average values from HSV components, nuclei concentration, basement concentration, and stroma average concentration determined at output of the pink colour filter. Some of these parameters are graphically displayed in Figure 7.

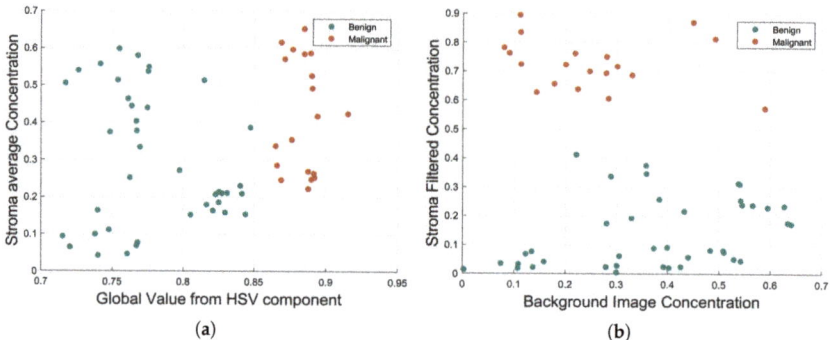

Figure 7. Morphological relationship between the four strongest correlated parameters. (**a**) Global value from HSV component and Stroma average Concentration. (**b**) Background Image Concentration and Stroma Filtered Concentration. In both cases, the benign and malignant cells are highlighted with different colours, which indicate a clear separation.

2.6. Training of Machine Learning Algorithms

Machine learning algorithms were trained with the parameter vector of size 22 determined by the statistical correlation analysis. From the training set, 4533 segmented cells were processed and its corresponding extracted parameters were used to generate a prediction function that classifies nuclei cells between malignant and normal cells. Three algorithms were tested: Support Vector Machines, Nearest K-Network, and AdaBoost. The accuracy of training process for every selected method with the training data showed values up to 0.99 due to a high correlation selected features used for training. TPR achieved are 0.97 for SVM, 0.95 for AdaBoost, and 0.97 for KNN (Figure 8). Support Vector Machines (SVM) is a training algorithm for optimal margin classifier [41], and it is based on a determination of a decision function of pattern vectors x of dimension n classifying in either A or B, in our case benign or malignant cells. The input is a set of p examples of x_i, i.e., the 22 strongest correlated features extracted. K-Nearest Neighbour method [42] was also selected, because it is one of the most well known algorithms within clustering and data classification, in our case between benign and malignant classes. AdaBoost [43] is a decision tree type learning algorithm that starts from observations of a certain item that is represented by branches and goes to conclusions about item target value or leaves. It has a best performance on binary classification problems.

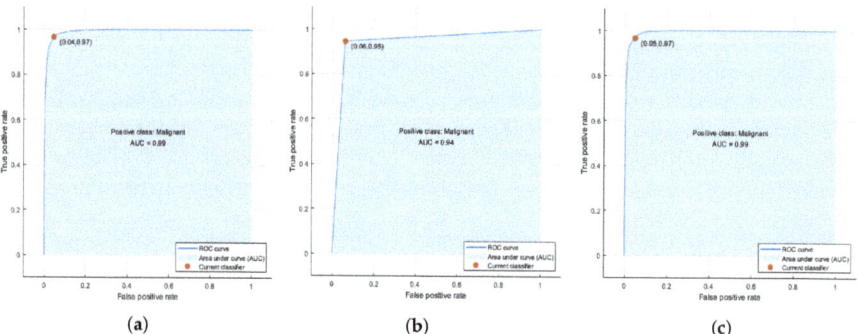

Figure 8. (**a**) Receiver operating characteristic (ROC) curves obtained during training phase for the three selected algorithms. (**a**) Support Vector Machines (SVM), (**b**) AdaBoost , and (**c**) K-Nearest Neighbour (KNN). The higher accuracy value achieved is obtained only with the training set that is highly correlated with Tumour Cellularity (TC).

2.7. Assessment of Tumour Cellularity

The methodology to estimate TC is illustrated in Figure 9, with three representative images with increasing TC from top to bottom in each row. In Figure 9a the nuclei are segmented and their corresponding parameters are extracted. Subsequently, the prediction function classifies every cell in either benign (green) or malignant (red), as illustrated in Figure 9b. Next, an estimation of full cell cytoplasm is done by morphological dilation drawn as the white circles around malignant cells (Figure 9c). The full cellularity that is detected region is shown in Figure 9d. TC is computed as the ratio of the area that is covered by cellularity (white in the figure) over the total area (white and black in figure).

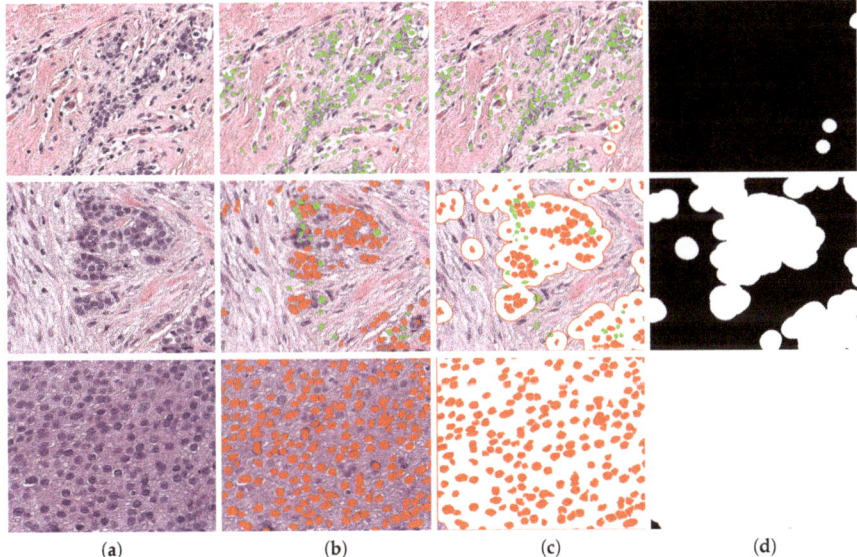

Figure 9. Visual description of the method. Three TC cases are presented in each row: 0, 0.5 and 1. (a) The original image, the image is segmented and key parameters are computed, then a classification predictor estimates either malignant or benign cells, shown in red and green, respectively in (b). A dilation of segmented malignant nuclei estimates full cytoplasm of every detected malignant cell (c) and TB region is shown in white in (d). The cellularity metrics calculated by the proposed methodology are: $TC = 0.0113$, $TC = 0.5181$ and $TC = 0.9936$.

3. Results

An automated estimation of TC was computed from two test data sets. Three prediction functions that were trained by machine learning algorithms were determined to be used with the automated processing software of breast cancer images that classifies cells and computes TC. The method was tested with a training set of 2579 images that were already classified by a pathologist with a TC value. Additionally, it was tested with the 1119 images for submission of SPIE Breast Challenge, with an unknown TC value. Figure 10 shows the statistical behaviour of the method's result for the training set as boxplots.

Dispersion plot indicates the method for approximating to the pathologist classification assignment. The results have a better approximation at higher cellularity values ($TC > 0.70$) and performs well with KNN algorithm. Additionally, around the middle region ($0.4 < TC < 0.6$) has a good approximation with AdaBoost. At low cellularity values ($TC < 0.3$), three methods present deviation, with its higher at cellularity zero, which correspond to images with only benign nuclei cells. According to Minimum Square Error (MSE), SVM performs better overall in the cellularity region.

This result can be validated by a visual inspection of boxplots of Figure 10 in the three cases there is a positive correlation between the actual cellularity (horizontal) and the estimated cellularity (vertical). However, SVM shows less dispersion, especially in the lower values of cellularity as compared with the other two techniques.

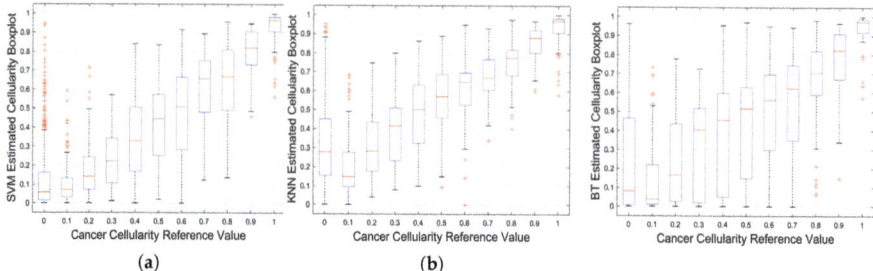

Figure 10. Results of implementation on Training Data. Boxplots for the Cancer Cellularity Reference Value against: (**a**) SVM estimation, (**b**) KNN estimation and (**c**) BT Estimation. It should be noted that large boxplots correspond to large variations of the estimations and as such, SVM shows the lowest variability

In order to analyse the limitations of the algorithm, the TC assessment outcomes with the highest errors were analysed. Figure 11 presents three cases where the TC was incorrectly calculated. All three cases in the figure are of benign tissue with no cellularity; this means that most of the segmented cells should be marked as benignant (green), but several of them are shown in red (b–d), which corresponds to false-positive cases. The expanded area around the cell (e) yields a high TC value instead of the correct value which should have been zero. We assume that this problem is because of the limited amount of cells used to train the algorithm. This problem also explains some of the outliers on the boxplots presented in Figure 10, which are mainly observed at low cellularity. Additionally, this suggests that other classification algorithms should be evaluated.

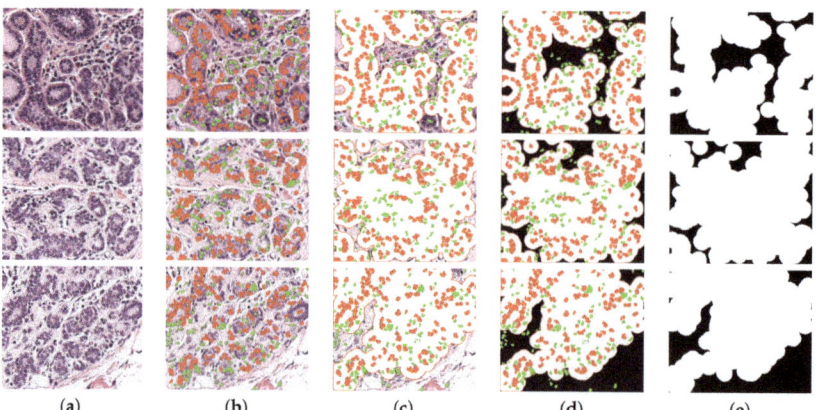

Figure 11. Three cases where the TC was incorrectly calculated. Each row corresponds to a patch with incorrect TC. Column (**a**) illustrates the original image, and columns (**b**–**e**) show the step by step process to assess cellularity. (**b**) Corresponds to the segmented image and classified into benign (green) and malignant (red). Columns (**c**,**d**) show expanded region of malignant cells. Column (**e**) corresponds to cancer cell region in white, used to compute TC. Three worst cases correspond to a TC of zero; this means there would not be any malignant cell and TC image must be completely black. Several cells were miss classified which yields to a TC wrong assessment. Estimated TC values are: 0.75, 0.81, and 0.75, instead of zero.

Statistical analysis of the training set revealed 22 key parameters that have a strong correlation to TC. The Stroma concentration (r = −0.9786), global Value of HSV component (r = −0.9728), regional histogram bins (r = −0.9659), and minor axis (r = 0.8939) from nuclei morphology were the strongest parameters, as shown in Figure 2.

This result revealed that the stroma region has a significant relation to TC, which is in agreement with the results of the hand engineering method by [45] that was trained by a 125-dimensional feature vector reported a 0.75 ICC (first column of Table 2). Lower and upper-bounds are shown in square brackets. Our methodology is also a hand engineering, but trained with only 22 key morphological parameters (second column of Table 2), indicates a 0.78 ICC. This result outperformed those that were obtained by the method of Peikari. The results based on Deep Learning techniques like a combined hand engineering Deep Neural Network reported by Akbar [20] is slightly above the proposed methodology (third column of Table 2). Finally, the methodology proposed was used to process the test set and the results were submitted to the challenge contest. The prediction probability result obtained from contest was $P_k = 0.76$.

Table 2. Comparison of the Intra-class Correlation Coefficients (ICC) of the proposed methodology against a Hand Engineering Methodology (Peikari [45]) and a combined deep learning and hand engineering methodology (Akbar [20]). Lower and upper bounds are shown in square brackets. Notice the closeness of the results of the proposed methodology against the Deep Learning approach.

	Hand Engineering (Peikari)	Key Parameters (Our methodology)	Combined Deep Network (Akbar)
ICC	0.75	0.78	0.79
[L,U]	[0.71, 0.79]	[0.75, 0.80]	[0.76, 0.81]

4. Discussion

A computer methodology that automatically processes H&E histopathology digital images based in the extraction of main morphological parameters at a cell, regional, and global level is presented in this paper. The methodology processed a training set of breast cancer images under NAT treatment and the results indicate 22 key morphological parameters are strongly correlated with cellularity. Interesting results were revealed from the correlation analysis of the morphological parameters. The strongest related parameter was stroma density, in agreement with Beck et al. [16], which is, the histology of stroma correlates with prognostic in breast cancer. Three different machine learning algorithms for cell classification were evaluated and compared in order to determine tumour regions. The best result was obtained with Support Vector Machines (SVM) algorithm. The relevance of this paper is a selection of a key parameters to train the algorithms, which results in a better performance of similar techniques; however, the reported deep learning algorithms outperform this result, which is a motivation to explore these techniques in the future.

Author Contributions: Conceptualisation, M.A.O.-R. and C.C.R.-A.; methodology, M.A.O.-R. and C.C.R.-A.; software, M.A.O.-R.; validation, M.A.O.-R., V.G.G. and C.C.R.-A.; formal analysis, M.A.O.-R. and C.C.R.-A.; investigation, M.A.O.-R. and C.C.R.-A.; resources, M.A.O.-R. and C.C.R.-A.; data curation, M.A.O.-R. and C.C.R.-A.; writing—original draft preparation, M.A.O.-R., C.K. and C.C.R.-A.; writing—review and editing, M.A.O.-R., C.K., V.G.G. and C.C.R.-A.; visualisation, M.A.O.-R. and C.C.R.-A.; supervision, V.G.G. and C.C.R.-A. All authors have read and agreed to the published version of the manuscript.

Funding: This research received no external funding.

Acknowledgments: The authors would like to thank Sunnybrook Health Sciences Centre, Toronto, for the breast cancer NAT images. We also would like to thank Kenny H. Chan for validating our test results which were submitted to SPIE Breast Challenge contest.

Conflicts of Interest: The authors declare no conflict of interest. The funders had no role in the design of the study; in the collection, analyses, or interpretation of data; in the writing of the manuscript, or in the decision to publish the results.

Abbreviations

The following abbreviations are used in this manuscript:

TC	Tumour Cellularity
NAT	Neo-Adjuvant treatment
WSIs	Whole slide images
H&E	Hematoxylin and Eosin
ICC	Intraclass correlation coefficient
ML	Machine Learning
IHC	Immunohistochemistry
CAD	Computer-assisted diagnosis
RCB	Residual Cancer Burden
pCR	Pathological complete response
TB	Tumour Bed
GT	Ground Truth
HSV	Hue, Saturation, Value
RGB	Red, Green, Blue
SVM	Support Vector Machines

References

1. Irshad, H.; Veillard, A.; Roux, L.; Racoceanu, D. Methods for nuclei detection, segmentation, and classification in digital histopathology: A review-current status and future potential. *IEEE Rev. Biomed. Eng.* **2013**, *7*, 97–114. [CrossRef] [PubMed]
2. Gurcan, M.N.; Boucheron, L.E.; Can, A.; Madabhushi, A.; Rajpoot, N.M.; Yener, B. Histopathological Image Analysis: A Review. *IEEE Rev. Biomed. Eng.* **2009**, *2*, 147–171. [CrossRef] [PubMed]
3. Madabhushi, A.; Lee, G. Image analysis and machine learning in digital pathology: Challenges and opportunities. *Med. Image Anal.* **2016**, *33*, 170–175. [CrossRef] [PubMed]
4. Kather, J.N.; Krisam, J.; Charoentong, P.; Luedde, T.; Herpel, E.; Weis, C.A.; Gaiser, T.; Marx, A.; Valous, N.A.; Ferber, D.; et al. Predicting survival from colorectal cancer histology slides using deep learning: A retrospective multicenter study. *PLoS Med.* **2019**, *16*, e1002730. [CrossRef] [PubMed]
5. Chan, J.K.C. The Wonderful Colors of the Hematoxylin–Eosin Stain in Diagnostic Surgical Pathology. *Int. J. Surg. Pathol.* **2014**, *22*, 12–32. [CrossRef] [PubMed]
6. Di Cataldo, S.; Ficarra, E.; Macii, E. Computer-aided techniques for chromogenic immunohistochemistry: Status and directions. *Comput. Biol. Med.* **2012**, *42*, 1012–1025. [CrossRef]
7. Okamura, S.; Osaki, T.; Nishimura, K.; Ohsaki, H.; Shintani, M.; Matsuoka, H.; Maeda, K.; Shiogama, K.; Itoh, T.; Kamoshida, S. Thymidine kinase-1/CD31 double immunostaining for identifying activated tumor vessels. *Biotech. Histochem. Off. Publ. Biol. Stain Comm.* **2019**, *94*, 60–64. [CrossRef]
8. Mohamed, S.Y.; Mohammed, H.L.; Ibrahim, H.M.; Mohamed, E.M.; Salah, M. Role of VEGF, CD105, and CD31 in the Prognosis of Colorectal Cancer Cases. *J. Gastrointest. Cancer* **2019**, *50*, 23–34. [CrossRef]
9. Reyes-Aldasoro, C.C.; Williams, L.J.; Akerman, S.; Kanthou, C.; Tozer, G.M. An automatic algorithm for the segmentation and morphological analysis of microvessels in immunostained histological tumour sections. *J. Microsc.* **2011**, *242*, 262–278. [CrossRef]
10. Maltby, S.; Wohlfarth, C.; Gold, M.; Zbytnuik, L.; Hughes, M.R.; McNagny, K.M. CD34 is required for infiltration of eosinophils into the colon and pathology associated with DSS-induced ulcerative colitis. *Am. J. Pathol.* **2010**, *177*, 1244–1254. [CrossRef]
11. Blanchet, M.R.; Bennett, J.L.; Gold, M.J.; Levantini, E.; Tenen, D.G.; Girard, M.; Cormier, Y.; McNagny, K.M. CD34 is required for dendritic cell trafficking and pathology in murine hypersensitivity pneumonitis. *Am. J. Respir. Crit. Care Med.* **2011**, *184*, 687–698. [CrossRef] [PubMed]
12. Chen, W.J.; He, D.S.; Tang, R.X.; Ren, F.H.; Chen, G. Ki-67 is a valuable prognostic factor in gliomas: Evidence from a systematic review and meta-analysis. *Asian Pac. J. Cancer Prev.* **2015**, *16*, 411–420. [CrossRef] [PubMed]

13. Ishibashi, N.; Nishimaki, H.; Maebayashi, T.; Hata, M.; Adachi, K.; Sakurai, K.; Masuda, S.; Okada, M. Changes in the Ki-67 labeling index between primary breast cancer and metachronous metastatic axillary lymph node: A retrospective observational study. *Thorac. Cancer* **2019**, *10*, 96–102. [CrossRef] [PubMed]
14. Sen, A.; Mitra, S.; Das, R.N.; Dasgupta, S.; Saha, K.; Chatterjee, U.; Mukherjee, K.; Datta, C.; Chattopadhyay, B.K. Expression of CDX-2 and Ki-67 in different grades of colorectal adenocarcinomas. *Indian J. Pathol. Microbiol.* **2015**, *58*, 158–162. [CrossRef]
15. Komura, D.; Ishikawa, S. Machine learning methods for histopathological image analysis. *Comput. Struct. Biotechnol. J.* **2018**, *16*, 34–42. [CrossRef]
16. Beck, A.H.; Sangoi, A.R.; Leung, S.; Marinelli, R.J.; Nielsen, T.O.; van de Vijver, M.J.; West, R.B.; van de Rijn, M.; Koller, D. Systematic analysis of breast cancer morphology uncovers stromal features associated with survival. *Sci. Transl. Med.* **2011**, *3*, 108ra113. [CrossRef]
17. DeSantis, C.E.; Ma, J.; Goding Sauer, A.; Newman, L.A.; Jemal, A. Breast cancer statistics, 2017, racial disparity in mortality by state. *CA A Cancer J. Clin.* **2017**, *67*, 439–448. [CrossRef]
18. Siegel, R.L.; Miller, K.D.; Jemal, A. Cancer statistics, 2019. *CA A Cancer J. Clin.* **2019**, *69*, 7–34. [CrossRef]
19. Veta, M.; Pluim, J.P.W.; Diest, P.J.V.; Viergever, M.A. Breast Cancer Histopathology Image Analysis: A Review. *IEEE Trans. Biomed. Eng.* **2014**, *61*, 1400–1411. [CrossRef]
20. Akbar, S.; Peikari, M.; Salama, S.; Panah, A.Y.; Nofech-Mozes, S.; Martel, A.L. Automated and manual quantification of tumour cellularity in digital slides for tumour burden assessment. *Sci. Rep.* **2019**, *9*, 1–9. [CrossRef]
21. Nahleh, Z.; Sivasubramaniam, D.; Dhaliwal, S.; Sundarajan, V.; Komrokji, R. Residual cancer burden in locally advanced breast cancer: A superior tool. *Curr. Oncol.* **2008**, *15*, 271–278. [CrossRef] [PubMed]
22. Kaufmann, M.; Hortobagyi, G.N.; Goldhirsch, A.; Scholl, S.; Makris, A.; Valagussa, P.; Blohmer, J.U.; Eiermann, W.; Jackesz, R.; Jonat, W.; et al. Recommendations from an international expert panel on the use of neoadjuvant (primary) systemic treatment of operable breast cancer: An update. *J. Clin. Oncol. Off. J. Am. Soc. Clin. Oncol.* **2006**, *24*, 1940–1949. [CrossRef] [PubMed]
23. Symmans, W.F.; Peintinger, F.; Hatzis, C.; Rajan, R.; Kuerer, H.; Valero, V.; Assad, L.; Poniecka, A.; Hennessy, B.; Green, M.; et al. Measurement of residual breast cancer burden to predict survival after neoadjuvant chemotherapy. *J. Clin. Oncol. Off. J. Am. Soc. Clin. Oncol.* **2007**, *25*, 4414–4422. [CrossRef]
24. Kumar, S.; Badhe, B.A.; Krishnan, K.; Sagili, H. Study of tumour cellularity in locally advanced breast carcinoma on neo-adjuvant chemotherapy. *J. Clin. Diagn. Res.* **2014**, *8*, FC09. [PubMed]
25. Peintinger, F.; Kuerer, H.M.; McGuire, S.E.; Bassett, R.; Pusztai, L.; Symmans, W.F. Residual specimen cellularity after neoadjuvant chemotherapy for breast cancer. *Br. J. Surg.* **2008**, *95*, 433–437. [CrossRef]
26. Okines, A.F. T-DM1 in the Neo-Adjuvant Treatment of HER2-Positive Breast Cancer: Impact of the KRISTINE (TRIO-021) Trial. *Rev. Recent Clin. Trials* **2017**, *12*, 216–222. [CrossRef]
27. van Zeijl, M.C.T.; van den Eertwegh, A.J.; Haanen, J.B.; Wouters, M.W.J.M. (Neo)adjuvant systemic therapy for melanoma. *Eur. J. Surg. Oncol. J. Eur. Soc. Surg. Oncol. Br. Assoc. Surg. Oncol.* **2017**, *43*, 534–543. [CrossRef]
28. Tann, U.W. Neo-adjuvant hormonal therapy of prostate cancer. *Urol. Res.* **1997**, *25*, S57–S62. [CrossRef]
29. Bourut, C.; Chenu, E.; Mathé, G. Can neo-adjuvant chemotherapy prevent residual tumors? *Bull. Soc. Sci. Medicales Grand-Duche Luxemb.* **1989**, *126*, 59–63.
30. Stolwijk, C.; Wagener, D.J.; Van den Broek, P.; Levendag, P.C.; Kazem, I.; Bruaset, I.; De Mulder, P.H. Randomized neo-adjuvant chemotherapy trial for advanced head and neck cancer. *Neth. J. Med.* **1985**, *28*, 347–351.
31. Rastogi, P.; Wickerham, D.L.; Geyer, C.E.; Mamounas, E.P.; Julian, T.B.; Wolmark, N. Milestone clinical trials of the National Surgical Adjuvant Breast and Bowel Project (NSABP). *Chin. Clin. Oncol.* **2017**, *6*, 7. [CrossRef]
32. Fatakdawala, H.; Xu, J.; Basavanhally, A.; Bhanot, P.; Ganesan, S.; Feldman, M.; Tomaszewski, J.E.; Madabhushi, A. Expectation–Maximization-Driven Geodesic Active Contour With Overlap Resolution (EMaGACOR): Application to Lymphocyte Segmentation on Breast Cancer Histopathology. *IEEE Trans. Biomed. Eng.* **2010**, *57*, 1676–1689. [CrossRef] [PubMed]
33. Veta, M.; van Diest, P.J.; Kornegoor, R.; Huisman, A.; Viergever, M.A.; Pluim, J.P.W. Automatic Nuclei Segmentation in H&E Stained Breast Cancer Histopathology Images. *PLoS ONE* **2013**, *8*, e70221. [CrossRef]
34. Al-Kofahi, Y.; Lassoued, W.; Lee, W.; Roysam, B. Improved Automatic Detection and Segmentation of Cell Nuclei in Histopathology Images. *IEEE Trans. Biomed. Eng.* **2010**, *57*, 841–852. [CrossRef] [PubMed]

35. Yamada, M.; Saito, A.; Yamamoto, Y.; Cosatto, E.; Kurata, A.; Nagao, T.; Tateishi, A.; Kuroda, M. Quantitative nucleic features are effective for discrimination of intraductal proliferative lesions of the breast. *J. Pathol. Inform.* **2016**, *7*. [CrossRef]
36. Fondón, I.; Sarmiento, A.; García, A.I.; Silvestre, M.; Eloy, C.; Polónia, A.; Aguiar, P. Automatic classification of tissue malignancy for breast carcinoma diagnosis. *Comput. Biol. Med.* **2018**, *96*, 41–51. [CrossRef]
37. De Lima, S.M.L.; da Silva-Filho, A.G.; dos Santos, W.P. Detection and classification of masses in mammographic images in a multi-kernel approach. *Comput. Methods Programs Biomed.* **2016**, *134*, 11–29. [CrossRef]
38. Araújo, T.; Aresta, G.; Castro, E.; Rouco, J.; Aguiar, P.; Eloy, C.; Polónia, A.; Campilho, A. Classification of breast cancer histology images using Convolutional Neural Networks. *PLoS ONE* **2017**, *12*, e0177544. doi:10.1371/journal.pone.0177544. [CrossRef]
39. Niu, Q.; Jiang, X.; Li, Q.; Zheng, Z.; Du, H.; Wu, S.; Zhang, X. Texture features and pharmacokinetic parameters in differentiating benign and malignant breast lesions by dynamic contrast enhanced magnetic resonance imaging. *Oncol. Lett.* **2018**, *16*, 4607–4613. [CrossRef]
40. Dong, F.; Irshad, H.; Oh, E.Y.; Lerwill, M.F.; Brachtel, E.F.; Jones, N.C.; Knoblauch, N.W.; Montaser-Kouhsari, L.; Johnson, N.B.; Rao, L.K.F.; et al. Computational Pathology to Discriminate Benign from Malignant Intraductal Proliferations of the Breast. *PLoS ONE* **2014**, *9*, e114885. [CrossRef]
41. Boser, B.E.; Guyon, I.M.; Vapnik, V.N. A Training Algorithm for Optimal Margin Classifiers. In Proceedings of the 5th Annual ACM Workshop on Computational Learning Theory, Pittsburgh, PA, USA, 27–29 July 1992; ACM Press New York, NY, USA, 1992; pp. 144–152.
42. Cover, T.; Hart, P. Nearest neighbor pattern classification. *IEEE Trans. Inf. Theory* **1967**, *13*, 21–27. [CrossRef]
43. Schapire, R.E.; Singer, Y. Improved boosting algorithms using confidence-rated predictions. *Mach. Learn.* **1999**, *37*, 297–336. [CrossRef]
44. Romagnoli, G.; Wiedermann, M.; Hübner, F.; Wenners, A.; Mathiak, M.; Röcken, C.; Maass, N.; Klapper, W.; Alkatout, I. Morphological Evaluation of Tumor-Infiltrating Lymphocytes (TILs) to Investigate Invasive Breast Cancer Immunogenicity, Reveal Lymphocytic Networks and Help Relapse Prediction: A Retrospective Study. *Int. J. Mol. Sci.* **2017**, *18*, 1936. [CrossRef] [PubMed]
45. Peikari, M.; Salama, S.; Nofech-Mozes, S.; Martel, A.L. Automatic cellularity assessment from post-treated breast surgical specimens. *Cytom. Part A J. Int. Soc. Anal. Cytol.* **2017**, *91*, 1078–1087. [CrossRef] [PubMed]
46. Soffer, S.; Ben-Cohen, A.; Shimon, O.; Amitai, M.M.; Greenspan, H.; Klang, E. Convolutional Neural Networks for Radiologic Images: A Radiologist's Guide. *Radiology* **2019**, *290*, 590–606. [CrossRef] [PubMed]
47. Kumar, N.; Gupta, R.; Gupta, S. Whole Slide Imaging (WSI) in Pathology: Current Perspectives and Future Directions. *J. Digit. Imaging* **2020**. [CrossRef]
48. Sirinukunwattana, K.; Raza, S.E.A.; Tsang, Y.W.; Snead, D.R.J.; Cree, I.A.; Rajpoot, N.M. Locality Sensitive Deep Learning for Detection and Classification of Nuclei in Routine Colon Cancer Histology Images. *IEEE Trans. Med. Imaging* **2016**, *35*, 1196–1206. [CrossRef]
49. Huang, L.; Xia, W.; Zhang, B.; Qiu, B.; Gao, X. MSFCN-multiple supervised fully convolutional networks for the osteosarcoma segmentation of CT images. *Comput. Methods Programs Biomed.* **2017**, *143*, 67–74. [CrossRef]
50. Arjmand, A.; Angelis, C.T.; Christou, V.; Tzallas, A.T.; Tsipouras, M.G.; Glavas, E.; Forlano, R.; Manousou, P.; Giannakeas, N. Training of Deep Convolutional Neural Networks to Identify Critical Liver Alterations in Histopathology Image Samples. *Appl. Sci.* **2020**, *10*, 42. [CrossRef]
51. Xu, J.; Luo, X.; Wang, G.; Gilmore, H.; Madabhushi, A. A Deep Convolutional Neural Network for segmenting and classifying epithelial and stromal regions in histopathological images. *Neurocomputing* **2016**, *191*, 214–223. [CrossRef]
52. Pei, Z.; Cao, S.; Lu, L.; Chen, W. Direct Cellularity Estimation on Breast Cancer Histopathology Images Using Transfer Learning. *Comput. Math. Methods Med.* **2019**, *2019*, 3041250. [CrossRef]
53. Bankhead, P.; Loughrey, M.B.; Fernández, J.A.; Dombrowski, Y.; McArt, D.G.; Dunne, P.D.; McQuaid, S.; Gray, R.T.; Murray, L.J.; Coleman, H.G.; et al. QuPath: Open source software for digital pathology image analysis. *Sci. Rep.* **2017**, *7*, 16878. [CrossRef]
54. Arthur, D.; Vassilvitskii, S. K-means++: The advantages of careful seeding. In Proceedings of the 18th Annual ACM-SIAM Symposium on Discrete Algorithms, New Orleans, LA, USA, 7–9 January 2007; pp. 1027–1035.
55. Otsu, N. A Threshold Selection Method from Gray-Level Histograms. *IEEE Trans. Syst. Man Cybern.* **1979**, *9*, 62–66. [CrossRef]

56. Yang, X.; Li, H.; Zhou, X. Nuclei Segmentation Using Marker-Controlled Watershed, Tracking Using Mean-Shift, and Kalman Filter in Time-Lapse Microscopy. *IEEE Trans. Circuits Syst. I* **2006**, *53*, 2405–2414. [CrossRef]
57. Jaccard, P. Étude comparative de la distribution florale dans une portion des Alpes et des Jura. *Bull. Soc. Vaudoise Sci. Nat.* **1901**, *37*, 547–579.

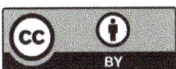 © 2020 by the authors. Licensee MDPI, Basel, Switzerland. This article is an open access article distributed under the terms and conditions of the Creative Commons Attribution (CC BY) license (http://creativecommons.org/licenses/by/4.0/).

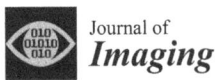

Article

Comparative Study of First Order Optimizers for Image Classification Using Convolutional Neural Networks on Histopathology Images

Ibrahem Kandel [1,*], Mauro Castelli [1] and Aleš Popovič [2]

[1] Nova Information Management School (NOVA IMS), Campus de Campolide, Universidade Nova de Lisboa, 1070-312 Lisboa, Portugal; mcastelli@novaims.unl.pt
[2] School of Economics and Business, University of Ljubljana, Kardeljeva Ploščad 17, 1000 Ljubljana, Slovenia; ales.popovic@ef.uni-lj.si
* Correspondence: d20181143@novaims.unl.pt

Received: 26 August 2020; Accepted: 6 September 2020; Published: 8 September 2020

Abstract: The classification of histopathology images requires an experienced physician with years of experience to classify the histopathology images accurately. In this study, an algorithm was developed to assist physicians in classifying histopathology images; the algorithm receives the histopathology image as an input and produces the percentage of cancer presence. The primary classifier used in this algorithm is the convolutional neural network, which is a state-of-the-art classifier used in image classification as it can classify images without relying on the manual selection of features from each image. The main aim of this research is to improve the robustness of the classifier used by comparing six different first-order stochastic gradient-based optimizers to select the best for this particular dataset. The dataset used to train the classifier is the PatchCamelyon public dataset, which consists of 220,025 images to train the classifier; the dataset is composed of 60% positive images and 40% negative images, and 57,458 images to test its performance. The classifier was trained on 80% of the images and validated on the rest of 20% of the images; then, it was tested on the test set. The optimizers were evaluated based on their AUC of the ROC curve. The results show that the adaptative based optimizers achieved the highest results except for AdaGrad that achieved the lowest results.

Keywords: image classification; convolutional neural networks; deep learning; medical images; transfer learning; optimizers

1. Introduction

To evaluate whether tissue is cancerous, a sample is taken from the suspicious area and then evaluated, under an optical microscope, by the pathologist. This procedure is very time-consuming and extremely complicated [1], and therefore, it requires an expert pathologist with years of experience. Depending on the particular task, even an expert pathologist could make errors. This complicated procedure often demands a second opinion or even assistance, which is where artificial intelligence assumes a role. Artificial intelligence (AI) can provide significant help, whether through a lot it is automation or to furnish the pathologist with a second opinion. AI can be defined as using a computer to generate a prediction of each image by training a deep neural network model. The training process consists of feeding the system labeled pathology images, after which the algorithm seeks; first, to map a function between the input label and the prediction and second, measures the error and tries to minimize it. The state-of-the-art algorithm used in the image classification is the convolutional neural network.

In the context of image classification, deep learning may be defined as a computer program is said to learn from experience E, like pathology images, concerning some task T, like image classification that differentiates between cancerous and non-cancerous images, and is capable of recognizing the relevant image without being explicitly programmed to do so, and using a performance measure like the AUC of the ROC curve. The algorithm's performance on the image classifier, as measured by the AUC, improves by adding more images. Practically speaking, machine learning is the task of recognizing patterns from training images and applying these patterns to identify an image with an unknown label.

The convolutional neural network (CNN) has been used as an image classification algorithm for nearly two decades [2]. The real power of CNN was rediscovered in the context of the ImageNet competition, where millions of images, with thousands of labels, were classified with 85% accuracy; at that time, CNN resumed its former role as one of the most important algorithms for image classification [3]. CNN has been applied in different image classification domains, such as agriculture [4–6] and traffic detection [7,8]. With the rapid improvements in GPU cards and the increasing size of datasets, many influential and robust architectures, like AlexNet [9], VGG16 [10], VGG19 [10], ResNet50 [11], and InceptionV3 [12], were introduced. Transfer learning is a deep learning technique, which allows the knowledge acquired during training on previous models to be applied to new tasks. Transfer learning has many advantages. It saves time by starting from the end point of the most recent training, instead of training the new model from scratch; it extends the knowledge it acquired from previous models; transfer learning is particularly useful when the size of the new training dataset is small. Transfer learning has made significant contributions to the fields of computer vision, audio classification, and natural language processing.

The difference between the predicted label and the correct label is called the cost function; the whole point of the algorithm is to minimize this cost function. As the algorithm most commonly used to minimize the cost function, backpropagation is an iterative algorithm, where each of its iterations consists of two passes: A forward pass throughout the entire network, where the inputs are propagated from the input layer to the output layer. At this point, the cost function is be calculated to measure the performance of the network; then there is the backward pass, where the weights are backpropagated from the output to the input of the network. The optimizers are used to minimize this cost function.

This work evaluates different first-degree optimizers used to classify pathology images as cancerous or non-cancerous. Each optimizer is evaluated based on its performance and convergence time. Four CNN architectures will be used to compare the performance of each optimizer to those of the others.

2. Related Works

Many works compared the performance of different optimizers in the context of different neural network architectures; the reported approaches differ in relation to the network architecture, datasets, and the optimizers under study.

In a study by Dogo et al. [13], the authors evaluated the performance of seven optimizers on three image datasets: Natural Images dataset, Cats and Dogs dataset, and Fashion MNIST dataset. The authors evaluated the performance of each optimizer based on accuracy achieved and the convergence time, where convergence consists of reaching the minimum of the function. To determine the performance quality of each optimizer, the authors proposed a simple CNN architecture, with three convolutional layers, and one dense layer with 64 neurons. For the Cats and Dogs dataset, the Nadam optimizer achieved the best performance, and the Adadelta optimizer produced the most mediocre performance; the RMSProp represents the shortest convergence time, and the Nadam optimizer achieved the longest convergence. For the Fashion dataset, the Adam optimizer achieved the highest degree of accuracy, and the Adadelta optimizer displayed the lowest accuracy; the Adamax optimizer achieved the shortest convergence time, and the Adadelta optimizer had the longest convergence time was the Adadelta optimizer. For the Natural dataset, the Nadam optimizer was the best performer, and the Adagrad optimizer exhibited the most inferior accuracy; the SGD algorithm achieved the shortest convergence time, and the Adadelta algorithm had the longest convergence time. The authors concluded that the Nadam optimizer was the best of all tested optimizer, due to its combined mastery of the momentum and the adaptive gradient estimation.

The authors Prilianti et al. [14] compared the performance of seven optimizers on the digital plant dataset. To evaluate each optimizer, the authors used three CNN architectures; the first was a shallow network with only one convolutional layer and without any dense layers; the second CNN architecture used was the LeNet architecture, which was introduced by Lecun et al., [15]; and the third CNN architecture was the AlexNet [9]. The authors evaluated the performance of each optimizer on each CNN architecture, based on the mean square error (MSE). The Adam optimizer achieved the lowest MSE for the shallow net architecture, as well as the LeNet architecture, while the Adadelta achieved the lowest MSE on the AlexNet architecture. The authors concluded that Adam optimizer achieved the best performance.

Jangid and Srivastava [16] assessed the performance of three optimizers on handwritten Devanagari characters. The optimizers tested were Adam, Adamax, and RMSProp. To evaluate each optimizer, the authors introduced a CNN architecture with three convolutional layers and one dense layer with 1000 neurons. For this architecture, RMSProp achieved the best accuracy. Swastika et al. [17] evaluated three optimizers to classify vehicle types: Adam, Adadelta, and SGD. The authors used three CNN architectures to evaluate each optimizer: a shallow network, LeNet, and MiniVGGNet. The optimizers were evaluated based on their accuracy, which meant that the Adadelta optimizer was the best for the Mini VGGNet architecture.

This study uses four CNN architectures to perform a comparative evaluation of six first-degree stochastic gradient descent optimizers: the optimizers tested are Nesterov gradient descent, Adagrad, Adam, Adamax, Nadam, and RMSProp; and the CNN architectures tested are VGG16, InceptionV3, DenseNet, and ResNet50. The optimizers are evaluated based on their AUC of the ROC curve and their convergence time. All the optimizers' default hyperparameters were kept constant throughout the experiment, except the learning rate, which was set to three values 0.001, 0.0001, and 0.0001. Fine-tuning was applied to each network to adjust its weight to the new dataset.

3. Methodology

3.1. Dataset

The public available PatchCamelyon dataset [18,19] was used in this study. The images represent sentinel axillary lymph nodes to investigate the spread of breast cancer. The dataset was sampled from two hospitals in the Netherlands, experienced pathologists from the Netherlands annotated the dataset labels. The dataset was acquired from the Kaggle platform [20]. The dataset consists of 220,025 images to train the classifier; the dataset is composed of 60% positive images and 40% negative images, and it includes 57,458 unlabeled images to test the classifier performance. All images have dimensions of 96 × 96 pixels. Eighty percent of the dataset is used to train the classifier, which is subsequently evaluated with the other 20% of the dataset images; the classifier is also tested on the online set of 57,458 images, and the results are uploaded to the Kaggle platform to detect the model performance. A sample of images is presented in Figure 1.

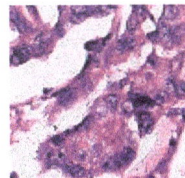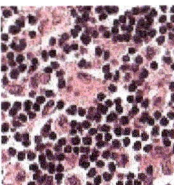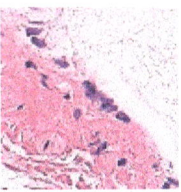

Figure 1. Example of images available in the PatchCamelyon dataset [20].

3.2. Convolutional Neural Networks

CNN is the most used algorithm in image classification, where it is understood to be a deep learning algorithm that serves as a feed-forward neural network with more than one hidden layer. The CNN for image classification was introduced by Fukushima [2] to mimic the biological visual cortex of the brain. CNN combines sophisticated features obtained from the higher layers of the network with the generic features obtained from the lower layers of the network. The most critical layer of CNN is the convolution layer, which is responsible for capturing the temporal and spatial information of each image; the convolutional layer must conduct the convolution operation, which is a mathematical operation performed between the input and the filter to produce the feature map. Equation (1) shows the convolution operation,

$$O[u,v] = F[m,n] * I[u,v] = \sum_m \sum_n F[m,n] \cdot I[u+m, v+n] \tag{1}$$

where $F[m,n]$ is the convolution filter, $I[u,v]$ is the input image and $O[u,v]$ is the output feature map.

A filter is convolved over the input image to produce a feature map. Another CNN layer is the activation function, which is used to present non-linearity because usually, the image classification task is highly non-linear. To reduce overfitting and to reduce the spatial footprint of each filter, two main techniques can be used to extract the essential pixels and removing the noise. The first involves using a stride value larger than 1, which reduces the output of each filter. The second technique is called pooling, where a pooling layer usually follows the activation layer. Pooling layers can strengthen network spatial invariance [21]. The two main types of pooling layers are the maximum pooling layer and the average pooling layer.

Then, fully connected layers follow, usually defined at the end of the network, which takes the output of the feature extraction layers. The primary purpose of the dense layer is to consider all the features extracted from the previous layers and employ these features to classify the output. The dense layers are followed by an activation function, which usually consists of a rectified linear unit (ReLU) layer; finally, at the end of the network, a softmax or sigmoid function is used to output the target probability.

3.3. Optimizers

The model learns (trains) on a given dataset by comparing the actual label of the input (available in the training set) to the predicted label, thereby, minimizing the cost function. Hypothetically, if the cost function is zero, the model has learned the dataset correctly. However, an optimization algorithm is needed to achieve the minimum of a cost function. The next section discusses different optimization algorithms, introduced in the literature, to minimize the cost function.

3.3.1. Vanilla Gradient Descent Optimizers

Gradient descent is the primary class of optimizers capable of finding the minimum value of the cost function. The literature has introduced three versions of gradient descent.

Batch Gradient Descent

The first optimization algorithm was the batch gradient descent optimization algorithm (BGD), which updates the network weights after scanning the whole training dataset; in the case of images, convergence takes much time, as there may be millions of weights to optimize and the whole dataset needs to be reevaluated at every step (i.e., epoch). For convex loss function, it is guaranteed that the BGD will converge to the global minimum, while it converges to a local minimum for non-convex functions. The weights are updated based on Equation (2):

$$w_{t+1} = w_t - \eta \frac{\partial C}{\partial w_t} \tag{2}$$

$$\frac{\partial C}{\partial w_t} = \nabla_w C(w_t) \tag{3}$$

where Equation (3) is the gradients update equation, and η is the learning rate hyperparameter. w_t are the weights at step t, $C(.)$ is the cost function and $\nabla_w C(w_t)$ is the gradient of weight parameters w_t.

Stochastic Gradient Descent

To overcome the shortcomings of BGD, stochastic gradient descent (SGD) was introduced. SGD allows to update the network weights per each training image, that is why SGD is sometimes called online training. However, such updates engender massive fluctuation in the loss function, due to the high variance between different images, which can create much noise in the training phase:

$$w_{t+1} = w_t - \eta \frac{\partial C}{\partial w_t} \tag{4}$$

$$\frac{\partial C}{\partial w_t} = \nabla_w C\left(w_t; x^{(i)}; y^{(i)}\right) \tag{5}$$

The weights are updated based on Equation (4), where Equation (5) is the gradient update equation, and η is the learning rate hyperparameter. w_t are the weights at step t, $C(.)$ is the cost function, and $\nabla_w C(w_t)$ is the gradient of weight parameters w_t for image x and its corresponding label y.

Mini-Batch Gradient Descent

Mini-batch gradient descent was introduced to overcome the shortcomings of the previous two algorithms, because it allows for the weights to be updated per batch, and not per image. As such, mini batch gradient descent may be regarded as a particular case of SGD, where the number of samples is more than one. In the literature and it follows, in this paper, the mini-batch is referred to as stochastic gradient descent (SGD):

$$w_{t+1} = w_t - \eta \frac{\partial C}{\partial w_t} \tag{6}$$

$$\frac{\partial C}{\partial w_t} = \nabla_w C\left(w_t; x^{(i:i+n)}; y^{(i:i+n)}\right) \tag{7}$$

The weights are updated based on Equation (6), and Equation (7) is the gradient update equation. η is the learning rate hyperparameter, w_t are the weights at step t, n is the number of data points, $C(.)$ is the cost function and $\nabla_w C(w_t)$ is the gradient of weight parameters w_t for image x and its corresponding label y.

3.3.2. Momentum-Based Gradient Descent Optimizers

The main drawback of using mini-batch SGD is the presence of oscillations during the updating of the weights. These oscillations usually result in a long time to reach convergence. Momentum, also known as moving average gradients, was introduced, in order to overcome this issue and to fix the gradients' direction.

Momentum Gradient Descent

Understanding the right direction for the gradient avoids oscillations in the wrong directions, and knowing the right direction relies on using the previous position for guidance. Considering the previous position, the updating rule adds a fraction of the previous update, which gives the optimizer the momentum needed to continue moving in the right direction. The weights are updated based on Equation (10),

$$V_t = \lambda V_{t-1} + \eta \frac{\partial C}{\partial w_t} \tag{8}$$

$$\frac{\partial C}{\partial w_t} = \nabla_w C\left(w_t; x^{(i:i+n)}; y^{(i:i+n)}\right) \tag{9}$$

$$w_{t+1} = w_t - V_t \tag{10}$$

where V is the velocity, and it is initialized to 0. λ is used to select the amount of information needed from the previous update. η is the learning rate hyperparameter, w_t are the weights at step t, n is the number of data points, $C(.)$ is the cost function, and $\nabla_w C(w_t)$ is the gradient of weight parameters w_t for image x and its corresponding label y.

Nesterov Momentum Gradient Descent

If the momentum is sufficiently high, close to the minimum, the optimizer may overshoot the minimum. The previous optimization algorithms take the current and the previous gradients into account for updating the weights. However, to make the optimization algorithm more robust, we must take the future gradients into account as well, to approximate the gradients' direction. The weights are updated based on Equation (13),

$$V_t = \lambda V_{t-1} + \eta \frac{\partial C}{\partial w_t} \tag{11}$$

$$\frac{\partial C}{\partial w_t} = \nabla_w C\left(w_t - \lambda V_{t-1}; x^{(i:i+n)}; y^{(i:i+n)}\right) \tag{12}$$

$$w_{t+1} = w_t - V_t \tag{13}$$

where V is the velocity, and it is initialized to 0, λ is used to select the amount of information needed from the previous update. While, η is the learning rate hyperparameter, w_t are the weights at step t, n is the number of data points, $C(.)$ is the cost function, and $\nabla_w C(w_t)$ is the gradient of weight parameters w_t for image x and its corresponding label y. $(w_t - \lambda V_{t-1})$ is the look-ahead position that is capable of approximating the next gradient position, thereby allowing it to slow down if it threatens to overshoot the minimum.

3.3.3. Adaptive Gradient Descent Optimizers

All the optimization mentioned above has a fixed learning rate, while, in practice, deep learning algorithms are non-convex problems. That may be a problem, as we may face a sparse weight matrix, where we require different updates for different weights, especially for infrequent weights, where significant updates are needed to reach to avoid oscillating.

AdaGrad Optimizer

To scale the learning rate for each weight, the AdaGrad optimization algorithm [22] was introduced to establish different updates for different weights. The learning rate is tuned automatically, by dividing the learning rate by the sum of squares of all previous gradients. The weights are updated based on Equation (14),

$$w_t^i = w_{t-1}^i - \frac{\eta}{\sqrt{\sum_{\mathcal{T}=1}^{t}\left(\nabla_w C\left(w_\mathcal{T}^i\right)\right)^2 + \epsilon}} \cdot \nabla_w C\left(w_t^i\right) \tag{14}$$

where η is the learning rate hyperparameter, w_t are the weights at step t, $C(.)$ is the cost function, and $\nabla_w C(w_t)$ is the gradient of weight parameters w_t for image x and its corresponding label y. The sum of squares $\sqrt{\sum_{\mathcal{T}=1}^{t}\left(\nabla_w C\left(w_\mathcal{T}^i\right)\right)^2}$ is used to scale the learning rate; it gives a high learning rate for the least frequent gradients and a low learning rate for the more frequent gradients.

RMSProp Optimizer

The main drawback of AdaGrad is that the learning rate decreases monotonically because every added term is positive. After many epochs, the learning rate is so small that it stops updating the weights. RMSProp was introduced to address the problem of the monotonically decreasing learning rate [23]. The weights are updated based on Equation (17),

$$G = \nabla_w C(w_t) \tag{15}$$

$$E[G^2]_t = \lambda E[G^2]_{t-1} + (1-\lambda)G_t^2 \tag{16}$$

$$w_t^i = w_{t-1}^i - \frac{\eta}{\sqrt{E[G^2]_t + \epsilon}} \cdot \nabla_w C(w_t^i) \tag{17}$$

where η is the learning rate hyperparameter, w_t are the weights at step t, $C(.)$ is the cost function, and $\nabla_w C(w_t)$ is the gradient of weight parameters w_t for image x and its corresponding label y. λ is used to select the amount of information needed from the previous update. $E[G^2]_t$ is the running average of the squared gradients, which has been used to avoid the monotonically decreasing gradients of the AdaGrad optimizer.

Adam Optimizer

The Adam optimization [24] algorithm was introduced to combine the benefits of Nesterov momentum, AdaGrad, and RMSProp algorithms. The weights are updated based on Equation (18):

$$w_t^i = w_{t-1}^i - \frac{\eta}{\sqrt{\hat{v}_t} + \epsilon} \cdot \hat{m}_t \tag{18}$$

where:

$$\hat{m}_t = \frac{m_t}{1-\beta_1^t} \tag{19}$$

$$\hat{v}_t = \frac{v_t}{1-\beta_2^t} \tag{20}$$

$$m_t = \beta_1 m_{t-1} + (1-\beta_1)G \tag{21}$$

$$v_t = \beta_2 v_{t-1} + (1-\beta_2)[G]^2 \tag{22}$$

$$G = \nabla_w C(w_t) \tag{23}$$

where η is the learning rate hyperparameter, w_t are the weights at step t, $C(.)$ is the cost function, and $\nabla_w C(w_t)$ is the gradient of weight parameters w_t for image x and its corresponding label y, β_i is used to select the amount of information needed from the previous update, where $\beta_i \in [0,1]$, m_t is the running average of the gradients, also known as the first moment, v_t is the running average of the squared gradients, and known as the second moment. If the first and second moments get initialized at zero, they are biased toward it, to solve this zero-biased problem, these moments are bias-corrected by dividing them by their respective β.

Adamax Optimizer

Adamax [24] is the update of the Adam algorithm, where the uncentered variance tends to ∞. The weights are updated based on Equation (24):

$$w_t^i = w_{t-1}^i - \frac{\eta}{v_t + \epsilon} \cdot \hat{m}_t \tag{24}$$

where:

$$\hat{m}_t = \frac{m_t}{1-\beta_1^t} \tag{25}$$

$$v_t = \max(\beta_2 \cdot v_{t-1}, |G_t|) \tag{26}$$

$$m_t = \beta_1 m_{t-1} + (1-\beta_1)G \tag{27}$$

$$G = \nabla_w C(w_t) \quad (28)$$

where η is the learning rate hyperparameter, w_t are the weights at step t, $C(.)$ is the cost function, and $\nabla_w C(w_t)$ is the gradient of weight parameters w_t for image x and its corresponding label y. β_i is used to select the amount of information needed from the previous update, where $\beta_i \in [0,1]$. m_t is the first moment, v_t is the second moment.

Nadam Optimizer

Nadam [25] is an extension of the Adam algorithm by combining it with Nesterov momentum gradient descent. The weights are updated based on Equation (29):

$$w_t^i = w_{t-1}^i - \frac{\eta}{\sqrt{v_t + \epsilon}} \cdot \widetilde{m}_t \quad (29)$$

where:

$$\widetilde{m}_t = \beta_1^{t+1} \hat{m}_t + (1-\beta_1^t)\hat{g}_t \quad (30)$$

$$\hat{m}_t = \frac{m_t}{1 - \prod_{i=1}^{t} \beta_1^i} \quad (31)$$

$$\hat{g}_t = \frac{g_t}{1 - \prod_{i=1}^{t} \beta_1^i} \quad (32)$$

where η is the learning rate hyperparameter, and w_t are the weights at step t. While, β_i is used to select the amount of information needed from the previous update, where $\beta_i \in [0,1]$, m_t is the first moment.

Fine-Tuning

According to [26,27] transfer learning can be formalized as follows: by having a domain D, where $D = \{X, P(X)\}$, in which X is the feature space and $P(X)$ is the marginal probability distribution and task $\mathcal{T} = \{Y, f(.)\}$, where Y is the label space and $f(.)$ is the predictive function which models $P(y|x)$ for $y \in Y$ and $x \in X$. By having a source domain D_S and learning task $\mathcal{T}_S$ and a target domain D_T and learning task $\mathcal{T}_T$, by using weights from D_S and $\mathcal{T}_S$, learning the target predictive function $f(.)$ in $\mathcal{T}_T$ can be improved a lot, where $D_S \neq D_T$, $\mathcal{T}_S \neq \mathcal{T}_T$, or both. Fine-tuning is very important in the classification of medical images, because the neural network usually needs many images to be trained. However, in the medical field, for many reasons, labeled medical images are scarce. Instead of initializing the weights from scratch, ImageNet weights can be used. In this paper, the networks were trained on ImageNet dataset and all the networks blocks were fine-tuned using the PatchCamelyon dataset [18,19].

3.3.4. VGG16 Network

VGG16 [10] was introduced in 2014 by the researchers at Oxford's Visual Geometry Group. It was one of the top algorithms involved in the ImageNet classification challenge, and it had an 8.1% error rate. VGG16 consists of five convolution blocks, where the first block contains two convolution layers, stacked together with 64 filters. The second block consists of two stacked convolution layers with 128 filters, where the second convolution block is separated from the first block by a max pool layer. The third block consists of three convolution layers, stacked together with 256 filters and separated from the second block by another max pool layer. The fourth and fifth layers have the same architecture, but instead, have 512 filters. The convolution filter used throughout this network is of size 3 × 3 and stride of 1. Then, a flatten layer is added between the convolution blocks and the dense layers, converting the 3D vector into a 1D vector. The last block consists of three dense layers, each of which has 4096 neurons, to classify each image. The last layer is a softmax layer, which is used to ensure that the probability summation of the output is one. ReLU was used as an activation layer throughout the network. This network was trained on the ImageNet dataset for three weeks on four GPUs to detect the ImageNet classification task. A summary of VGG16 network is presented in Table 1.

Table 1. Number of layers and parameters of the CNNs used in this study.

Networks	Number of Layers	Number of Parameters
VGG16	16	14,714,688
InceptionV3	48	21,802,784
ResNet50	50	23,587,712
DenseNet121	121	7,037,504

3.3.5. InceptionV3 Network

The authors Szegedy et al. [28] introduced a novel architecture, called Inception, to participate in the ImageNet competition in 2015; Inception had an accuracy rate of 92.2%. The architecture consists of 48 layers and total parameters of 22,000,000. This architecture has a concatenated layer of convolutions, stacked in parallel to decrease the size of the architecture while maintaining its complexity. InceptionV3 network architecture is shown in Figure 2. A summary of InceptionV3 network is presented in Table 1.

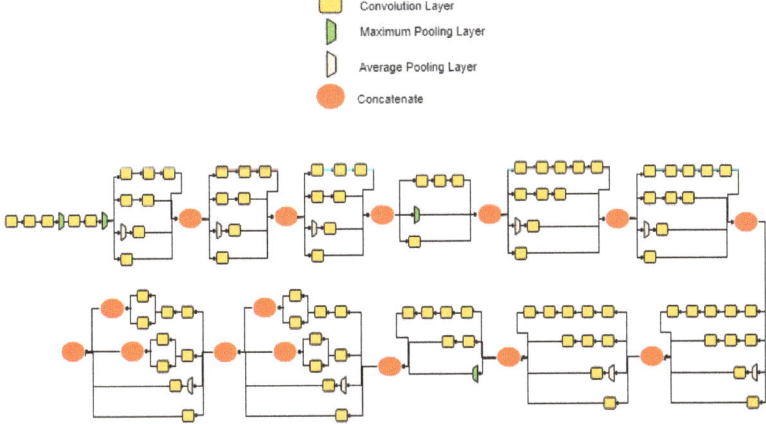

Figure 2. InceptionV3 network architecture.

3.3.6. ResNet Network

The authors, He et al. [11], investigated the effect of increasing the depth of the convolutional neural network and its impact on network performance. The authors noticed that increasing the depth of the network decreases the generalizability of the network, which means that the test error of the network is higher than a shallow network. This may be due to the vanishing gradients, where the weights are not updated in deep layers. Therefore, He et al. [11] introduced a novel architecture called ResNet, where Res signifies the application of a residual connection between the convolutional layers, which is then passed to the ReLU activation layer. One of the main benefits of adding the residual connection is that the weights learned from the previous layers can be carried to the next layers during the backpropagation step. ResNet won the ImageNet competition in 2015 with Top-5 accuracy of 94.29%. It has a total of 23,587,712 parameters, and its ImageNet weights are available in the Keras package. A summary of ResNet network is presented in Table 1.

3.3.7. DenseNet Network

DenseNet network [29] was inspired by the residual connection of the ResNet architecture. All the layers are connected to all their subsequent layers, meaning that a residual connection is established between all the layers. Merging will be used instead of adding to combine the layers. DenseNet has many variants depends on the number of layers; some of the variants are DenseNet 121, DenseNet169, and DenseNet201. In this paper, we opted for the DenseNet121 network. A summary of DenseNet network is presented in Table 1.

3.4. Overcoming Overfitting

Overfitting generally consists of memorization of the training dataset and usually leads to poor performance on the test dataset. This means that the performance on the training set can be excellent, but the performance on the test set is quite poor. The loss of the generalizability of the network may be due to many issues, such as the capacity of the network or the nature of the training dataset itself. Many measures have been introduced in the literature to overcome overfitting. Below are some techniques that were used in this research to overcome overfitting.

3.4.1. Dropout

A regularization layer introduced by [30] can be applied to any layer in the network. During network training, some neurons are disabled with a pre-defined dropout-rate probability P. This can be understood as a sort of bagging for neural networks.

3.4.2. Image Augmentation

Increasing the size of the training set improves the performance of the network. For image datasets, many duplicates can be created with simple changes to the original dataset, including rotation, flipping, zooming, and cropping. These transformations make the network more robust in defending against overfitting, and it enhances network performance as well. In our case, the original images are flipped, rotated, zoomed, and shifted. The rotation range used was 180°; and the images were randomly flipped horizontally and vertically; the shifting range used was 25%; and the zoom range used was 40%.

3.4.3. Early Stopping

Early stopping is a precautionary measure used to prevent the network from overfitting, which may be defined as stopping the training phase of the network when the performance on the validation set stops improving for a pre-defined number of epochs. This pre-defined number usually ranges from 10–50 epochs. In our case, the number of epochs is 10.

3.5. Evaluation Metrics

To assess the quality of the trained CNN, many measures have been developed. For classification tasks, a confusion matrix is constructed to assess the model quality; it categorizes the model predictions, according to whether they match the correct label of the image. It has four central values:

TP: True positive (A positive example, classified as a positive example)
TN: True negative (A negative example, classified as a negative example)
FP: False positive (A negative example, but classified as a positive example)
FN: False-negative (A positive example, but classified as a negative example)

To visualize the model performance, the ROC curve was introduced to examine the trade-off between sensitivity and specificity visually. The main idea of the ROC curve is to plot the specificity of the algorithms, which is the percentage of the correctly classified negatives against the sensitivity, which is the percentage of the correctly classified positives of the algorithm [31]. The ROC curve has a diagonal line, which represents a random guess model. It means that the model cannot differentiate between true positives and false positives; this diagonal line can be considered as the baseline where models can be judged. The best model has a curve that passes through the top left corner for "100%

Sensitivity" and has a 0% false-positive rate. To measure the quality of the model using the ROC curve, a statistic known as AUC or "Area under the ROC curve," is used; this treats the ROC diagram as a two-dimensional square and measures the area under the curve. AUC has a minimum value of 0.5 and a maximum value of 1, where 0.5 represents a model with no predictive power, and 1 represents a model with 100% predictive power. According to Vuk [32], the AUC is calculated by Equation (33):

$$AUC = \int_0^1 \frac{TP}{P} d\frac{FP}{N} = \frac{1}{PN} \int_0^N TP \, dFP \qquad (33)$$

where $TP + FN = P$ and $TN + FP = N$.

4. Results

The following section details the results obtained from training the four network architectures using the six selected optimizers with three learning rates, namely, 1×10^{-3}, 1×10^{-4}, and 1×10^{-5}. Many experiments have been conducted on this dataset, to determine the behavior of each optimizer with each network architecture to determine the best combination. The performance of each optimizer with the VGG16 architecture is presented in Table 2, with the InceptionV3 architecture in Table 3, with the ResNet architecture in Table 4, and with the DenseNet architecture in Table 5. To test the performance of each configuration, two types of evaluation were used; the first consists of splitting the training dataset into 80%/20% to train and validate the dataset. After training, the model is used to predict the class of the images in the test set, and the result is submitted to the Kaggle platform to assess the performance of each model. The AUC of the ROC curve measured the performance. The optimizers are ranked based on their test AUC that was acquired from the Kaggle platform.

In all the experiments, the default settings of each optimizer were chosen, except the learning rate, and image augmentation used for rotating, flipping, and cropping all the images. The size of the images was kept constant at 96 × 96; a batch size of 64 images was used, and early stopping was applied with the number of epochs equal to 10.

4.1. VGG16 Architecture Result

Table 2 shows the results for the VGG16 architecture, which shows that the highest AUC was achieved by Adam optimizer, which also took the shortest time to achieve convergence. At the same time, the lowest test AUC was achieved by RMSProp and Adamax optimizers that did not converge at all. For the highest learning rate (1×10^{-3}) the highest AUC achieved was by the Adam optimizer, and the lowest AUC achieved was by the RMSProp and Adamax optimizers. For the medium learning rate (1×10^{-4}) the highest AUC achieved was by NAG optimizer, and the lowest AUC achieved was by both AdaGrad and Adam optimizers. For the lowest learning rate (1×10^{-5} The AdaGrad optimizer achieved), the highest AUC achieved by the Adam optimizer and the lowest AUC. Overall, the medium learning rate achieved the best results, followed by the lowest learning rate. Adam optimizer was the most stable optimizer with high results and low variance between different learning rates.

Table 2. Results obtained with the VGG16 architecture. Where LR stands for learning rate; NAG represents Nesterov momentum; AdaGrad represents the adaptive gradient optimizer; RMSProp represents the root mean square propagation optimizer; Adam represents adaptive moment estimation optimizer; AdaMax represents maximum adaptive moment estimation optimizer; and Nadam represents Nesterov and Adam optimizer.

Optimizers	LR = 10^{-3}	LR = 10^{-4}	LR = 10^{-5}
NAG	89.45%	94.64%	94.25%
AdaGrad	88.50%	87.40%	88.07%
RMSProp	50.00%	94.33%	93.45%
Adam	90.88%	90.39%	95.01%
Adamax	50.00%	94.02%	94.20%
Nadam	85.00%	91.14%	94.33%

4.2. InceptionV3 Architecture Result

Table 3 shows the results for the InceptionV3 architecture, which shows that the highest AUC was achieved by the RMSProp optimizer, which also took the shortest time to achieve convergence. At the same time, the lowest test AUC was achieved by AdaGrad optimizer, which also took the longest time to convergence. For the highest learning rate (1×10^{-3}), the AdaGrad optimizer achieved the highest AUC, while, the Adam optimizer achieved the lowest AUC. For the medium learning rate (1×10^{-4}) the highest AUC achieved was by the RMSProp optimizer, and the lowest AUC achieved was by the AdaGrad optimizer. For the lowest learning rate (1×10^{-5} The AdaGrad optimizer achieved), the highest AUC achieved by the AdaMax optimizer and the lowest AUC. Overall, the medium learning rate achieved the best results, followed by the lowest learning rate. Adamax optimizer was the most stable optimizer with high results and low variance between different learning rates.

Table 3. Results obtained with the InceptionV3 architecture. Where LR stands for learning rate; NAG represents Nesterov momentum; AdaGrad represents the adaptive gradient optimizer; RMSProp represents the root mean square propagation optimizer; Adam represents adaptive moment estimation optimizer; AdaMax represents maximum adaptive moment estimation optimizer; and Nadam represents Nesterov and Adam optimizer.

Optimizers	LR = 10^{-3}	LR = 10^{-4}	LR = 10^{-5}
NAG	93.18%	93.25%	90.81%
AdaGrad	93.64%	90.46%	86.32%
RMSProp	91.41%	94.91%	92.65%
Adam	90.44%	92.53%	93.22%
Adamax	93.44%	93.11%	93.95%
Nadam	91.97%	91.33%	92.46%

4.3. ResNet Architecture Result

Table 4 shows the results for the ResNet architecture, which shows that the best AUC was achieved by the Nadam optimizer, while the AdaGrad optimizer achieved the lowest AUC. For the highest learning rate (1×10^{-3}) the highest AUC achieved was by the AdaGrad optimizer, and the lowest AUC achieved was by the RMSProp optimizer. For the medium learning rate (1×10^{-4}) the highest AUC achieved was by the NAG optimizer, and the lowest AUC achieved was by the AdaGrad optimizer. For the lowest learning rate (1×10^{-5} The AdaGrad optimizer achieved), the highest AUC achieved by the Nadam optimizer and the lowest AUC. Overall, the medium learning rate achieved the best results, followed by the lowest learning rate. Adamax optimizer was the most stable optimizer with high results and low variance between different learning rates.

Table 4. Results obtained with the ResNet architecture. Where LR stands for learning rate; NAG represents Nesterov momentum; AdaGrad represents the adaptive gradient optimizer; RMSProp represents the root mean square propagation optimizer; Adam represents adaptive moment estimation optimizer; AdaMax represents maximum adaptive moment estimation optimizer; and Nadam represents Nesterov and Adam optimizer.

Optimizers	LR = 10^{-3}	LR = 10^{-4}	LR = 10^{-5}
NAG	90.07%	93.84%	89.00%
AdaGrad	93.04%	89.11%	83.46%
RMSProp	89.56%	89.62%	93.04%
Adam	90.24%	90.24%	93.84%
Adamax	90.24%	92.24%	93.70%
Nadam	91.91%	89.36%	93.85%

4.4. DenseNet Architecture Result

Table 5 shows the results for the DenseNet architecture, where the best AUC was achieved by Adamax optimizer, while the Adam optimizer achieved the lowest AUC. For the highest learning rate (1×10^{-3}) the highest AUC achieved was by the AdaGrad optimizer, and the lowest AUC achieved was by the Adam optimizer. For the medium learning rate (1×10^{-4}) the highest AUC achieved was by Adamax optimizer, and the lowest AUC achieved was by the Adam optimizer. For the lowest learning rate $(1 \times 10^{-5}$ The AdaGrad optimizer achieved), the highest AUC was achieved by the RMSProp optimizer and the lowest AUC. Overall, the medium learning rate achieved the best results, followed by the lowest learning rate. Adamax optimizer was the most stable optimizer with high results and low variance between different learning rates.

Table 5. Results obtained with the DenseNet architecture. Where LR represents learning rate; NAG represents Nesterov momentum; AdaGrad represents the adaptive gradient optimizer; RMSProp represents the root mean square propagation optimizer; Adam represents adaptive moment estimation optimizer; AdaMax represents maximum adaptive moment estimation optimizer; and Nadam represents Nesterov and Adam optimizer.

Optimizers	LR = 10^{-3}	LR = 10^{-4}	LR = 10^{-5}
NAG	93.08%	94.31%	91.64%
AdaGrad	93.89%	93.57%	87.70%
RMSProp	88.19%	93.98%	94.61%
Adam	84.18%	89.69%	94.43%
Adamax	90.62%	95.12%	93.91%
Nadam	86.77%	94.21%	93.77%

Overall, in terms of performance across all four networks, the highest results were achieved by the adaptive learning optimizers, like Adam, Adamax, Nadam, and RMSProp. However, these optimizers needed a lower learning rate to be able to converge, while the high learning rate did not achieve good results. One exception was the AdaGrad optimizer that did not achieve high results with a low learning rate; on the contrary, it needed a high learning rate to be able to converge to an acceptable result. From our results and the results obtained by Prilianti et al. [14], it is apparent that every combination of network and optimizer will produce a unique combination. However, the general behavior of each optimizer can be noted, which can be concluded from the results. Overall, NAG optimizer did achieve high results overall the four architectures and overall the three learning rates used with the medium learning rate (1×10^{-4}) achieved the best results. The AdaGrad optimizer did not achieve high results compared to other optimizers used, especially when trained using low learning rates. RMSProp optimizer did achieve high results with a low learning rate but was unstable with high learning rates. Adam optimizer needed a low learning rate to be able to converge to high results. While, the AdaMax optimizer behaved similarly to the Adam optimizer, except for a high learning rate with the VGG16, where it did not converge at all, one reason may be the shallow depth of the VGG16 network. Nadam optimizer did achieve high results with both the medium learning rate and the low learning rate.

5. Discussion

Taking into account the results achieved from the experimental campaign, it is possible to draw some interesting observations of the behavior of the CNNs and optimizers considered in this paper. By focusing on the choice of the optimizer and its relation with the learning rate, the experimental results confirm that the choice of the learning rate may result in an unstable behavior of the training process. This is particularly evident, for some of the considered networks and optimizers, when considering the smallest learning rate used in the experiments. As one can see, when $LR = 10^{-3}$, the training process of VGG16 with both RMSProp and Adamax optimizer result in a poor performance of the model. As explained in the previous sections, this can be motivated by the fact that the weights of the network change abruptly from one epoch to the next. Moving to lower LR values allows the convergence of the training process in all the configurations that were investigated. Overall, the results match the theoretical expectation: A lower LR value allows for a smoother convergence, but it requires more time with respect to a greater LR value.

Another interesting observation relates to the importance of the hyperparameters. While this is a topic of fundamental importance in the area of deep learning, it is particularly evident from the results of the experimental phase. In particular, all the considered architecture produced a comparable performance when the best configuration of the learning rate and optimizer (that is different for each type of architecture) was considered. In other words, it seems that the choice of the hyperparameters not only plays an essential role in determining the performance of the model, but the CNNs under exam are indistinguishable in terms of performance. We believe that this is an interesting observation that should further stress the importance of the tuning of the hyperparameters.

Focusing on the optimizers, AdaGrad produces the best performance with $LR = 10^{-3}$ and, under this aspect, it behaves differently with respect to the other optimizers under analysis. Conversely, Adam, Adamax, and Nadam obtained the best performance on the considered CNNs when $LR = 10^{-5}$ (except Adamax on the DenseNet architecture, where the best performance is obtained with $LR = 10^{-4}$).

Globally, the best result on the considered dataset was achieved by Adamax optimizer and DenseNet network. Anyway, the differences in terms of performance among the best configurations of each network, are not statistically significant. Overall, every optimizer behaved differently according to the particular architecture. For instance, for the deep architectures like ResNet, AdaGrad outperformed Adam and Adamax. For the shallow architectures like VGG16, AdaMax and NAG had the same performance. Given a specific network, each optimizer requires a different amount of time for converging (i.e., concluding ten epochs). In particular, RMSProp was the fastest optimizer, whereas training a CNN with AdaGrad resulted in the slowest training process. This result is coherent with respect to the one discussed proposed by Dogo et al. [13], in which the authors investigated the effect of different optimizers in terms of required time to reach. More in detail, training the VGG16 architecture requires a minimum of 90 min (RMSProp optimizer and learning rate of 10^{-3}) and a maximum of nine hours (AdaGrad optimizer and learning rate of 10^{-5}). InceptionV3 requires approximately one hour more than VGG16; in this case, the use of RMSProp (with a learning rate of 10^{-3}) resulted in the fastest training process (approximately 150 min), while the use of AdaGrad (with a learning rate of 10^{-5}) required approximately 10 h to finish. An identical pattern was observed for ResNet and DenseNet, that are requiring approximately two hours more than VGG16 for concluding the training process.

Finally, it is important to compare the results achieved with transfer learning against the ones obtained with CNNs that were specifically built for classifying the images of the PatchCamelyon dataset. The winner of the Kaggle competition obtained an AUC of 1, while the second-best performing network obtained an AUC of 0.98. On the other hand, the best performing network obtained with transfer learning (DenseNet architecture, with Adamax optimizer, and a learning rate of 10^{-4}) was able to obtain an AUC of 0.95. This result confirms the suitability of transfer learning for the task at hand. More in detail, we believe that, by considering deeper architectures and more epochs, it could be possible to improve the results of this study, thus equaling the performance achieved by the winner of the Kaggle competition. On the other hand, we highlight a fundamental difference between the best performance reported in the present study and the best performance of the Kaggle competition: The former was obtained using an existing network (used for addressing different computer vision tasks) and by fine-tuning it, while the latter was achieved by designing an ad hoc CNN, a time-consuming task that requires some expertise.

6. Conclusions

CNN represents an analysis of images created using current computation techniques. This is mostly due to their ability to obtain a performance that is similar to, or better than, the one achieved by human beings. Nevertheless, similarly to other deep learning models, training a CNN is a task that usually requires a vast amount of images. This is an essential limitation in all the domains, like the medical one, in which data are scarce and difficult to obtain. In such a situation, transfer learning may provide a viable option. The idea of transfer learning is to use a model trained over thousands of observations (i.e., images in this study) to provide an initial architecture and set of weights for addressing a similar problem over a different domain. Motivated by the success of transfer learning in the analysis of medical images, and for further studying this promising research area, this paper compared the performance optimizers used in popular CNNs for the classification of histopathology images. In particular, four network architectures were used in the evaluation process. These networks were trained on the ImageNet dataset, which consists of millions of images, and their weights were fine-tuned to suit the considered histopathology images dataset. The results obtained from the experimental phase, in which different combinations of network, optimizer, and learning rate were considered, corroborated the initial hypothesis on the importance of the optimizer and the learning rate. While the choice of CNN is essential, it is clear that by fixing the value of the learning rate, the results obtained using different optimizers could be significantly different. On the other hand, once a particular optimizer is selected, the choice of the learning rate plays an essential role in determining the final performance of CNNs.

Interestingly, for each of the different CNNs under exam, it is possible to notice that the best performing configuration of optimizer and learning rate produces an AUC that is approximately 94%. This result strengthens the importance of selecting the hyperparameters of the network, and, in a future investigation, we will extend this work to include additional hyperparameters and datasets aiming at providing formal guidelines for medical experts that want to use CNN models to support their daily work.

Author Contributions: Conceptualization, I.K. and M.C.; methodology, I.K.; software, I.K.; validation, I.K., M.C.; formal analysis, I.K.; investigation, I.K., M.C.; resources, M.C.; data curation, I.K.; writing—original draft preparation, I.K.; writing—review and editing, I.K. and M.C; visualization, I.K.; supervision, M.C. and A.P.; project administration, M.C. and A.P.; funding acquisition, M.C. and A.P. All authors have read and agreed to the published version of the manuscript.

Funding: This work was partially supported by FCT, Portugal, through projects GADgET (DSAIPA/DS/0022/2018) and AICE (DSAIPA/DS/0113/2019) and by the financial support from the Slovenian Research Agency (research core funding No. P5-0410).

Conflicts of Interest: The authors declare no conflict of interest.

References

1. Jukić, D.M.; Drogowski, L.M.; Martina, J.; Parwani, A.V. Clinical examination and validation of primary diagnosis in anatomic pathology using whole slide digital images. *Arch. Pathol. Lab. Med.* **2011**, *135*, 372–378. [CrossRef] [PubMed]

2. Fukushima, K. Neocognitron: A self-organizing neural network model for a mechanism of pattern recognition unaffected by shift in position. *Biol. Cybern.* **1980**, *36*, 193–202. [CrossRef] [PubMed]
3. Tajbakhsh, N.; Shin, J.Y.; Gurudu, S.R.; Hurst, R.T.; Kendall, C.B.; Gotway, M.B.; Liang, J. Convolutional Neural Networks for Medical Image Analysis: Full Training or Fine Tuning? *IEEE Trans. Med Imaging* **2016**, *35*, 1299–1312. [CrossRef] [PubMed]
4. Fuentes, A.; Yoon, S.; Kim, S.C.; Park, D.S. A Robust Deep-Learning-Based Detector for Real-Time Tomato Plant Diseases and Pests Recognition. *Sensors* **2017**, *17*, 2022. [CrossRef] [PubMed]
5. Mohanty, S.P.; Hughes, D.P.; Salathé, M. Using Deep Learning for Image-Based Plant Disease Detection. *Front. Plant Sci.* **2016**, *7*, 1419. [CrossRef] [PubMed]
6. Singh, A.K.; Ganapathysubramanian, B.; Sarkar, S.; Singh, A. Deep Learning for Plant Stress Phenotyping: Trends and Future Perspectives. *Trends Plant Sci.* **2018**, *23*, 883–898. [CrossRef] [PubMed]
7. John, V.; Yoneda, K.; Qi, B.; Liu, Z.; Mita, S. Traffic light recognition in varying illumination using deep learning and saliency map. In *17th International IEEE Conference on Intelligent Transportation Systems (ITSC)*; Institute of Electrical and Electronics Engineers (IEEE): Piscataway, NJ, USA, 2014; pp. 2286–2291. [CrossRef]
8. Tae-Hyun, H.; In-Hak, J.; Seong-Ik, C. *Detection of Traffic Lights for Vision-Based Car Navigation System BT-Advances in Image and Video Technology*; Springer: Berlin/Heidelberg, Germany, 2006; pp. 682–691.
9. Krizhevsky, A.; Sutskever, I.; Hinton, G.E. ImageNet Classification with Deep Convolutional Neural Networks. *Neural Inf. Process. Syst.* **2012**, *25*. [CrossRef]
10. Simonyan, K.; Zisserman, A. Very Deep Convolutional Networks for Large-Scale Image Recognition. *arXiv* **2014**, arXiv:1409.1556.
11. He, K.; Zhang, X.; Ren, S.; Sun, J. Deep Residual Learning for Image Recognition. In *2016 IEEE Conference on Computer Vision and Pattern Recognition (CVPR)*; Institute of Electrical and Electronics Engineers (IEEE): Piscataway, NJ, USA, 2016; pp. 770–778. [CrossRef]
12. Szegedy, C.; Vanhoucke, V.; Ioffe, S.; Shlens, J.; Wojna, Z. Rethinking the Inception Architecture for Computer Vision. In *IEEE Conference on Computer Vision and Pattern Recognition (CVPR)*; Institute of Electrical and Electronics Engineers (IEEE): Piscataway, NJ, USA, 2016; pp. 2818–2826. [CrossRef]
13. Dogo, E.M.; Afolabi, O.J.; Nwulu, N.I.; Twala, B.; Aigbavboa, C.O. Aigbavboa, A Comparative Analysis of Gradient Descent-Based Optimization Algorithms on Convolutional Neural Networks. In Proceedings of the 2018 International Conference on Computational Techniques, Electronics and Mechanical Systems (CTEMS), Belgaum, India, 21–22 December 2018.
14. Prilianti, K.R.; Brotosudarmo, T.H.P.; Anam, S.; Suryanto, A. *Performance Comparison of the Convolutional Neural Network Optimizer for Photosynthetic Pigments Prediction on Plant Digital Image*; AIP Publishing: University Park, MA, USA, 2019.
15. LeCun, Y.; Bottou, L.; Bengio, Y.; Haffner, P. Gradient-based learning applied to document recognition. In Proceedings of the IEEE; IEEE: Piscataway, NJ, USA, 1998; Volume 86, pp. 2278–2324. [CrossRef]
16. Jangid, M.; Srivastava, S. Deep ConvNet with different stochastic optimizations for handwritten devanagari character. In Proceedings of the IC4S 2017, Patong Phuket, Thailand, 11–12 October 2017; Volume 1, pp. 51–60.
17. Swastika, W.; Ariyanto, M.F.; Setiawan, H.; Irawan, P.L.T. Appropriate CNN Architecture and Optimizer for Vehicle Type Classification System on the Toll Road. *J. Phys. Conf. Ser.* **2019**, *1196*, 012044. [CrossRef]
18. Bejnordi, B.E.; Veta, M.; Van Diest, P.J.; Van Ginneken, B.; Karssemeijer, N.; Litjens, G.; Van Der Laak, J.A.W.M.; The CAMELYON16 Consortium; Hermsen, M.; Manson, Q.F.; et al. Diagnostic Assessment of Deep Learning Algorithms for Detection of Lymph Node Metastases in Women With Breast Cancer. *JAMA* **2017**, *318*, 2199–2210. [CrossRef] [PubMed]
19. Veeling, B.S.; Linmans, J.; Winkens, J.; Cohen, T.; Welling, M. *Rotation Equivariant CNNs for Digital Pathology BT-Medical Image Computing and Computer Assisted Intervention–MICCAI 2018*; Springer: Berlin/Heidelberg, Germany, 2018; pp. 210–218.
20. Kaggle. PatchCamelyon. Available online: https://www.kaggle.com/c/histopathologic-cancer-detection/data (accessed on 1 September 2020).
21. Scherer, D.; Müller, A.; Behnke, S. Evaluation of Pooling Operations in Convolutional Architectures for Object Recognition. *Computer Vision* **2010**, *6354*, 92–101.
22. Duchi, J.C.; Hazan, E.; Singer, Y. Adaptive Subgradient Methods for Online Learning and Stochastic Optimization. *J. Mach. Learn. Res.* **2011**, *12*, 2121–2159.

23. Hinton, G.; Srivastava, N.; Swersky, K. Neural Networks for Machine Learning, Lecture 6a Overview of Mini-Batch Gradient Descent. Available online: http://www.cs.toronto.edu/-hinton/coursera/lecture6/lec6.pdf (accessed on 24 August 2020).
24. Kingma, D.; Ba, J. Adam: A Method for Stochastic Optimization. Available online: https://arxiv.org/abs/1412.6980 (accessed on 22 August 2020).
25. Dozat, T. Incorporating Nesterov Momentum into Adam. In Proceedings of the 4th International Conference on Learning Representations, Workshop Track, San Juan, Puerto Rico, 2–4 May 2016.
26. SPan, S.J.; Yang, Q. A Survey on Transfer Learning. *IEEE Trans. Knowl. Data Eng.* **2009**, *22*, 1345–1359. [CrossRef]
27. Xie, M.; Jean, N.; Burke, M.; Lobell, D.; Ermon, S. Transfer learning from deep features for remote sensing and poverty mapping. In Proceedings of the 30th AAAI Conference on Artificial Intelligence, AAAI 2016, Phoenix, AZ, USA, 12–17 February 2016; pp. 3929–3935.
28. Szegedy, C.; Liu, W.; Jia, Y.; Sermanet, P.; Reed, S.; Anguelov, D.; Erhan, D.; Vanhoucke, V.; Rabinovich, A. Going deeper with convolutions. In Proceedings of the 2015 IEEE Conference on Computer Vision and Pattern Recognition (CVPR), Boston, MA, USA, 7–12 June 2015; pp. 1–9. [CrossRef]
29. Huang, G.; Liu, Z.; Van Der Maaten, L.; Weinberger, K.Q. Densely Connected Convolutional Networks. In Proceedings of the 2017 IEEE Conference on Computer Vision and Pattern Recognition (CVPR), Honolulu, HI, USA, 21–26 July 2017; pp. 2261–2269. [CrossRef]
30. Srivastava, N.; Hinton, G.; Krizhevsky, A.; Sutskever, I.; Salakhutdinov, R. Dropout: A Simple Way to Prevent Neural Networks from Overfitting. *J. Mach. Learn. Res.* **2014**, *15*, 1929–1958.
31. Fawcett, T. ROC Graphs: Notes and Practical Considerations for Data Mining Researchers. Available online: https://www.hpl.hp.com/techreports/2003/HPL-2003-4.pdf (accessed on 27 August 2020).
32. Vuk, M. ROC Curve, Lift Chart and Calibration Plot. *Comput. Sci.* **2006**, *3*, 89–108.

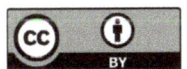

© 2020 by the authors. Licensee MDPI, Basel, Switzerland. This article is an open access article distributed under the terms and conditions of the Creative Commons Attribution (CC BY) license (http://creativecommons.org/licenses/by/4.0/).

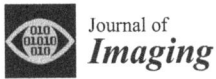

Article

Detection of HER2 from Haematoxylin-Eosin Slides Through a Cascade of Deep Learning Classifiers via Multi-Instance Learning

David La Barbera [1], António Polónia [2,3], Kevin Roitero [1], Eduardo Conde-Sousa [3,4] and Vincenzo Della Mea [1,*]

1. Department of Mathematics, Computer Science and Physics, University of Udine, 33100 Udine, Italy; labarbera.david@spes.uniud.it (D.L.B.); roitero.kevin@spes.uniud.it (K.R.)
2. Department of Pathology, Ipatimup Diagnostics, Institute of Molecular Pathology and Immunology, University of Porto, 4169-007 Porto, Portugal; apolonia@ipatimup.pt
3. i3S—Instituto de Investigação e Inovação em Saúde, Universidade do Porto, 4169-007 Porto, Portugal; econdesousa@gmail.com
4. INEB—Instituto de Engenharia Biomédica, Universidade do Porto, 4169-007 Porto, Portugal
* Correspondence: vincenzo.dellamea@uniud.it

Received: 1 July 2020; Accepted: 18 August 2020; Published: 23 August 2020

Abstract: Breast cancer is the most frequently diagnosed cancer in woman. The correct identification of the HER2 receptor is a matter of major importance when dealing with breast cancer: an over-expression of HER2 is associated with aggressive clinical behaviour; moreover, HER2 targeted therapy results in a significant improvement in the overall survival rate. In this work, we employ a pipeline based on a cascade of deep neural network classifiers and multi-instance learning to detect the presence of HER2 from Haematoxylin–Eosin slides, which partly mimics the pathologist's behaviour by first recognizing cancer and then evaluating HER2. Our results show that the proposed system presents a good overall effectiveness. Furthermore, the system design is prone to further improvements that can be easily deployed in order to increase the effectiveness score.

Keywords: digital pathology; whole slide image processing; multiple instance learning; convolutional neural networks; deep learning classification; HER2

---

1. Introduction

Breast cancer is the most frequently diagnosed cancer in women. As shown by Siegel et al. [1], breast cancer in 2020 is expected to account for 30% of female cancer in United States. The diagnosis of breast cancer, including its morphological subtypes, is that was carried out by a pathologist by examining a microscope histologic slide obtained from a breast biopsy or from a surgical sample. The slide is stained with a two-colors staining, called Haematoxylin-Eosin (HE), which enables the recognition of morphological features of the cancer. Haematoxylin-Eosin (HE) is universally used for histologic diagnosis. In addition to that, further sections are prepared and stained with immunohistochemical techniques (IHC) to evidentiate the expression of specific proteins. In the case of breast cancer, routine examination includes oestrogen and progesterone receptors, MIB2, and HER2. Visually, HE-stained slides show blue (for nuclei) and pink (for cytoplasm), while IHC slides are brown where the investigated protein is expressed, and counterstained in blue by means of haematoxylin.

According to current guidelines of the College of American Pathologists for HER2 testing in breast cancer [2], Human Epidermal growth factor Receptor 2 (HER2) quantification must be routinely tested, in invasive breast cancer, recurrences, and metastases. HER2 is a trans-membrane protein receptor with tyrosine kinase activity; studies have shown that HER2 is amplified and/or over-expressed in about 25% of breast cancer cases [3]. The over-expression and/or amplification of the HER2 receptor have been associated with aggressive clinical behaviour; nevertheless, the accurate assessment of the HER2 receptor has proven to be essential for identifying breast cancer patients who will benefit from HER2-targeted therapy [4]. It has been demonstrated by many clinical trials that the HER2-targeted therapy (both when administrated during and/or after chemotherapy) results in a significant improvement in both disease-free and overall survival in patients who have shown either an amplification or over-expression of the HER2 receptor [4]. Consequently, the correct identification of the HER2 receptor lead to select patients who are expected to benefit from the targeted therapy; this makes HER2 a helpful marker for the therapy decision making process.

Many researchers tried to develop IHC techniques that are able to identify HER2 with a sufficient precision and therefore be able to help the pathologist with the characterization of breast cancer [5–13]. The current approach to HER2 testing consists in cutting an additional section for the IHC evaluation of the positivity, negativity, or uncertain status of HER2 expression. In uncertain cases, a further examination has to be done based on In-Situ Hybridization, increasing costs and time. This, in addition to the HE stained slide, which is always prepared because needed for morphological diagnosis of cancer and of its subtypes. In the context of digital pathology, there is an increasing interest in developing Deep Learning (DL) techniques that can support the decision making process of the pathologist, especially when dealing with cancer related topics [10]. The practical use of deep learning in the context of breast cancer diseases is mainly due the performance achieved by deep learning algorithms over the last decade in the field of image recognition [14–16].

The recent HEROHE challenge proposed a peculiar research question: is it possible to identify HER2 from Hematoxylin–Eosin images of invasive breast cancer? In case of success, this would allow obtaining HER2 status without the corresponding IHC image, thus reducing time and costs. In fact, it is known that HER2 positivity is associated with aggressiveness of the tumour, which, in turn, is associated with certain morphological features, such as high histological grade. Thus, the idea is to exploit such morphological features as a proxy for HER2 status. For this, the Challenge organizers provided a set of 400 digitized haematoxylin-eosin slides accompanied by their HER2 status, and subsequently 150 slides for testing.

The objective of our study is the same behind the HEROHE challenge: to find a method to recognize the therapeutically useful HER2 status from the morphological aspects of the breast cancer only, as recognisable in the HE slides that are already used for diagnosis.

More in detail, our approach is based on deep learning algorithms employed in the setting of image recognition and Multiple Instance Learning (MIL) [17–21].

Digitized microscope slides, normally called digital slides or Whole Slide Images (WSI), correspond to huge scanned images that are difficult to process with standard Machine Learning (ML) or Deep Learning (DL) approaches due to hardware limitations [22]. A technique that is used to overcome such limitations is represented by MIL [23,24]. Opposed to the classical ML and DL classification setting where the learning algorithm receives in input a set of individually labelled instances, in MIL the learning algorithm receives a set of labelled instances (in our case, each instance is a WSI), each of these containing many unlabelled instances (in our case, the WSI is divided into tiles). Subsequently, the final class for the instance (i.e., the WSI) is decided upon the predicted classes of the unlabelled instances (i.e., the tiles). For example, in the simplest case, the main instance may be labelled as negative if all its unlabelled instances in it are labelled as negative negative [25].

We now detail some work related to the work of this paper.

MIL has been proven to be effective in the setting of image recognition and, in particular, in the context of cancer detection: Campanella et al. [26] used MIL to tackle the problem of prostate cancer detection, basal cell carcinoma, and breast cancer metastases to axillary lymph nodes. Their approach resulted in areas under the ROC curve (AUC) above 0.98 for the cancer types considered in the study.

MIL has also been used in the setting of breast cancer image detection. P J et al. [27] conducted experiments on a public dataset of biopsy images of benign and malignant breast cancers; according to their findings, MIL provides better results than state-of-the-art approaches in the setting of the detection of breast cancer in images. A more relevant work to our setting is the study conducted by Couture et al. [28], which investigated a method to predict cancer subtypes from histologic images. Couture et al. used MIL to model the problem and account for intra-cancer variations in cancer subtypes, improving the correct classification of cancer subtypes with reference to the state of the art approaches, and providing also insights about cancer heterogeneity.

Other researchers tried to detect HER2 from HER2 stained digital slides, using ML or not ML methods [29–34]; we do not detail their methodology, since they are out of scope for this work.

Thus, our specific contribution is a pipeline based on a cascade of deep neural network classifiers and multi-instance learning, which partly mimics the pathologist' behaviour by first recognizing cancer and then evaluating HER2, and able to currently provide state-of-the-art performance for the novel problem of detecting HER2 from Haematoxylin–Eosin slides.

2. Materials and Methods

2.1. Dataset and Materials

In our study, we used the dataset made available from the Instituto de Investigação and Inovação em Saúde and Instituto de Engenharia de Sistemas e Computadores, Tecnologia e Ciência from Porto University in Porto, Portugal, who together organized the HEROHE Grand Challenge for ECDP2020 (see https://ecdp2020.grand-challenge.org). The classification of this dataset used the latest American Society of Clinical Oncology/College of American Pathologists (ASCO/CAP) classification of breast cancer (Focused Update 2018) [2]. The HEROHE training dataset is composed of 144 positive slides (i.e., WSI of cases which are labelled as HER2 positive) and 216 negative slides (i.e., WSI of cases that are labelled as HER2 negative). Figure 1 shows an example of positive and negative slides present in the dataset.

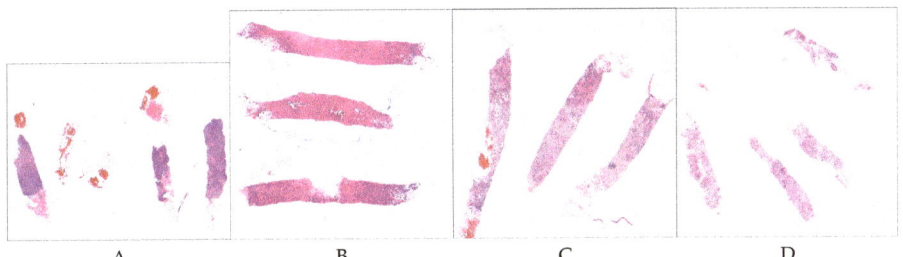

Figure 1. Example of tiles from the HEROHE dataset. The left-most two slides (**A**,**B**) have been labelled as positive for HER2; The right-most two slides (**C**,**D**) have been labelled as negative.

After implementing the proposed solution (as detailed in the next section), we tested it on the HEROHE Grand Challenge test set that is composed of 60 positive and 90 negative slides. The training, validation, and testing phase has been carried out using either a Titan XP GPU or using the Google Cloud Platform. The proposed solution has been implemented on the fast.ai Framework. Due to the nature of the data used in this study, we cannot publicly release the images used to train our algorithms. However, we release all of the code used to conduct the experiments as well as the trained models (Supplementary Materials).

2.2. Our Approach: A Cascade of Deep Learning Classifiers

The idea behind this work is to build a system that mimics the actions a pathologist performs when detecting the presence of the HER2 receptor. The actions include to divide each slide into tiles under the "divide et impera" principle, filter the tiles in order to keep only the most informative ones for the purpose of HER2 detection (i.e., only the tiles containing cancer), check for the presence of

HER2 into the individual tiles, and finally aggregate the tile information at the slide level to perform the decision whether the whole slide expresses or not the HER2 receptor.

To this aim, we developed a multi-stage pipeline as graphically represented in Figure 2. We considered a multi-stage system because this architectural design allowed us to try different techniques (or different variants of a single technique) for each stage, and then deploy to the final version of the system using only the most effective combination of stages. Furthermore, a multi-stage pipeline is the ideal scenario to test different approaches and compare single techniques at different levels of the pipeline. The pipeline we implemented is composed, as follows: the first stage extracts the tiles (Section 2.2.1), second stage considers either all tiles (Section 2.2.2), or a subset of them (Section 2.2.3), third stage details the main classifier architecture (Section 2.2.4), fourth stage formalize the features considered (Section 2.2.5), and fifth stage consider the post-training aggregation by means of either majority voting (Section 2.2.6) or a Tabular learner (Section 2.2.7). In the following sections, we discuss the role of each stage in detail.

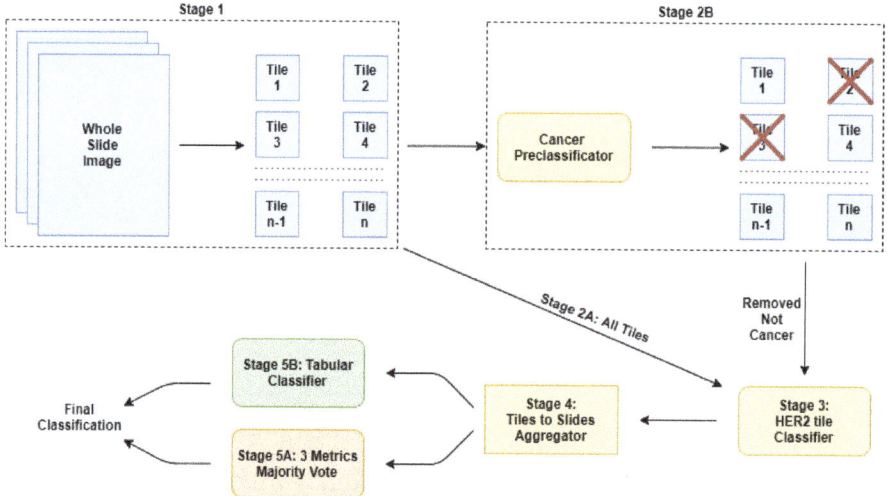

Figure 2. Graphical overview of the multi-stage deep learning pipeline.

2.2.1. Stage 1: The Tiles Extractor

The first stage of our pipeline is devoted to extract the tiles from every WSI present in the dataset. We consider each tile to be an instance necessary? (using the DL nomenclature) of our problem formulation. Slides provided by the HEROHE challenge were scanned at 40× magnification (which corresponds to a pixel size of 0.25 µm/pixel), with a 3DHistech Pannoramic 1000 scanner, and stored in their proprietary format. For the present work, slides were subsampled to 20× magnification (which has proven to reduce the computational complexity, but not decrease the overall accuracy with reference to the 40× magnification [26]) and converted to TIFF format. Therefore, the pixel size of the used slides corresponds to 0.50 µm/pixel.

After such process, each slide is then decomposed into squares (i.e., the tiles) of 512 × 512 pixels, with no stride. Figure 3 shows an example of the decomposition of two slides into tiles. Note that the slides in the dataset might have different dimensions, thus each of them is decomposed in a variable number of tiles.

Subsequently, in order to increase the overall accuracy model and preserve salient features [35], we dropped the tiles that have an average grey-scale value (i.e., the pixel value that represents the brightness of the pixel; the lower the value, the darker the pixel) greater than 0.8. This allows to discard background slides, including those presenting very small amounts of tissue.

After this stage, we considered two different approaches: the former consists in passing forward to the next stage all of the tiles; the latter in considering only an informative subset of tiles. Such approaches are detailed respectively in Sections 2.2.2 and 2.2.3.

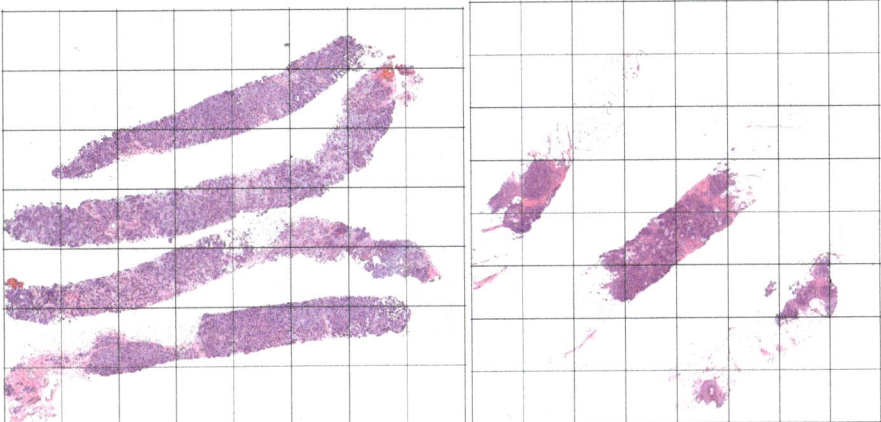

Figure 3. An example of slides from our dataset in which we applied a rectangular grid (shown with the continuous black lines) to show the division of a slide in tiles.

2.2.2. Stage 2A: Using All the Tiles

This stage simply consists in keeping all the tiles, without discarding any, and forwarding them without any modification to the next stage. The rationale behind this stage is that by maintaining all of the tiles we do not discard any potentially useful information, and we delegate to (the classifier of) the next stages the task to discern between relevant and not relevant information (i.e., noise) for all of the tiles considered.

2.2.3. Stage 2B: Using a Subset of Tiles

This stage takes in input all of the tiles from Stage 1 (see Section 2.2.1) and filters them, under the rationale that a subset of tiles is more informative for the model than the whole set of (potentially noisy) tiles. Moreover, this process simulates the real case scenario; in fact, when looking for the presence of HER2 in slides, the pathologist focus the search only in the part of slides (similar to our tiles) containing cancer, and more specifically in the tiles containing invasive cancer. One additional reason is that HER2 might also be expressed outside the cancer tissue, in normal ducts, or as extracellular accumulation, or also as staining artifacts. While we might expect that DL is able to cope with these situations too, we did not want to expose the network to spurious data, or at least to reduce the amount of noise. We perform a pre-classification task, with the purpose of discerning between the tiles that contain cancer and those that do not, in order to filter the input tiles. To this aim, we developed a model based on a Convolutional Neural Network (CNN), relying on the model detailed by Della Mea and Pilutti [36], which is based on the densenet-201 architecture [37–39] pretrained on the ImageNet dataset [40]. However, the HEROHE data set did not include annotations for identifying cancer areas inside the slides, which may as well contain normal tissue or tissue representing other not tumoral diseases. Thus, although not optimal, we had to exploit a different set of training images. For this aim, we fine-tuned the model on 400 images from the BACH Challenge Part A (see https://iciar2018-challenge.grand-challenge.org/) [41] dataset. These images are 2048 × 1536; by means of SlideJ [42] we extracted tiles of 512 × 512 size, with a stride of 256, obtaining 35 tiles per image. Thus, we trained for three epochs to fine-tune the last layer, plus three epochs for the whole network. We applied the default fast.ai data augmentation transforms, including random mixtures of flips, rotations, moderate zoom (up to 1.1×), warping, luminosity, and contrast variations. We collapsed the original labels (i.e., "normal", "benign", "in situ carcinoma", and "invasive carcinoma", 100 images for each class, corresponding to 3500 tiles) into two binary categories, as follows: we mapped the original labels "normal" and "benign" into the label "no cancer", and the labels "in situ carcinoma" and "invasive carcinoma" into the label "cancer". Note that we also consider tiles that contain in-situ cancer because, at high resolution, it would be impossible to distinguish them from the ones with invasive cancer.

After the training phase, we fed all of the tiles considered in this work to the fine-tuned classifier, and we removed the tiles classified as not containing cancer. Overall, we fed the model with 90.068 test tiles, and we removed 29.429 tiles (32.68%), maintaining 60.639 (67.32%). On average, we removed the 29.27% of tiles from each slide; more in detail, on average, we removed 32.02% of tiles from negative slides and 25.16% from positive slides. Figure 4 shows an example of the classification outcome in term of slides.

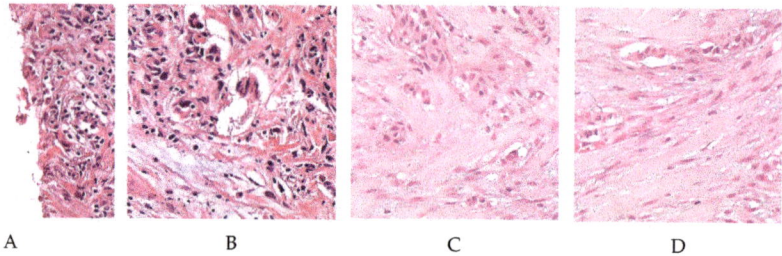

Figure 4. Tiles identified by the cancer classifier as: positive (first two tiles, tile (**A**) is a true positive, tile (**B**) is a false positive), and negative (last two tiles, tile (**C**) is a true negative, tile (**D**) is a false negative).

2.2.4. Stage 3: The Main Classifier

After the second stage, we trained the main classifier, either with all tiles (from stage 2A) or with the subset of tiles labelled as containing cancer (from stage 2B). Our main architecture is as follows. We trained a classifier based on the ResNet152 architecture [43], a well-known architecture for image recognition [43–46] based on the concept of residual learning [43]. Figure 5 provides a schema of the model architecture and the block for residual learning. We fed the classifier each tile with the associated HER2 status. We did not expect to obtain high accuracy, because in a positive slide HER2 is not expressed everywhere; on the other side, in a negative slide, we expect HER2 not to be expressed, although it is known that it could also be present in normal tissue, which is one reason why we wanted to discard not cancer tiles. We trained the classifier using the HEROHE training set for three epochs while using precision as loss function. For data augmentation, we applied the same transforms as the first classifier. Learning rate has been set according the One-cycle policy developed by L.Smith [47].

Figure 6 shows an example of the classification outcome in terms of tiles.

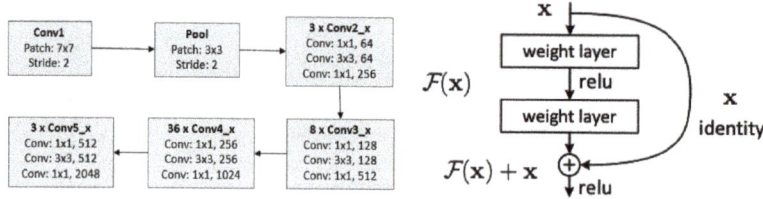

Figure 5. The basic architecture of Resnet152 (**left**, from [48]), and the building block for the residual learning (**right**, from [43]).

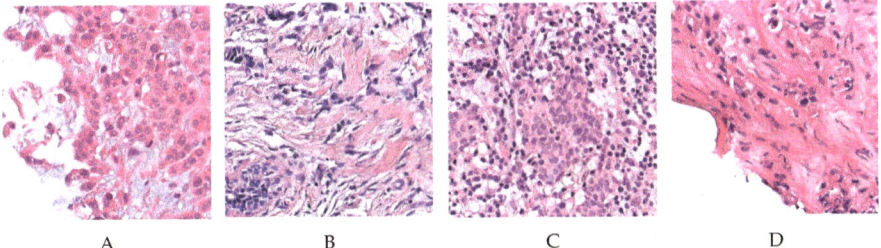

Figure 6. Tiles identified by the HER2 classifier as positive (first two tiles, tile (**A**) is a true positive, tile (**B**) is a false positive), and negative (last two tiles, tile (**C**) is a true negative, and tile (**D**) is a false negative).

2.2.5. Stage 4: Computing the Features

The classifier detailed in the previous stage returns as output, for each test instance, the probability that the test instance belongs to a given class, for all of the classes. In our setting, the classifier returns a probability value in the $[0,1]$ range that denotes the probability of each tile in be positive for the HER2 receptor. Those are the probabilities we will consider in this section. After training our main classifier to determine for each tile its probability of containing the HER2 receptor, we aggregated the results at the tile level to determine the overall classification outcome, which correspond to assess whether the whole slide contains or not the HER2 receptor. To this aim, we used two strategies detailed in the following, which take advantage of the features described in this section.

Suppose that we have S slides, and that each slide is divided into T tiles. We denote with p_i^j is the probability of the i-th tile (belonging to the j-th slide) to be tested positive for HER2.

Subsequently, in the first case we compute the binary positivity $P_1(s_i)$ of the slide s_i by considering the simple arithmetic average of the probabilities p_i^j for all of the tiles; formally:

$$P_1(s_i) = \begin{cases} 1 & \text{if } \frac{1}{T}\sum_{i=1}^{T} p_i^j \geq 0.5, \\ 0 & \text{otherwise.} \end{cases}$$

In the second case, we compute the binary positivity $P_2(s_i)$ of the slide s_i by considering the simple arithmetic average of the probabilities p_i^j for tiles having probability $p_i^j \geq 0.5$; formally:

$$P_2(s_i) = \begin{cases} 1 & \text{if } \frac{1}{T}\sum_{i=1}^{T} p_i^j \cdot G(p_i^j) \geq 0.66, \\ 0 & \text{otherwise,} \end{cases}$$

where

$$G(p_i^j) = \begin{cases} 1 & \text{if } p_i^j \geq 0.5, \\ 0 & \text{otherwise.} \end{cases}$$

In the third case, we compute the binary positivity $P_3(s_i)$ of the slide s_i by considering the slide positive if at least the 35% of its tiles have a probability $p_i^j \geq 0.5$; formally:

$$P_3(s_i) = \begin{cases} 1 & \text{if } \frac{1}{T}\sum_{i=1}^{T} G(p_i^j) \geq 0.35, \\ 0 & \text{otherwise.} \end{cases}$$

Apart from the three positivity indices $P_1(s_i)$, $P_2(s_i)$, and $P_3(s_i)$ of each slide, we consider, as additional set of features, the frequency of the probabilities p_i^j for each slide, for each interval $[h, h+0.1]$, $h \in \{0.5, 0.6, 0.7, 0.8, 0.9\}$; formally,

$$F_h(s_i) = \frac{1}{T} \sum_{i=1}^{T} C(p_i^j, h),$$

where

$$C(p_i^j, h) = \begin{cases} 1 & \text{if } p_i^j \in [h, h+0.1), \\ 0 & \text{otherwise.} \end{cases}$$

After computing the positivity indices $P_1(s_i)$, $P_2(s_i)$, and $P_3(s_i)$, and the set of features $F_h(s_i)$, $h \in \{0.5, 0.6, 0.7, 0.8, 0.9\}$, we aggregate such indices to compute the overall positivity of the i-th slide. To do so, we adopt two strategies, detailed in the following.

2.2.6. Stage 5A: Post-Trainer Aggregation Using Majority Vote

The first strategy we adopt to compute the overall positivity of each slide is to simply compute the majority vote of the $P_1(s_i)$, $P_2(s_i)$, and $P_3(s_i)$ indices. In this way, we assume that all of the features are equally informative for the final decision.

2.2.7. Stage 5B: Post-Trainer Aggregation Using a Tabular Learner

The second strategy we adopt to the overall positivity of each slide consists in train a classifier to learn the best weights for the indices. More in detail, in this phase, we use the $P_1(s_i)$ probabilities not binarized, denoted as $P_1^*(s_i)$ (i.e., $\frac{1}{T}\sum_{i=1}^T p_i^j$), as well as the set of features $F_h(s_i), h \in \{0.5, 0.6, 0.7, 0.8, 0.9\}$ to build the feature matrix detailed in Table 1. Following this approach, we delegate to the algorithm the task of learning how to combine the features in the best possible way. We trained the Tabular learning while using an architecture with three layers composed by respectively 500, 250, and 125 fully connected layers, and we used accuracy as loss function. We did some experiments to include all the $P_1(s_i)$, $P_2(s_i)$, and $P_3(s_i)$ indices in the feature matrix, but we found that the additional indices did not provide a significant increase in the effectiveness scores.

Table 1. Training matrix for the Tabular Learner. $P_1^*(s_i)$ represents the non binarized $P_1(s_i)$ probability. $P(s_i)$ represents the true positivity for the i-th tile (used only for the training phase).

	P_1^*	$F_{0.5}$	$F_{0.6}$	$F_{0.7}$	$F_{0.8}$	$F_{0.9}$	P
s_1	$P_1^*(s_1)$	$F_{0.5}(s_1)$	$F_{0.6}(s_1)$	$F_{0.7}(s_1)$	$F_{0.8}(s_1)$	$F_{0.9}(s_1)$	$P(s_1)$
s_2	$P_1^*(s_2)$	$F_{0.5}(s_2)$	$F_{0.6}(s_2)$	$F_{0.7}(s_2)$	$F_{0.8}(s_2)$	$F_{0.9}(s_2)$	$P(s_2)$
⋮	⋮	⋮	⋮	⋮	⋮	⋮	⋮
s_i	$P_1^*(s_i)$	$F_{0.5}(s_i)$	$F_{0.6}(s_i)$	$F_{0.7}(s_i)$	$F_{0.8}(s_i)$	$F_{0.9}(s_i)$	$P(s_i)$
⋮	⋮	⋮	⋮	⋮	⋮	⋮	⋮
s_S	$P_1^*(s_S)$	$F_{0.5}(s_S)$	$F_{0.6}(s_S)$	$F_{0.7}(s_S)$	$F_{0.8}(s_S)$	$F_{0.9}(s_S)$	$P(s_S)$

3. Results

Table 2 reports the effectiveness of our approach measured on the HEROHE Grand Challenge test set. To the best of our knowledge, there are no other published results (up to current date) that investigate our same problem or use the same test data as we do. For this reason, Table 2 reports the effectiveness scores of our method and the leaderboard of the HEROHE challenge only. Note that the leaderboard has been chosen by the organising committee of the HEROE challenge on the basis of the F1 score alone.

Table 2. Evaluation metrics for our two approaches and the leaderboard of the HEROHE challenge. In bold we highlight the best result obtained for each evaluation metric.

	All Tiles		Subset of Tiles		Best
	Majority Vote	Tabular Classifier	Majority Vote	Tabular Classifier	HEROHE
Accuracy	0.687	0.673	0.667	**0.707**	-
Precision	0.570	0.560	0.580	**0.603**	0.5682
Recall	**0.883**	0.864	0.783	0.797	0.8333
F1-Score	**0.693**	0.680	0.667	0.687	0.6757

As we can see from the table, if we consider the variants of our approach separately, it is always the case that our system outperforms the leaderboard of the HEROHE challenge, even though different metrics are maximized by different algorithms. The only variant that outperforms the leaderboard of the HEROHE challenge on all the considered metrics is the "All Tiles–Majority Vote" variant.

Turning to compare the different approaches that we propose, we see that it is not always the case that employing the Tabular classifier lead to obtain higher effectiveness scores; more in detail, we see that for precision oriented metrics (i.e., Accuracy and Precision) consider a subset of tiles lead to higher effectiveness scores, and for the metrics affected by recall (i.e., Recall and F1) when considering all of the tiles lead to higher effectiveness scores.

Investigating the most effective approach for each metric separately, we see that our approach leads to obtain an accuracy score of about 0.7 and a precision score of about 0.6, suggesting that our model is able to correctly identify positives in the majority of positive cases. We also see that our model finds almost all positive cases in our dataset (recall of 0.88). When considering the metric used to rank systems in the HEROHE challenge, we see that our model has an F1 score of about 0.7, indicating a good overall balance between precision and recall.

4. Discussion and Conclusions

By looking at the results, we can draw different remarks. First, we see that recall (and F1 as result) is maximized when all the tiles are kept in the dataset; this an expected outcome. It is natural that by keeping all of the tiles (i.e., by keeping more data) we obtain a higher recall score. Nevertheless, this behaviour suggests that, when considering the effectiveness metrics all together, it is not straightforward to choose whether to remove or not a subset of tiles, as some tiles might be more informative than others for some metrics, but not for all of them. Finally, this behaviour can be caused not only by the fact that we keep more data, but also by complex interactions between the classification algorithm and some particular feature of the tile. We plan to address this matter in future work. When considering that our problem is a high recall problem, we can say that the best variant of our approach is the "All Tiles–Majority Vote" one. In other terms, considering our setting we want to find all of the patients that actually are positive for HER2, and we can accept a lower precision if the effort to conduct a clinical test to detect HER2 is not significant, which we believe is a more than reasonable assumption to make: we are willing to spend a little more in clinical testing but be able to save more lives. Summarising the remarks drawn from the results section, we can state that our results indicate that our multi-stage pipeline is indeed effective in detecting HER2. Furthermore, the results indicate that our approach is not over- nor under-dimensioned, given that both the filtering of tiles and the post classifier aggregation done with learners boost the results for some evaluation metric. Finally, we remark that a multi-stage pipeline has the advantage of being easily maintainable, and the accuracy of the single levels can be increased independently.

In this paper, we tackled the problem of classification of the HER2 status on HE slides of invasive breast cancer. Our approach based on a cascade of deep learning classifiers and multi instance learning shows good effectiveness scores for different evaluation metrics. We show that pre-filtering tiles lead to remove potentially noisy tiles and overall leads to an improvement of some effectiveness metrics. We also found that combining different predictors by means of a Tabular classifier is more effective than doing that by the means of a majority voting scores for precision oriented metrics, indicating that, indeed, different predictors need to be weighted and provide signals of different importance for the overall task. However, the overall effectiveness if far from being usable in clinical practice a substitution of the traditional IHC- and ISH-based testing. While this could be due to the intrinsic independency of the information provided by morphology and by HER2 expression, it is also surely conditioned by the relatively low number of slides used for training. In fact, while the overall number of images is high, they correspond to the about 400 cases provided by the Challenge, which are likely too few for Multiple Instance Learning. While no direct comparison is possible about HER2 detection, in other MIL-based related works on digital slides, larger data sets have been used with better results than ours. In particular, in [26] a dataset of about 44,000 slides has been used; although not directly comparable, they reached an AUC of 0.99. In the work of Couture et al. [28] the dataset is closer in size (571 slides) to ours, but also measures of effectiveness, while higher, are not too dissimilar (e.g., 0.80 accuracy for estrogen receptor status, which is a similar but not identical problem as HER2 status). Overall, we think that our work is an important step towards the development of a supervised approach that can serve the purpose of helping medical experts in the delicate task of selecting the appropriate treatment when dealing with clinical cases of breast cancer. For future work, we plan to develop the presented pipeline in order to increase the effectiveness metrics by increasing the impact and the effectiveness of the different stages of the pipeline. One way is to include further case details in the last stage of the pipeline, e.g., the other IHC results, patient data, etc. The other relatively easy enhancement will come from training the cancer classifier on slides acquired with the same setup as the other classifier. In fact, as is the cancer classifier is sub-optimal. In this way, we can provide even more information to the medical experts with the aim of providing a more sound and robust tool that can be practically used in the clinical decision making process.

Supplementary Materials: The software and trained models are available online at https://github.com/MITEL-UNIUD/HE2HER2/.

Author Contributions: (In alphabetical order within each category) Conceptualization, V.D.M., D.L.B., and K.R.; methodology, V.D.M., D.L.B., and K.R.; validation, V.D.M., D.L.B., and K.R.; formal analysis, D.L.B.; investigation, V.D.M., and D.L.B.; resources, V.D.M., A.P. and E.C.-S.; data curation, D.L.B., A.P. and E.C.-S.; writing—original draft preparation, V.D.M., D.L.B., and K.R.; writing—review and editing, V.D.M., D.L.B., K.R., A.P. and E.C.-S.; visualization, D.L.B.; supervision, V.D.M. and K.R.; project administration, V.D.M., A.P. and E.C.-S.; funding acquisition, V.D.M. and A.P. All authors have read and agreed to the published version of the manuscript.

Funding: Eduardo Conde-Sousa was supported by the project PPBI-POCI-01-0145-FEDER-022122, in the scope of Fundação para a Ciência e Tecnologia, Portugal (FCT) National Roadmap of Research Infrastructures.

Acknowledgments: The digital slides of breast cancer tissue samples stained with HE were digitized at IPATIMUP Diagnostics, University of Porto, Portugal. We thank Nvidia for providing the GPU used to train the models, and Google for providing the grant consisting in Google Cloud credits used to carry out the experiments detailed in this paper.

Conflicts of Interest: The authors declare no conflict of interest.

Abbreviations

The following abbreviations are used in this manuscript:

CNN	Convolutional Neural Network
DL	Deep Learning
HER2	Human Epidermal growth factor Receptor 2
MIL	Multiple Instance Learning
ML	Machine Learning
WSI	Whole Slide Image

References

1. Siegel, R.L.; Miller, K.D.; Jemal, A. Cancer statistics, 2020. *CA A Cancer J. Clin.* **2020**, *70*, 7–30. [CrossRef] [PubMed]
2. Wolff, A.C.; Hammond, M.E.H.; Allison, K.H.; Harvey, B.E.; Mangu, P.B.; Bartlett, J.M.S.; Bilous, M.; Ellis, I.O.; Fitzgibbons, P.; Hanna, W.; et al. Human Epidermal Growth Factor Receptor 2 Testing in Breast Cancer: American Society of Clinical Oncology/College of American Pathologists Clinical Practice Guideline Focused Update. *Arch. Pathol. Lab. Med.* **2018**, *142*, 1364–1382. [CrossRef] [PubMed]
3. Dean-Colomb, W.; Esteva, F.J. Her2-positive breast cancer: Herceptin and beyond. *Eur. J. Cancer* **2008**, *44*, 2806–2812. [CrossRef] [PubMed]
4. Nahta, R.; Esteva, F.J. HER-2-Targeted Therapy. *Clin. Cancer Res.* **2003**, *9*, 5078–5084.
5. Gutierrez, C.; Schiff, R. HER2: Biology, detection, and clinical implications. *Arch. Pathol. Lab. Med.* **2011**, *135*, 55–62.
6. Al-Khafaji, Q.; Harris, M.; Tombelli, S.; Laschi, S.; Turner, A.; Mascini, M.; Marrazza, G. An electrochemical immunoassay for HER2 detection. *Electroanalysis* **2012**, *24*, 735–742. [CrossRef]
7. Riethdorf, S.; Müller, V.; Zhang, L.; Rau, T.; Loibl, S.; Komor, M.; Roller, M.; Huober, J.; Fehm, T.; Schrader, I. Detection and HER2 expression of circulating tumor cells: Prospective monitoring in breast cancer patients treated in the neoadjuvant GeparQuattro trial. *Clin. Cancer Res.* **2010**, *16*, 2634–2645. [CrossRef]
8. Gevensleben, H.; Garcia-Murillas, I.; Graeser, M.K.; Schiavon, G.; Osin, P.; Parton, M.; Smith, I.E.; Ashworth, A.; Turner, N.C. Noninvasive detection of HER2 amplification with plasma DNA digital PCR. *Clin. Cancer Res.* **2013**, *19*, 3276–3284. [CrossRef]
9. Gohring, J.T.; Dale, P.S.; Fan, X. Detection of HER2 breast cancer biomarker using the opto-fluidic ring resonator biosensor. *Sens. Actuators B Chem.* **2010**, *146*, 226–230. [CrossRef]
10. Vandenberghe, M.E.; Scott, M.L.; Scorer, P.W.; Söderberg, M.; Balcerzak, D.; Barker, C. Relevance of deep learning to facilitate the diagnosis of HER2 status in breast cancer. *Sci. Rep.* **2017**, *7*, 45938. [CrossRef]
11. Yaziji, H.; Goldstein, L.C.; Barry, T.S.; Werling, R.; Hwang, H.; Ellis, G.K.; Gralow, J.R.; Livingston, R.B.; Gown, A.M. HER-2 testing in breast cancer using parallel tissue-based methods. *JAMA* **2004**, *291*, 1972–1977. [CrossRef] [PubMed]
12. Basavanhally, A.N.; Ganesan, S.; Agner, S.; Monaco, J.P.; Feldman, M.D.; Tomaszewski, J.E.; Bhanot, G.; Madabhushi, A. Computerized image-based detection and grading of lymphocytic infiltration in HER2+ breast cancer histopathology. *IEEE Trans. Biomed. Eng.* **2009**, *57*, 642–653. [CrossRef] [PubMed]
13. Cruz-Roa, A.; Gilmore, H.; Basavanhally, A.; Feldman, M.; Ganesan, S.; Shih, N.N.; Tomaszewski, J.; González, F.A.; Madabhushi, A. Accurate and reproducible invasive breast cancer detection in whole-slide images: A Deep Learning approach for quantifying tumor extent. *Sci. Rep.* **2017**, *7*, 46450. [CrossRef]
14. Ravì, D.; Wong, C.; Deligianni, F.; Berthelot, M.; Andreu-Perez, J.; Lo, B.; Yang, G.Z. Deep learning for health informatics. *IEEE J. Biomed. Health Inform.* **2016**, *21*, 4–21. [CrossRef] [PubMed]
15. Litjens, G.; Kooi, T.; Bejnordi, B.E.; Setio, A.A.A.; Ciompi, F.; Ghafoorian, M.; Van Der Laak, J.A.; Van Ginneken, B.; Sánchez, C.I. A survey on deep learning in medical image analysis. *Med Image Anal.* **2017**, *42*, 60–88. [CrossRef]
16. Shen, D.; Wu, G.; Suk, H.I. Deep learning in medical image analysis. *Annu. Rev. Biomed. Eng.* **2017**, *19*, 221–248. [CrossRef]
17. Zha, Z.J.; Hua, X.S.; Mei, T.; Wang, J.; Qi, G.J.; Wang, Z. Joint multi-label multi-instance learning for image classification. In Proceedings of the 2008 IEEE Conference on Computer Vision and Pattern Recognition, Anchorage, AK, USA, 23–28 June 2008; pp. 1–8.
18. Zhou, Z.H.; Xu, J.M. On the relation between multi-instance learning and semi-supervised learning. In Proceedings of the 24th International Conference on Machine Learning, Corvallis, OR, USA, 20–24 June 2007; pp. 1167–1174.
19. Zhou, Z.H.; Zhang, M.L. Neural networks for multi-instance learning. In Proceedings of the International Conference on Intelligent Information Technology, Beijing, China, 22–25 September 2002; pp. 455–459.
20. Zhou, Z.H. Multi-instance learning: A survey. *Dep. Comput. Sci. Technol. Nanjing Univ. Tech. Rep.* **2004**, *2*.
21. Zhou, Z.H.; Zhang, M.L. Ensembles of multi-instance learners. In Proceedings of the 14th European Conference on Machine Learning, Cavtat-Dubrovnik, Croatia, 22–26 September 2003; Springer: Berlin/Heidelberg, Germany, 2003; pp. 492–502.

22. Sze, V.; Chen, Y.H.; Emer, J.; Suleiman, A.; Zhang, Z. Hardware for machine learning: Challenges and opportunities. In Proceedings of the 2017 IEEE Custom Integrated Circuits Conference (CICC), Austin, TX, USA, 30 April–3 May 2017; pp. 1–8.
23. Carbonneau, M.A.; Cheplygina, V.; Granger, E.; Gagnon, G. Multiple Instance Learning: A Survey of Problem Characteristics and Applications. *Pattern Recognit.* **2016**. [CrossRef]
24. Herrera, F.; Ventura, S.; Bello, R.; Cornelis, C.; Zafra, A.; Sanchez Tarrago, D.; Vluymans, S. *Multiple Instance Learning. Foundations and Algorithms*; Springer: Berlin/Heidelberg, Germany, 2016. [CrossRef]
25. Foulds, J.; Frank, E. A Review of Multi-Instance Learning Assumptions. *Knowl. Eng. Rev.* **2010**, *25*. [CrossRef]
26. Campanella, G.; Hanna, M.; Geneslaw, L.; Miraflor, A.; Silva, V.; Busam, K.; Brogi, E.; Reuter, V.; Klimstra, D.; Fuchs, T. Clinical-grade computational pathology using weakly supervised deep learning on whole slide images. *Nat. Med.* **2019**, *25*, 1. [CrossRef]
27. P J, S.; Petitjean, C.; Spanhol, F.; Oliveira, L.; Heutte, L.; Honeine, P. Multiple Instance Learning for Histopathological Breast Cancer Image Classification. *Expert Syst. Appl.* **2018**. [CrossRef]
28. Couture, H.D.; Williams, L.A.; Geradts, J.; Nyante, S.J.; Butler, E.N.; Marron, J.S.; Perou, C.M.; Troester, M.A.; Niethammer, M. Image analysis with deep learning to predict breast cancer grade, ER status, histologic subtype, and intrinsic subtype. *NPJ Breast Cancer* **2018**. [CrossRef]
29. Qaiser, T.; Mukherjee, A.; Reddy Pb, C.; Munugoti, S.D.; Tallam, V.; Pitkäaho, T.; Lehtimäki, T.; Naughton, T.; Berseth, M.; Pedraza, A.; et al. HER2 challenge contest: A detailed assessment of automated HER2 scoring algorithms in whole slide images of breast cancer tissues. *Histopathology* **2017**, *72*, 227–238. [CrossRef] [PubMed]
30. Jakobsen, M.R.; Teerapakpinyo, C.; Shuangshoti, S.; Keelawat, S. Comparison between digital image analysis and visual assessment of immunohistochemical HER2 expression in breast cancer. *Pathol.-Res. Pract.* **2018**, *214*, 2087–2092. [CrossRef] [PubMed]
31. Mukundan, R. Analysis of Image Feature Characteristics for Automated Scoring of HER2 in Histology Slides. *J. Imaging* **2019**, *5*, 35. [CrossRef]
32. Qaiser, T.; Rajpoot, N.M. Learning Where to See: A Novel Attention Model for Automated Immunohistochemical Scoring. *IEEE Trans. Med. Imaging* **2019**, *38*, 2620–2631. [CrossRef]
33. Yim, K.; Park, H.S.; Kim, D.M.; Lee, Y.S.; Lee, A. Image Analysis of HER2 Immunohistochemical Staining of Surgical Breast Cancer Specimens. *Yonsei Med. J.* **2019**, *60*, 158. [CrossRef]
34. Li, A.C.; Zhao, J.; Zhao, C.; Ma, Z.; Hartage, R.; Zhang, Y.; Li, X.; Parwani, A.V. Quantitative digital imaging analysis of HER2 immunohistochemistry predicts the response to anti-HER2 neoadjuvant chemotherapy in HER2-positive breast carcinoma. *Breast Cancer Res. Treat.* **2020**, *180*, 321–329. [CrossRef]
35. Güneş, A.; Kalkan, H.; Durmuş, E. Optimizing the color-to-grayscale conversion for image classification. *Signal Image Video Process.* **2016**, *10*, 853–860. [CrossRef]
36. Della Mea, V.; Pilutti, D. Classification of Histologic Images Using a Single Staining: Experiments With Deep Learning on Deconvolved Images. *Stud. Health Technol. Inform.* **2020**, *270*, 1223–1224.
37. Iandola, F.; Moskewicz, M.; Karayev, S.; Girshick, R.; Darrell, T.; Keutzer, K. Densenet: Implementing efficient convnet descriptor pyramids. *arXiv* **2014**, arXiv:1404.1869.
38. Yu, X.; Zeng, N.; Liu, S.; Zhang, Y.D. Utilization of DenseNet201 for diagnosis of breast abnormality. *Mach. Vis. Appl.* **2019**, *30*, 1135–1144. [CrossRef]
39. Yilmaz, F.; Kose, O.; Demir, A. Comparison of two different deep learning architectures on breast cancer. In Proceedings of the 2019 Medical Technologies Congress (TIPTEKNO), Izmir, Turkey, 3–5 October 2019; pp. 1–4.
40. Deng, J.; Dong, W.; Socher, R.; Li, L.J.; Li, K.; Fei-Fei, L. Imagenet: A large-scale hierarchical image database. In Proceedings of the 2009 IEEE Conference on Computer Vision and Pattern Recognition, Miami, FL, USA, 20–25 June 2009; pp. 248–255.
41. Aresta, G.; Araújo, T.; Kwok, S.; Chennamsetty, S.S.; Safwan, M.; Alex, V.; Marami, B.; Prastawa, M.; Chan, M.; Donovan, M. Bach: Grand challenge on breast cancer histology images. *Med. Image Anal.* **2019**, *56*, 122–139. [CrossRef] [PubMed]
42. Della Mea, V.; Baroni, G.L.; Pilutti, D.; Loreto, C.D. SlideJ: An ImageJ plugin for automated processing of whole slide images. *PLoS ONE* **2017**, *12*, e0180540. [CrossRef]

43. He, K.; Zhang, X.; Ren, S.; Sun, J. Deep residual learning for image recognition. In Proceedings of the 29th IEEE Conference on Computer Vision and Pattern Recognition, Las Vegas, NV, USA, 27–30 June 2016; pp. 770–778.
44. Szegedy, C.; Ioffe, S.; Vanhoucke, V.; Alemi, A.A. Inception-v4, inception-resnet and the impact of residual connections on learning. In Proceedings of the Thirty-First AAAI Conference on Artificial Intelligence, San Francisco, CA, USA, 4–9 February 2017.
45. Targ, S.; Almeida, D.; Lyman, K. Resnet in resnet: Generalizing residual architectures. *arXiv* **2016**, arXiv:1603.08029.
46. Wu, Z.; Shen, C.; Van Den Hengel, A. Wider or deeper: Revisiting the resnet model for visual recognition. *Pattern Recognit.* **2019**, *90*, 119–133. [CrossRef]
47. Smith, L.N. A disciplined approach to neural network hyper-parameters: Part 1—Learning rate, batch size, momentum, and weight decay. *arXiv* **2018**, arXiv:1803.09820.
48. Nguyen, L.D.; Lin, D.; Lin, Z.; Cao, J. Deep CNNs for microscopic image classification by exploiting transfer learning and feature concatenation. In Proceedings of the 2018 IEEE International Symposium on Circuits and Systems (ISCAS), Florence, Italy, 27–30 May 2018; pp. 1–5.

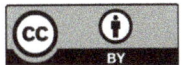

© 2020 by the authors. Licensee MDPI, Basel, Switzerland. This article is an open access article distributed under the terms and conditions of the Creative Commons Attribution (CC BY) license (http://creativecommons.org/licenses/by/4.0/).

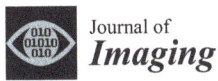

Article

Full 3D Microwave Breast Imaging Using a Deep-Learning Technique

Vahab Khoshdel *, Mohammad Asefi, Ahmed Ashraf and Joe LoVetri

Department of Electrical and Computer Engineering, University of Manitoba, Winnipeg, MB R3T 5V6, Canada; masefi@151research.com (M.A.); ahmed.ashraf@umanitoba.ca (A.A.); Joe.LoVetri@umanitoba.ca (J.L.)
* Correspondence: khoshdev@myumanitoba.ca

Received: 18 July 2020; Accepted: 5 August 2020; Published: 11 August 2020

Abstract: A deep learning technique to enhance 3D images of the complex-valued permittivity of the breast obtained via microwave imaging is investigated. The developed technique is an extension of one created to enhance 2D images. We employ a 3D Convolutional Neural Network, based on the U-Net architecture, that takes in 3D images obtained using the Contrast-Source Inversion (CSI) method and attempts to produce the true 3D image of the permittivity. The training set consists of 3D CSI images, along with the true numerical phantom images from which the microwave scattered field utilized to create the CSI reconstructions was synthetically generated. Each numerical phantom varies with respect to the size, number, and location of tumors within the fibroglandular region. The reconstructed permittivity images produced by the proposed 3D U-Net show that the network is not only able to remove the artifacts that are typical of CSI reconstructions, but it also enhances the detectability of the tumors. We test the trained U-Net with 3D images obtained from experimentally collected microwave data as well as with images obtained synthetically. Significantly, the results illustrate that although the network was trained using only images obtained from synthetic data, it performed well with images obtained from both synthetic and experimental data. Quantitative evaluations are reported using Receiver Operating Characteristics (ROC) curves for the tumor detectability and RMS error for the enhancement of the reconstructions.

Keywords: microwave breast imaging; image reconstruction; tumor detection; convolutional neural networks; deep learning

1. Introduction

Microwave Imaging (MWI) techniques that have been applied to the detection of breast cancer come in two forms: Radar-based techniques that attempt to detect tumors within the breast's interior [1], and inverse-scattering based methods that attempt to reconstruct complex permittivity maps corresponding to the distribution of different breast tissues [2]. The quantitative techniques, which are of interest herein, rely on the fact that different breast tissues (e.g., skin, adipose, fibroglandular and cancerous tumors) have different dielectric properties in the microwave frequency band [3,4].

Successfully implementing the inverse-scattering approach requires that one has a good numerical electromagnetic field model for the MWI system being used to acquire scattered-field data, including the antennas and the breast, but more importantly, requires that one solves a non-linear ill-posed inverse scattering problem. This is usually accomplished using computationally expensive iterative methods where the inversion model consists of a numerical solution of an electromagnetic forward scattering problem [5]. One challenge in using MWI for breast imaging is that the breast is a high-contrast object-of-interest (OI) having complicated internal structures and this produces unique artifacts in the quantitative reconstructions of the complex-valued permittivity of the breast tissue.

Both the non-linearity and the ill-posedness of the inverse scattering problem become more difficult to deal with for high contrast OIs having such complicated internal structure because they lead to multiple reflections within the OI.

The MWI technique we use in the work reported herein is the Contrast Source Inversion (CSI) method [6–8]. Although this is a state-of-the-art MWI technique it still succumbs to artifacts even when prior information is utilized to try to alleviate the non-linearity and ill-posedness of the problem [9,10]. Note that all MWI techniques, qualitative and quantitative alike, currently have difficulties with imaging artifacts [1,2,5,11].

Recently, there has been intense interest in the use of deep learning techniques in a broad range of applications such as natural language processing, computer vision and speech recognition [12]. In medical imaging, utilizing deep learning techniques for segmentation [13,14], as well as detection and classification [15–17] has been well investigated, at least for the more common modalities. Studies have shown that there is significant potential in applying deep learning techniques for the purpose of removing artifacts from biomedical images generated using some common modalities. Kang et al. proposed a deep Convolutional Neural Networks (CNNs) using directional wavelets for low dose x-ray computed tomography (CT), and results illustrate that a deep CNN using directional wavelets was more efficient in removing low dose-related CT noise [18]. Han et al. [19] and Jin et al. [20] independently proposed multi-scale residual learning networks using U-Net to remove these global streaking artifacts, In addition, domain adaptation from CT to MRI has been successfully demonstrated [21].

MWI researchers are also trying to use machine learning techniques to improve the performance of microwave imaging. For instance, researchers combined a neural network with microwave imaging to learn the forward model for a complex data-acquisition system [22]. Rekanos et al. proposed radial basis function neural network to estimate the position and size of proliferated marrow inside bone tissue with microwave imaging [23]. Le et al. tried to take the benefit of a deep neural network to enhance the constructed images [24]. Their deep neural network was trained to take microwave images created using the back-projection (BP) method as an input and have the network output a much-improved image. In fact, they tried to by-pass the use of iterative techniques for solving the full nonlinear electromagnetic inverse problem. Most recently, we have investigated utilizing deep learning techniques to improve 2D microwave imaging for the breast imaging application [25]. Researchers employing radar-based techniques have also been investigating machine learning approaches for the detection of breast lesions [26].

In this paper, we utilize a deep learning technique, based on CNNs, to enhance full 3D MWI reconstructions obtained using a 3D CSI algorithm that uses the Finite Element Method (FEM) to solve the electromagnetic forward problem [27]. The enhancement removes reconstruction artifacts and improves the accuracy of the resulting images. We utilize a 3D 10-channel U-Net architecture for the CNN where the input and output are both 3D images, and each channel corresponds to the real and imaginary parts of the complex-valued permittivity images created using five different microwave frequencies.

In Section 2 we start by providing a brief description of the CSI-based methodology that we use, as well as the numerical phantoms and MWI parameters utilized to generate training images. We also provide details of our chosen deep learning approach. In Section 3 we describe the training data set as well as the parameters used for the network training. In the following, quantitative assessment and assessment of robustness for numerical experiments are described. Section 4 provides a brief description of our experimental setup and also the result of trained CNN for the experimental data. Finally, in Section 5 we give our conclusion and explain our future work.

2. 3D CSI-Deep-Learning Methodology

In microwave data acquisition processes, electromagnetic fields scatter from, and propagate through, the tissue in a three-dimensional (3D) space. However, to accelerate the image reconstruction process and reduce the computational complexity, researchers are trying to represent electromagnetic waves in 3D space as a simplified 2D model. However, studies have shown that simplifying 3D problems to 2D models can increase the level of artifacts in the recovered dielectric properties [28]. Moreover, in 2D imaging when the object of interest is small, there is a chance that it place between two consecutive imaging slice, then the reconstruction algorithm would not discover the target precisely. Hence, utilizing a viable 3D microwave image reconstruction will enhance the accuracy and quality of reconstruction [29]. While iterative methods have improved dramatically over the years, providing improved resolution and accuracy of the reconstructed properties, as well as more efficient implementations, there are still many fundamental trade-offs between these three aspects due to operational, financial, and physical constraints.

Lower resolution in comparison with other modalities, as well as the many reconstruction artifacts that are related to the nonlinearity and ill-posedness of the associated inverse problem, are the main reasons that MWI is not clinically accepted yet. Although it has been shown that using accurate prior information will reduce the Root-Mean-Squared (RMS) reconstruction error over the whole image [9,10,30–32], artifacts and reconstruction errors near the tumor can translate to poor tumor detection results [33].

2.1. Microwave Imaging via Contrast Source Inversion

The first part of the proposed 3D CSI-Deep-Learning methodology consists of quantitatively generating the complex-valued permittivity images using a MWI technique. Quantitative MWI requires that one solve a non-linear ill-posed inverse scattering problem. A plethora of algorithms have been developed during the past 40 years to solve this problem. They generally involve computationally expensive iterative methods to locally minimize a specially designed functional that incorporates a numerical inversion model approximating the relevant electromagnetic phenomena of the problem [5,11]. In the past, different MWI techniques have utilized tailored optimization algorithms with various functionals. Some of the most prominent techniques have been the Distorted Born Iterative Method [34], Gauss–Newton Inversion [35], the Levenberg–Marquardt method [36] and the Contrast Source Inversion technique [6]. Innovations on these foundational algorithms have allowed improvements to the obtainable imaging accuracy and resolution, especially in the area of breast imaging, e.g., [37,38]. Being an ill-posed problem, regularization techniques are required to solve the inverse scattering problem [39,40].

As previously mentioned, to solve the electromagnetic inverse scattering problem associated with microwave breast imaging we employ the CSI method. The numerical inversion model utilized within the CSI algorithm is based on a full-vectorial 3D electromagnetic model of the MWI system that includes a quasi-resonant flat-faceted chamber [41,42]. The 3D FEM-CSI algorithm is utilized with prior information in the form of an inhomogeneous background as was done in [27]. Breast images reconstructed from both synthetic and experimental scattered-field data are utilized in this work. The experimental data is collected using the same air-based quasi-resonant imaging chamber described in [27]. Thus, the forward model for creating the synthetic data and the inversion model, both utilize a 3D finite element model of the same imaging chamber.

We consider both synthetic and actual experimental breast phantoms with three tissue types: fat, fibroglandular and tumor. These breast phantoms are formed using a simple outer fat layer, and an interior fibroglandular region that contains one or more embedded tumors. The breast phantoms are positioned within the chamber as depicted in Figure 1.

The phantoms are interrogated using microwave energy with magnetic-field probes located on the conductive chamber walls. The same probes are used as those in receivers. As described in [42], the 24 transmitters and receivers are ϕ-polarized. Data were collected at single frequencies and for every transmitter, 23 magnetic fields were recorded at the receiver locations. Thus, 552 complex numbers (magnitude and phase) were utilized to reconstruct the breast phantom that was located within the chamber. That is, the real and imaginary parts of the complex permittivity of the breast phantom were reconstructed using the CSI algorithm.

The forward data were obtained using a 3D-FEM electromagnetic field solver. Before inverting the data using the FEM-CSI algorithm, we added 5 % noise as is usual in creating synthetic data [8]. This procedure was performed at individual frequencies and for the work considered herein, the frequency band of 1.1 GHz to 1.5 GHz was used. It has been shown that reconstruction artifacts appear at different locations of the imaging domain when different frequencies are used, whereas the tumor is typically reconstructed at approximately the same location [27]. In that work, it was shown that this feature can improve the tumor detection by using the intersection of thresholded images.

For the synthetically generated data and inversions, the permittivity was assumed to be constant over frequency. The complex permittivity values that were used are given in Table 1. For the experimental test case considered herein, the permittivities of the utilized tissue-mimicking liquids do vary with frequency (see [27] for details).

Table 1. Complex permittivity for different tissues.

	Permittivity		
Air	Fat	Fibroglandular	Tumor
$1 - 0.001j$	$3 - 0.6j$	$20 - 21.6j$	$56.3 - 30j$

It has been shown that successful CSI reconstructions can be obtained if one introduces a fat and fibroglandular region as prior information in the CSI algorithm. This prior information is in the form of an inhomogeneous numerical background against which the contrast is defined. That is, if $\epsilon_n(r)$ and $\epsilon(r)$ represent the background information and the desired complex permittivity, as functions of position, then the contrast $\chi(r) = (\epsilon(r) - \epsilon_n(r))/\epsilon_n(r)$ is one of the variables solved for in the CSI algorithm (the other variable being the contrast sources generated for each transmitter). Full details of the CSI algorithm, used in this way, are provided in [9,10].

Introducing an inhomogeneous background in this way is a form of regularizing the inverse problem, but as was already mentioned, various reconstruction artifacts are still present in the CSI-reconstructed images. These artifacts increase the false-positive and reduce the true-positive tumor detection rates. For the case of 2D imaging, it was recently shown that using a deep-learning technique ameliorates this problem [25]. This has motivated the interest in using a similar deep-learning technique to improve 3D MWI. However, in addition to artifacts, 3D MWI also suffers from the problem of producing reconstructions that do not reach the maximum permittivity values of the true phantom model. This was noted in [27] and therefore the detection threshold was based on 85% of the maximum reconstructed value. Fortunately, the tumor permittivity values are at the extreme end of the scale, so such a procedure is successful. Improving the CSI reconstructions by correcting the reconstructed permittivity values, in addition to removing artifacts is the sought after goal of using a deep learning technique.

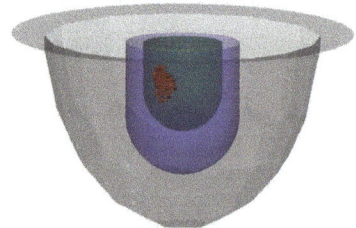

Figure 1. Simulated Breast Model. Gray, blue, green, and red regions represent air, fat, fibroglandular, and tumor, respectively.

2.2. Machine Learning Approach to Reconstruction

Combining the CSI technique with a deep learning approach is accomplished by learning a data-driven mapping, $\mathcal{G}$, from a CSI reconstruction to the true permittivity ($\mathcal{G} : \epsilon^{CSI} \to \epsilon^{true}$).

In this study, we learn a mapping from the real and imaginary parts of the permittivities in CSI reconstructions at several frequencies to a single real permittivity image. Thus, if the CSI complex permittivity map is an $L \times M \times N$ 3D image, and reconstructions at five frequencies are utilized, then each of the learned functions maps $5 \times L \times M \times N$ complex domain to $L \times M \times N$ real domain (e.g., $\mathcal{G}_R : \mathbb{C}^{5 \times L \times M \times N} \mapsto \mathbb{R}^{L \times M \times N}$). The complex output of CSI at the five selected frequencies can be treated as a 10-channel image. We realized this mapping through a deep neural network as follows.

The desired mapping for our task at hand is an image-to-image transformation; there are multiple neural architectures that can implement this mapping. For instance, a naive choice could be a fully-connected single layer neural network which takes in CSI reconstruction as input and is trained to output the ground truth permittivity. However, such an architecture would be very prone to overfitting [12]. We, therefore, use a hierarchical convolutional neural network for our image-to-image transformation task. A good template for such a task is the U-Net architecture which is one of the most successful deep neural networks for image segmentation and reconstruction problems [13]. The architecture consists of successive convolutional and downsampling layers, followed by successive deconvolutional and upsampling layers. Moreover, the skip connections between the corresponding contractive and expansive layers keep the gradients from vanishing that helps in the optimization process [13,43]. To use a U-Net for reconstruction, the original objective of the U-Net is replaced with the sum of pixelwise squared reconstruction errors between the true real part of permittivity and the output of U-Net [13]. In our problem, the network input is the 3D CSI reconstructed complex images (after 500 iterations). Thus, there are two options for choosing the U-Net architecture, U-Net with complex weights and U-Net with real weights. Very few studies have been done on the training of U-Net with complex weights, although very recently Trabelsi et al. tried to train the neural network with complex weights for convolutional architectures [44]. In this paper, we decided to use a U-Net architecture having real-valued weights. A schematic representation of our architecture is shown in Figure 2. The motivation for choosing the neural network parameters (the number of convolutional layers, size and number of filters) is as follows. In a hierarchical multi-scale CNN, the effective receptive field of the convolution filters is variable at each layer, i.e., through successive sub-sampling it is possible to have a larger receptive field even by using filters of smaller kernel size [12,45]. As mentioned above, the input to our neural network is $L \times M \times N \times 10$; in particular, for each frequency, the dimension of our input image volume is $64 \times 64 \times 64$ (i.e., $L = M = N = 64$). If we start with a 3D receptive field of $3 \times 3 \times 3$, after four layers of successive convolutions and subsampling (by a factor of $1/2$), the receptive field would effectively span the entire image volume. We, therefore, use four convolutional layers with a 3D filter kernel size of $3 \times 3 \times 3$. Since after each convolutional layer the size of the image volume is reduced, we can increase the number of filters at each successive layer to enhance the representational power of the neural network [12]. In particular, we start with 32 filters for the first layer and successively double the number of filters after each layer (number of filters after the fourth layer is 512). This defines the encoder part of the U-net i.e., the part of a neural network consisting of contractive convolutions. For the decoder part, we follow a symmetric architecture consisting of expansive convolutions [13].

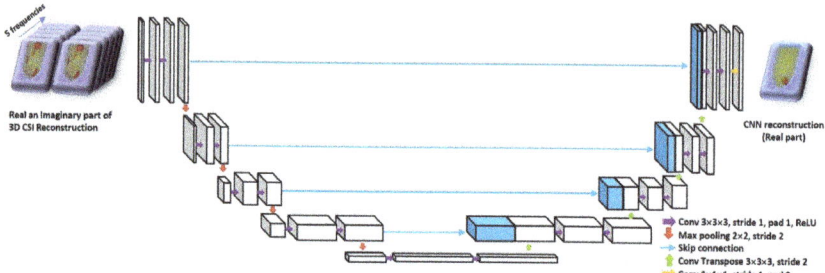

Figure 2. Schematic for the proposed U-Net to reconstruct the real part of permittivity. The input to the network is the 3D Contrast-Source Inversion (CSI) reconstruction, and the network is trained to output the corresponding true 3D permittivity map.

3. Numerical Experiments

3.1. Datasets

While we tested our neural network on both experimental and synthetic data, for training we only used a synthetically generated dataset. The training dataset consisted of 600 numerical breast phantoms; tumors were randomly generated within the fibroglandular region of the phantom. Starting from a random initial position, tumor pixels were grown randomly until the maximum diameter reached a threshold. To have variability in the dataset, the threshold for the maximum diameter was also randomly sampled from the range: 1.1–1.5 cm. One half the dataset consisted of breast phantoms with one tumor, while the other half had phantoms with two tumors. We then employed a forward solver [8] to generate the scattered field data corresponding to the phantoms. CSI reconstructions were performed at five frequencies: 1.1, 1.2, 1.3, 1.4, and 1.5 GHz. These CSI reconstructions together with the corresponding ground-truth permittivity values for the phantoms formed our training data for the U-Net input and output respectively.

3.2. Network Training

All the CNNs were implemented using Python 3.6 and Keras 2.0.6 with Tensorflow backend. We used a Windows 10 computer with a Tesla P100-PCIE-12GB graphic processor and Intel(R) CPU(3.50 GHz). We used the popular Xavier initialization for the convolutional layer weights to obtain an appropriate scale [46]. We trained with a batch size of 10, for 200 epochs with Adam optimization. Four-fold cross-validation strategy has been utilized to evaluate the proposed deep neural network for all experiments. The U-net wastrained using the real and imaginary parts for five different frequencies as inputs. With 600 phantoms in our dataset, each fold in four-fold cross-validation consisted of 150 examples. For every fold, training was done using 450 cases, while the testing set consisted of the held-out 150 examples. Thus all 600 cases featured as test examples when they were not part of the training set. For the loss function, we use pixel wise mean squared error between the ground truth 3D image and the CNN 3D reconstructed image as follows:

$$RMSError = \frac{1}{LMN} \sum_{x=1}^{L} \sum_{y=1}^{M} \sum_{z=1}^{N} (I_{x,y,z}^{GT} - I_{x,y,z}^{CNN})^2 \qquad (1)$$

where $I_{x,y,z}^{CNN}$ represents a 3D image reconstructed by the CNN and $I_{x,y,z}^{GT}$ represents a 3D ground truth image.

3.3. Quantitative Assessment

The CNN-enhanced reconstruction performance and the subsequent tumor segmentation based on thresholding was evaluated quantitatively. The Root Mean Squared (RMS) reconstruction error between the network output and the true permittivity values was used to evaluate the reconstruction quality. The performance of a detection algorithm is often assessed in terms of two types of error i.e., False Positive Rate (FPR) and False Negative Rate (FNR). FPR and FNR will vary depending on the decision threshold used on the output score of the detection algorithm. To quantify the ability of the output score to separate the two classes, we need to analyze the two errors for all possible thresholds. In particular, we performed Receiver Operating Characteristics (ROC) analysis to assess the ability of the reconstructed complex permittivity to distinguish between tumor and non-tumor pixels. The ROC curve is a plot of True Positive Rate ($TPR = \frac{TP}{TP+FN}$) against the False Positive Rate ($FPR = \frac{FP}{FP+TN}$) for all thresholds. The Area Under the Curve (AUC) for the ROC is a metric quantifying the separability between tumor and non-tumor pixels [47]. For comparison we also computed RMS reconstruction error and performed ROC analysis on CSI-only reconstructions. ROC carries information about the relation of the true positives vs. the false positives. However, the information about the distributions of thresholds at which the different ratios fall would be lost in this curve. Therefore, the distance from any location on the ROC curve to the top-left corner of the plot is also an informative metric (we call this the "Distance-to-MaxTD" or "DMTD" plot). We use the DMTD curve as a complementary metric to display/analyze the relation between the true positive detection as well as the threshold at which a certain true positive to negative ratio happens. This will especially help us better understand the performance of the overlapping (or very similar) ROC curves for different scenarios. The depth of the curve tells us about the quality of the reconstruction; the lower the dip, the better the performance of the algorithm. The location of the dip carries information about the separation of the tumor relative to the background; for instance, the further the dip of the DMTD curve is to the left, the higher the separation between the background and tumor. Additionally, the width of the dip gives us information about the robustness of the algorithm; the wider the dip of the curve, the higher the chances of having a tumor with no artifacts (false positives) for the proper reconstruction of the tumor size and shape. The results of this quantitative evaluation by using four-fold cross-validation strategy for all 600 images are shown in Figure 3 and Table 2.

Figure 4 illustrates the performance of the trained U-Net in comparison with CSI reconstruction for an arbitrary example with two tumors. Based on the AUC and RMS error metrics, it could be concluded that the proposed CNN is successful in term of reconstruction and tumor detection. However, in a previous study [27], it was shown that taking the intersection of multi-frequency thresholded 3D images performs the best at detecting tumors. Therefore, we compared our trained CNN with the intersection of multi-frequency thresholded 3D images in terms of detection. The superiority of the trained CNN to CSI results as well as to multi-frequency thresholded results are shown in Figure 3. For this same example, the CSI reconstructions at the remaining four other frequencies are shown in Figure 5. The resulting images for the real and imaginary parts of the permittivity after taking the intersection of the reconstructions that were thresholded at 85% of the maximum reconstructed permittivity value are also shown in the figure. Note that results using a CNN trained to reconstruct the imaginary part of the complex permittivity (not shown) are very similar to those using the CNN trained to reconstruct the real part in terms of tumor detection (ROC Curve) and reconstruction performance (RMS error). Thus, the ROC curve in Figure 3 and RMS error in Table 2, were computed using only reconstructions of the real part of the permittivity.

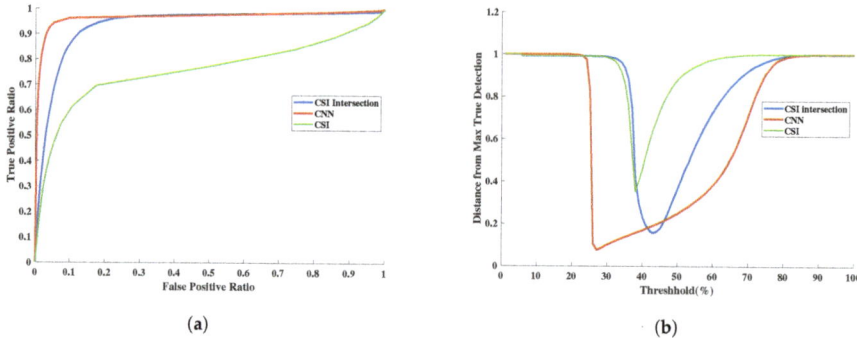

Figure 3. The detection performance using the reconstructed outputs of the Convolutional Neural Network (CNN) and CSI as well as the intersection of CSI reconstructions at the five chosen frequencies. (**a**) Receiver Operating Characteristics (ROC) curves derived from the reconstructions. (**b**) The DMTD curve.

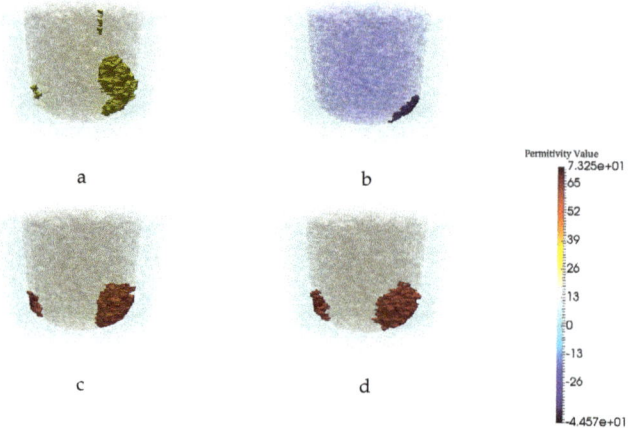

Figure 4. Reconstruction results for a particular example with two tumors. The real (**a**) and imaginary (**b**) part of CSI reconstruction at 1.1 GHz. (**c**) CNN reconstruction. (**d**) Ground truth.

Table 2. Comparison of reconstruction and tumor detection performance.

	RMS Error		AUC	
	CSI	CNN	CSI	CNN
Synthetic Data	1.4356	1.161	0.935	0.957
Exprimental Data	1.250	1.172	0.794	0.938

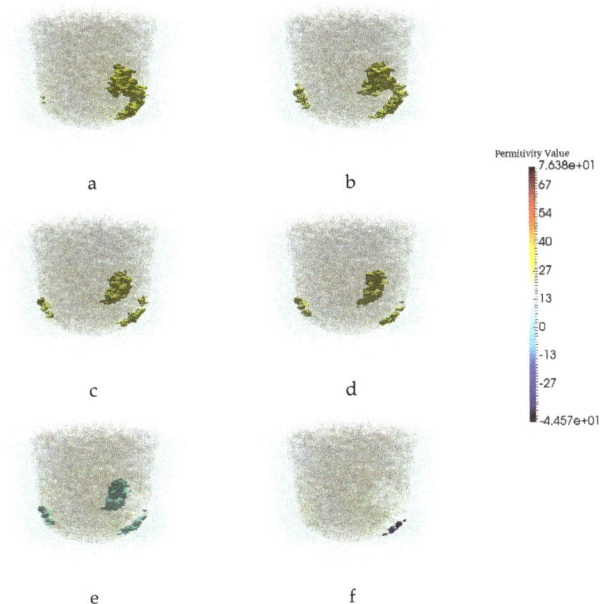

Figure 5. CSI reconstructions at four remaining frequencies for the same example as in Figure 4 and resulting images after intersecting images thresholded at 85% of the maximum reconstructed permittivity. (**a**–**d**) The real part of CSI reconstructions at 1.2, 1.3, 1.4, and 1.5 GHz. (**e**) Intersection of real part of CSI reconstructions. (**f**) Intersection of imaginary part of CSI reconstructions.

3.4. Assessment of Robustness

It is important to assess the robustness of our trained neural network when being tested on images different from those used during training. We investigate four aspects of variation in test data as compared to the training data: (i) changes in frequencies used to generate CSI reconstructions, (ii) changes in breast phantom geometry, (iii) changes in prior-information, and (v) breast phantom with no tumor.

3.4.1. Robustness to Changes in Frequency

First, given that the CNN was trained utilizing images created at 1.1 GHz, 1.2, 1.3, 1.4, and 1.5 GHz, the performance of the trained network was checked qualitatively by testing with CSI reconstructions that were created using data obtained at five arbitrarily chosen frequencies: 1.05, 1.15, 1.25, 1.35 and 1.45 GHz. Therefore, CSI reconstructions at chosen frequencies for five different breast phantoms have been created. These tests indicated that the trained U-Net was indeed superior to the CSI-only case. Results for one test example of the CSI and CNN outputs, from data obtained at 1.05 GHz, are shown in Figure 6. This suggests that the CNN is robust to testing images reconstructed using frequencies in the same bandwidth as used for training (one does not have to rely on using the exact same frequencies). As will be seen shortly, however, this is not the case once much higher frequencies are used.

3.4.2. Robustness to Changes in Breast Phantom Geometry

The next test for the network's robustess is to check against geometric changes of the breast phantom model. Thus, a new model which has the same dimensions for the fat region but has a smaller fibroglandular region (the height of fibroglandular region is decreased by 0.9 cm) was generated. By using this new small model, five different breast phantoms with a random tumor have been generated to evaluate the trained CNN. Figure 7 demonstrates the performance of the trained CNN for a particular example when the input images were CSI reconstructed images for this new model. As can be seen, the CNN significantly alters the CSI reconstructions (row 1) to bring them closer to the ground truth (row 2).

3.4.3. Robustness to Imperfections in Prior Information

In order to understand the U-Net's ability to remove artifacts, the next test case artificially induces artifacts into the CSI reconstructions by utilizing incorrect, or imperfect, prior information. Clearly, using perfect prior information results in very good CSI reconstructions; however, perfect prior information regarding the structural shape of the fibroglandular region as well as the permittivity of the fibroglandular tissue is difficult to obtain in practical circumstances. It is well known that using CSI with imperfect prior information produces various reconstruction artifacts. To evaluate this aspect of robustness we introduced 10% error in the permittivity of the fibroglandular tissue used as prior information. Figure 8 shows the performance of the CNN when tested with CSI reconstructions using imperfect permittivity in a structurally perfect fibroglandular region. The ROC curves created from the CSI and CNN outputs corresponding to this case shown in the plots of Figure 9. From the green colored curves we see that the CNN-enhanced reconstructions do provide an improvement over the CSI reconstructions. The distance-to-maxTD curve in Figure 9 clearly shows that the range in the threshold that could be used for good detection for the CNN-enhanced reconstructions is much wider than that could be used for the CSI reconstructions. When imperfect structural prior was used for a test case it was found that neither the CSI nor the CNN reconstructions performed well. This is the last test performed using synthetically generated images.

3.4.4. Robustness to Breast Phantom with No Tumor

Lastly, given that the CNN was trained only on breast phantom in presence of tumor, the last test in this section has been done to check the performance of the trained CNN for breast phantom with no tumor. Note that to prevent having zero scattered field data, we have to use imperfect prior information. We introduced 5% error in the permittivity of the fibroglandular tissue used as prior information. Figure 10 demonstrates the performance of the trained network when the input images were CSI reconstructed images with no tumor.

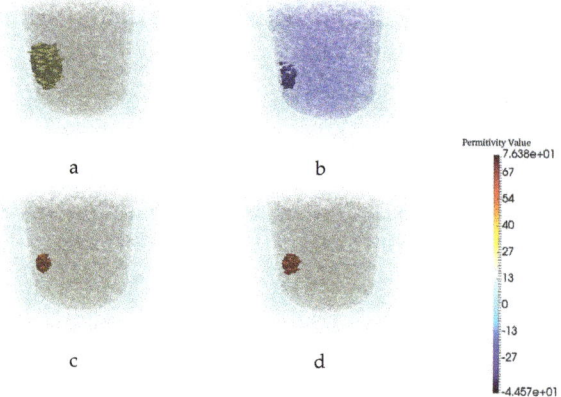

Figure 6. Reconstruction results for a particular example with one tumor at 1.05 GHz. The real (**a**) and imaginary (**b**) part of CSI reconstruction. (**c**) CNN reconstruction. (**d**) Ground truth.

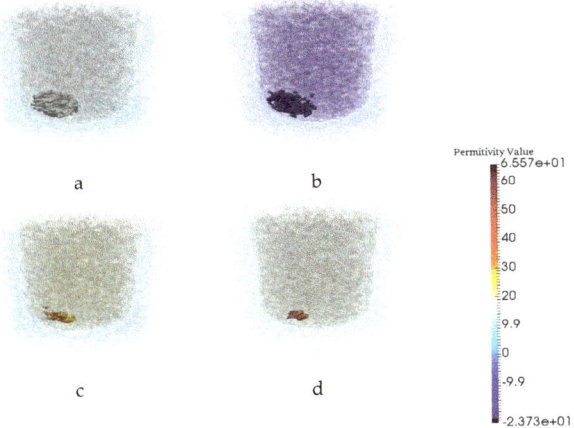

Figure 7. Reconstruction results for a particular example when the test images are CSI results for a breast phantom having a smaller fibroglandular region than those of the training set. The (**a**) real and (**b**) imaginary parts of the CSI reconstructions. (**c**) CNN reconstruction. (**d**) Ground truth.

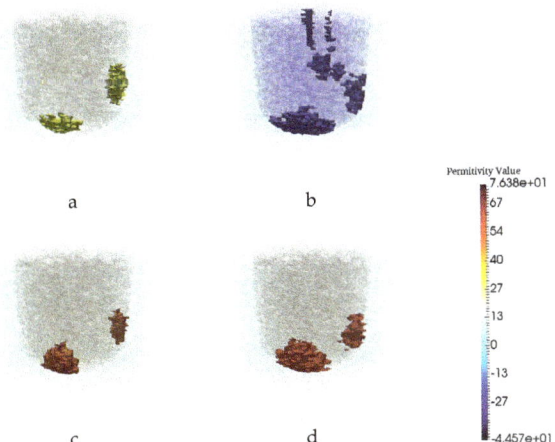

Figure 8. Reconstruction results for a particular example with two tumor when the training images are CSI results with perfect prior information, but the neural net was tested on imperfect prior information. The real (**a**) and imaginary (**b**) part of CSI reconstruction. (**c**) CNN reconstruction. (**d**) Ground truth.

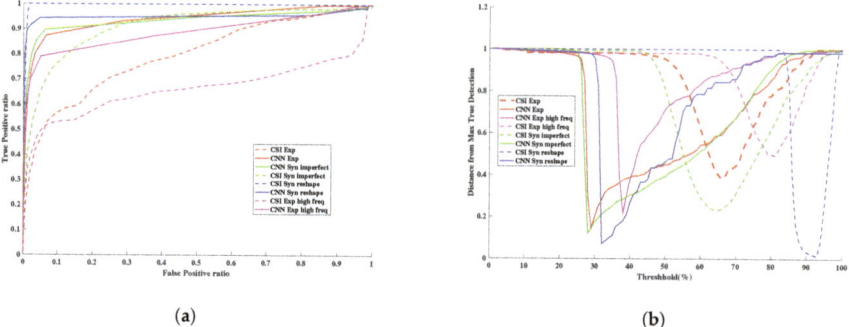

(a) (b)

Figure 9. Detection performance based on the reconstructed outputs of CNN and CSI. (**a**) ROC curves derived from the reconstructed real part of the permittivity from CSI and CNN. (**b**) The DMTD. test cases are: synthetic: imperfect permittivity prior, and true breast phantom with elongated fibroglandular region. Experimental: using data within the frequency band and much higher than the training frequency band.

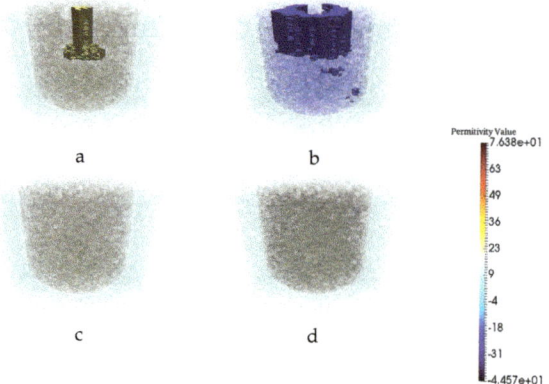

Figure 10. Reconstruction results for a particular example when the training images are CSI results with one or two tumors but the neural net was tested on a phantom with no tumor. The real (**a**) and imaginary (**b**) part of CSI reconstruction. (**c**) CNN reconstruction. (**d**) Ground truth.

4. Experimental Tests and Results

The experimental setup described in [27,42] was used to collect data to test the described neural network. A depiction of the imaging chamber and the breast phantom used in the experiment is shown in Figure 11. This chamber has 44 facets and contains 24 magnetic field probes and the breast phantom used in the chamber has three regions with similar sizes and properties to those of the numerical breast phantom described earlier for the fat and fibro regions; a 2 cm spherical phantom was used as the tumor region with properties similar to that of the tumor described in the numerical test cases. To mimic the properties close to those of a realistic breast, the fat region was filled with canola oil while a 20:80 ratio of water to glycerin is used to fill the fibroglanduar shell, and a 10:90 ratio of water to glycerin is used to fill the spherical inclusion representing a tumor. For these ratios, the permittivities of the canola oil and water/glycerin mixture are measured as $3.0 - j0.193$, $23.3 - j18.1$ and $50 - j25$ respectively for fat, fibrogladular, and tumor at 1.1 GHz [27]. It is worth noting that this simplistic phantom is used as a simple proof of concept target for inverting a high contrast multilayered medium in an air background and not testing the system against realistic breast phantoms.

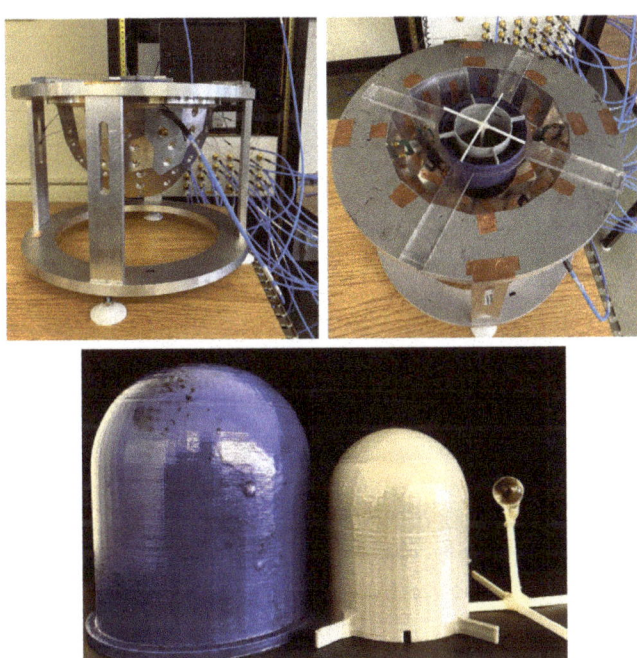

Figure 11. The experimental system including the three region breast phantom (Diameter of fat, fibroglanduar and tumor regions are 10 , 8 and 2 CM respectively).

In medical imaging, sometimes it is difficult to build a large experimental training data set. Therefore, it is desirable that a neural network trained on synthetic data generalizes well when tested on experimental data. To investigate this, we collected experimental data using a wide range of frequencies (1.1 to 2.9 GHz). The performance of the trained network for experimental data is evaluated and shown in Figure 12. Results illustrate that trained CNN improved the experimental CSI reconstructed images when frequencies similar or close to those for training data were used. However, when we tested the trained CNN with experimental images created with frequencies well beyond the band of frequencies used to create the training data, it is observed that CNN is not able to detect the tumor. Figure 13. One reason for this can be the significant change in the nature of the artifacts. In general, for the results presented in this manuscript, the artifacts at almost all lower frequency reconstructions have a lower permittivity compared to the value of the reconstructed tumor. However, the permittivities of the reconstructed artifacts at higher frequencies are higher than those of the reconstructed tumor.

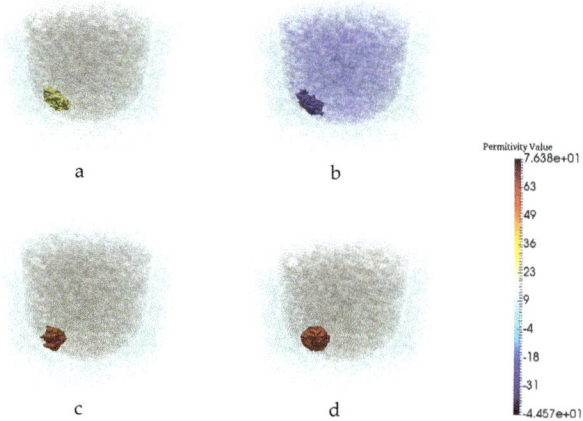

Figure 12. CNN performance for experimental result when the neural net was trained on Synthetic data. The real (**a**) and imaginary (**b**) part of CSI reconstruction. (**c**) CNN reconstruction. (**d**) Ground truth.

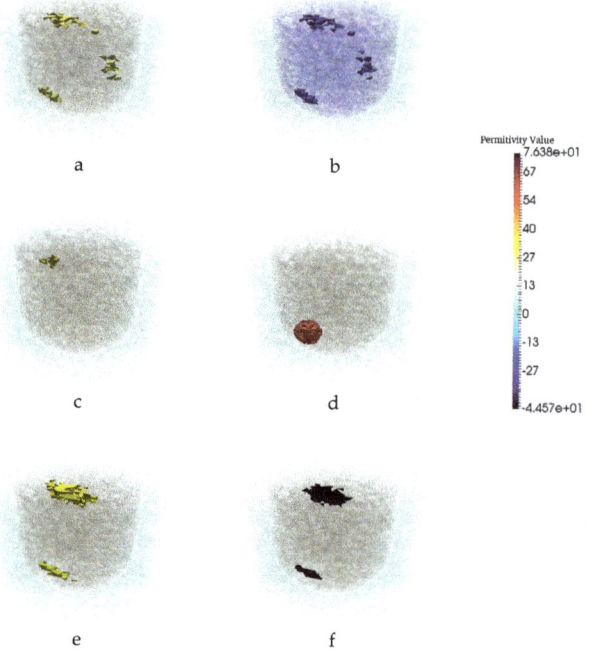

Figure 13. Reconstruction results for a particular example when the test images are CSI results in high frequencies but the neural net was trained on low frequencies. The real (**a**) and imaginary (**b**) part of CSI reconstruction. (**c**) CNN reconstruction. (**d**) Ground truth. (**e**) Intersection of real part of CSI reconstruction at all frequencies.(**f**) Intersection of imaginary part of CSI reconstruction at all frequencies(two intersection images are binary image).

5. Conclusions

A deep learning technique using a 3D CNN was developed to improve the imaging performance of 3D MWI of the breast. The improvement manifests as the removal of artifacts in the 3D reconstructions of the complex-valued permittivity of the breast being imaged. These reconstruction artifacts are specific to the MWI system wherein the microwave scattered-field data is collected as well as to the numerical inversion algorithm, in our case CSI, being used to create the images. Using synthetic 3D images that take both these factors into account, a CNN was trained with the goal to reproduce the true permittivity image of the breast from the artifact-laden 3D reconstructions. The trained CNN was tested with synthetic images as well as with images created using experimentally obtained microwave scattered-field data from an MWI system: the same MWI system for which a numerical model was utilized in the creation of the synthetic 3D images.

The RMS error between the CNN-reconstructed images and the true images are improved over the corresponding error between the CSI-only reconstructions and the true images. In addition, tumor detection was evaluated using ROC-AUC metrics and these are much improved for the CNN-reconstructed images over the ROC-AUC results for the CSI-only reconstructions. The results show that this deep learning technique has the ability to improve 3D CSI reconstructions in three interdependent ways. First, and foremost, the CNN has shown its ability to remove reconstruction artifacts which are a great challenge for quantitative MWI. Secondly, the trained CNN successfully corrects the permittivity values which tend to be undershot in the CSI reconstructions. Finally, from a qualitative perspective, the tumor location is more accurately reconstructed with respect to its true position and size.

There are several limitations of this work, but the most critical is that numerical phantoms with a single, relatively simple, fibroglandular region were utilized for training and testing. This same region was reproduced in the physical phantom utilized for the experimental results. Our experience with utilizing a similar technique with 2D images showed that this limitation can be removed by training with breast models having several types of fibroglandular regions. Similarly, this work has shown that when the artifacts are due to reconstructions obtained from data generated with MWI system parameters that were not utilized in the training set, for example artifacts generated by using microwave frequencies that are much higher than what the MWI system was designed for, then the trained CNN was not able to identify these as artifacts. In fact, some of these artifacts were identified as tumors. This result limits the robustness of the trained CNN but this study has provided a good understanding of that robustness. We further note that due to the significant level of computational resources required during the generation of forward data and inverse 3D CSI reconstructions, we generated only a moderately sized dataset consisting of 600 phantoms. Being aware of the limited number of training examples, we made extensive use of cross-validation and regularization techniques to avoid the possibility of model overfitting, which is evidenced by the generalization our CNN demonstrates on unseen examples. That said, having more training data would potentially help us to train a more robust CNN with better generalization properties. Techniques for overcoming some of these limitations will be investigated in planned future work.

Author Contributions: All four authors (V.K., M.A., A.A., J.L.) contributed to Methodology, Validation, Investigation, Writing (review and editing). V.K. and J.L. have contributed to Writing (original draft preparation), Conceptualization and Resources. J.L. contributed to Project administration and Supervision. V.K. contributed to Software and Visualization. All authors have read and agreed to the published version of the manuscript.

Funding: This research was funded by the Natural Sciences and Engineering Research Council (NSERC) and the Canadian Cancer Society, grant number 300028. All authors have read and agreed to the published version of the manuscript.

Conflicts of Interest: The authors declare no conflict of interest.

References

1. O'Loughlin, D.; O'Halloran, M.J.; Moloney, B.M.; Glavin, M.; Jones, E.; Elahi, M.A. Microwave Breast Imaging: Clinical Advances and Remaining Challenges. *IEEE Trans. Biomed. Eng.* **2018**, *65*, 2580–2590. [CrossRef]
2. Bolomey, J.C. Crossed Viewpoints on Microwave-Based Imaging for Medical Diagnosis: From Genesis to Earliest Clinical Outcomes. In *The World of Applied Electromagnetics: In Appreciation of Magdy Fahmy Iskander*; Lakhtakia, A., Furse, C.M., Eds.; Springer International Publishing: Cham, Switzerland, 2018; pp. 369–414.
3. Lazebnik, M.; Popovic, D.; McCartney, L.; Watkins, C.B.; Lindstrom, M.J.; Harter, J.; Sewall, S.; Ogilvie, T.; Magliocco, A.; Breslin, T.M.; et al. A large-scale study of the ultrawideband microwave dielectric properties of normal, benign and malignant breast tissues obtained from cancer surgeries. *Phys. Med. Biol.* **2007**, *52*, 6093. [CrossRef]
4. Halter, R.J.; Zhou, T.; Meaney, P.M.; Hartov, A.; Barth, R.J., Jr.; Rosenkranz, K.M.; Wells, W.A.; Kogel, C.A.; Borsic, A.; Rizzo, E.J.; et al. The correlation of in vivo and ex vivo tissue dielectric properties to validate electromagnetic breast imaging: Initial clinical experience. *Physiol. Meas.* **2009**, *30*, S121. [CrossRef]
5. Pastorino, M. *Microwave Imaging*; John Wiley & Sons: Hoboken, NJ, USA, 2010.
6. Van den Berg, P.M.; Kleinman, R.E. A contrast source inversion method. *Inverse Probl.* **1997**, *13*, 1607–1620. [CrossRef]
7. Abubakar, A.; van den Berg, P.M.; Mallorqui, J.J. Imaging of biomedical data using a multiplicative regularized contrast source inversion method. *IEEE Trans. Microw. Theory Tech.* **2002**, *50*, 1761–1771. [CrossRef]
8. Zakaria, A.; Gilmore, C.; LoVetri, J. Finite-element contrast source inversion method for microwave imaging. *Inverse Probl.* **2010**, *26*, 115010. [CrossRef]
9. Kurrant, D.; Baran, A.; LoVetri, J.; Fear, E. Integrating prior information into microwave tomography Part 1: Impact of detail on image quality. *Med. Phys.* **2017**, *44*, 6461–6481. [CrossRef] [PubMed]
10. Baran, A.; Kurrant, D.; Fear, E.; LoVetri, J. Integrating prior information into microwave tomography part 2: Impact of errors in prior information on microwave tomography image quality. *Med. Phys.* **2017**, *44*, 6482–6503.
11. Chen, X. *Computational Methods for Electromagnetic Inverse Scattering*; Wiley Online Library: Hoboken, NJ, USA, 2018.
12. Goodfellow, I.; Bengio, Y.; Courville, A. *Deep Learning*; MIT Press: Cambridge, MA, USA, 2016; Available online: http://www.deeplearningbook.org (accessed on 10 August 2020).
13. Ronneberger, O.; Fischer, P.; Brox, T. U-Net: Convolutional Networks for Biomedical Image Segmentation. *arXiv* **2015**, arXiv:1505.04597.
14. Wang, G.; Li, W.; Zuluaga, M.A.; Pratt, R.; Patel, P.A.; Aertsen, M.; Doel, T.; David, A.L.; Deprest, J.; Ourselin, S.; et al. Interactive Medical Image Segmentation Using Deep Learning With Image-Specific Fine Tuning. *IEEE Trans. Med. Imaging* **2018**, *37*, 1562–1573. [CrossRef]
15. Shin, H.; Roth, H.R.; Gao, M.; Lu, L.; Xu, Z.; Nogues, I.; Yao, J.; Mollura, D.; Summers, R.M. Deep Convolutional Neural Networks for Computer-Aided Detection: CNN Architectures, Dataset Characteristics and Transfer Learning. *IEEE Trans. Med Imaging* **2016**, *35*, 1285–1298. [CrossRef]
16. McCann, M.T.; Jin, K.H.; Unser, M. Convolutional Neural Networks for Inverse Problems in Imaging: A Review. *IEEE Signal Process. Mag.* **2017**, *34*, 85–95. [CrossRef]
17. Xie, Y.; Xia, Y.; Zhang, J.; Song, Y.; Feng, D.; Fulham, M.; Cai, W. Knowledge-based Collaborative Deep Learning for Benign-Malignant Lung Nodule Classification on Chest CT. *IEEE Trans. Med. Imaging* **2019**, *38*, 991–1004. [CrossRef] [PubMed]
18. Kang, E.; Min, J.; Ye, J.C. A deep convolutional neural network using directional wavelets for low-dose X-ray CT reconstruction. *Med. Phys.* **2017**, *44*, e360–e375. [CrossRef] [PubMed]
19. Han, Y.; Yoo, J.J.; Ye, J.C. Deep Residual Learning for Compressed Sensing CT Reconstruction via Persistent Homology Analysis. *arXiv* **2016**, arXiv:1611.06391.
20. Jin, K.H.; McCann, M.T.; Froustey, E.; Unser, M. Deep Convolutional Neural Network for Inverse Problems in Imaging. *IEEE Trans. Image Process.* **2017**, *26*, 4509–4522. [CrossRef]
21. Han, Y.; Yoo, J.; Kim, H.H.; Shin, H.J.; Sung, K.; Ye, J.C. Deep learning with domain adaptation for accelerated projection-reconstruction MR. *Magn. Reson. Med.* **2018**, *80*, 1189–1205. [CrossRef]

22. Rahama, Y.A.; Aryani, O.A.; Din, U.A.; Awar, M.A.; Zakaria, A.; Qaddoumi, N. Novel Microwave Tomography System Using a Phased-Array Antenna. *IEEE Trans. Microw. Theory Tech.* **2018**, *66*, 5119–5128. [CrossRef]
23. Rekanos, I.T. Neural-network-based inverse-scattering technique for online microwave medical imaging. *IEEE Trans. Magn.* **2002**, *38*, 1061–1064. [CrossRef]
24. Li, L.; Wang, L.G.; Teixeira, F.L.; Liu, C.; Nehorai, A.; Cui, T.J. DeepNIS: Deep Neural Network for Nonlinear Electromagnetic Inverse Scattering. *IEEE Trans. Antennas Propag.* **2019**, *67*, 1819–1825. [CrossRef]
25. Khoshdel, V.; Ashraf, A.L.J. Enhancement of Multimodal Microwave-Ultrasound Breast Imaging Using a Deep-Learning Technique. *Sensors* **2019**, *19*, 4050. [CrossRef] [PubMed]
26. Rana, S.P.; Dey, M.; Tiberi, G.; Sani, L.; Vispa, A.; Raspa, G.; Duranti, M.; Ghavami, M.; Dudley, S. Machine learning approaches for automated lesion detection in microwave breast imaging clinical data. *Sci. Rep.* **2019**, *9*, 1–12. [CrossRef] [PubMed]
27. Asefi, M.; Baran, A.; LoVetri, J. An Experimental Phantom Study for Air-Based Quasi-Resonant Microwave Breast Imaging. *IEEE Trans. Microw. Theory Tech.* **2019**, *67*, 3946–3954. [CrossRef]
28. Meaney, P.M.; Paulsen, K.D.; Geimer, S.D.; Haider, S.A.; Fanning, M.W. Quantification of 3-D field effects during 2-D microwave imaging. *IEEE Trans. Biomed. Eng.* **2002**, *49*, 708–720. [CrossRef]
29. Golnabi, A.H.; Meaney, P.M.; Epstein, N.R.; Paulsen, K.D. Microwave imaging for breast cancer detection: Advances in three–dimensional image reconstruction. In Proceedings of the 2011 Annual International Conference of the IEEE Engineering in Medicine and Biology Society, Boston, MA, USA, 30 August–3 September 2011; pp. 5730–5733.
30. Golnabi, A.H.; Meaney, P.M.; Geimer, S.D.; Paulsen, K.D. 3-D Microwave Tomography Using the Soft Prior Regularization Technique: Evaluation in Anatomically Realistic MRI-Derived Numerical Breast Phantoms. *IEEE Trans. Biomed. Eng.* **2019**, *66*, 2566–2575. [CrossRef]
31. Abdollahi, N.; Kurrant, D.; Mojabi, P.; Omer, M.; Fear, E.; LoVetri, J. Incorporation of Ultrasonic Prior Information for Improving Quantitative Microwave Imaging of Breast. *IEEE J. Multiscale Multiphys. Comput. Tech.* **2019**, *4*, 98–110. [CrossRef]
32. Gil Cano, J.D.; Fasoula, A.D.L.; Bernard, J.G. Wavelia Breast Imaging: The Optical Breast Contour Detection Subsystem. *Appl. Sci.* **2020**, *10*, 1234. [CrossRef]
33. Odle, T.G. Breast imaging artifacts. *Radiol. Technol.* **2015**, *89*, 428.
34. Chew, W.C.; Wang, Y.M. Reconstruction of two-dimensional permittivity distribution using the distorted Born iterative method. *IEEE Trans. Med. Imaging* **1990**, *9*, 218–225. [CrossRef]
35. Joachimowicz, N.; Pichot, C.; Hugonin, J.P. Inverse scattering: An iterative numerical method for electromagnetic imaging. *IEEE Trans. Antennas Propag.* **1991**, *39*, 1742–1753. [CrossRef]
36. Franchois, A.; Pichot, C. Microwave imaging-complex permittivity reconstruction with a Levenberg-Marquardt method. *IEEE Trans. Antennas Propag.* **1997**, *45*, 203–215. [CrossRef]
37. Bulyshev, A.; Semenov, S.; Souvorov, A.; Svenson, R.; Nazarov, A.; Sizov, Y.; Tatsis, G. Computational modeling of three-dimensional microwave tomography of breast cancer. *IEEE Trans. Biomed. Eng.* **2001**, *48*, 1053–1056. [CrossRef] [PubMed]
38. Meaney, P.M.; Geimer, S.D.; Paulsen, K.D. Two-step inversion with a logarithmic transformation for microwave breast imaging. *Med. Phys.* **2017**, *44*, 4239–4251. [CrossRef]
39. Mojabi, P.; LoVetri, J. Overview and classification of some regularization techniques for the Gauss-Newton inversion method applied to inverse scattering problems. *IEEE Trans. Antennas Propag.* **2009**, *57*, 2658–2665. [CrossRef]
40. Van den Berg, P.; Abubakar, A.; Fokkema, J. Multiplicative regularization for contrast profile inversion. *Radio Sci.* **2003**, *38*. [CrossRef]
41. Zakaria, A.; Jeffrey, I.; LoVetri, J.; Zakaria, A. Full-Vectorial Parallel Finite-Element Contrast Source Inversion Method. *Prog. Electromagn. Res.* **2013**, *142*, 463–483. [CrossRef]
42. Nemez, K.; Baran, A.; Asefi, M.; LoVetri, J. Modeling Error and Calibration Techniques for a Faceted Metallic Chamber for Magnetic Field Microwave Imaging. *IEEE Trans. Microw. Theory Techn.* **2017**, *65*, 4347–4356. [CrossRef]
43. He, K.; Zhang, X.; Ren, S.; Sun, J. Deep Residual Learning for Image Recognition. In Proceedings of the 2016 IEEE Conference on Computer Vision and Pattern Recognition (CVPR), Las Vegas, NV, USA, 27–30 June 2016; pp. 770–778.

44. Trabelsi, C.; Bilaniuk, O.; Zhang, Y.; Serdyuk, D.; Subramanian, S.; Santos, J.F.; Mehri, S.; Rostamzadeh, N.; Bengio, Y.; Pal, C. Deep Complex Networks. *arXiv* **2018**, arXiv:1705.09792.
45. Krizhevsky, A.; Sutskever, I.; Hinton, G.E. ImageNet Classification with Deep Convolutional Neural Networks. In *Advances in Neural Information Processing Systems 25*; Pereira, F., Burges, C.J.C., Bottou, L., Weinberger, K.Q., Eds.; Curran Associates, Inc.: Red Hook, NY, USA, 2012; pp. 1097–1105.
46. Glorot, X.; Bengio, Y. Understanding the difficulty of training deep feedforward neural networks. In Proceedings of the International Conference on Artificial Intelligence and Statistics (AISTATS'10), Society for Artificial Intelligence and Statistics, Tübingen, Germany, 21–23 April 2010.
47. Hanley, J.; McNeil, B. The meaning and use of the area under a receiver operating characteristic (ROC) curve. *Radiology* **1982**, *43*, 29–36. [CrossRef]

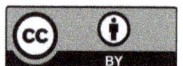

© 2020 by the authors. Licensee MDPI, Basel, Switzerland. This article is an open access article distributed under the terms and conditions of the Creative Commons Attribution (CC BY) license (http://creativecommons.org/licenses/by/4.0/).

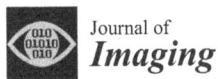

Article

Analyzing Age-Related Macular Degeneration Progression in Patients with Geographic Atrophy Using Joint Autoencoders for Unsupervised Change Detection

Guillaume Dupont [1], Ekaterina Kalinicheva [1], Jérémie Sublime [1,2,*], Florence Rossant [1,*] and Michel Pâques [3]

[1] ISEP, DaSSIP Team, 92130 Issy-Les-Moulineaux, France; guillaume.dupont@isep.fr (G.D.); ekaterina.kalinicheva@isep.fr (E.K.)
[2] Université Paris 13, LIPN - CNRS UMR 7030, 93430 Villetaneuse, France
[3] Clinical Imaging Center 1423, Quinze-Vingts Hospital, INSERM-DGOS Clinical Investigation Center, 75012 Paris, France; mpaques@15-20.fr
* Correspondence: jeremie.sublime@isep.fr or sublime@lipn.univ-paris13.fr (J.S.); florence.rossant@isep.fr (F.R.); Tel.: +33-1-4954-5262 (F.R.)

Received: 6 May 2020; Accepted: 23 June 2020; Published: 29 June 2020

Abstract: Age-Related Macular Degeneration (ARMD) is a progressive eye disease that slowly causes patients to go blind. For several years now, it has been an important research field to try to understand how the disease progresses and find effective medical treatments. Researchers have been mostly interested in studying the evolution of the lesions using different techniques ranging from manual annotation to mathematical models of the disease. However, artificial intelligence for ARMD image analysis has become one of the main research focuses to study the progression of the disease, as accurate manual annotation of its evolution has proved difficult using traditional methods even for experienced practitioners. In this paper, we propose a deep learning architecture that can detect changes in the eye fundus images and assess the progression of the disease. Our method is based on joint autoencoders and is fully unsupervised. Our algorithm has been applied to pairs of images from different eye fundus images time series of 24 ARMD patients. Our method has been shown to be quite effective when compared with other methods from the literature, including non-neural network based algorithms that still are the current standard to follow the disease progression and change detection methods from other fields.

Keywords: ARMD; change detection; unsupervised learning; medical imaging

1. Introduction

Dry age-related macular degeneration (ARMD or sometimes AMD), a degenerative disease affecting the retina, is a leading cause of intractable visual loss. It is characterized by a centrifugal progression of atrophy of the retinal pigment epithelium (RPE), a cellular layer playing a key role in the maintenance of the photoreceptors. Blindness may occur when the central part of the eye, the fovea, is involved. The disease may be diagnosed and monitored using fundus photographs: ophthalmologists can observe pathologic features such as drusen that occur in the early stages of the ARMD, and evaluate the geographic atrophic (GA) progression in the late stages of degeneration (Figure 1).

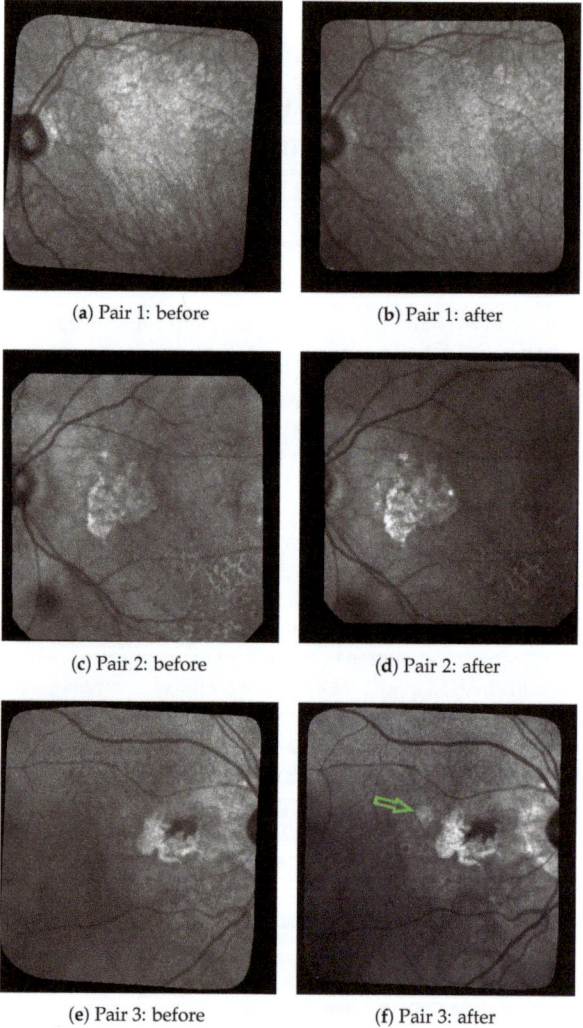

Figure 1. 3 of pairs of images acquired six months apart, the GA corresponds to the bright areas. The green arrow in (**f**) shows a new lesion.

Automatic analysis of fundus images with dry ARMD is of high medical interest [1] and this has been an important research field for two decades, for diagnosis [2] or follow up [3,4] purposes. Imaging modalities are most often color eye fundus images [5–7], fundus autofluorescence (FAF) [4,8,9], and, to a lesser extent, confocal scanning laser ophthalmoscopy (cSLO) in infrared (IR), or optical coherence tomography (OCT) [10]. In this work, we process cSLO images in IR: this modality is comfortable for the patient, and it has higher resolution and higher contrast than color imaging, an older technology. Our goal is to detect the appearance of new atrophic areas and quantify the growth of GA from pairs of images acquired at regular time intervals to ultimately propose predictive models of the disease progress.

Figure 1 shows three pairs of consecutive images, taken at 6-month intervals. The lesions (GA) are the brighter regions in the fundus and around the optical disk. Automatic processing to follow up these areas is obviously very challenging given the quality of the images: uneven illumination, saturation issues, illumination distortion between images, GA poorly contrasted with retinal structures interfering (vessel, optical disk), blur, etc. The difficulty also lies in the high variability of the lesions in terms of shape, size, and number. The lesion boundary is quite smooth in some cases (c and d) and very irregular in others (a and b). At any time, new spots can appear (as shown by the green arrow between e and f) and older lesions can merge. All these features make the segmentation task very difficult, and especially long and tedious to perform manually. It is worth noting that even experts cannot be sure of their manual delineation in all cases.

Modeling ARMD evolution from a series of eye fundus images requires segmenting the GA in each image and/or to perform a differential analysis between consecutive images to get the lesion growth. In this paper, we propose a differential analysis method based on a joint convolutional fully convolutional autoencoder. Our model is fully unsupervised and does not require labeled images that are difficult to come by in quantity and quality high enough to train a supervised neural network. Our method is applied to pairs of images of a patient eye fundus time series and aims at efficiently segmenting medically significant changes between the two images: meaningless differences caused by image quality or lighting issues are ignored while changes related to GA lesion evolution are extracted.

The remainder of the paper is organized as follows: In Section 2, we review works dedicated to automated processing of images of eye fundus with ARMD and we present approaches for change detection applied to medical image analysis as well as other fields. In Section 3, we present briefly our data and the way we process our images. Then, we detail our proposed method and the architecture of our neural network (Section 4). Section 5 shows our experimental results. Finally, we draw some conclusions in Section 6 and give some possible future perspectives of this work.

2. Related Works

This state-of-the-art section is split into three sections presenting methods closest to this work and also based on the differential approach first. Then, we will introduce a few methods also developed for the study of ARMD or other eye diseases but that rely on a segmentation based approach on individual images. In addition, we will finish this state of the art with some examples of other change detection methods from outside the field of medical imaging.

Before we start, we remind our readers that this work introduces a fully unsupervised method for change detection in ARMD images. The main difference between supervised and unsupervised learning is the following:

- In supervised learning, Machine Learning algorithms are trained using data that have been pre-classified or annotated by human with the goal of building a model based on these data. This model is then applied to new data with the goal of providing a classification for them. While this type of Machine Learning is considered to be the most powerful, its main weakness is that it cannot be used if no or not enough annotated data are available.
- In unsupervised learning, on the other hand, all data are provided raw and without any annotation or classification, and the algorithm must find by itself different classes called clusters of elements that are similar. Since the process is not guided, hence the name "unsupervised", the cluster found using this process may or may not match the classes expected by the users, and the performances of unsupervised learning are expected to be lower than these of supervised learning. Unsupervised Learning is usually used as an exploratory task or when there are no available annotated data (or not enough), both of which are the case for our application to ARMD image time series.

With this related work section, we hope to demonstrate that providing fully automated tools reaching the required level of performance for medical application is a difficult task, especially in an unsupervised context with few annotated images.

2.1. Differential Approaches Applied to ARMD

The following works are most related to our proposed algorithm as they are unsupervised algorithms applied to various eye disease images, including ARMD: In [11], Troglio et al. published an improvement of their previous works realized with Nappo [12] where they use the Kittler and Illingworth (K&I) thresholding method. Their method consists of applying the K&I algorithm on random sub-images of the difference image obtained between two consecutive eye fundus images of a patient with retinopathy. By doing so, they obtain multiple predictions for each pixel and can then make a vote to decide the final class. This approach has the advantage that it compensates for the non-uniform illumination across the image; however, it is rather primitive since it does not actually use any Machine Learning and rely on different parameters of the thresholding method to then make a vote. To its credit, even if it achieves a relatively weak precision, it is fully unsupervised like our method. In [6], the authors tackle a similar problematic to ours where they correct eye fundus images by pairs, by multiplying the second image by a polynomial surface whose parameters are estimated in the least-squares sense. In this way, illumination distortion is lessened and the image difference enhances the areas of changes. However, the statistical test applied locally at each pixel is not reliable enough to get an accurate map of structural changes.

2.2. Segmentation First Approaches Applied to ARMD and Other Eye Diseases

Other works related with eye diseases take the different approach of segmenting lesions in individual images instead of looking for changes in pairs of images. In [5], Köse et al. proposed an approach where they first segment all healthy regions to get the lesions as the remaining areas. This approach also requires segmenting separately the blood vessels, which is known to be a difficult task. This method involves many steps and parameters that need to be supervised by the user. In [4], Ramsey et al. proposed a similar but unsupervised method for the identification of ARMD lesions in individual images: They use an unsupervised algorithm based on fuzzy c-means clustering. Their method achieves good performances for FAF images, but it performs less well for color fundus photographs. We can also mention the work of Hussain et al. [13] in which the authors are proposing another supervised algorithm to track the progression of drusen for ARMD follow-up. They first use U-Nets to segment vessels and detect the optic disc with the goal of reducing the region of interest for drusen detection. After this step, they track the drusen using intensity ratio between neighbor pixels.

Using the same approach of segmenting the lesions first and then tracking the changes, there are a few supervised methods available. We can, for instance, mention [14] in which the authors propose another related work in which they use a pre-trained supervised neural network to detect ARMD lesions with good results. In addition, in [15], the same team uses another supervised convolutional neural network (CNN) to assess the stage of ARMD based on the lesions.

Other traditional more machine learning approaches have also been used for GA segmentation such as the k-nearest neighbor classifiers [9], random forests [7], as well as combinations of Support Vector Machines and Random Forests [16]. Feature vectors for these approaches typically include intensity values, local energy, texture descriptors, values derived from multi-scale analysis and distance to the image center. Nevertheless, these algorithms are supervised: they require training the classifier from annotated data, which brings us back to the difficulty of manually segmenting GA areas.

Related to other medical images, in [17], the authors show that the quantization error (QE) of the output obtained with the application of Self Organized Maps [18] is an indicator of small local changes in medical images. This work is also unsupervised but has the defaults that the SOM algorithm cannot provide a clustering on its own and must be coupled with another algorithm such as K-Means to do so. Furthermore, since there is no feature extraction done, this algorithm would most likely be very sensitive to the lighting and contrast issues that are present in most eye fundus time series. Lastly, the use of SOM based methods on monochromatic images is discouraged since no interesting topology may be found from a single attribute.

Finally, the literature also contains a few user-guided segmentation frameworks [19,20] that are valuable when it is possible to get a user input.

2.3. Change Detection Methods from Other Fields

Apart from medicine, change detection algorithms have been proposed for many different applications such as remote sensing or video analysis. In [21], the authors reveal a method combining principal component analysis (PCA) and K-means algorithm on the difference image. In [22], an architecture relying on joint auto-encoders and convolutional neural networks is proposed to detect non-trivial changes between two images. In [23], the authors propose an autoencoder architecture for anomaly detection in videos.

Finally, as we have seen that quite a few methods rely on segmentation first and change detection after, we can also mention a few noteworthy unsupervised segmentation algorithms used outside the field of medicine: Kanezaki et al. [24] used CNN to group similar pixels together with consideration of spatial continuity as a basis of their segmentation method. In addition, Xia and Kulis [25] developed W-Net using a combination of two U-Nets with a soft Normalized-Cut Loss.

In Table 1, we sum up the main methods presented in this related work section. The first column specifies if the method is supervised or unsupervised. The second column indicates if the method uses the directly pairs of images (or their difference), or if it uses individual images to segment them first and then compare the segmentations. The "Algorithm" column details which algorithm is used. The last column gives the application field.

Table 1. Summary of the state-of-the-art methods for change detection that are mentioned in this work.

Authors	Supervised	Images Used	Algorithm	Application
Troglio, Napo et al. [11,12]	No	Pairs	K&I Thresholding	ARMD
Marrugo et al. [6]	No	Pairs	Image correction	ARMD
Köse et al. [5]	semi	Individual	Raw segmentation	ARMD
Ramsey et al. [4]	No	Individual	Fuzzy C-Means	ARMD
Hussain et al. [13]	Yes	Individual	U-Nets	ARMD
Burlina et al. [14,15]	Yes	Individual	pre-trained CNN	ARMD
Kanezaki et al. [24]	No	Individual	CNN	Image Processing
Sublime et al. [26]	No	Pairs	Joint-AE & KMeans	Remote Sensing
Celik et al. [21]	No	Pairs	PCA & KMeans	Remote Sensing
Our Method	No	Pairs	Joint-AE	ARMD

3. Dataset Presentation

In this section, we will provide some details on the image time series used in this work in terms of their characteristics, flaws, and how we pre-processed them before comparing different methods for change detection on them.

Our images whose main characteristics can be found in Table 2 were all acquired at the Quinze–Vingts National Ophthalmology Hospital in Paris, in cSLO with IR illumination. This modality has the advantage of being one of the most common and cheapest legacy method of image acquisition for eye fundus images, thus allowing to have lots of images and to follow the patients for several years. However, it is infrared only and therefore all images are monochromatic and may contain less information than images acquired from other techniques with multiple channels (that are less common for this type of exam and more difficult to find in numbers).

Table 2. Description of the data.

Number of patients	15
Number of image time series	18
Average number of images per series	13
Total number of images	336
Acquisition period	2007–2019
Average time between two images	6 months

While some 3D OCT and 2D FAF images were available, the infrared light penetrates better than blue light through media opacities and requires pupil dilation hence IR imaging is more robust (and better supported by patients). Although OCT is becoming the preferred imaging modality to appreciate the progression of GA, it requires a standard acquisition modality at each exam to ensure comparability, hence a lot of data acquired during routine follow-up cannot be used. On the other hand, the 30° IR imaging is the default mode of fundus image acquisition and hence most patients have such image taken whatever the OCT protocol has been done. Thus, we stick to cSLO with infrared only so that we could have longer and more homogeneous series, and therefore all images are monochromatic and may contain less information than images acquired from other techniques with multiple channels (that are less common for this type of exam and more difficult to find in numbers).

Patients have been followed-up during a few years, hence we have a series of retinal fundus images, sometimes for both eyes (hence the number of series and patients being different in Table 2), showing the progression of the GA. The average number of images in each series is 13. The images are dated from 2007 for the oldest to 2019 for the most recent. All pictures are in grayscale and vary greatly in size, but the most common size is 650 × 650 pixels.

As mentioned previously, we notice many imperfections such as blur, artifacts and, above all, non-uniform illumination inside the images and between them (see Figure 2). All images were spatially aligned with i2k software (https://www.dualalign.com/retinal/image-registration-montage-software-overview.php). In every image, the area of useful data does not fill the entire image and is surrounded by black borders. The automatic detection of these black zones in each image gives a mask of the useful data, and the intersection of all masks the common retinal region where changes can be searched for.

We also designed a new method to compensate for illumination distortion between the images (not published yet). This algorithm is based on an illumination/reflectance model and corrects all images of a series with respect to a common reference image. Uneven illumination generally remains present in every processed image (Figure 2), but the smooth illumination distortions are compensated. The calculus of the absolute value of the difference between two consecutive images demonstrates the benefit of this algorithm (Figure 2, last column).

We used five different series of images to evaluate quantitatively our method of change detection: they feature different characteristics in terms of disease progress, lesion shape and size. We developed several user-guided segmentation tools to make the ground truth, based on classical segmentation algorithms: thresholding applied locally on a rectangle defined by the user, parametric active contour model initialized by the user, and simple linear interpolation between points entered by the user. The user can use the most appropriate tool to locally delimit the lesion border, and thus progresses step by step. Local thresholding or active contour algorithm makes it possible to obtain segmentations that depend less on the user than the use of interpolation, which is applied when the two previous methods fail. However, the segmentation remains mostly manual, user-dependent, and tedious. An ophthalmologist realized all segmentation used in our experiments. Finally, the binary change mask between two consecutive images was obtained by subtraction of the segmentation masks.

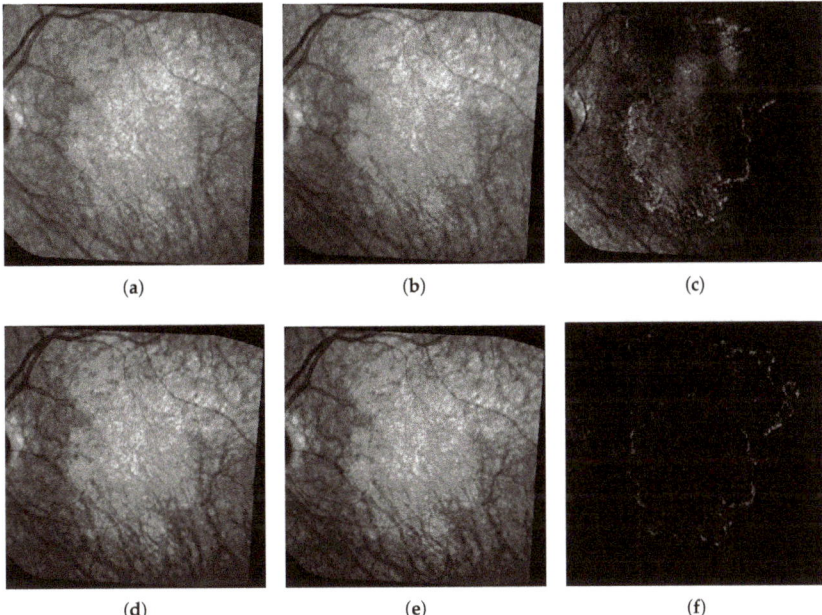

Figure 2. Example of Illumination correction. The three images on the top row represent the two original consecutive images (**a**,**b**), and their raw difference in absolute value (**c**); on the bottom row: the same images after illumination correction (**d**,**e**), and the new difference (**f**).

It is worth noting that the manual segmentation of a single image by expert ophthalmologists takes on average 13 min for a single image, and that many disagreements as to what the ideal segmentation should be arise when comparing the segmentations made by different experts for the same image: In particular, many doctors disagree on which internal changes are interesting or not (and therefore should or should not be in the ground truth), and they may also have different advice for the borders of particularly difficult lesions. For these reasons, and because we kept the results of only a single ophthalmologist, the ground-truth provided for our images have to be taken with caution as they are not always reliable, and, as we will see in later sections, they may feature defects that will affect dices' indexes computed based on them. Furthermore, for the same reason that it takes a lot of time to produce reliable change maps, our test set is relatively small in size compared to other applications that features much larger data sets, and in particular larger test sets.

4. Description of Our Proposed Architecture

Our algorithm is inspired from earlier works from remote sensing [22,26], where the authors applied an unsupervised deep autoencoder to automatically map non-trivial changes between pairs of satellite images to detect meaningful evolutions such as new constructions or changes in landcover while discarding trivial seasonal changes.

In our paper, we use the similarities between satellite images and our medical ARMD eye fundus to adapt their method: both types of images may suffer from lighting issues, noise issues, blurry elements, complex objects present in the images, various time gaps between two images of the same series, and most importantly the common goal of detecting meaningful changes despite all these issues.

While they share similarities, our medical images and satellite images are also quite different: they do not have the same number of channels, they have very different sizes, and the nature of the objects and changes to detect is also quite different. For these reasons, the following subsection will detail how we modified their architecture, and it will explain all steps of our algorithm.

4.1. Joint Autoencoder Architecture

As mentioned earlier, in this research, we use a fully convolutional autoencoder. Autoencoders [27] are a type of neural networks whose purpose is to make the output as close as possible to the input. During the learning process, the encoder learns some meaningful representation of the initial data that is transformed back with the decoder. Hence, in a fully convolutional AE, a stack of convolutive layers is applied to the input image in order to extract feature maps (FM) which will then be used to reconstruct the input image.

Usually, AEs with dense layers are used to perform a dimensionality reduction followed by a clustering or segmentation. However, in computer vision, fully convolutional AEs are preferred for their ability to extract textures. Examples of such networks include fully convolutional networks (FCNs) [28] or U-Nets [29]. However, in our case, we do not use Max-pooling layers, and so we keep the same dimensions as the input and only the depth increases.

Our network (Figure 3) is made of four convolutional layers in the encoder of size 16, 16, 32, and 32, respectively, and in the same way as four convolutional layers of size 32, 32, 16, and 16, respectively, in the decoder side. We apply a batch normalization and a ReLU activation function at each step of the network except for the last layer of the encoder where we only add the L2 normalization, and also for the last layer of the decoder where we apply a Sigmoid function (see in Figure 3).

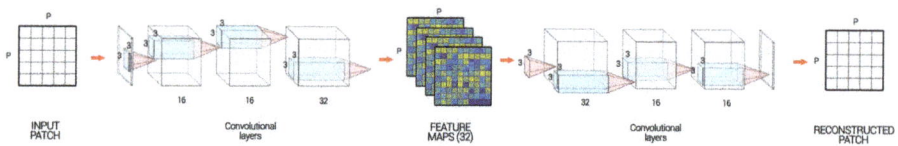

Figure 3. Autoencoder architecture for our algorithm.

4.2. Algorithm Steps

Our algorithm is made of four steps. We start by dividing the images into several patches. Then, we build the joint autoencoder where it learns how to reconstruct the images, and after we tweak the method by learning the autoencoder to reconstruct not the image itself but the precedent or the future image. The neural networks will learn easily the changes due to the non-uniform illumination or noise but will fail on ARMD progression generating a high reconstruction error (RE), consequently making it possible to detect them. The next subsections will detail some of these steps:

4.2.1. Patches Construction

One of the issues with the retinal fundus images we have is their shape. Indeed, our images are not necessarily square and differ from one set to another. This is why we use an approach based on patches that allows us to manage several sizes of images but also several forms of useful areas thanks to a simple manipulation that we explain right away.

As mentioned in Section 3, the area of useful data are not rectangular and is generally surrounded by black borders, which can be detected by a simple logic test. As can be seen in Figure 4, we solve this problem by using the Inpainting function of the library *scikit-image* [30] to complete this background. This inpainting function is based on the biharmonic equation [31,32], and it exploits the information in the connected regions to fill the black zones with consistent gray level values. Let us denote by $P \times P$ the size of the patches. The image is also padded with $\frac{P}{2}$ pixels along all dimensions and directions before applying the inpainting. Thanks to this operation, we can extract patches from the whole image, i.e., patches centered on every useful pixel, without any cropping, and so we can exploit all our available data without border effects.

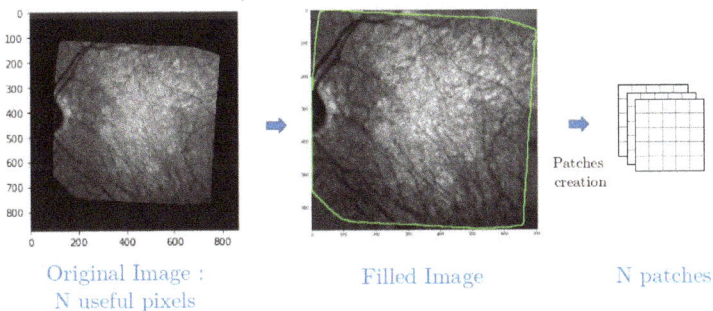

Figure 4. Patches construction, useful pixels are inside the green area.

4.2.2. Pre-Training

Let us consider a series of M images representing the progression of ARMD in a patient's eye. After the pre-processing and once the images have been aligned and cropped, all images from the same series have the same number of N useful patches. From there, to pre-train or network, we sample $\left\lfloor \frac{N}{M} \right\rfloor$ of the patches for every image hence, regardless of the size of the series, we use a total of N patches. This allows us to build a unique autoencoder AE that works for all pairs in the series, and to prevent overfitting.

As an example, for a series of 16 images and 600×600 useful patches per image, we would randomly sample $\frac{1}{16}$ of the patches for each image of the series (22,500 patches per image), and use a total of 360,000 patches to pre-train our network.

When processing the patches, our network applies a Gaussian filter in order to weight the pixels by giving more importance to the center of the patch in the RE calculus.

During the encoding pass of the AE, the model extracts feature maps of N patches of chosen samples with convolutional layers (Figure 5), and then, during the decoding pass, it reconstructs them back to the initial ones.

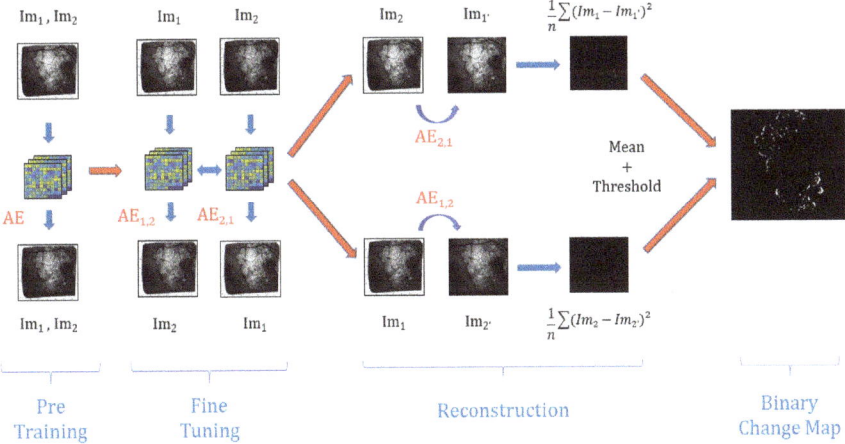

Figure 5. Structure of the algorithm. Example for set of two images Im_1 and Im_2 and n the number of patches.

4.2.3. Fine-Tuning

For every consecutive pair $i, i+1$ with $i \in [\![1; M-1]\!]$ of images, we are going to build two autoencoders initialized with the weights found in the pre-training part. On one hand, $AE_{i,i+1}$ aims to reconstruct patches of Im_{i+1} from patches of Im_i and, on the other hand, $AE_{i+1,i}$ is going to reconstruct patches of Im_i from patches of Im_{i+1}.

The whole model is trained to minimize the difference between: the decoded output of $AE_{i,i+1}$ and Im_{i+1}, the decoded output of $AE_{i+1,i}$ and Im_i, and the encoded outputs of $AE_{i,i+1}$ and $AE_{i+1,i}$, see Figure 5.

This joint configuration where the learning is done in both temporal directions, using joint backpropagation, has empirically proven to be much more robust than using a regular one-way autoencoder. To optimize the parameters of the model, we use the mean squared error (MSE) of the reconstructed patches.

For the fine-tuning, we stop iterating and running epochs when the MSE of the reconstructed patches stabilizes, as is standard for the training of Deep Learning networks.

4.2.4. Reconstruction and Thresholding

Once the models are trained and stabilized, we perform the image reconstruction. For each pair, we note $Im_{i+1'}$ the reconstruction of Im_{i+1} from Im_i with $AE_{i,i+1}$ and likewise we note $Im_{i'}$ the reconstruction of Im_i from Im_{i+1} with $AE_{i+1,i}$. Then, we calculate the reconstruction error RE for every patch between Im_i and $Im_{i'}$ on one side and between Im_{i+1} and $Im_{i+1'}$ on another side. This gives us two images for each pair representing the average REs for $Im_{i'}$ and $Im_{i+1'}$ that we average to get only one. The model will easily learn the transformation of unchanged areas from one image to the other: changes in luminosity and blurring effects. At the same time, because the changes caused by the disease progression are unique, they will be considered as outliers by the model, and thus will have a high RE. Hence, we apply Otsu's thresholding [33] that requires no parameters and enables us to produce a binary change map (BCM).

If we sum up, our algorithm uses the strengths of joint auto-encoders to map the light changes, contrast defects, and texture changes from one image to another. This way, most of the image defects and noise issues will be removed. In addition, then, we use the inability of the auto-encoder to predict structural changes in the lesions through time (this algorithm is not designed to do this), as is the inability of the algorithm to generate a high reconstruction error in areas where the lesions have progressed when comparing the encoded reconstructed images with the real images. This way, we have a fully unsupervised way to remove noise and detect changes in the lesions. The full process is explained in Figure 5.

5. Experimental Results

5.1. Experimental Setting

We chose to compare our methods presented in Section 4.1 with three other methods, all on the preprocessed images. We applied all the methods to three of our series for which we have a ground truth.

The following parameters were chosen for all convolutional layers of our method: kernel size to 3, stride to 1, and padding to 1. The Adam algorithm was used to optimize the models. We set the number of epochs to 8 for the pre-training phase and just 1 for the fine-tuning phase. These parameters were chosen as they are the limit after which the reconstruction error generally does not improve anymore. More epochs during the pre-training phase led to more required epochs to adjust the model to each couple during the fine-tuning phase without much improvements on the results. In addition, more epochs on the fine-tuning phase did not lead to any significant improvement in the results and sometimes resulted in overfitting. Therefore, we fix these parameters both to ensure quality results and to avoid running extra unneeded epochs for both the pre-training and fine-tuning phase.

For both phases, the learning rate was set to 0.0001 and the batch size to 100.

The first method that we use for comparison is a simple subtraction of two consecutive images with an application of Otsu's thresholding on the result. The second comparison is a combination of principal component analysis (PCA) and K-means algorithm on the difference image proposed by Celik et al. in [21], and we apply it to medical images with blocks of size 5. To finish, we take a Deep-Learning based approach [24] which uses CNN to group similar pixels together with consideration of spatial continuity. This work by Kanezaki et al. was initially made for unsupervised segmentation; consequently, we apply the algorithm to our images and then do the segmentation substractions to get binary change maps. The convolution layers have the same configuration than for our network and we set the parameter for the *minimum number of labels* to 3.

As it is common practice, even for unsupervised algorithms, we assess the results of the different methods using classical binary indexes intended for supervised classification: accuracy, precision, recall, and F1-Score. All formulas are given in Equations (1)–(4), where we used the change areas as the positive class and no change as the negative class. The notations "TP", "TN", "FP", and "FN" are used for true positive, true negative, false positive, and false negative, respectively.

Accuracy refers to the proportion of correct predictions made by the model. It is sensitive to class imbalance:

$$Accuracy = \frac{TP + TN}{TP + TN + FP + FN} \quad (1)$$

Precision is the proportion of identifications classified as positive by the model that is actually correct:

$$Precision = \frac{TP}{TP + FP}. \quad (2)$$

Recall is the proportion of positive results that are correctly identified. It can be thought of as the proportion of progression of the lesion correctly identified:

$$Recall = \frac{TP}{TP + FN}. \quad (3)$$

F1-Score also known as the F-Measure, or balanced F Score, is the harmonic mean between the precision and the recall and is computed as follows:

$$F1 = \frac{2 \times precision \times recall}{precision + recall} \quad (4)$$

5.2. Parameters' Fine-Tuning

The fully convolutional AE model for change detection is presented in Section 4.1.

There are two main parameters in our algorithm. The first one is the the patch size P. As we can see in Figure 6, a smaller value of P will increase our precision and, on the contrary, a high value of P will increase our recall. Thus, the challenge is to find a trade-off value between both scores in order to get the best F1 score possible. In order to improve the performances, we decided to introduce a second parameter: sigma σ. This one refers to Gaussian weights which are applied to the patches to give more importance to central pixels and less to pixels closer to the sides of the patches during the RE loss computation. For each series, we did experiments such as the one shown in Figure 7 to find the best patch size P and value σ. In general, we got that a high size of the patch gave us a relatively good recall and the Gaussian weights allow us to regain precision. Two pairs of values came up more often: patch size $P = 13$ and a value $\sigma = 12$ for patients with larger lesions, and patch size $P = 7$ and a value $\sigma = 5$ for patients with smaller lesions.

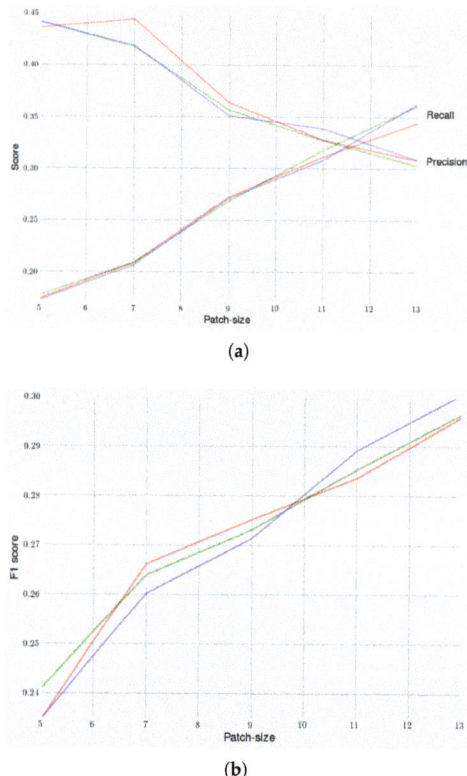

(a)

(b)

Figure 6. Average recall, Precision, and F1 Score depending on the patch size and sigma: $\sigma = 5$ in red $\sigma = 7$ in green $\sigma = 9$ in blue. (**a**) Recall and Precision depending on the patch size; (**b**) F1 Score depending on the Patch size.

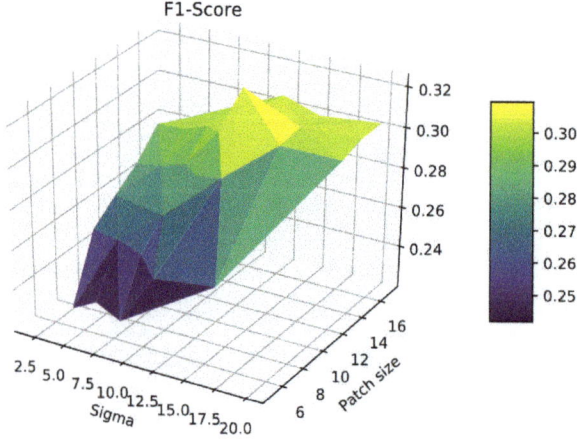

Figure 7. F1-Score as a function of the patch size and the value of sigma σ on patient 005.

All of the algorithm steps were executed on an Nvidia GPU (RTX TITAN) with 64 GB of RAM and an Intel 9900 k. It took about 20 min for a series of 8 frames with a patch size P of 13, with the execution time increasing with it.

5.3. Results

The results for patients 1, 3, 5, 10, and 115 are shown in Table 3, as well as Figures 8–11 that we added for visual inspection purposes. Additional images for patient 18 are available in some of the figures. Other patients were not added to Table 3 or the figures because we do not have reliable enough change map ground-truths to compute the dice indexes, or because we do not have them at all. Note that the scores presented in Table 3 are for the complete series (15 to 20 pairs per patient), while the scores shown in the figures are for the individual couples of images used in each example. The bottom line of Table 3 shows the weighted mean values for all indexes and all methods for all series.

When looking at Table 3, we can see that the simple difference coupled with Otsu thresholding achieves the best recall results on average that there is no clear winner for the Precision, and that our proposed method on average has the best F1 Score.

Please note that we did not display the Accuracy because of the strong class imbalance, with a large majority of "no change class" pixels leading to results over 85% for Kanezaki's approach and the simple differentiating with Otsu thresholding, and over 95% for our approach and Celik approach. Since these figures are obviously very biased and given that we are more interested in "change" pixels than "no change" pixels, we did not report them in Table 3 and preferred to focus on commenting on the Precision, Recall, and F1-score that are less affected by class imbalance.

Table 3. Results and comparison of the different approaches. It contains the means of the recall, the precision, and the F1 score for each time series. For each patient, the best dice results are in bold.

Patient ID	Method	Authors	Recall	Precision	F1 Score
001 15 images	Diff + Otsu CNN PCA + KMeans Joint-AE	- Kanezaki et al. Celik et al. Our method	0.68 0.32 0.48 0.44	0.11 **0.29** 0.28 0.21	0.16 0.18 **0.3** 0.26
003 5 images	Diff + Otsu CNN PCA + KMeans Joint-AE	- Kanezaki et al. Celik et al. Our method	0.55 0.2 0.24 0.29	0.1 0.27 **0.33** 0.28	0.17 0.07 0.27 **0.28**
005 8 images	Diff + Otsu CNN PCA + KMeans Joint-FCAE	- Kanezaki et al. Celik et al. Our method	0.46 0.2 0.26 0.33	0.2 **0.43** 0.37 0.34	0.26 0.21 0.28 **0.32**
010 6 images	Diff + Otsu CNN PCA + KMeans Joint-FCAE	- Kanezaki et al. Celik et al. Our method	0.68 0.32 0.47 0.38	0.06 0.03 0.23 **0.35**	0.10 0.05 0.29 **0.36**
115 9 images	Diff + Otsu CNN PCA + KMeans Joint-FCAE	- Kanezaki et al. Celik et al. Our method	0.53 0.33 0.24 0.33	0.25 0.15 0.38 **0.39**	0.29 0.16 0.25 **0.34**
Total (patients' mean—43 images)	Diff + Otsu CNN PCA + KMeans Joint-AE	- Kanezaki et al. Celik et al. Our method	0.58 0.27 0.33 0.35	0.16 0.27 **0.32** 0.32	0.20 0.14 0.27 **0.31**

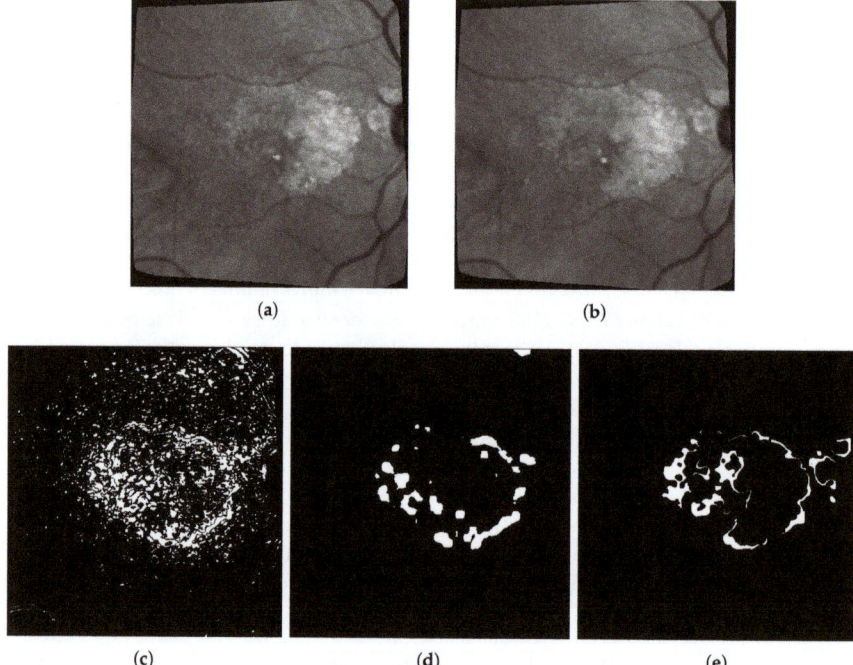

Figure 8. Difference + Otsu thresholding vs. our approach (AE) on patient 003. (**a**) Image at $t = 0$; (**b**) Image at $t + 3$ months; (**c**) Raw difference and Otsu thresholding, F1 score = 0.26; (**d**) Our method, F1 score = 0.36; (**e**) Proposed ground truth.

Our interpretation of these results is the following: Otsu thresholding applied to the difference between two images has the best recalls because it detects most real change pixels. However, the binary change map is also very noisy, corresponding to a high number of false positives (wrongly detected changes), which is confirmed by the very low precision score. This can also be observed in Figures 8c and 11d, which are examples of the high number of false positives detected using Otsu thresholding compared with the ground truth in Figure 8c, or our method results in Figure 8e.

In Figures 9–11, we compare our approach with the two other algorithms relying on more advanced Machine Learning techniques. First, we can see that, like in Table 3, our approach gets the best F1-score for both patients and pairs of images. Then, we can see that the Kanezaki et al. approach achieves over-segmentation in Figure 9d and under-segmentation in Figure 10d, which highlights that it is more difficult to parametrize properly and may require different parameters for each pair of image, which is not the case for both our approach and the Celik et al. approach. Finally, regarding the comparison between the Celik et al. approach and our proposed method, we can see from Figures 9e,f, 10e,f, and 11e,f that also, like in Table 3, the Celik et al. approach achieves overall good results that are comparable to the ones of our method. However, in the same way that we have better F1-score and accuracy results, the visual results for our methods are also better as the changes we detect in the lesions are cleaner and overall less fragmented into very small elements compared with the ones found by the Celik et al. approach.

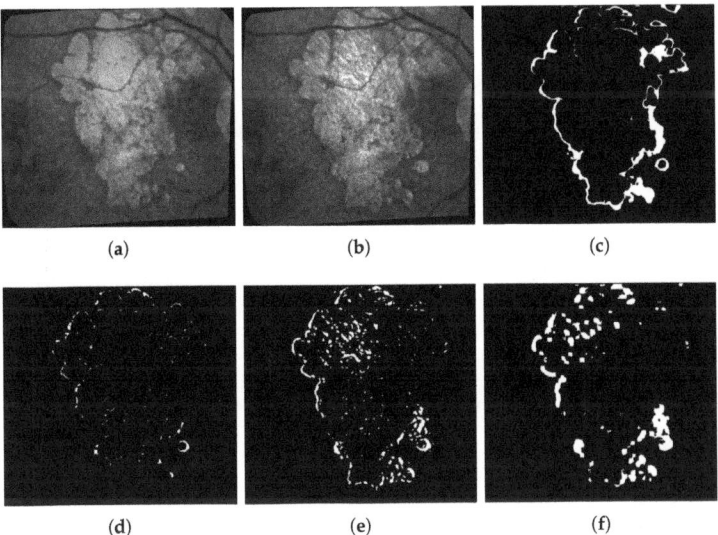

Figure 9. Comparison example of the three methods on patient 005. (**a**) Corrected Image from October 2017; (**b**) Corrected Image from June 2018; (**c**) Proposed ground truth; (**d**) Asako Kanezaki's approach, F1 score = 0.15; (**e**) Turgay Celik's approach, F1 score = 0.35; (**f**) Our Fully Convolutional AE, F1 score = 0.4.

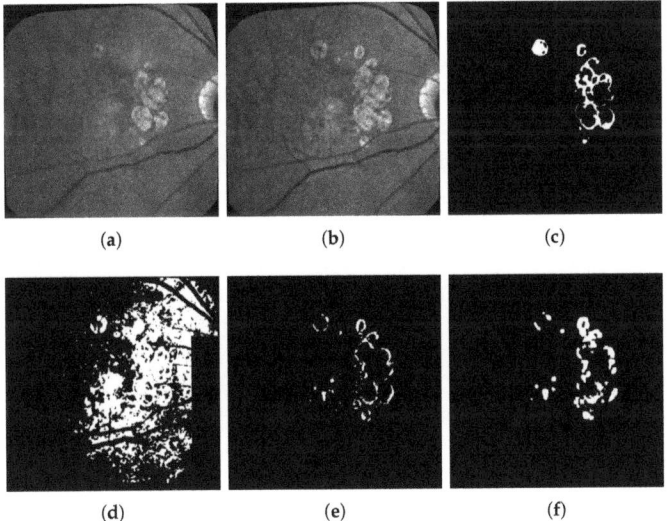

Figure 10. Comparison example of the three methods on patient 001. (**a**) Corrected Image from April 2017; (**b**) Corrected Image from October 2017; (**c**) Proposed ground truth; (**d**) Asano Kanezaki's approach, F1 score = 0.17; (**e**) Turgay Celik's approach, F1 score = 0.43; (**f**) Our Fully convolutional AE, F1 score = 0.43.

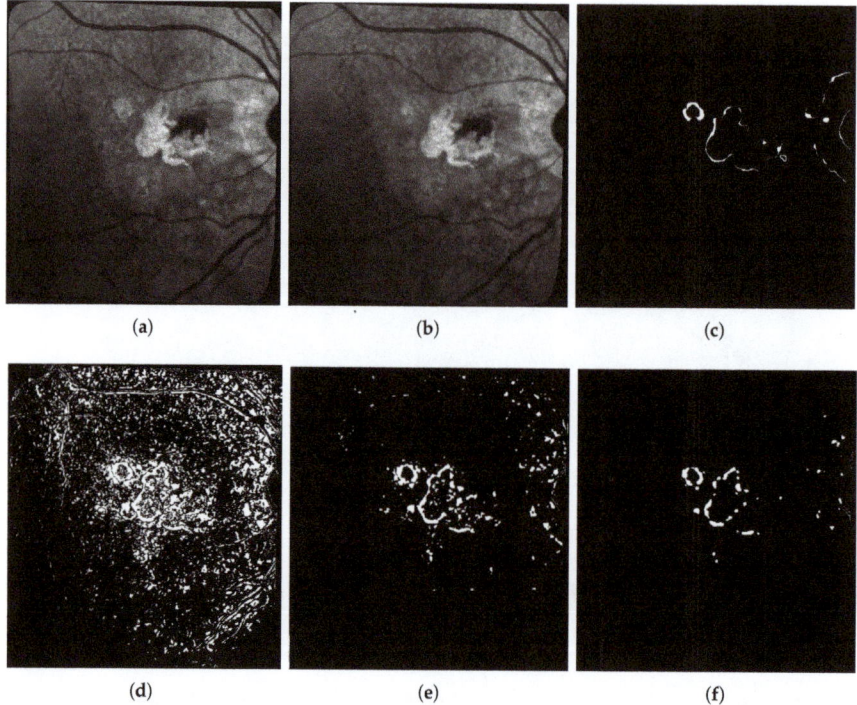

Figure 11. Comparison example of the three methods on patient 010. (**a**) Corrected Image from November 2017; (**b**) Corrected Image from May 2018; (**c**) Proposed ground truth; (**d**) Otsu thresholding, F1 score = 0.05; (**e**) Turgay Celik's approach, F1 score = 0.253; (**f**) Our Fully convolutional AE, F1 score = 0.38.

When looking at the figures and areas where the changes are detected, we can see that our method finds changes that are more in the peripheral areas of the lesions, while the Celik et al. approach tends to find lots of noisy elements inside existing lesions (see Figure 10e). From a medical point of view and to study the progression of ARMD, we are of course more concerned with lesion growth and therefore with what is going on in the peripheral areas of the lesions, thus giving an advantage to our methods, since it is better at capturing these peripheral changes. However, it does not mean that changes deep inside the lesions have no values and could not be used to better understand the mechanisms of the disease in another study.

5.4. Discussion

Overall, we can conclude that both Otsu thresholding and Kanezaki's approach suffer from risks of over-segmentation detecting a lot of noise, or under-segmentation detecting nothing, both of which are impossible to exploit from a medical point of view. On the other hand, despite somewhat mild recall and precision scores, the Celik approach and our method are visually much better at detecting meaningful changes in ARMD lesions' structures. Moreover, we can see that, despite the strong class imbalance that we mentioned earlier, our proposed method has a slightly higher F1-Score and finds structures that are visually better and more interesting from a medical point of view since they tend to be more on the outside and at the limits of existing lesions instead of inside them, and are also less fragmented.

To conclude this experimental section, we would like to discuss some of the main weaknesses and limitations of our proposed approach and of this study overall.

The first limitation that is not inherent to our approach is the difficulty to get accurate ground-truths to assess the quality of the results (hence why unsupervised learning should be preferred). In particular, all the ground-truths we have completely ignore possible textural changes within existing areas of geographic atrophy, and they don't always have the level of accuracy we hope for when it comes to subtle small changes in the lesions. This is due to the fact that most of these ground truths are built by subtracting masks of segmented lesions during two consecutive exams as shown in Figure 12: Doing so results in ground-truths that ignore most of the changes happening inside the lesions. It is worth mentioning that series with larger lesions are more affected by this issue as these lesions are more likely to have internal changes.

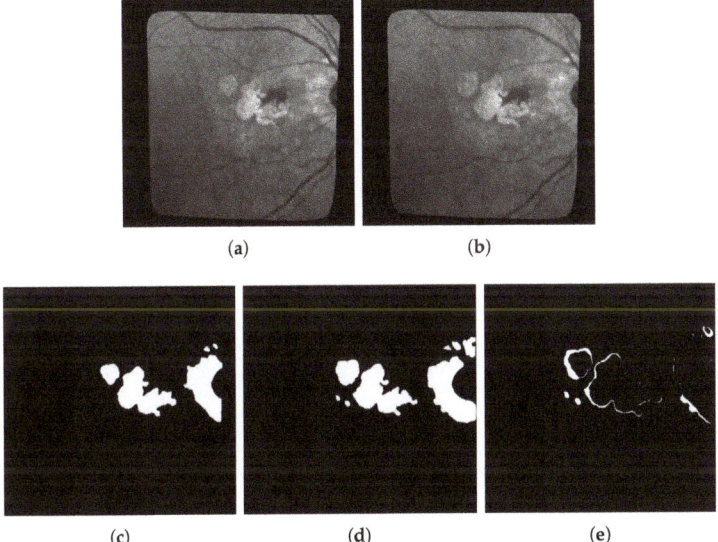

Figure 12. Example of ground-truth build for patient 010 based on two consecutive masks of segmented lesions at time t and $t + 1$: All changes inside the lesions, textural or otherwise, are ignored. (**a**) Image t; (**b**) Image $t + 1$; (**c**) segmentation mask t; (**d**) segmentation mask $t + 1$; (**e**) Ground truth built from Mask t and $t + 1$.

This explains some of the low dice scores from Table 3 since in many cases there are internal changes (textural, structural, or both) happening within ARMD lesions, and some of them will be detected by the algorithms used in this paper. However, almost all of these changes detected inside the lesions will be classified as false positive since they are not present on the ground truth. One example of such issue is shown in Figure 13 where all pixels in red in sub-figure (d) will be classified as false positive despite some of them being actual changes (seeing some internal structural changes is possible by zooming in on sub-figures a and b).

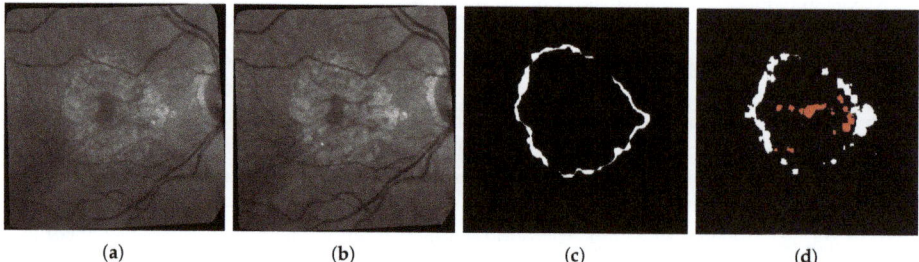

Figure 13. Example of a segmentation in (**d**) where all changes detected in red will be considered false positive since the ground truth does not consider changes within existing lesions regardless of if they are structural of textural. (**a**) Image of patient 018 at time t; (**b**) Image of patient 018 at time $t + 1$; (**c**) Proposed Ground truth; (**d**) Proposed segmentation.

The second obvious weakness of our approach is also related to the difficulty of finding reliably annotated data and ground-truth. Because it is difficult to find them, we propose an unsupervised approach. In addition, unfortunately, unsupervised approaches are known to produce results that are less impressive than their supervised counterparts. A fully unsupervised framework which has the advantage that it does not require any annotated data to be trained—which is a real strength when very few are available—but has the weakness that its performances are weaker. In future works, we hope to refine our method so that we can improve the quality indexes a bit, but, even with better ground-truths, we expect the performances to remain limited so long as the framework is fully unsupervised.

A third limitation that can be mentioned and comes more from the data and experimental protocol than the methods is the following: Given that our method is fully unsupervised, and since we use change maps made by experts ophthalmologists that are not always reliable due to disagreements between experts on what is an interesting change or not, we have both a test set problem (as mentioned before), and a choice of metric problem as dice indexes while commonly used are probably not ideal to evaluate unsupervised methods, especially when there is uncertainty on the quality of the expert change maps. Two solutions that we plan to use on our future works are the following:

- To have several experts rating the proposed change maps, and use the average mark as a quality index. This method has the advantage that it is the fairest, but it is inconvenient that it is very time consuming and does not scale with large datasets as it takes on average 13 min for an ophthalmologist to do a quality segmentation on a single image.
- Using unsupervised quality indexes alongside the accuracy and the three dice indexes that we already use, so that we have a more fair evaluation of all methods. While this has the advantage of scaling well, it is probably a weaker quality argument than supervised indexes and experts' ratings for an application in the field of medicine.

The fourth limitation of our method that can be pointed out is that, as it stands, our algorithm does not yet achieve the goal of predicting how the pathology evolves: Our method detects changes and how the ARMD lesions evolved from one image to the next, but it does not provide any growth model or any interpretation of why it grew this way. Furthermore, while our algorithm detects changes fairly well, it is yet unable to predict future changes and therefore to tell in advance how the lesions might evolve on the short or long term for a given patient. While prediction was not the goal of the method proposed in this paper, it is certainly a future evolution that we are interested in. In fact, we hope that we will be able to use the results provided by our method on how the lesions grow and change from one image to the next to build predictive models based on this information. Some leads on approaches with which to combine our algorithm include other deep learning approaches such as long short term memory [34], gated recurrent units [35], or generative adversarial networks [36], all of which have shown to be useful for time series prediction or long term predictions.

Finally, even if our work does not lead to a huge leap forward in result quality due to various issues that we previously mentioned, the fact that we proposed a deep learning architecture will make it a lot easier in the future to couple our approach with predicting architectures such as the ones we just mentioned.

6. Conclusions

In this paper, we have presented a new fully unsupervised deep learning architecture based on a joint autoencoder that detects the evolution of ARMD lesions in an eye fundus series of images. With a pre-cleaning of the series to remove as many lighting issues as possible, our proposed method is based on an auto-encoder architecture that can detect non-trivial changes between pairs of images, such as the evolution of a lesion, while discarding more trivial changes such as lighting problems or slight texture changes due to different image angles. Our proposed method was applied to three real sets of images, and was compared with three methods from the state of the art. Despite mild F1-Score results due to various issues, our method has been shown to give good enough results for a fully unsupervised algorithm and to perform better than the other methods from the state of the art, and may prove useful to assist doctors in properly detecting the evolution of ARMD lesions by proposing a first raw segmentation of the evolution.

While our results are not perfect and cannot yet be used for a fully automated diagnosis, it is obvious to us that our proposed algorithm may prove useful to assist doctors in properly detecting the evolution of ARMD lesions by proposing a first raw segmentation of the evolution that is a lot better than what can be done with the existing methods.

In our future works, our priority will be to solve our ground-truth and test set issues by trying to have more experts producing and rating our results. This is an important pre-requisite as we plan on working on approaches that can work on full time series rather than pairs of images. This would also require both better lighting correction algorithms but may lead to more interesting models to predict the evolution of ARMD. Developing long-term prediction algorithms is another goal of ours that could be achieved using a combination of this work on longer series with other deep approaches that are more adapted for prediction.

Finally, as there are other modalities of images available to study ARMD, some of which have colors, but with different resolutions, one of our other goals would be to combine several of these types of images to globally improve our prediction scores. This future work of combining images with different scales, alignments, and color bands shall prove to be very challenging and will hopefully yield more interesting results while still using a fully unsupervised approach.

Author Contributions: M.P. and the Clinical Imaging Center of Paris Quinze-Vingts hospital provided the data after a first preprocessing step. M.P. also provided the medical knowledge necessary to interpret our algorithm's results. F.R. and M.P. worked together to produce and validate ground truths as reliable as possible. F.R. worked on data curation and the preprocessing algorithm for lighting correction. Most of the software programming, investigation, and experiments, as well as the result visualization were done by G.D. during his internship. J.S. and E.K. worked on the problem analysis and conceptualization, as well as domain adaptation from Remote Sensing to Medical Imaging. All authors participated in the validation of the experimental results. G.D. and E.K. wrote the original manuscript draft. J.S. revised and edited the manuscript. F.R. and J.S. conducted the project and were G.D. advisors for his internship. All authors have read and agreed to the published version of the manuscript.

Funding: This research was made possible through an internship funded by ISEP, France.

Acknowledgments: This study has been approved by a French ethical committee (Comité de Protection des Personnes) and all participants gave informed consent. The authors would like to thank M. Clément Royer who helped us during the revision phase of this paper.

Conflicts of Interest: The authors declare no conflict of interest.

Abbreviations

The following abbreviations are used in this manuscript:

AE	Autoencoder
ARMD or AMD	Age Related Macular Degeneration
BCM	Binary Change Map
CNN	Convolutional Neural Networks
cSLO	confocal Scanning Laser Ophthalmoscopy
FAF	Fundus Autofluorescence
GA	Geographic Atrophy
IR	Infrared
OCT	Optical Coherence Tomography
PCA	Principal Component Analysis
RE	Reconstruction Error
RPE	Retinal Pigment Epithelium

References

1. Kanagasingam, Y.; Bhuiyan, A.; Abràmoff, M.D.; Smith, R.T.; Goldschmidt, L.; Wong, T.Y. Progress on retinal image analysis for age related macular degeneration. *Prog. Retin. Eye Res.* **2014**, *38*, 20–42. [CrossRef]
2. Priya, R.; Aruna, P. Automated diagnosis of Age-related macular degeneration from color retinal fundus images. In Proceedings of the 2011 3rd International Conference on Electronics Computer Technology, Kanyakumari, India, 8–10 April 2011; Volume 2, pp. 227–230.
3. Köse, C.; Sevik, U.; Gençalioglu, O. Automatic segmentation of age-related macular degeneration in retinal fundus images. *Comput. Biol. Med.* **2008**, *38*, 611–619. [CrossRef]
4. Ramsey, D.J.; Sunness, J.S.; Malviya, P.; Applegate, C.; Hager, G.D.; Handa, J.T. Automated image alignment and segmentation to follow progression of geographic atrophy in age-related macular degeneration. *Retina* **2014**, *34*, 1296–1307. [CrossRef]
5. Köse, C.; Sevik, U.; Gençalioğlu, O.; Ikibaş, C.; Kayikiçioğlu, T. A Statistical Segmentation Method for Measuring Age-Related Macular Degeneration in Retinal Fundus Images. *J. Med. Syst.* **2010**, *34*, 1–13. [CrossRef]
6. Marrugo, A.G.; Millan, M.S.; Sorel, M.; Sroubek, F. Retinal image restoration by means of blind deconvolution. *J. Biomed. Opt.* **2011**, *16*, 116016. [CrossRef]
7. Feeny, A.K.; Tadarati, M.; Freund, D.E.; Bressler, N.M.; Burlina, P. Automated segmentation of geographic atrophy of the retinal epithelium via random forests in AREDS color fundus images. *Comput. Biol. Med.* **2015**, *65*, 124–136. [CrossRef]
8. Lee, N.; Laine, A.F.; Smith, R.T. A hybrid segmentation approach for geographic atrophy in fundus auto-fluorescence images for diagnosis of age-related macular degeneration. In Proceedings of the 2007 29th Annual International Conference of the IEEE Engineering in Medicine and Biology Society, Lyon, France, 22–26 August 2007; pp. 4965–4968.
9. Hu, Z.; Medioni, G.G.; Hernandez, M.; Sadda, S.R. Automated segmentation of geographic atrophy in fundus autofluorescence images using supervised pixel classification. *J. Med. Imaging* **2015**, *2*, 014501. [CrossRef]
10. Hu, Z.; Medioni, G.G.; Hernandez, M.; Hariri, A.; Wu, X.; Sadda, S.R. Segmentation of the geographic atrophy in spectral-domain optical coherence tomography and fundus autofluorescence images. *Investig. Ophthalmol. Vis. Sci.* **2013**, *54*, 8375–8383. [CrossRef]
11. Troglio, G.; Alberti, M.; Benediktsson, J.; Moser, G.; Serpico, S.; Stefánsson, E. Unsupervised Change-Detection in Retinal Images by a Multiple-Classifier Approach. In *International Workshop on Multiple Classifier Systems*; Springer: Berlin/Heidelberg, Germany, 2010; pp. 94–103.
12. Troglio, G.; Nappo, A.; Benediktsson, J.; Moser, G.; Serpico, S.; Stefánsson, E. Automatic Change Detection of Retinal Images. In Proceedings of the World Congress on Medical Physics and Biomedical Engineering, Munich, Germany, 7–12 September 2009; Volume 25, pp. 281–284.

13. Hussain, M.A.; Govindaiah, A.; Souied, E.; Smith, R.; Bhuiyan, A. Automated tracking and change detection for Age-related Macular Degeneration Progression using retinal fundus imaging. In Proceedings of the 2018 Joint 7th International Conference on Informatics, Electronics & Vision (ICIEV) and 2018 2nd International Conference on Imaging, Vision & Pattern Recognition (icIVPR), Kitakyushu, Japan, 25–29 June 2018; pp. 394–398. [CrossRef]
14. Burlina, P.; Freund, D.E.; Joshi, N.; Wolfson, Y.; Bressler, N.M. Detection of age-related macular degeneration via deep learning. In Proceedings of the 2016 IEEE 13th International Symposium on Biomedical Imaging (ISBI), Prague, Czech Republic, 13–16 April 2016; pp. 184–188.
15. Burlina, P.M.; Joshi, N.; Pekala, M.; Pacheco, K.D.; Freund, D.E.; Bressler, N.M. Automated Grading of Age-Related Macular Degeneration From Color Fundus Images Using Deep Convolutional Neural Networks. *JAMA Ophthalmol.* **2017**, *135*, 1170–1176. [CrossRef]
16. Phan, T.V.; Seoud, L.; Cheriet, F. Automatic Screening and Grading of Age-Related Macular Degeneration from Texture Analysis of Fundus Images. *J. Ophthalmol.* **2016**, *2016*, 5893601. [CrossRef]
17. Wandeto, J.; Nyongesa, H.; Rémond, Y.; Dresp, B. Detection of small changes in medical and random-dot images comparing self-organizing map performance to human detection. *Inform. Med. Unlocked* **2017**, *7*, 39–45. [CrossRef]
18. Kohonen, T. (Ed.) *Self-Organizing Maps*; Springer: Berlin/Heidelberg, Germany, 1997.
19. Lee, N.; Smith, R.T.; Laine, A.F. Interactive segmentation for geographic atrophy in retinal fundus images. In Proceedings of the 2008 42nd Asilomar Conference on Signals, Systems and Computers, Pacific Grove, CA, USA, 26–29 October 2008; pp. 655–658.
20. Deckert, A.; Schmitz-Valckenberg, S.; Jorzik, J.; Bindewald, A.; Holz, F.; Mansmann, U. Automated analysis of digital fundus autofluorescence images of geographic atrophy in advanced age-related macular degeneration using confocal scanning laser ophthalmoscopy (cSLO). *BMC Ophthalmol.* **2005**, *5*, 8. [CrossRef]
21. Celik, T. Unsupervised change detection in satellite images using principal component analysis and *k*-means clustering. *IEEE Geosci. Remote Sens. Lett.* **2009**, *6*, 772–776. [CrossRef]
22. Kalinicheva, E.; Sublime, J.; Trocan, M. Change Detection in Satellite Images Using Reconstruction Errors of Joint Autoencoders. In *Artificial Neural Networks and Machine Learning—ICANN 2019: Image, Processings of the 8th International Conference on Artificial Neural Networks, Munich, Germany, 17–19 September 2019*; Proceedings, Part III; Lecture Notes in Computer Science 11729; Springer: Cham, Switzerland, 2019; pp. 637–648, ISBN 978-3-030-30507-9. [CrossRef]
23. Chong, Y.S.; Tay, Y.H. Abnormal Event Detection in Videos Using Spatiotemporal Autoencoder. In *Advances in Neural Networks—ISNN 2017, Proceedings of the 14th International Symposium, ISNN 2017, Sapporo, Hakodate, and Muroran, Hokkaido, Japan, 21–26 June 2017*; Proceedings, Part II; Cong, F., Leung, A.C., Wei, Q., Eds.; Springer: Berlin/Heidelberg, Germany, 2017; Volume 10262, pp. 189–196. [CrossRef]
24. Kanezaki, A. Unsupervised Image Segmentation by Backpropagation. In Proceedings of IEEE International Conference on Acoustics, Speech, and Signal Processing (ICASSP), Calgary, AB, Canada, 15–20 April 2018 .
25. Xia, X.; Kulis, B. W-Net: A Deep Model for Fully Unsupervised Image Segmentation. *arXiv* **2017**, arXiv:1711.08506.
26. Sublime, J.; Kalinicheva, E. Automatic Post-Disaster Damage Mapping Using Deep-Learning Techniques for Change Detection: Case Study of the Tohoku Tsunami. *Remote Sens.* **2019**, *11*, 1123. [CrossRef]
27. Hinton, G.E.; Salakhutdinov, R.R. Reducing the Dimensionality of Data with Neural Networks. *Science* **2006**, *313*, 504–507. [CrossRef]
28. Long, J.; Shelhamer, E.; Darrell, T. Fully Convolutional Networks for Semantic Segmentation. *arXiv* **2014**, arXiv:1411.4038.
29. Ronneberger, O.; Fischer, P.; Brox, T. U-net: Convolutional networks for biomedical image segmentation. In *International Conference on Medical Image Computing and Computer-Assisted Intervention*; Springer: Berlin/Heidelberg, Germany, 2015; pp. 234–241.
30. Van der Walt, S.; Schönberger, J.L.; Nunez-Iglesias, J.; Boulogne, F.; Warner, J.D.; Yager, N.; Gouillart, E.; Yu, T. scikit-image: Image processing in Python. *PeerJ* **2014**, *2*, e453. [CrossRef] [PubMed]
31. Chui, C.; Mhaskar, H. MRA contextual-recovery extension of smooth functions on manifolds. *Appl. Comput. Harmon. Anal.* **2010**, *28*, 104–113. [CrossRef]
32. Damelin, S.B.; Hoang, N.S. On Surface Completion and Image Inpainting by Biharmonic Functions: Numerical Aspects. *Int. J. Math. Math. Sci.* **2018**, *2018*, 1–8. [CrossRef]

33. Otsu, N. A Threshold Selection Method from Gray-Level Histograms. *IEEE Trans. Syst. Man Cybern.* **1979**, *9*, 62–66. [CrossRef]
34. Gers, F.A.; Schmidhuber, J.; Cummins, F.A. Learning to Forget: Continual Prediction with LSTM. *Neural Comput.* **2000**, *12*, 2451–2471. [CrossRef] [PubMed]
35. Cho, K.; van Merrienboer, B.; Gülçehre, Ç.; Bahdanau, D.; Bougares, F.; Schwenk, H.; Bengio, Y. Learning Phrase Representations using RNN Encoder-Decoder for Statistical Machine Translation. In Proceedings of the 2014 Conference on Empirical Methods in Natural Language Processing, EMNLP 2014, Doha, Qatar, 25–29 October 2014; pp. 1724–1734. [CrossRef]
36. Goodfellow, I.J.; Pouget-Abadie, J.; Mirza, M.; Xu, B.; Warde-Farley, D.; Ozair, S.; Courville, A.C.; Bengio, Y. Generative Adversarial Nets. In *Advances in Neural Information Processing Systems 27, Proceedings of the Annual Conference on Neural Information Processing Systems 2014, Montreal, QC, Canada, 8–13 December 2014*; Ghahramani, Z., Welling, M., Cortes, C., Lawrence, N.D., Weinberger, K.Q., Eds.; 2014; pp. 2672–2680.

Sample Availability: Sample images and the source code are available from https://github.com/gouzmi/Unsupervised-Change-Detection and https://github.com/gouzmi/Env_DMLA (for the other methods and extra samples). Please note that since we are dealing with medical images, we are only allowed to disclose a limited number of them and not the full time series.

© 2020 by the authors. Licensee MDPI, Basel, Switzerland. This article is an open access article distributed under the terms and conditions of the Creative Commons Attribution (CC BY) license (http://creativecommons.org/licenses/by/4.0/).

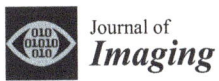

Article

Classification Models for Skin Tumor Detection Using Texture Analysis in Medical Images

Marcos A. M. Almeida [1,*] **and Iury A. X. Santos** [2]

[1] Departamento de Eletrônica e Sistemas, Centro de Tecnologia, Universidade Federal de Pernambuco, Recife-PE 50670-901, Brazil
[2] Departamento de Física, Universidade Federal Rural de Pernambuco, Recife-PE 52171-900, Brazil; iuryadones@gmail.com
* Correspondence: marcos.almeida@ufpe.br; Tel.: +55-81-2126-7129

Received: 13 May 2020; Accepted: 16 June 2020; Published: 19 June 2020

Abstract: Medical images have made a great contribution to early diagnosis. In this study, a new strategy is presented for analyzing medical images of skin with melanoma and nevus to model, classify and identify lesions on the skin. Machine learning applied to the data generated by first and second order statistics features, Gray Level Co-occurrence Matrix (GLCM), keypoints and color channel information—Red, Green, Blue and grayscale images of the skin were used to characterize decisive information for the classification of the images. This work proposes a strategy for the analysis of skin images, aiming to choose the best mathematical classifier model, for the identification of melanoma, with the objective of assisting the dermatologist in the identification of melanomas, especially towards an early diagnosis.

Keywords: texture analysis; melanoma; glcm matrix; machine learning; classifiers

1. Introduction

The skin cancer is among the most common types of cancer in the world [1]. Melanoma is the most dangerous type of skin cancer, caused by over production of melanin pigments that change the color and texture of skin, resulting as a dark area on the skin [2]. Data indicate that the incidence of melanoma, which is a type of cancer that metastasizes rapidly, has increased alarmingly [3].

However, visual analysis is limited by human visual ability, as well as human perception and sensitivity, in addition to the fact that not all melanomas have the same characteristics. The tumor is an exceptional expansion of human cells that reproduce in an unrestricted way and that can be identified by a variation of color and texture of the human tissue under study, making information contained in the images extremely valuable. Textures are visual patterns, which have brightness, color, slope, size and other attributes. When partitioned into sub-images by regions of interest, they are able to be properly classified.

Color is one of the significant features in the examination of skin lesion. The distribution of texture and color features presents significant information, as Figure 1 shows.

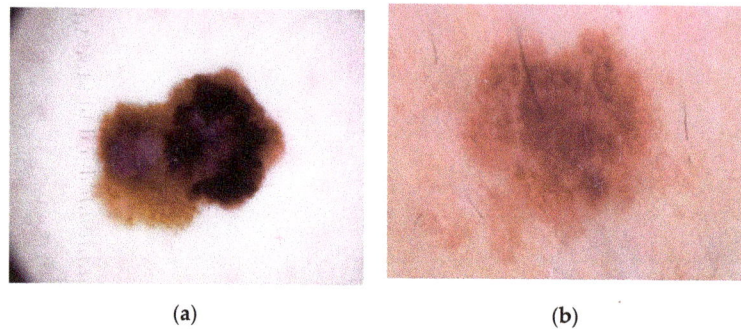

Figure 1. Images of melanoma and nevus tissues: (**a**) Skin lesion from melanoma image; (**b**) Nevus Skin.

A technique of analysis that focuses on the extraction of intrinsic characteristics of the image such as—brightness and color, providing an idea of the roughness or smoothness, among other characteristics, is texture analysis. Digital image texture analysis refers to techniques that use image processing in order to extract representative features of the images studied which can have importance in the discrimination between images.

This makes it possible to accelerate decisions concerning diagnosis. In these cases, image quality is essential, relying on bandwidth, sensitivity, resolution and signal-to-noise ratio of the image systems. Artificial intelligence can be very useful in assisting oncologists and radiologists in making early diagnoses of tissue regions with melanoma [4].

In Figure 2 a graphical representation of nearly 300,000 cases predicted indicates melanoma was the 19th most-incident tumor in the world in 2018 and will continue rising, according to the World Health Organization's (WHO) International Agency for Research on Cancer (IARC) study Globocan [5].

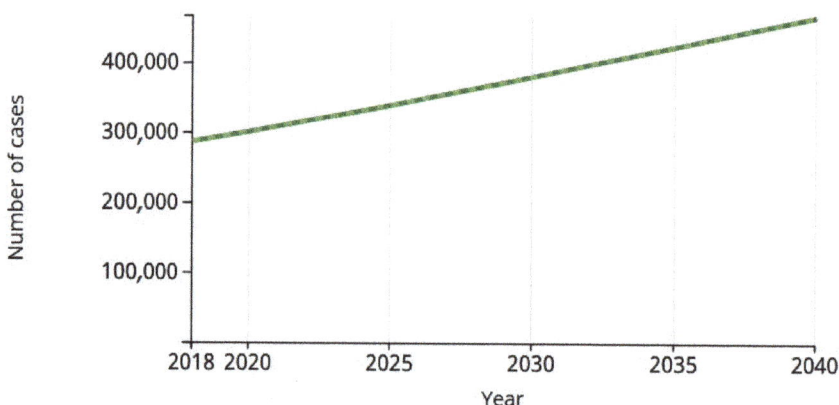

Figure 2. Estimated of incident cases from 2018 to 2040, melanoma of skin, both sexes, all ages. Source: International Agency for Research on Cancer of World Health Organization.

The estimate foresees that, this year, 2020, 1.81 million new cases of cancer and 9.5 million deaths due to neoplasia will occur. One in five men and one in six women are predicted to develop the disease over a lifetime. This is in contrast to the last survey published, in 2012, when the International Agency for Research on Cancer (IARC of WHO) predicted 14.1 million new cases and 8.2 million deaths.

According to the IARC, by 2020 there are expected to be 300,000 new cases of melanoma in the world.

In 2018, the number of melanoma cases was 287,723. The estimate for 2040 will be 466,914. Estimated number of deaths from 2018 to 2040 will be 42,208, melanoma of skin, both sexes, all ages.

Given the growth of demand for early diagnosis, a tool such as computer vision with a machine learning tool could help radiologists to produce relevant diagnoses more quickly and provide quantitative measures for regions suspected of having melanoma cancer. The works related to this research reveal this trend.

In this article, the new strategy is proposed through the addition of texture information, through the red, green and blue color channels, called here RGB components. In the process of acquiring the characteristics of the textures, using the Python syntax and the algorithms in the Python library to pinpoint the location of the region of interest (ROI) in the skin image, regardless of the image position.

Artificial intelligence when applied to the set of data representative of characteristic textures of the images, can assist oncologists and radiologists in identifying suspicious skin regions. Adequate experimental results have shown how this strategy can provide an accurate measure of quality that correspond to the subjective assessments by clinical experts [6].

The human eye, despite its perfection, is not able to capture certain details in an image or to distinguish small differences between certain micro-textures. Using Machine Learning, these differences can be measured, evaluated and compared to standard images and thus identify microtextural differences in medical examination images. Different parameters of texture reflect different properties within the image.

The purpose of resource extraction is to choose a data set representative of the original image measuring certain properties or resources that can distinguish a pattern between one sub-image and another.

This is a problem of binary classification, since the samples belonged to two classes—nevus tissue or melanoma, so the proposal for a solution for this new strategy for detecting melanoma is presented. All experimental simulations were implemented and executed using the Python language.

The paper is organized as follows—Section 2 presents the studies related to research, introducing the most common techniques used for the detection of tumors.

Section 3, deals with the theoretical framework in first and second order statistics.

Section 4 proposes strategies and solutions using a machine learning application for the detection of skin cancer.

Section 5 is dedicated to presenting the results of the experiments. Some discussions are presented in Section 6 and in Section 7 we make conclusions from the results of this study, with suggestions for new lines of research and future work.

2. Related Works

Some research works are related to our study because they use convergent techniques for texture analysis.

The diagnosis of skin lesions was studied by Zhang [7]. The analysis considered Convolutional Neural Networks (CNN) for automatic detection of skin cancer, comparing this with other research methods. The proposed method called CNN/WOA achieved an accuracy of 91.00%, with a sensitivity of 95.00% and specificity of 91.00%.

Pathan [8] reviewed the cutting-edge techniques declared in the literature, summarizing these state of art approaches. The steps included dermoscopic image pre-processing, segmentation, extraction and selection of peculiar characteristics and disposition of the skin lesions. The study also evaluated the consequences of the methodologies reported in the literature in addition to the results and future directions of research. The best result from the listed methods and algorithms was the Otsu threshold with Active Contour using a Sparse-Field level-set method, with a precision ability of 97.50% for the detection of melanomas.

Lee et al. [9] proposed the skin disease classification solution using Fine-tuned Neural Networks. The model achieved an accuracy of 89.90% and 78.50% in the validation set and the test set, respectively.

Using the technique of aggregating robust convolutional neural networks (CNNs) into a structure, Harangi [10] achieved classification results in three classes of injuries. The experimental results concluded that the average area under the receiver operating characteristic curve (AUC) was 89.10% for the task of categorizing the 3 classes.

Li [11] proposed two deep learning methods to address three main tasks emerging in the area of skin lesion image processing, that is, lesion segmentation (task 1), lesion dermoscopic feature extraction (task 2) and lesion classification (task 3). The proposed deep learning frameworks were evaluated on the ISIC 2017 dataset. Experimental results show the promising accuracies of these frameworks, that is, 75.30% for task 1, 84.80% for task 2 and 91.20% for task 3 were achieved.

A method proposed by Abbadi [12], takes into account the techniques known as ABCD—Asymmetry, Edge, Color and Diameter. For the detection of melanoma, the metric TDS (Total Dermoscopy Score) was calculated to perform the classification. The accuracy found in the results was 95.45%.

Fernandez [3] proposed in his research the extraction of characteristics that appear in the image of the lesion and treated with the Gray Level Co-occurrence Matrix (GLCM) method. Then, during the detection phase, a set of classifiers determined the occurrence of a malignant tumor. The experiments were carried out on images obtained from the ISIC repository. The proposed system provides skin cancer detection accuracy above 88.00%.

Ansari [13] proposed a skin cancer detection framework using SVM for early detection of skin cancer. The dermoscopic image of skin cancer was obtained and submitted to different pre-processing strategies using filtering images. The GLCM system was used to select specific highlights on the image which were then used to help establish the classifier. The classification determined whether the image was of a cancerous or non-cancerous tissue. The accuracy of the proposed structure is 95.00%.

The following are references from other authors with their respective works and applications, using similar techniques for extracting characteristics in medical images.

The diagnosis of breast cancer subtypes using image texture analysis was studied by Waugh [14]. The analysis considered the distribution of the pixel intensities in the magnetic resonance images. The entropy parameters of the GLCM matrix resulted in significant contributions to image classification, which can be useful in the treatment and monitoring of breast cancer therapeutics.

Recently, Vamvakas [15] proposed the solution of a challenge in the diagnosis of magnetic resonance images, using advanced techniques such as Diffusion Tensor Imaging—distinguishing ambiguous images in the appearance of Glioblastoma Multiforme and solitary metastasis, using 3D textural resources with GLCM.

Jennitta [16] using GLCM and Local Standard Descriptor parameters, applied to magnetic resonance images of the brain, showed a promising approach to medical diagnosis.

Hiba Asri [17], with the objective of diagnosing breast cancer, used machine learning techniques, such as—Support Vector Machine (SVM), Decision Tree, Naive Bayes and K closest neighbors, in the Wisconsin Breast Cancer database. The results proved that the SVM had the best accuracy—97.13%.

In a recent study on lung cancer, Yoon et al. [18], selected parameters for texture analysis in magnetic resonance images. Correlation between tumor area and size was calculated by linear regression. The injection of contrast material was used to check the MRI images and improvements were recorded in the selected texture parameters, in a time window between 120–180 s.

A predictive and two probabilistic model for detecting cancer in the human liver using computed tomography images was shown by Seal [19]. Haralick [20] calculated parameters in the GLCM of images of the liver with injury and without injury, as made available with several classification models such as—Logistic Regression (LR), Linear Discriminant Analysis (LDA) and a predictive model using Multilayer Perceptron (MLP), to estimate the likelihood of a patient having liver cancer or not. It was proved that logistic regression (96.67%) obtained the best accuracy when compared to LDA (95.00%) and MLP (94.40%).

Harshavardhan [21] used the SVM (Support Vector Machine) to classify data extracted from brain images to characterize benign or malignant tumors. To evaluate the performance of these resources, several texture methods were used, such as the histogram, Gray Level Co-occurrence Matrix (GLCM), gray level execution length matrix (GRLM), all analyzed separately. Performance results ranged from 82.97% to 92.83%.

Bahadure [22] demonstrated an efficient proposal to identify normal and abnormal tissues from MRI images of the brain. The experimental results identified one classified with an accuracy of 96.51%, specificity of 94.20% and sensitivity of 97.72%. Machine learning techniques were used, with data on texture, color, contrast and GLCM of the studied images.

Abdel-Nasser et al. [23] proposed a method that generates a set of compact representations of infrared breast images, with competitive results (AUC = 0.989), able to differentiate between normal and cancerous cases.

3. Materials and Methods

There follows a general description of the statistical parameters used in the proposal of this work, for the extraction of characteristics from the images. These characteristics make up the co-occurrence matrix (GLCM) and are part of the keypoints, applied to each image.

Let f (x, y) be a function of two discrete variables x and y, $x = 0, 1, \ldots, N - 1$ and $y = 0, 1, \ldots, M - 1$. The discrete function f (x, y) can assume values for $i = 0, 1, \ldots, L - 1$, where L is the number of grayscale levels. The intensity-level histogram is a function showing (for each intensity level) the number of pixels in the whole image, which have this intensity:

$$h(i) = \sum_{x=0}^{N-1} \sum_{y=0}^{M-1} \delta(f(x,y), j), \tag{1}$$

where $\delta(i, j)$ is the Kronecker delta function

$$\delta(i, j) = \begin{cases} 1. & i = j \\ 0. & i \neq j \end{cases}. \tag{2}$$

The probability of occurrence of each pixel in the image that will appear in the histogram is given by:

$$p(i) = \frac{h(i)}{M}, \quad i = 0, 1, \ldots, L - 1. \tag{3}$$

These resources are determined automatically, constituting the first order statistics (Equations (4)–(7)) and used at keypoints. The average intensity of the grayscale is calculated by:

$$\mu = \sum_{i=0}^{L-1} ip(i). \tag{4}$$

The variance shows the degree of variability around the average grayscale distribution:

$$\sigma^2 = \sum_{i=0}^{L-1} (i - \mu)^2 p(i). \tag{5}$$

Skewness measures the asymmetry of the histogram:

$$\mu_3 = \sigma^{-3} \sum_{i=0}^{L-1} (i - \mu)^3 p(i). \tag{6}$$

Kurtosis is a measure of whether the data are heavy-tailed or light-tailed relative to the normal distribution. The kurtosis is a measure of flatness of the histogram.

$$\mu_4 = \sigma^{-4} \sum_{i=0}^{L-1} (i-\mu)^4 p(i) - 3. \tag{7}$$

The second-order histogram is defined as that Gray-Level Co-occurrence Matrix, that is a square matrix is formed by elements that indicate the probability of occurrence for a pair of pixels with intensities that depend on the distance d and the angle θ. Equations (8) through (14) make up the second-order statistics set.

$$p(i,j,d,\theta) = \{((x_1, y_1), (x_2, y_2)) : h(x_1, y_1) = i, h(x_2, y_2) = j\}, \tag{8}$$

where

$$(x_2, y_2) = (x_1, y_1) + (d\cos\theta, d\sin\theta). \tag{9}$$

In this study, the distances considered were d = 1, 2, ..., 5, with angles θ = 0°, 45°, 90° and 135°.

Energy derived from the second angular momentum measures the local uniformity of the shades of gray.

$$E = \sum_i \sum_j [p(i,j)]^2. \tag{10}$$

Entropy measures the degree of clutter between the image pixels:

$$H = -\sum_i \sum_j p(i,j) \log_2[p(i,j)]. \tag{11}$$

Correlation is a measure of how a pixel is associated with its neighbor across the image and assumes values ranging from ±1.

$$\rho = \sum_{i=0}^{L-1} \sum_{j=0}^{L-1} p(i,j) \frac{(i-\mu_X)(j-\mu_Y)}{\sigma_X \sigma_Y}. \tag{12}$$

Contrast is a difference moment of the GLCM and measures the amount of local variations in an image:

$$C = \sum_{i=0}^{L-1} \sum_{j=0}^{L-1} (i-j)^2 p(i,j). \tag{13}$$

Haralick [20] proposed a set of scalar quantities for summarizing the information contained in a GLCM. Originally these comprised a total of 14 features namely, angular second moment, contrast, correlation, sum of variance, inverse difference moment, sum average, sum variance, sum entropy, entropy, difference variance, difference entropy, information measures of correlation and maximal correlation coefficient. In order to obtain texture features, the normalized GLCM was computed for each of four orientations (0°, 45°, 90° and 135°).

GLCM expresses the texture feature according to the calculation of the conditional probability of the pixel pair of the gray intensities, for the different spatial positions [24].

$$p(i,j|d,\theta) = \frac{p(i,j,d,\theta)}{\sum_i \sum_j p(i,j|d,\theta)}. \tag{14}$$

The next step was to format a proposal, containing the extraction of characteristics from medical images to build a classification based on several state-of-the-art classifiers.

4. Proposed Strategy

The present study investigates the best strategy for aiding in the diagnosis of the presence or absence of melanoma through skin imaging. In the proposed strategy, what differentiates it from other methods of texture analysis is the inclusion of RGB components, adding texture information to the keypoints.

The developed strategy involves the following steps:

1. Random selection of a set of images with melanoma and nevus.
2. Generation of keypoints containing:

    a. first order statistics information;
    b. second order statistics parameters;
    c. RGB component information.

3. Extraction of characteristics from all training images.
4. Classification phase with the modeling using the training database.
5. Application of the selected model to a test image database.
6. Result of the model applied to the test database.

In addition, the algorithm used to read the keypoints does not depend on the image position, when capturing information in the region of interest—ROI.

The block diagram in Figure 3 shows the proposed strategy.

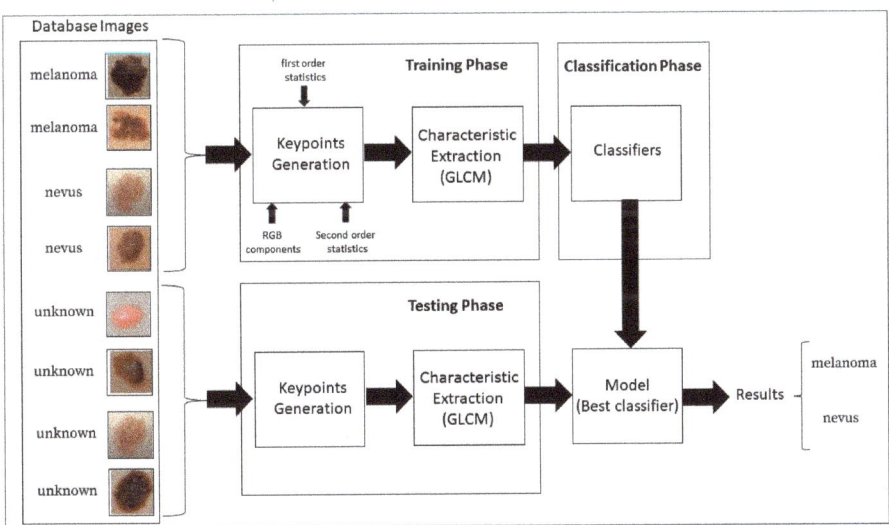

Figure 3. Block Diagram of the proposed strategy.

All data sets used are available in the Skin Lesion Analysis Towards Melanoma—International Skin Imaging Collaboration (ISIC) 2019 [25].

The database was formed by 2000 jpeg skin images, selected at random. The learning process was performed on 75% of the database, as in this research, 10 samples were used per image, the learning process analyzed a total of 15,000 samples. In the testing process, the remaining 25% of the images in the database were used, making a total of 5000 samples in the testing phase. Each sample had a dimension of 6 pixels × 6 pixels.

To increase the efficiency in extracting characteristics for differentiation of the tissues, it was necessary to add parameters as first and second order statistics into keypoints, such as—mean, variance, kurtosis, skewness, contrast, correlation, entropy, energy, maximum and minimum value, as well as RGB components.

After extracting the characteristics of the images, modeling was performed through training the database, using the best-known classifiers and their variations, as found in the academic literature:

- Stochastic Gradient Classifier. The basic idea of this classifier method is straightforward—iteratively adjust the parameters θ in the direction where the gradient of the cost function is large and negative. In this way, the training procedure ensures the parameters flow towards a local minimum of the cost function.
- Naïve Bayes Classifier. A Naive Bayes classifier is a simple probabilistic classifier based on applying Bayes' theorem (from Bayesian statistics) with strong (naive) independence assumptions. This classifier is among those common learning methods grouped by similarities which makes use of Bayes' theorem of probability to build ML models, especially those related to disease prediction and document classification.
- Decision Tree Classifier. A decision tree is a decision support tool that uses a tree-like graph and its possible results. It is a way to display the algorithm.
- Random Forest Classifier. Random forests are an ensemble learning method for classification, regression and other tasks, that operate by constructing a multitude of decision trees at training time. As a result, the classes (classification) or average forecast (regression) of these individually generated trees are grouped. This method aims at averaging many approximately unbiased but noisy trees to obtain low variances results. Is a collection of decisions tress, which, together, forms a forest.
- KNN Classifier. Classification is achieved by identifying the nearest neighbors to a query example and using those neighbors to determine the class of the query.
- Support Vector Machine Classifier. The objective of the SVM classifier is to find the hyperplane that separates the points of classes C_1 and C_2 with a maximum margin, linearly penalizing points within the margin through a regularization parameter selected by the user. Support vector machines bring a new option to the pattern recognition problem with clear connections in statistical learning theory. They differ radically from other methods, for example, neural networks—the training of an SVM always finds a global minimum and its simple geometric interpretation provides much scope for deeper investigations.
- Model Logistic Regression Classifier. Logistic regression classifies by using the log-ratios between the probability of groups given the data. For the groups g_1 and g_2:

$$\log \frac{P(G = g_1|X = x)}{P(G = g_2|X = x)} = \beta_0 + x\,\beta_x = 0. \tag{15}$$

The decision boundary is the value where the probability of the group given the data is equal. To find it, the likelihood function of β is maximized:

$$L(\beta) = \sum_{i=1}^{N} \log P g_i(x|\beta). \tag{16}$$

In machine learning, the classification identifies to which Class a set of observed data belongs. Classification is an example of pattern recognition. Some variants of the classifiers cited and available in the library of the Python environment were used, to increase the set of classifiers tested:

1. sklearn.linear_model.SGDClassifier;
2. sklearn.naive_bayes.GaussianNB;
3. sklearn.naive_bayes.BernoulliNB;

4. sklearn.naive_bayes.MultinomialNB;
5. sklearn.tree.DecisionTreeClassifier;
6. sklearn.ensemble.ExtraTreesClassifier;
7. sklearn.ensemble.RandomForestClassifier;
8. sklearn.ensemble.GradientBoostingClassifier;
9. sklearn.neighbors.KNeighborsClassifier;
10. sklearn.svm.LinearSVC;
11. sklearn.svm.SVC;
12. sklearn.linear_model.LogisticRegression.

After the computational effort using the twelve classifiers, the five best ones were selected, based on the area under the Receiver Operating Characteristics:

1. Linear Model Logistic Regression.
2. Gradient Boosting (Stochastic Gradient Boosting).
3. SVM Linear SVC (Support Vector Machine Linear—Support Vector Classification).
4. Linear Model Stochastic Gradient Descendent (Linear Model SGD).
5. SVM SVC (Support Vector Machine—Support Vector Clustering).

The results of the database simulation are provided in detail in the following sections.

5. Results

First-order statistics concern the distribution of gray levels in an image, where the first-order histogram is used as the basis for extracting its characteristics, such as—mean, standard deviation, kurtosis and skewness, as shown in Table 1. These are not sufficient, however, for decision making between what is melanoma tissue and what is healthy tissue. The Mann-Whitney U test applied to the parameters in Table 1 show that ($p < 0.05$), therefore, the null hypothesis is rejected. Meaning that the distributions of both samples (melanoma and nevus) are not the same.

Table 1. First-order statistics.

Parameters	Nevus Tissue	Melanoma Tissue	p-Value
Mean Intensity	0.4514 ± 0.14340	0.4204 ± 0.1543	0.000
Kurtosis	3.0953 ± 5.4136	3.6476 ± 6.7590	0.003
Skewness	0.1935 ± 1.7280	0.2479 ± 1.8501	0.022

The boxplot in Figure 4 shows that it is not possible to differentiate nevus tissue from tissue with melanoma by only observing the average intensity values.

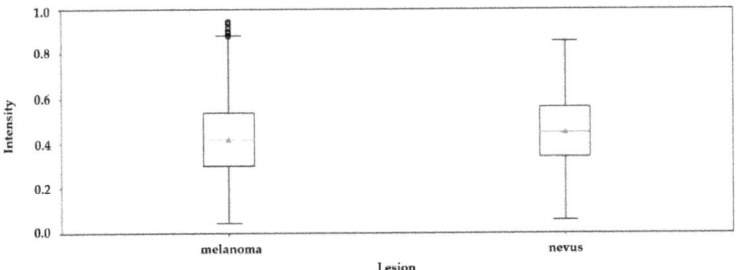

Figure 4. Boxplot with average intensities of grayscale images with melanoma and nevus.

Performance Metrics for Classifiers

In academic medical literature, instances are designated as positive, indicating the existence of the disease and negative, indicating the absence of the disease; thus, four possibilities arise when medical images are submitted to the classifiers:

- TP-True Positive: correctly classified positive cases.
- TN-True Negative: correctly classified negative cases.
- FP-False Positive: incorrectly classified negative cases.
- FN-False Negative: incorrectly classified positive cases.

The metrics that were considered to evaluate the classifiers for these were:

1. Accuracy is the ratio of the number of instances correctly classified to the number of all instances in the test suite.

$$Accuracy = \frac{TP + TN}{TP + TN + FP + FN} \qquad (17)$$

2. Sensitivity, also known as recall, is the ratio of positives predicted correctly relative to the actual number of positives in the test set.

$$Sensitivity = \frac{TP}{TP + FN} \qquad (18)$$

3. Specificity is the version of the sensitivity for negatives and indicates the proportion of negatives correctly predicted relative to the actual number of negatives.

$$Specificity = \frac{TN}{TP + FP} \qquad (19)$$

4. The F score is a metric that considers both precision and sensitivity by taking their harmonic mean.

$$F-score = 2 * \frac{recall * precision}{recall + precision} \qquad (20)$$

The ideal limit for all metrics is to reach the unit value.

Table 2 shows the five best classifiers in descending order by Area Under the Receiver Operating Characteristics (AUC); these presented the best performance, of the twelve tested.

In this study, considering the test database, the AUC of this set of classifiers, reached levels between 95.04% and 97.46%. All experiments were conducted under the same Python software setup.

Having a unique metric evaluation facilitates the decision-making process for selection of the best classifier from a set of the top five. This metric is the AUC. It provides a clear classification of preferences among all of them and therefore a clear choice of direction. Thus, the best classifier was the Linear Logistic Regression Model.

Table 2. Classifiers ordered by Area Under the Receiver Operating Characteristics (AUC).

	Classifiers	AUC	Precision	Recall	F1-Score	Support
1.	Logistic Regression	0.9746				
	Melanoma		0.98	0.97	0.98	269
	Nevus		0.96	0.98	0.97	231
	Accuracy				0.97	
	Weighted average		0.97	0.98	0.97	500
2.	Gradient Boosting	0.9699				
	Melanoma		0.97	0.97	0.97	269
	Nevus		0.97	0.97	0.97	231
	Accuracy				0.97	
	Weighted average		0.97	0.97	0.97	500
3.	SVM Linear SVC	0.9659				
	Melanoma		0.99	0.94	0.97	269
	Nevus		0.93	0.99	0.96	231
	Accuracy				0.96	
	Weighted average		0.96	0.97	0.96	500
4.	Linear Model SGD	0.9551				
	Melanoma		0.95	0.97	0.96	269
	Nevus		0.96	0.94	0.95	231
	Accuracy				0.96	
	Weighted average		0.96	0.96	0.96	500
5.	SVM SVC	0.9504				
	Melanoma		0.94	0.97	0.96	269
	Nevus		0.96	0.93	0.95	231
	Accuracy				0.95	
	Weighted average		0.95	0.95	0.95	500

[1] Linear Model Logistic Regression. [2] Stochastic Gradient Boosting. [3] Support Vector Machine Linear—Support Vector Classification. [4] Linear Model Stochastic Gradient Descendent. [5] Support Vector Machine—Support Vector Clustering.

The receiver operating curve (ROC) in Figure 5 is another common tool used with the binary classifier. It clarifies resource selection and the accuracy of the logistic regression classifier. The blue dotted line represents the ROC curve of a purely random classifier. A good classifier stays as far away from that line as possible, as here, in the upper left corner.

A suitable overall measure for the curve is the area under the curve (AUC).

The confusion matrix of the Logistic Regression method that describes the complete performance of the model is shown in Figure 6. This generates a sensitivity and specificity of 0.97.

The accuracy of a classification can be evaluated by computing the number of correctly recognized class examples (true positives), the number of correctly recognized examples that do not belong to the class (true negatives) and examples that either were incorrectly assigned to the class (false positives) or that were not recognized as class examples (false negatives) [26].

In the Linear Logistic Regression model, the recall for identification of melanoma was 97%. So, of the 500 medical images in the test database, 269 images were of melanoma and the classifier was 97% correct, that is, it identified TP = 261 images correctly, wrongly classifying FN = 8 of the images as nevus.

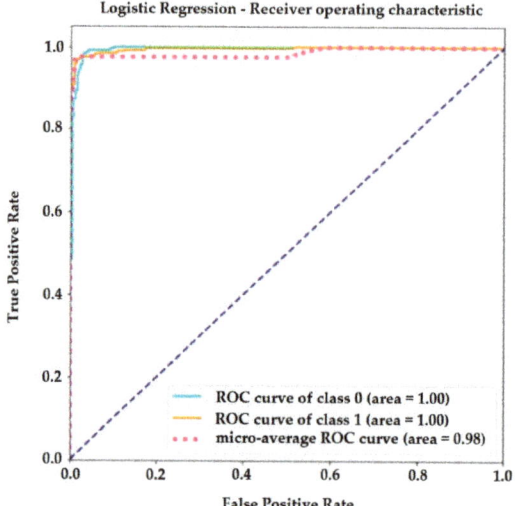

Figure 5. Receiver operating curve (ROC) curve of logistic regression.

Similarly, the recall for nevus identification was 98.00%. The classifier recognized TN = 226 images as nevus, classifying FP = 5 images as melanoma, for a total of 231 nevus medical images. The same reasoning can be made for the other classifiers listed in Table 2.

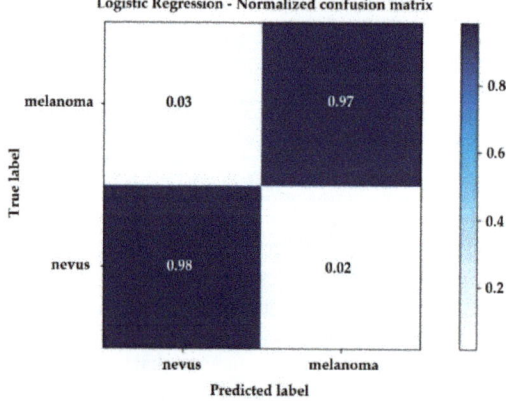

Figure 6. Confusion Matrix considering the Logistic Regression Model.

For the best performance model, the probability curve is shown through the sigmoid curve showed in Figure 7.

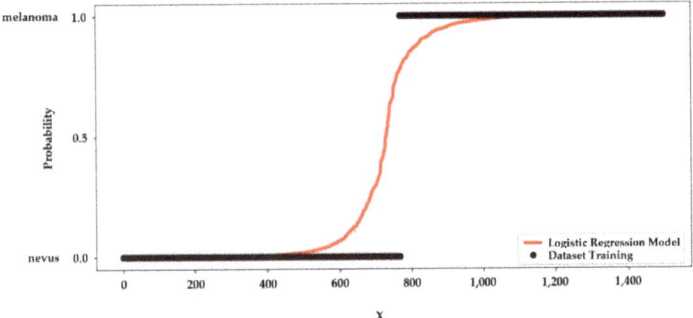

Figure 7. Logistic Regression Model of the Proposed Strategy.

Just as linear regression uses the least common square method to minimize error and to attain the best possible solution, logistic regression achieves the best results using the maximum likelihood method, plotting the probability curve as a function of the number of samples tested. The steeper this curve, the smaller the sample range that leads to the probability curve $0 < p < 1$, for diagnosis detection, $p > 0.5$ probably the tissue will be melanoma, if $p < 0.5$ the tissue will be nevus.

A ROC curve is a graphical tool used to understand the performance of a classification model. For a logistic regression model, a prediction can either be positive or negative. Also, this prediction can either be correct or incorrect.

$$False\ Positive\ Rate = \frac{FP}{TN+FP} = 1 - Specificity. = 84.01\%. \tag{21}$$

The Specificity is 15.99%. The number of positive and negative outcomes change as we change the threshold of probability values to classify a probability value as a positive or negative outcome. Thus, the Sensitivity and Specificity will change as well [27].

6. Discussion

Although the results were satisfactory with the use of statistical techniques, for future studies, it should be noted that when second order GLCM parameters were used, it is necessary to take some precautions regarding the size of the region of interest.

In some cases, the size of the ROI can change values in some parameters. For example, parameters describing the image homogeneity and complexity (angular second moment, entropy, sum entropy and difference entropy) are examples of parameters that depend on the ROI size, especially with small ROI sizes that approach a limit value [28].

The AUC found in this study, as shown in Table 2, considering the test database, reached levels between 95.04% and 97.46%, which corresponds to an accuracy between 95.00% and 97.00%, respectively. The Linear Model Logistic Regression classifiers were the most accurate.

This shows the effectiveness of second-order statistics and the inclusion of RGB components in the composition of keypoints in improving performance of the proposed strategy.

7. Conclusions

The proposed mechanism of identifying and classifying skin tissue is general; in future work it can be applied to other medical images to verify the results, since the strategy analyzes the texture of the images and reveals their differences according to the parameters set, enabling the image classification.

Texture analysis utilizes the changes in the grey value of image pixels and their distribution pattern, which can reflect microscopic pathological changes that are not visible to the human eye and can be used in the analysis of various images. Thus, texture analysis in medical imaging can be a substantial support for the clinical decision-making process in the diagnosis and classification of tumors. This methodology is expected to become more accurate than the human eye in detecting minute deviations in cell and tissue structures.

Statistical methods using GLCM features, associated with red, green and blue color information to perform micro-texture analyzes of human tissues and image classification for tumor detection showed great efficiency in the results presented.

The results show that for the detection of melanoma in human tissues, the logistic regression model was the best model with 97.00% of accuracy and precision on benchmark dataset and also a sensitivity and specificity of 97.00%.

The second-best method of classifying the data of the evaluated medical images was the Classification of the Gradient Boosting.

Author Contributions: M.A.M.A. and I.A.X.S. contributed in equal proportion to the development of the algorithm presented in this paper, which was written by the first author. I.A.X.S. was responsible for the Python implementation of the proposed algorithm. All authors have read and agreed to the published version of the manuscript.

Funding: This research received no external funding.

Acknowledgments: We would like to thank the International Skin Imaging Collaboration (ISIC), sponsored by the International Society for Digital Skin Imaging (ISDIS) for making publicly available databases on the ISIC Archive containing the largest publicly available collection of quality controlled dermoscopic images of skin lesions.

Conflicts of Interest: The authors declare no conflict of interest.

References

1. World Cancer Research Fund—American Institute for Cancer Research. Available online: https://www.wcrf.org/dietandcancer/cancer-trends/skin-cancer-statistics (accessed on 1 June 2020).
2. Karabulut, E.M.; Ibrikci, T. Texture Analysis of Melanoma Images for Computer-aided Diagnosis. In Proceedings of the Annual Int'l Conference on Intelligent Computing, Computer Science and Information Systems (ICCSIS-16), Pattaya, Thailand, 28–29 April 2016; Volume 1, pp. 26–29.
3. Fernandez, H.C.; Ortega, O.L. Félix Castro-Espinozaa and Volodymyr Ponomaryov. An Intelligent System for the Diagnosis of Skin Cancer on Digital Images taken with Dermoscopy. *Acta Polytech. Hung.* **2017**, *14*, 169–185.
4. Almeida, M.A.M. Use of Statistical Techniques to Analyze Textures in Medical Images for Tumor Detection and Evaluation. *Adv. Mol. Imaging Interv. Radiol.* **2018**, *1*, 1–6.
5. World Health Organization's (WHO); International Agency for Research on Cancer (IARC). Available online: https://www.iarc.fr (accessed on 2 May 2020).
6. Singh, P.; Mukundan, R.; De Ryke, R. Texture Based Quality Analysis of Simulated Synthetic Ultrasound Images Using Local Binary Patterns. *J. Imaging* **2017**, *4*, 3. [CrossRef]
7. Zhang, L.; Gao, H.J.; Zhang, J.; Badami, B. Optimization of the Convolutional Neural Networks for Automatic Detection of Skin Cancer. *Open Med.* **2020**, *15*, 27–37. [CrossRef] [PubMed]
8. Pathan, S.; Prabhu, G.; Siddalingaswamy, P. Techniques and algorithms for computer aided diagnosis of pigmented skin lesions—A review. *Biomed. Signal Process. Control.* **2018**, *39*, 237–262. [CrossRef]
9. Lee, Y.C.; Jung, S.H.; Won, H.H. WonDerM: Skin Lesion Classification with Fine-tuned Neural Netwporks. In *ISIC 2018 Lesion Analysis Towards Melanoma Detection*; Cornell University: Ithaca, NY, USA, 2018; pp. 1–4.
10. Harangi, B. Skin lesion classification with ensembles of deep convolutional neural networks. *J. Biomed. Inform.* **2018**, *86*, 25–32. [CrossRef]
11. Li, Y.; Shen, L. Skin Lesion Analysis towards Melanoma Detection Using Deep Learning Network. *Sensors* **2018**, *18*, 556. [CrossRef]
12. Abbadi, N.K.; Faisal, Z. Detection and Analysis of Skin Cancer from Skin Lesions. *Int. J. Appl. Eng. Res.* **2017**, *12*, 9046–9052.
13. Ansari, U.B. Skin Cancer Detection Using Image Processing. *Int. Res. J. Eng. Technol.* **2017**, *4*, 2875–2881.
14. Waugh, S.; Purdie, C.; Jordan, L.B.; Vinnicombe, S.; Lerski, R.A.; Martin, P.; Thompson, A.M. Magnetic resonance imaging texture analysis classification of primary breast cancer. *Eur. Radiol.* **2015**, *26*, 322–330. [CrossRef]

15. Vamvakas, A.; Tsougos, I.; Arikidis, N.; Kapsalaki, E.; Fountas, K.; Fezoulidis, I.; Costaridou, L. Exploiting morphology and texture of 3D tumor models in DTI for differentiating glioblastoma multiforme from solitary metastasis. *Biomed. Signal Process. Control.* **2018**, *43*, 159–173. [CrossRef]
16. Jenitta, A.; Ravindran, R.S. Image Retrieval Based on Local Mesh Vector Co-occurrence Pattern for Medical Diagnosis from MRI Brain Images. *J. Med Syst.* **2017**, *41*, 1–10. [CrossRef] [PubMed]
17. Asri, H.; Mousannif, H.; Al Moatassime, H.; Noel, T. Using Machine Learning Algorithms for Breast Cancer Risk Prediction and Diagnosis. *Procedia Comput. Sci.* **2016**, *83*, 1064–1069. [CrossRef]
18. Yoon, S.H.; Park, C.M.; Park, S.J.; Yoon, J.-H.; Hahn, S.; Goo, J.M. Tumor Heterogeneity in Lung Cancer: Assessment with Dynamic Contrast-enhanced MR Imaging. *Radiol.* **2016**, *280*, 940–948. [CrossRef] [PubMed]
19. Seal, A.; Bhattacharjee, D.; Nasipuri, M. Predictive and probabilistic model for cancer detection using computer tomography images. *Multimedia Tools Appl.* **2017**, *77*, 3991–4010. [CrossRef]
20. Haralick, R.M. Statistical and structural approaches to texture. *Proc. IEEE* **1979**, *67*, 786–804. [CrossRef]
21. Harshavardhan, A.; Babu, S.; Venugopal, T. Analysis of Feature Extraction Methods for the Classification of Brain Tumor Detection. *Int. J. of Pure Appl. Math.* **2017**, *117*, 147–154.
22. Bahadure, N.; Ray, A.K.; Thethi, H.P. Image Analysis for MRI Based Brain Tumor Detection and Feature Extraction Using Biologically Inspired BWT and SVM. *Int. J. Biomed. Imaging* **2017**, *2017*, 1–12. [CrossRef]
23. Abdel-Nasser, M.; Moreno, A.; Puig, D. Breast Cancer Detection in Thermal Infrared Images Using Representation Learning and Texture Analysis Methods. *Electron.* **2019**, *8*, 100. [CrossRef]
24. Ayyachamy, S. Registration Based Retrieval using Texture Measures. *Appl. Med Inform.* **2015**, *37*, 1–10.
25. International Skin Imaging Collaboration. Available online: https://challenge2019.isic-archive.com/ (accessed on 2 December 2019).
26. Ashish, K. *Learning Predictive Analytics with Phyton*; Packet Publishing—Open Source: Birmingham, UK, 2016; pp. 346–352.
27. Sokolova, M.; Lapalme, G. A systematic analysis of performance measures for classification tasks. *Inf. Process. Manag.* **2009**, *45*, 427–437. [CrossRef]
28. Sikiö, M.; Holli-Helenius, K.K.; Ryymin, P.; Dastidar, P.; Eskola, H.; Harrison, L. The effect of region of interest size on textural parameters. In Proceedings of the 2015 9th International Symposium on Image and Signal Processing and Analysis (ISPA), Zagreb, Croatia, 7–9 September 2015; Institute of Electrical and Electronics Engineers (IEEE): Piscataway, NJ, USA, 2015; pp. 149–153.

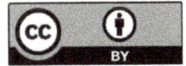 © 2020 by the authors. Licensee MDPI, Basel, Switzerland. This article is an open access article distributed under the terms and conditions of the Creative Commons Attribution (CC BY) license (http://creativecommons.org/licenses/by/4.0/).

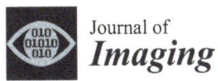

Article

Deep Multimodal Learning for the Diagnosis of Autism Spectrum Disorder

Michelle Tang [1], Pulkit Kumar [2], Hao Chen [2] and Abhinav Shrivastava [2,*]

[1] Science, Math, and Computer Science Magnet Program, Montgomery Blair High School, Silver Spring, MD 20901, USA; mtang@umiacs.umd.edu
[2] Institute for Advanced Computer Studies, University of Maryland College Park, College Park, MD 20742, USA; pulkit@cs.umd.edu (P.K.); chenh@cs.umd.edu (H.C.)
* Correspondence: abhinav@cs.umd.edu

Received: 5 May 2020; Accepted: 5 June 2020; Published: 10 June 2020

Abstract: Recent medical imaging technologies, specifically functional magnetic resonance imaging (fMRI), have advanced the diagnosis of neurological and neurodevelopmental disorders by allowing scientists and physicians to observe the activity within and between different regions of the brain. Deep learning methods have frequently been implemented to analyze images produced by such technologies and perform disease classification tasks; however, current state-of-the-art approaches do not take advantage of all the information offered by fMRI scans. In this paper, we propose a deep multimodal model that learns a joint representation from two types of connectomic data offered by fMRI scans. Incorporating two functional imaging modalities in an automated end-to-end autism diagnosis system will offer a more comprehensive picture of the neural activity, and thus allow for more accurate diagnoses. Our multimodal training strategy achieves a classification accuracy of 74% and a recall of 95%, as well as an F1 score of 0.805, and its overall performance is superior to using only one type of functional data.

Keywords: deep learning; multimodal learning; convolutional neural networks; autism; fMRI

1. Introduction

Autism spectrum disorder (ASD) is a lifelong neurological condition characterized by repetitive, restricted behavior as well as limitations in communication and social abilities, manifesting in a wide range of sensorimotor deficits [1]. Diagnostic processes for ASD are based on the assessment of social behaviors and language skills; however, there is limited understanding of the neural patterns behind the spectrum of autism behavior and the severity of the disease [2]. Recently, noninvasive brain imaging techniques have allowed for a better understanding of the neural circuitry underlying neurodeficiency disorders and their associated symptoms, such as ASD and its behavioral deficits. Specifically, functional magnetic resonance imaging (fMRI) allows physicians and medical experts to visually evaluate the functional characteristics or properties of a brain. This radioimaging procedure is able to assist neuroscientists in acquiring valuable and precise information on different neurological disorders [3]. For instance, in the diagnosis of ASD, instead of solely relying on observation and speaking with the patient, physicians analyze neuroimages for anomalies in brain activity, helping them more efficiently and precisely identify differences in their patients' neural pathways. Identifying the neural patterns of activation for ASD and associating these patterns with physiological and psychological features will aid scientists and medical practitioners in gaining more insight into the etiology of mental disorders [4].

Computational diagnosis: However, even with high-quality images, manual analysis is inefficient and at risk of human error, due to the variation between both doctors and patients. In an effort to make this process more objective, machine learning and computer vision techniques have frequently been applied in medical imaging problems to construct computer-assisted diagnosis systems [5]. State-of-the-art neuroimaging analysis uses activation maps, alternatively known as correlation matrices, which are constructed from the radiology scans. Activation maps provide information regarding the interaction between different areas of the brain by describing the relationship between their corresponding neural activity [6]. In doing so, the activation maps allow scientists to localize abnormal neural activity to specific regions of the brain and focus on those regions when manually analyzing the scans for anomalies.

Traditional machine learning in computer vision relies heavily on features pre-selected by medical experts. Early machine learning algorithms, e.g., support vector machines (SVM), k-nearest neighbors (KNN), decision trees, etc., analyze raw image data without any learning of hidden representations. On the other hand, deep learning (DL) algorithms in computer vision has shown significant advantage in capturing hidden representations and automatically extracting features from the given image data. Based on artificial neural networks structures, DL algorithms have multiple stages of non-linear feature transformation, which leads to hierarchical representations from pixels to edge, motif, part, and the entire object. State-of-the-art deep learning algorithms include convolutional neural networks (CNNs), recurrent neural networks (RNNs), long short term memory (LSTM) networks, generative adversarial networks (GANs), etc., which do not require manual processing or feature selection on raw data.

Related Work

The Autism Brain Imaginge Data Exchange (ABIDE) is a public, anonymized neuroimaging dataset that has been analyzed extensively in the past using various different techniques. Nielsen [7] analyzed ABIDE data to classify autism versus control subjects based on brain connectivity measurements. The study replicated earlier methods and implemented them on point-to-point connectivity data, and achieved roughly 60% accuracy with whole-brain classification.

Connectivity maps. The most common approach to fMRI analysis focuses on ROI mean time series data, since it is a representation of brain activity in distinct regions of the brain. Prior to analysis, pair-wise correlations are calculated between ROIs to form a functional connectivity matrix—each element of the matrix is a Pearson correlation coefficient representing the level of co-activation between the signals in the two ROI based on the time series data. The resulting matrix, also known as an activation map, is reshaped into a feature vector and then used as input into a classification algorithm [8,9].

Full-brain connectivity fingerprints. There are several arguments against exclusively using ROI time series data to analyze fMRI scans. The original form of each functional scan is a complete 3D scan of the brain across time (i.e., 4D matrix); thus, averaged ROI signal intensities only offers a partial representation of the fMRI scan, since by condensing the correlation matrix, one effectively loses the spatial structure of the connectome [10]. Khosla et. al. (2017) [9] proposed an alternative to relying exclusively on ROI data—instead of only computing the correlation between each region's signal intensities, they construct a full-brain connectivity "fingerprint" consisting of correlation coefficients between voxels from the fMRI scan and signal intensities from ROIs, incorporating both the spatial information offered by the original functional image volume along with the averaged time series data. The connectivity fingerprint is then used as input into a simple CNN architecture [8].

Multimodal learning. Computer vision and deep learning have been used extensively to achieve automatic disease diagnosis with medical imaging analysis [11,12]. Specifically, many machine learning problems involve the analysis of different forms of data to arrive at a result; as part of the classification problem, it is important to understand the relationship between these different data types, or modalities of data. Zhang et. al. (2018) [13] use generative adversarial networks (GANs) to translate between computed tomography (CT) and magnetic resonance imaging (MRI) data. Fukui et. al. (2016) [14] propose a new method for multimodal compact bilinear (MCB) pooling by computing the outer product of the different feature vectors from multiple modalities. MCB is based on previous compact bilinear pooling methods and allows for a more expressive and also efficient way of constructing a joint representation of both inputs [15]. The model was used to solve visual question answering (VQA) and visual grounding problems and outperforms state-of-the-art methods.

Our Approach. Previous studies on functional neuroimaging analysis use only one type of activation map in their evaluation [8,9,16]. In this study, we propose to include both activation maps in our analysis, and that by using two modalities instead of one, we will be able to create a more accurate and holistic representation of the functional imaging data, and thus achieve more accurate diagnoses. To do so, we propose a model architecture capable of analyzing both types of activation maps by combining different deep learning networks. Specifically, one of the inputs is the ROI time series activation map as described above, constructed by computing the correlation matrix between all pairs of ROI, and the second is the fMRI $\times$ ROI activation map. The pooling technique used in our model is a concatenation of the two feature vectors, which is then used as input to four fully-connected layers before the network outputs its prediction. The resulting classification system is a multimodal model, an automated disease classification system that uses two types of activation maps to predict whether the given patient is healthy or has autism. With both input modalities, the resulting diagnosis system is both more accurate and offers a more complete understanding of the functional data, and provides a powerful aid to physicians during the diagnostic process.

The main contributions of our method are highlighted as follows:

1. We propose an end-to-end deep neural network-based multimodal architecture that incorporates features from two different types of modalities. Our proposed architecture incorporates all connectomic information from the functional imaging data, which allows for a more comprehensive and holistic functional image analysis.
2. By incorporating both types of activation maps from the functional data, the overall performance of the classifier is improved and thus creates a more powerful diagnostic tool to assist doctors. Moreover, we also provide 'visual explanations' of the regions in fMRI images that our model utilizes to make diagnosis predictions. We believe this visualization offers transparency on the model and is crucial in providing effective assistance to the diagnostic process.

The remainder of this paper is organized as follows: in Section 2, we present the dataset and imaging modalities that were analyzed in our study, and our methods for analysis, including the preprocessing pipeline and network architectures; in Section 3, we discuss the details behind the training and testing of our constructed models; in Section 4, we present the results and performance metrics of each model and discuss them with respect to other publications in the field; and we present our conclusions and future work in Section 5.

2. Methods and Data

2.1. Data

In this study, we focus on the analysis of functional magnetic resonance imaging, or fMRI scans. The purpose of these images is to track changes in blood oxygen level-dependent (BOLD) signal in the brain across a period of time. Functional images are thus four-dimensional, where the dimensions (H, W, D, T) represent the height, width, depth, and time dimensions of the image volume, respectively [3]. fMRI scans can also be represented as regions of interest (ROI) mean time series data [17,18], which is constructed from the fMRI scan after preprocessing, and can be considered of as an abridged or summarized version of the complete multidimensional fMRI image volume. The ROI time series data is constructed by first segmenting the original fMRI scan functionally homogeneous regions (ROI), and then taking the average BOLD signal from each area. These ROIs are typically segmented using a functional parcellation brain atlas [19]; different atlases "segment" the full brain scan into different ROIs. For the purposes of our research, we chose to use the Automated Anatomical Labeling (AAL) atlas. After the regions have been specified, the BOLD signal intensities of each voxel are averaged across all voxels enclosed in the region, to return one intensity value for each time frame. The result is a T-dimensional vector for every ROI, where T represents the number of seconds for which the signal was measured. Thus, for each subject, one ROI mean time series volume is a 2D matrix with dimensions (N, T), where N represents the number of ROIs [8].

However, the BOLD signal measured by fMRI images represents changes in the blood oxygenation of brain tissue, and are not equivalent to neural activity [20]. Thus, it is not appropriate to directly use the fMRI scan of BOLD signals nor the ROI time series data as input for analysis. Instead, correlations between the time series data must be computed, either between voxels and ROIs or only pairs of ROIs—these correlations serve as the two different features used in our model. The resulting output from this step is a correlation matrix or activation map, which indicates points in the scan where there is neural activity.

This study was conducted on the ABIDE dataset [21], a multi-site open-access MRI study containing anonymized patient neuroimaging data. Data from the first phase of the study (ABIDE-I) was used in our analysis, which consisted of fMRI images and regions of interest (ROI) time series signals from both control and disease groups. The original ABIDE-I dataset consists of 1112 subjects; in this study, 77 subjects were removed from consideration due to low quality or missing scans. This yielded a total of 1035 subjects, with 505 individuals diagnosed with ASD and 530 typical controls, from 17 sites.

2.2. Preprocessing

Prior to classification, neuroimaging and connectomic data must be appropriately preprocessed in order to allow efficient and precise analysis. Preprocessing can be divided into two steps, as outlined in the following sections: (1) preparation and quality assessment of neuro-images and extraction of time series data and (2) feature preprocessing.

2.2.1. Preprocessing of Neuro-images

As previously mentioned (see Section 2.1), the dataset used in this study consists of images collected from 17 different sites [21]. The standard preprocessing steps were taken to prepare the neuroimages for analysis using the Configurable Pipeline for the Analysis of Connectomes (CPAC) toolbox [10], which compiles preprocessing tools from multiple state-of-the-art neuroimaging analysis libraries, such as AFNI, FSL, ANTs, etc. Namely, the preprocessing frameworks in this pipeline include slice timing correction, motion correction, global mean intensity normalization and standardization of functional data to MNI space ($3 \times 3 \times 3$ mm resolution). We used data extracted with global signal regression and band-pass filtering (0.01–10Hz) in our analysis. After preprocessing was complete with the CPAC pipeline, ROI time series data was then extracted from the resulting fMRI images using the Automated Anatomical Labeling (AAL) functional parcellation brain atlas, which consists of $N = 116$ labeled regions [19].

2.2.2. Feature Preprocessing

As previously described in Section 3.1, connectomic data consists of the fMRI image scan, as well as the ROI time series data. While most state-of-the-art neuroimaging analysis studies focus on only one form of functional data, we computed both ROI connectivity matrices, i.e., ROI × ROI activation maps, and full-brain connectivity fingerprints, i.e., fMRI voxels × ROI activation maps, using the fMRI scan and ROI signal intensities.

Activation map of fMRI and ROI. The connectivity fingerprints between the functional images and mean time series data were computed by calculating correlation coefficients between every pair of voxels from the fMRI scan and ROI from the time series data [9]. We first restructured the 4D fMRI scan into a 2D matrix, such that each row of the matrix corresponds to one voxel, and each column is one intensity value at a given time T. The reshaped matrix would have thus have dimensions $(H \times W \times D, T)$. We then compute a correlation matrix between the voxel intensities and the ROI time series data; the resulting matrix will be of dimensions $(H \times W \times D, N)$, where N is the number of ROI.

Activation map of only ROI. The ROI functional connectivity maps were constructed by computing a correlation matrix for each subject, where each cell of the matrix contains the correlation coefficient between a pair of regions, i.e., the level of co-activation in the signals between any two given regions. Since the resulting correlation matrix is symmetrical along its diagonal, we removed the values in the lower triangle to delete the duplicates, and also deleted the main diagonal of the matrix, which represents the correlations of each region with itself. The remaining matrix values were then reshaped into a vector of features to use as input into the model. The number of features in the final vector is given by $\frac{1}{2}((N-1)N)$, where N is the total number of regions [8]. Since the AAL brain atlas was used to extract the ROI time series data ($N = 116$), the resulting vector consisted of 6670 features. The entire feature extraction and connectivity matrix construction workflow is illustrated in Figure 1.

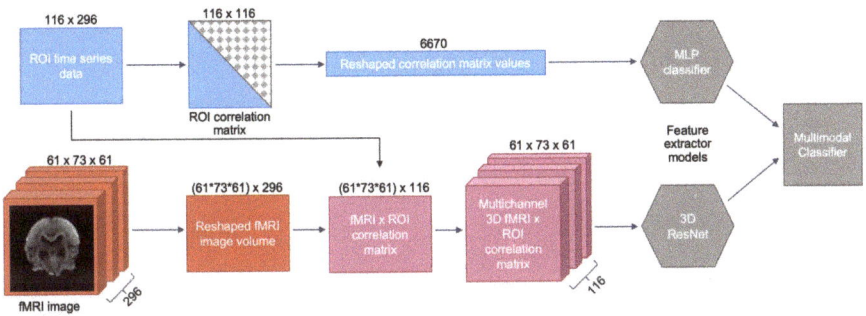

Figure 1. Preprocessing workflow. Construction of correlation matrices, or activation maps (terms are used interchangeably) between fMRI voxels × ROI time series and between pairs of ROI time series alone. Numbers on edges of the objects indicate matrix dimensions at the current step, e.g., the dimensions of the fMRI scan and ROI time series data are ($H = 61, W = 73, D = 61, T = 296$) and ($N = 116, T = 296$), respectively. For more detail on ResNet and MLP network architectures, refer to Figure 2.

2.3. Network Architectures

In this neuroimaging classification problem, the input to the model is an fMRI × ROI connectivity fingerprint and a vector of ROI correlation coefficients, and the goal is to diagnose the subject as either positive (with autism) or negative (healthy) based on both inputs. The proposed multimodal model extracts representations for both the fMRI scan and the ROI input, pools the feature vectors using simple vector concatenation, and arrives at a diagnosis using the combined features, which are propagated through four fully-connected layers before being classified into one of two classes.

We extracted features from fMRI × ROI correlation matrices using a modified 18-layer Residual Network (ResNet-18) [22]. All 2-dimensional convolution layers were replaced by their 3-dimensional equivalents in order to process the multichannel 3D correlation matrices. The correlation matrices were all uniformly of the dimensions (61, 73, 61, 116), corresponding to (H, W, D, T) respectively. During training, the data is reshaped to be (116, 61, 73, 61) so that the ROI dimension is used as the number of input channels into the first convolutional layer of the ResNet-18 network. Max-pooling is performed following the input convolutional layer over a $1 \times 3 \times 3$ pixel window, with a stride of (1, 2, 2). The stride attribute determines how far the window or filter is moved in each dimension after every computation; e.g., with a stride of 2, the filter moves 2 pixels in the specified dimension. The matrix is then passed through a stack of convolutional blocks (Res-blocks), each with multiple convolutional layers, where we pass filters across the image to convolve over the height, width, and depth dimensions. The filters have very small receptive fields: $3 \times 3 \times 3$ (which is the smallest size to capture the notion of left/right, up/down, center). In the first two convolutional blocks, we also use $1 \times 3 \times 3$ or convolution filters. The convolution stride varies between 1 and 2 pixels depending on the dimension. Following the convolutional blocks, average pooling is performed over a 32 × 3 × 2 window, and the resulting output is a 512-D vector. The vector is then passed through a fully connected layer before returning the final model output.

ROI × ROI connectivity map features were extracted using a multilayer perceptron (MLP) classifier, which was a simple fully-connected network. The MLP consisted of three hidden layers, each with 100 nodes. As stated above, the ROI correlation matrices were reshaped into 6670-D vectors, where each element represents a pairwise correlation coefficient between the averageBOLD signal of two ROIs.

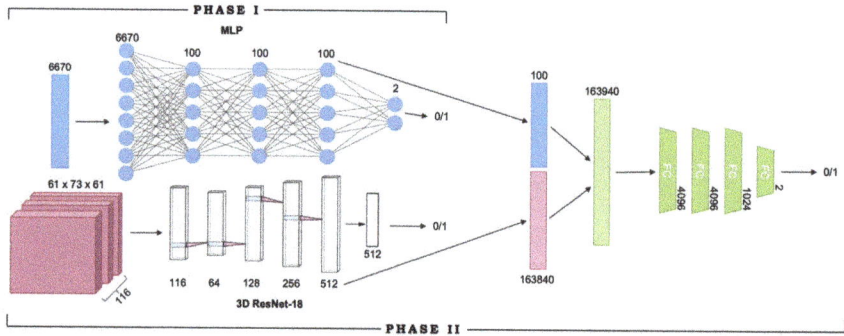

Figure 2. Multimodal network architectures and training phases. Visualization of the structure of the complete deep multimodal network. Numbers denote nodes or input channels in the labeled layer; FC implies fully connected layers. Phase I of training refers to the training of Resnet-18 and MLP for feature extraction; Phase II refers to the end-to-end training of the entire multimodal model after removing output layers from the feature extractors (as shown in the figure, the last 2-node layer of the MLP and the 512-channel layer of the ResNet are bypassed during Phase II of training.)

3. Experimental Details

Training occurred in two separate phases due to the nature of the model architecture, as described in Section 4.2. In Phase I, the feature extractors were separately trained as independent networks. Namely, the MLP was trained on ROI activation maps, and ResNet-18 was trained on fMRI × ROI activation maps. Upon completion of training for both networks, Phase II of training began. Both MLP and ResNet-18 models were truncated to remove their output layers to be used as feature extractors, and then combined with the four fully-connected layers to form the end-to-end model. The resulting multimodal network, built from the pretrained MLP and ResNet-18 models (the learned network weights of both models were saved and loaded into the multimodal network), was trained from scratch in Phase II, initialized with the learned weights from Phase I. After training is complete, we report performance metrics of classification accuracy, precision, recall, and F1 score for each feature extractor model, as well as the final end-to-end multimodal model. The full network architecture and the two training phases are visualized in Figure 2.

3.1. Training Details

Prior to training, the neuroimaging datasets was randomly split into the training and testing sets. 900 subjects were used to train the model, and the remaining 135 subjects were used to evaluate the trained model. The same training and testing sets were used in both phases of training, i.e., to train both the feature extractor models and the overall combined multimodal network to avoid polluting the test set with training data, or vice versa.

The ResNet-18 network used in this work is detailed in Table 1. We used a rectified linear unit (ReLU) activation function [23] after each layer and Softmax cross-entropy loss to train the network using minibatch stochastic gradient descent. We used a batch size = 8 and momentum = 0.9 to train both the feature extractor models and the end-to-end multimodal model. Both the feature extractor models were trained from scratch. To train the 3D CNN feature extractor, we used a learning rate of 1×10^{-2} for 30 epochs and dropped the learning rate after every 6 epochs by a factor of 1×10^{-1}; with the MLP, we used a learning rate of 1×10^{-2} across 50 epochs and dropped the learning rate by a factor of 1×10^{-1} after every 5 epochs. In the second phase of training for the end-to-end model, the feature extractor layers were initialized using the MLP and ResNet's weights learned during Phase I of training; the entire network was then trained end to end with a learning rate of 1×10^{-5} for 30 epochs. The learning rate was dropped after every 8 epochs for this network with a factor of 1×10^{-1}. All models were constructed using Pytorch [24] and were trained on a single Nvidia P6000 GPU. The end-to-end training process of both feature extractors and the complete multimodal model took roughly two hours.

Table 1. ResNet-18 architecture. Network architecture for 3D ResNet-18 model used for corr (fMRI, ROI) feature extraction. Building blocks are shown in brackets, with the numbers of blocks stacked.

Layer Name	3D ResNet-18	Output Size
conv1	$5 \times 5 \times 5$, 64, stride(2,2,2)	$32 \times 38 \times 32 \times 64$
Max Pool	$1 \times 3 \times 3$ max pool, stride(1,2,2)	$32 \times 19 \times 16 \times 64$
Res-block 1	$\begin{bmatrix} 1 \times 3 \times 3, 64, \text{stride}(1,1,1) \\ 1 \times 3 \times 3, 64, \text{stride}(1,1,1) \end{bmatrix} \times 2$	$32 \times 19 \times 16 \times 64$
Res-block 2	$\begin{bmatrix} 1 \times 3 \times 3, 128, \text{stride}(1,2,2) \\ 1 \times 3 \times 3, 128, \text{stride}(1,1,1) \end{bmatrix} \times 2$	$32 \times 10 \times 8 \times 128$
Res-block 3	$\begin{bmatrix} 3 \times 3 \times 3, 256, \text{stride}(1,2,2) \\ 3 \times 3 \times 3, 256, \text{stride}(1,1,1) \end{bmatrix} \times 2$	$32 \times 5 \times 4 \times 256$
Res-block 4	$\begin{bmatrix} 3 \times 3 \times 3, 512, \text{stride}(1,2,2) \\ 3 \times 3 \times 3, 512, \text{stride}(1,1,1) \end{bmatrix} \times 2$	$32 \times 3 \times 2 \times 512$
Average Pool	$32 \times 3 \times 2$ average pool	$1 \times 1 \times 1 \times 512$
Fully connected	512×2 fully connected layer	2

We present details of the ResNet-18 network architecture in Table 1 above.

4. Results

Due to the absence of any standardized benchmarks or training-testing set splits, it is difficult to compare against other published works in this field. Previous papers also do not evaluate networks using the same metrics, and thus do not all report precision, recall and F1 scores, and thus cannot be directly compared with our results. The following studies use different architectures and do not specify the data used for training and testing, and are meant to serve only as a reference to the present paper.

Previous studies on functional imaging analysis used only one type of correlation matrix or activation map as input. Khosla et. al. [9] analyzed the fMRI voxel and ROI time series activation map, and achieved 73% accuracy with their ensemble model. Guo et. al. [16] conducted studies on the ROI time series activation map, and achieved 81% accuracy using a fully-connected DNN network. Heinsfeld et. al. [8], also only used the ROI time series activation map, and report classification accuracies ranging from 52% to 70% using DNNs. They also studied the same data using support vector machines and random forests, which achieved 62% and 58% accuracy, respectively.

When trained on a random subset of 90% of the total ABIDE-I dataset and evaluated on the remaining patients, our proposed multimodal model is able to achieve an accuracy of 74% and an F1-score of 0.805. More importantly, we are able to reach a very high recall of 95%, which is crucial for a computer-assisted diagnosis system—when physicians diagnose patients for disease, a false negative can have extremely adverse consequences.

4.1. Ablation Results

We compare the performance of the feature extractor models and the combined multimodal model in Table 2. The ResNet-18 network, trained on fMRI × ROI activation maps, achieved a classification accuracy of 73.1%; the MLP classifier, trained on ROI × ROI activation maps, achieved a classification accuracy of 70.8%. When the feature vectors from both networks are pooled and used in the combined multimodal model, the resulting network has a higher classification accuracy of 74%, as well as a very high recall of 95% and an F1 score of 0.805, indicating that integrating both types of input in the model improves the overall network performance and be able to more accurately predict the correct diagnosis.

Table 2. Results and performance metrics. Classification accuracy, precision, recall, and F1 scores for both feature extractor networks and final end-to-end multimodal model.

Training Phase	Input	Model	Accuracy	Precision	Recall	F1 Score
Phase I	corr(fMRI, ROI)	ResNet-18	0.731	0.726	0.849	0.783
	corr(ROI, ROI)	MLP	0.708	**0.737**	0.759	0.749
Phase II	**Both** corr	Multimodal	**0.740**	0.699	**0.949**	**0.805**

4.2. Explanation of Model Predictions

Many medical imaging analysis techniques, especially those involving complex deep learning models, are difficult to interpret—it is difficult to decipher the inner workings of the networks or understand how they arrive at their predictions. To make our multimodal model more transparent, we visualized the regions of the fMRI images where the network focused on during the prediction process, as shown in Figure 3. Using gradient-weighted class activation mapping (Grad-CAM) as proposed by Selvaraju et. al. [25], we computed the activation gradients on the fMRI and ROI correlation matrices that were computed during the feature preprocessing stage of our study. We then overlaid these gradient-maps (heatmaps) on the original ABIDE fMRI scans to provide a clearer visual on which areas of the scan the model focuses on during the training and learning process. Through this visualization process, we were able to construct 'visual explanations' for the decisions made by our model by highlighting the important regions in the functional image for predicting the diagnosis. In doing so, we can clearly see the areas of the brain the model focuses on to identify differences between healthy control subjects and patients with autism. Moreover, this visualization will also aid doctors and physicians in the diagnostic process for ASD by assisting them in pinpointing the regions most likely to contain neural anomalies.

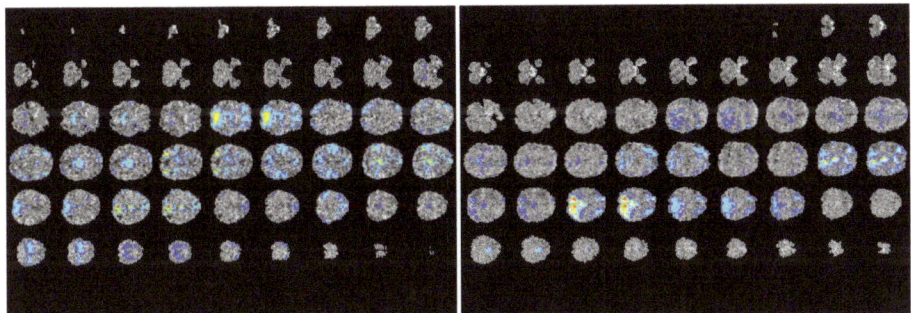

Figure 3. Explanations of model predictions. Cross-sections of fMRI scans indicating the regions that the network focused on when making predictions. Left: scans from a patient with autism; right: scans from a healthy individual with normal development. These images depict the regions the model used to predict the diagnosis of the scan, offering transparency on the model's decision-making process. The visualizations were produced using techniques proposed by Selvaraju et al. [25].

5. Conclusions

In this paper, we proposed a deep multimodal learning model for neuroimaging classification on the ABIDE dataset. Two types of functional imaging data, namely the activation maps calculated between fMRI image voxels × ROI time series and between only ROI time series, were used as input to two separate classifiers, a 3D ResNet-18 network and a multilayer perceptron classifier. The resulting feature vectors from these networks were pooled and used as input into several fully-connected layers to make the final prediction either control (healthy) or diseased (with autism). By proposing a model architecture that incorporates both types of activation maps, we use all the information provided by the functional data and demonstrate that the new model is capable of more accurate performance and thus makes for a better diagnosis system to assist doctors and medical practitioners.

However, at this point in time, the prediction accuracy of the multimodal model has only reached 74%, due to the limited amount of training data. This leads to the overfitting of our model. In the future, we plan to expand the training dataset by data augmentation and collecting more images to train our models in an effort to achieve higher accuracy. We hope that with further optimization and testing, we can eliminate any overfitting and reduce the amount of time needed for training. Moreover, we will be able to expand our analysis to other neuroimaging datasets, and demonstrate the generalizability of our methods by applying our automated system to diagnose more neurological diseases in addition to autism. With more testing and a larger quantity of data, we also hope to perform separate analysis on the visualizations of the model predictions, and to study the trends in which regions our model focuses on when making a diagnosis.

Author Contributions: M.T. conceptualized the research problem, collected and analyzed the data, and drafted the manuscript. A.S. supervised M.T., assisted development and edited the manuscript. All the authors have read and approved this version of the manuscript. Conceptualization, M.T. and A.S.; methodology, M.T.; validation, M.T., P.K.; visualization, P.K.; formal analysis, M.T.; investigation, M.T.; resources, A.S.; data curation, M.T., H.C.; writing–original draft preparation, M.T.; writing–review and editing, M.T., H.C., P.K., A.S.; visualization, P.K.; supervision, A.S.; project administration, M.T., A.S. All authors have read and agreed to the published version of the manuscript.

Funding: This research received no external funding.

Conflicts of Interest: The authors declare no conflict of interest.

Abbreviations

The following abbreviations are used in this manuscript:

MDPI	Multidisciplinary Digital Publishing Institute
DOAJ	Directory of open access journals
ABIDE	Autism Brain Imaging Data Exchange
CNN	convolutional neural network
Grad-CAM	gradient-weighted class activation mapping
ROI	regions of interest

References

1. Sparks, B.; Friedman, S.; Shaw, D.; Aylward, E.H.; Echelard, D.; Artru, A.; Maravilla, K.; Giedd, J.; Munson, J.; Dawson, G.; et al. Brain structural abnormalities in young children with autism spectrum disorder. *Neurology* **2002**, *59*, 184–192. [CrossRef] [PubMed]
2. Huerta, M.; Lord, C. Diagnostic evaluation of autism spectrum disorders. *Pediatr. Clin. N. Am.* **2012**, *59*, 103. [CrossRef] [PubMed]
3. Glover, G.H. Overview of functional magnetic resonance imaging. *Neurosurg. Clin.* **2011**, *22*, 133–139. [CrossRef] [PubMed]
4. Biswal, B.; Zerrin Yetkin, F.; Haughton, V.M.; Hyde, J.S. Functional connectivity in the motor cortex of resting human brain using echo-planar MRI. *Magn. Reson. Med.* **1995**, *34*, 537–541. [CrossRef] [PubMed]
5. Zhou, Y.; He, X.; Huang, L.; Liu, L.; Zhu, F.; Cui, S.; Shao, L. Collaborative Learning of Semi-Supervised Segmentation and Classification for Medical Images. In Proceedings of the IEEE Conference on Computer Vision and Pattern Recognition, Long Beach, CA, USA, 15–20 June 2019; pp. 2079–2088.
6. Friman, O.; Cedefamn, J.; Lundberg, P.; Borga, M.; Knutsson, H. Detection of neural activity in functional MRI using canonical correlation analysis. *Magn. Reson. Med.* **2001**, *45*, 323–330. [CrossRef]
7. Nielsen, J.A.; Zielinski, B.A.; Fletcher, P.T.; Alexander, A.L.; Lange, N.; Bigler, E.D.; Lainhart, J.E.; Anderson, J.S. Multisite functional connectivity MRI classification of autism: ABIDE results. *Front. Hum. Neurosci.* **2013**, *7*, 599. [CrossRef] [PubMed]
8. Heinsfeld, A.S.; Franco, A.R.; Craddock, R.C.; Buchweitz, A.; Meneguzzi, F. Identification of autism spectrum disorder using deep learning and the ABIDE dataset. *Neuroimage Clin.* **2018**, *17*, 16–23. [CrossRef] [PubMed]
9. Khosla, M.; Jamison, K.; Kuceyeski, A.; Sabuncu, M.R. 3D convolutional neural networks for classification of functional connectomes. In *Deep Learning in Medical Image Analysis and Multimodal Learning for Clinical Decision Support*; Springer: Berlin/Heidelberg, Germany, 2018; pp. 137–145.
10. Craddock, C.; Benhajali, Y.; Chu, C.; Chouinard, F.; Evans, A.; Jakab, A.; Khundrakpam, B.S.; Lewis, J.D.; Li, Q.; Milham, M.; et al. The Neuro Bureau Preprocessing Initiative: Open sharing of preprocessed neuroimaging data and derivatives. *Front. Neuroinf.* **2013**, *7*. [CrossRef]
11. Xu, Y.; Mo, T.; Feng, Q.; Zhong, P.; Lai, M.; Eric, I.; Chang, C. Deep learning of feature representation with multiple instance learning for medical image analysis. In Proceedings of the 2014 IEEE International Conference on Acoustics, Speech and Signal Processing (ICASSP), Florence, Italy, 4–9 May 2014; pp. 1626–1630.
12. Ayyachamy, S.; Alex, V.; Khened, M.; Krishnamurthi, G. Medical image retrieval using Resnet-18. In Proceedings of the Medical Imaging 2019: Imaging Informatics for Healthcare, Research, and Applications. International Society for Optics and Photonics, San Diego, CA, USA, 16–21 February 2019; Volume 10954, p. 1095410.
13. Zhang, Z.; Yang, L.; Zheng, Y. Translating and segmenting multimodal medical volumes with cycle-and shape-consistency generative adversarial network. In Proceedings of the IEEE Conference on Computer Vision and Pattern Recognition, Salt Lake City, UT, USA, 16–20 June 2018; pp. 9242–9251.
14. Fukui, A.; Park, D.H.; Yang, D.; Rohrbach, A.; Darrell, T.; Rohrbach, M. Multimodal compact bilinear pooling for visual question answering and visual grounding. *arXiv* **2016**, arXiv:1606.01847.
15. Gao, Y.; Beijbom, O.; Zhang, N.; Darrell, T. Compact bilinear pooling. In Proceedings of the IEEE Conference on Computer Vision and Pattern Recognition, Las Vegas, NV, USA, 26 June–1 July 2016; pp. 317–326.

16. Guo, X.; Dominick, K.C.; Minai, A.A.; Li, H.; Erickson, C.A.; Lu, L.J. Diagnosing autism spectrum disorder from brain resting-state functional connectivity patterns using a deep neural network with a novel feature selection method. *Front. Neurosci.* **2017**, *11*, 460. [CrossRef] [PubMed]
17. Logothetis, N.K. What we can do and what we cannot do with fMRI. *Nature* **2008**, *453*, 869. [CrossRef] [PubMed]
18. Arthurs, O.J.; Boniface, S. How well do we understand the neural origins of the fMRI BOLD signal? *Trends Neurosci.* **2002**, *25*, 27–31. [CrossRef]
19. Wang, J.; Wang, L.; Zang, Y.; Yang, H.; Tang, H.; Gong, Q.; Chen, Z.; Zhu, C.; He, Y. Parcellation-dependent small-world brain functional networks: A resting-state fMRI study. *Hum. Brain Mapp.* **2009**, *30*, 1511–1523. [CrossRef] [PubMed]
20. Smith, S.M. Overview of fMRI analysis. *Br. J. Radiol.* **2004**, *77*, S167–S175. [CrossRef] [PubMed]
21. Di Martino, A.; Yan, C.G.; Li, Q.; Denio, E.; Castellanos, F.X.; Alaerts, K.; Anderson, J.S.; Assaf, M.; Bookheimer, S.Y.; Dapretto, M.; et al. The autism brain imaging data exchange: Towards a large-scale evaluation of the intrinsic brain architecture in autism. *Mol. Psychiatry* **2014**, *19*, 659. [CrossRef] [PubMed]
22. He, K.; Zhang, X.; Ren, S.; Sun, J. Deep residual learning for image recognition. In Proceedings of the IEEE Conference on Computer Vision and Pattern Recognition, Las Vegas, NV, USA, 26 June–1 July 2016; pp. 770–778.
23. Nair, V.; Hinton, G.E. Rectified linear units improve restricted boltzmann machines. In Proceedings of the 27th International Conference on Machine Learning (ICML-10), Haifa, Israel, 21–24 June 2010; pp. 807–814.
24. Ketkar, N., Introduction to PyTorch. In *Deep Learning with Python, a Hands-on Introduction*, Apress ed.; Apress: New York, NY, USA, 2017; pp. 195–208. [CrossRef]
25. Selvaraju, R.R.; Cogswell, M.; Das, A.; Vedantam, R.; Parikh, D.; Batra, D. Grad-cam: Visual explanations from deep networks via gradient-based localization. In Proceedings of the IEEE International Conference on Computer Vision, Venice, Italy, 22–29 October 2017; pp. 618–626.

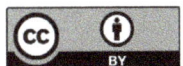

© 2020 by the authors. Licensee MDPI, Basel, Switzerland. This article is an open access article distributed under the terms and conditions of the Creative Commons Attribution (CC BY) license (http://creativecommons.org/licenses/by/4.0/).

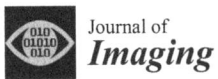

Article

Explainable Machine Learning Framework for Image Classification Problems: Case Study on Glioma Cancer Prediction

Emmanuel Pintelas [1,*], Meletis Liaskos [2], Ioannis E. Livieris [1], Sotiris Kotsiantis [1] and Panagiotis Pintelas [1]

1 Department of Mathematics, University of Patras, GR 265-00 Patras, Greece; livieris@upatras.gr (I.E.L.); sotos@math.upatras.gr (S.K.); ppintelas@gmail.com (P.P.)
2 Department of Biomedical Engineering, University of West Attica, GR 122-43 Egaleo Athens, Greece; melletis@hotmail.com
* Correspondence: ece6835@upnet.gr

Received: 30 April 2020; Accepted: 26 May 2020; Published: 28 May 2020

Abstract: Image classification is a very popular machine learning domain in which deep convolutional neural networks have mainly emerged on such applications. These networks manage to achieve remarkable performance in terms of prediction accuracy but they are considered as black box models since they lack the ability to interpret their inner working mechanism and explain the main reasoning of their predictions. There is a variety of real world tasks, such as medical applications, in which interpretability and explainability play a significant role. Making decisions on critical issues such as cancer prediction utilizing black box models in order to achieve high prediction accuracy but without provision for any sort of explanation for its prediction, accuracy cannot be considered as sufficient and ethically acceptable. Reasoning and explanation is essential in order to trust these models and support such critical predictions. Nevertheless, the definition and the validation of the quality of a prediction model's explanation can be considered in general extremely subjective and unclear. In this work, an accurate and interpretable machine learning framework is proposed, for image classification problems able to make high quality explanations. For this task, it is developed a feature extraction and explanation extraction framework, proposing also three basic general conditions which validate the quality of any model's prediction explanation for any application domain. The feature extraction framework will extract and create transparent and meaningful high level features for images, while the explanation extraction framework will be responsible for creating good explanations relying on these extracted features and the prediction model's inner function with respect to the proposed conditions. As a case study application, brain tumor magnetic resonance images were utilized for predicting glioma cancer. Our results demonstrate the efficiency of the proposed model since it managed to achieve sufficient prediction accuracy being also interpretable and explainable in simple human terms.

Keywords: interpretable/explainable machine learning; image classification; image processing; machine learning models; white box; black box; cancer prediction

---

1. Introduction

Image classification is a very popular machine learning domain in which Convolutional Neural Networks (CNNs) [1] have been successfully applied on wide range of image classification problems. These networks are able to filter out noise and extract useful information from the initial images' pixel representation and use it as input for the final prediction model. CNN-based models are able to achieve remarkable prediction performance although in general they need very large number of input instances. Nevertheless, this model's great limitation and drawback is that it is almost totally unable to interpret and explain its predictions, since its inner workings and its prediction function is not transparent due to its high complexity mechanism [2].

In recent days, interpretability/explainability in machine learning domain has become a significant issue, since much of real-world problems require reasoning and explanation on predictions, while it is also essential to understand the model's prediction mechanism in order to trust it and make decisions on critical issues [3,4]. The European Union General Data Protection Regulation (GDPR) which was enacted in 2016 and took effect in 2018, demanded a "right to explanation" for decisions performed by automated and artificial intelligent algorithmic systems. This new regulation promotes to develop algorithmic frameworks which will ensure an explanation for every Machine Learning decision while this demand will be legally mandated by the GDPR. The term right to explanation [5] refers to the explanation that an algorithm must give, especially on decisions which affect human individual rights and critical issues. For example, a person who applies for a bank loan and was not approved may ask for an explanation which could be "The bank loan was rejected because you are underage. You need to be over 18 years old in order to apply." It is obvious that there could be plenty of other reasons for his rejection, however the explanation has to be short and comprehensive [6], presenting the most significant reason for his rejection, while it would be very helpful if the explanation provides also a fast solution for this individual in order to counter the rejection decision.

Explainability can also assist in building efficient machine learning models and secures that they are reliable in practice [6]. For example, let assume that a model classified an image as a "cat" followed by explanations like "because there is a tree in image". In this scenario, the model associated the whole image as a cat based on a tree which is indeed pictured in the image, but the explanation is obviously based on an incorrect feature (the tree). Thus, explainability revealed some hidden weaknesses that this model may have even if its testing prediction accuracy is accidentally very high. An explainable model can reveal the significant features which affect a prediction. Subsequently, humans can then determine if these features are actually correct, based on their domain knowledge, in order to make the model reliable and generalize well in every new instance in real world applications. For example, a possible "correct" feature which would prove that the model makes reliable predictions could be "this image is classified as a cat because the model identified sharp contours" this explanation would reflect that the model associated the cat with its nails which is probably a unique and correct feature that represents a cat.

Medical applications such as cancer prediction, is another example where explainability is essential since it is considered a critical and a "life or death" prediction problem, in which high forecasting accuracy and interpretation are two equally essential and significant tasks to achieve. However, this is generally a very difficult task, since there is a "trade-off" between interpretation and accuracy [4]. Imaging (Radiology) tests for cancer is a medical area in which radiologists try to identify signs of cancer utilizing imaging tests, sending forms of energy such as magnetic fields, in order to take pictures of the inner human body. A radiologist is a doctor who specializes in imaging analysis techniques and is authorized to interpret images of these tests and write a report of his/her findings. This report finally is sent to the patient's doctor while a copy of this report is sent to the patient records. CNNs have proved that they are almost as accurate as these specialists on predicting cancer from images. However, reasoning and explanation of their predictions is one of their greatest limitations in contrast to the radiologists which are able (and obligated) to analyze, interpret and explain their decision based on the features they managed to identify in an image. For example, an explanation/reasoning of a diagnosis/prediction of a case image could probably be: "This image probably is classified as cancer because the tumor area is large, its texture color is white followed by high density and irregular shape."

Developing an accurate and interpretable model at the same time is a very challenging task as typically there is a trade-off between interpretation and accuracy [7]. High accuracy often requires developing complicated black box models while interpretation requires developing simple and less complicated models, which are often less accurate. Deep neural networks are some examples of powerful, in terms of accuracy, prediction models but they are totally non-interpretable (black box models), while decision trees and logistic regression are some classic examples of interpretable models (white box models) which are usually not as accurate. In general, interpretability methods can be divided into two main categories, intrinsic and post-hoc [6]. Intrinsic methods are considered the prediction models which are by nature interpretable, such as all the white box models like decision trees and linear models, while post-hoc methods utilize secondary models in order to explain the predictions of a black box model.

Local Interpretable Model-agnostic Explanations (LIME) [8], One-variable-at-a-Time approach [9], counterfactual explanations [10] and SHapley Additive exPlanations (SHAP) [6] are some state of the art examples of post-hoc interpretable models. Grad-CAM [11] is a very popular post-hoc explanation technique applied on CNNs models making them more transparent. This algorithm aims to interpret any CNN model by "returning" the most significant pixels which contributed to the final prediction via a visual heatmap of each image. Nevertheless, explainability properties such as fidelity, stability, trust and representativeness of explanations (some essential properties which define an explanation as "good explanation") constitute some of the main issues and problems of post hoc methods in contrast to intrinsic models. Our proposed prediction framework is intrinsic model able to provide high quality explanations (good explanations).

In a recent work, Pintelas et al. [7], proposed an intrinsic interpretable Grey-Box ensemble model exploiting black-box model's accuracy and white-box model's explainability. The main objective was the enlargement of a small initial labeled dataset via a large pool of unlabeled data adding black-box's most confident predictions. Then, a decision tree model (intrinsic interpretable model) was trained with the final augmented dataset while the prediction and explanation were performed by the white box model. However, one basic limitation is that the application of a decision tree classifier or any white box classifier on raw image data without a robust feature extraction framework would be totally inefficient since it would require an enormous amount of images in order to build an accurate and robust image classification model. In addition, the interpretation of this tree would be too complicated since the explanations would rely on individual pixels. Our proposed prediction framework would be able to provide stable/robust and accurate predictions followed by explanations based on meaningful high-level features extracted from every image.

This paper proposes an explainable machine learning prediction framework for image classification problems. In short, it is composed by a feature extraction and an explanation extraction framework followed by some proposed "conditions" which aim to validate the quality of any model's predictions explanations for every application domain. The feature extraction framework is based on traditional image processing tools and provides a transparent and well-defined high level feature representation input, meaningful in human terms, while these features will be used for training a simple white box model. These extracted features aim to describe specific properties found in an image based on texture and contour analysis. The feature explanation framework aims to provide good explanations for every individual prediction by exploiting the white box model's inner function with respect to the extracted features and our defined conditions. It is worth mentioning that the proposed framework is general and can potentially be applied to any image classification task. However, this work aims to apply this framework on tasks where interpretation and explainability are vitally and significantly prominent. To this end, it was chosen to perform a case study application on Magnetic Resonance Imaging (MRI) for brain cancer prediction. In particular, we aim to diagnose and interpret glioma, which is a very dangerous type of tumor, being in most cases a malignant cancer [12], versus other tumor types, which are most of the times benign. Some examples of extracted meta-features for this case study are tumor's size, tumor's shape, texture irregularity level and tumor's color.

The contribution of this work lies on the development of an accurate and robust prediction framework, being also intrinsic interpretable, able to make high quality explanations and make reasoning and justification on its predictions for image classification tasks. For this task, it is proposed a feature extraction framework which creates transparent and meaningful high level features from images and an explanation extraction framework which exploits a linear model's inner function in order to make good explanations. Furthermore, we propose and define some conditions which aim to validate the quality of any model's explanations on every application domain. In particular, if one model verifies all these conditions, then its predictions' explanations can be considered as good. Finally, 3 types of presentation forms are also proposed for the prediction's explanations with respect to the target audience and the application domain.

The remainder of this paper is organized as follows. Section 2 presents in a very detailed way our proposed research framework while Section 3 presents our experimental results, regarding the prediction accuracy and model interpretation/explanation. In Section 4, a brief discussion regarding our proposed framework is conducted. Finally, Section 5 sketches our conclusive remarks and possible future research.

2. Materials and Methods

2.1. Proposed Explainable Prediction Framework

Figure 1 presents the abstract architecture of our model which is composed by the feature extraction framework, which will be described in next subsection, a white box linear model and an explanation extraction framework. The great advantage of lineal models is that the identification of the most important features is very easy since it naturally comes out by the interpretation of their corresponding weights. A low weight's absolute value indicates low importance while in contrast a high, indicates high importance. We have to mention that although linear models are considered intrinsic interpretable models, this does not imply that they can also provide by default good explanations. Therefore, it was developed a new explanation extraction framework that will exploit the inner linear model's prediction function in such a way that will provide an easily understandable explanation output scheme which will satisfy all the proposed conditions that verify an explanation as good.

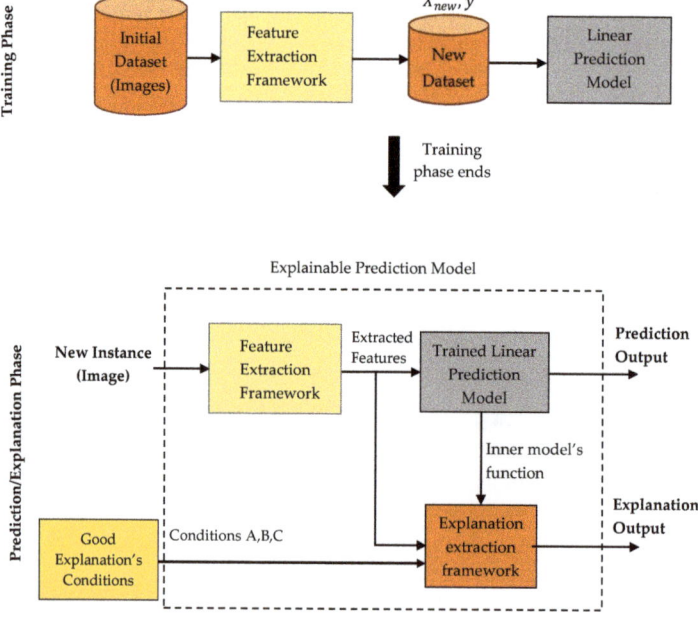

Figure 1. An abstract overview of our proposed explainable model.

2.2. Image Feature Extraction Methodology

In general, the input feature representation which a machine learning model uses to make predictions or the feature representation input that an explanation algorithm uses to make explanations (e.g., post hoc models) must be understandable to humans when the objective is the development of an explainable prediction model [8]. Therefore, we introduce a feature extraction framework which will create transparent and well-defined features from images by processing the pixel values from grayscale images based on traditional image analysis techniques, while these features will be also applied as an input on a prediction model. This feature extraction step is essential in order to convert the initial noisy pixel representation input of every image to a compressed, compact, robust and meaningful high-level feature representation input for the final prediction model while this representation will be meaningful to humans too. Following such approach, we can get rid of the black box approach of utilizing CNN models for image classification tasks and use instead simple, stable and intrinsic interpretable models as final predictors such as linear models.

It is worth mentioning that probably some of the utilized features will not be totally understandable to every human since the main audience domain which are directed to is for image analysts and therefore this fact points out our main approach's limitation. Based on this limitation, in Section 2.2.4 we provide a qualitative explanation in human understandable terms for some of these complex features in order to expand our model's explanations audience range. However, easily defined features such as size of object (e.g., tumor size in our case study), mean value of image pixels (e.g., tumor color tends to be black or white) and cyclic level (e.g., tumor shape tends to be cyclic or oval) are by default easily understandable to most humans but they may not be significant for the prediction problem which a machine learning model aims to solve. Therefore, identifying features understandable to humans being also informative and useful for the machine learning model, constitute a key factor for creating efficient and viable explainable prediction models.

2.2.1. Data Acquisition

As mentioned before, the main objective of this work is to apply the proposed framework on tasks where interpretation and explainability is vital and very significant. Therefore, we chose to perform a case study application on MRI for glioma tumor classification. The utilized dataset is publicly available [13]. In particular, it is consisted of 3064 head images with glioma (1426 slices), meningioma (708 slices) and pituitary (930 slices). The slices consist of 512×512 resolution, 0.49×0.49 mm^2 voxel size and tumor depicted in three planes (axial, coronal and sagittal). The main task of this case study is the identification of glioma tumor, since in most cases, the glioma lesion tends to be malignant while meningioma and pituitary (the other two main types of brain tumor) tend to be benign. Therefore, the images were separated in two groups. The first group includes glioma with 1426 instances and the other meningioma and pituitary with 1638 instances.

Our feature extraction procedure consists of two main image feature family types, texture and contour features. Texture features are extracted based on the image's pixel values intensities (e.g., gray levels) while contour features based on the shape of the Region of Interest (ROI) lied into the image. The final extracted dataset consists of 234 different features in total composed by 194 texture features and 40 contour features. Some examples of these extracted features from each image are area size of tumor, pixels mean value, intensity, variation, correlation, smoothness, coarseness and regularity [14].

The first step constitutes the identification of the ROI. The ROI was evaluated quantitatively using the manual segmentation by experts as ground truth. Figures 2 and 3 present some examples of extracted tumor areas.

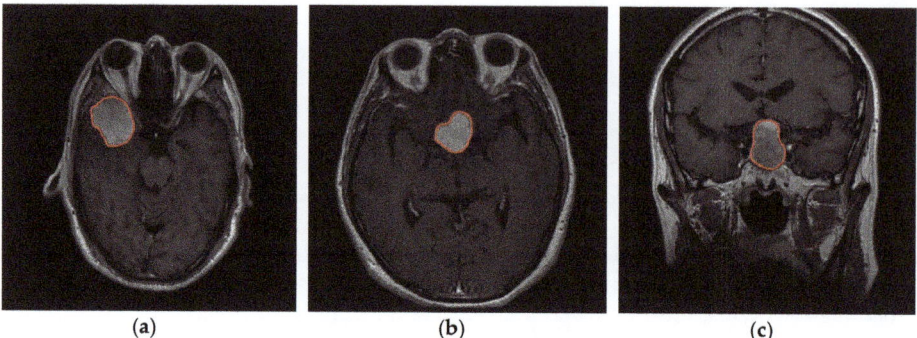

Figure 2. Head MRI examples. The red color illustrates the tumor area (**a**) glioma, (**b**) meningioma, (**c**) pituitary.

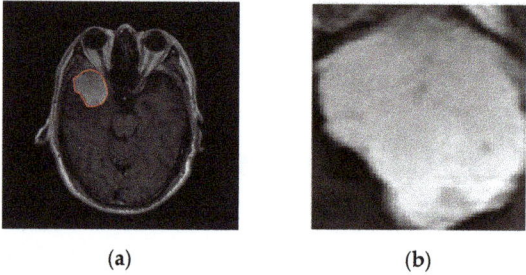

Figure 3. (**a**) Image with glioma, (**b**) Region of Interest (ROI) extraction.

The body of tumor is represented by pixels with different gray levels. Every pixel has significant information about the type of tumor. Furthermore, we normalized the images from 0 to 32 gray levels. The low values represent the dark color pixels and the high values the light white pixels.

2.2.2. Texture Features

Texture analysis is one of the high-speed feature extraction methods for image analysis and classification using the pixel's values. These methods mainly aim to describe the spatial distribution of intensities and the varying shades of pixels in images. In this study, three major approaches were utilized, the gray-level Co-Occurrence matrix, Run length and Statistical values from ROI matrix.

Co-Occurrence matrix [14] characterizes the texture of an image by capturing the gray-level values with spatial dependence from image, calculating how often pairs of pixel with specific values and in a specified spatial relationship occur in an image. In particular, we used the initial ROI matrix of every image and four more scales from wavelet transform [15] as pre-processing step, in order to find all pixel information. Then, the Co-occurrence matrices for every ROI image (initial plus four extracted filtered images) were calculated. The Co-Occurrence matrix is calculated by the following equation:

$$G = \begin{bmatrix} p(1,1) & p(1,2) & \cdots & p(1,N_g) \\ p(2,1) & p(2,2) & \cdots & p(2,N_g) \\ \vdots & \vdots & \ddots & \vdots \\ p(N_g,1) & p(N_g,2) & \cdots & p(N_g,N_g) \end{bmatrix}$$

N_g is the number of gray levels in the image and $p(i,j)$ is the probability that a pixel with value I will be found adjacent to a pixel of value j. Based on the Co-Occurrence matrix, meaningful features for every image can be extracted such as entropy, energy, contrast, homogeneity, variance and correlation. In total, we extracted 100 features via the Co-Occurrence approach. Some of the most significant identified features are presented in Table 1.

Table 1. Mathematic description of the most important identified features of Co-Occurrence approach.

Co-Occurrence Features	Formula
Correlation	$\frac{1}{\sigma_x \sigma_y} \left(\sum_{i=1}^{N_g} \sum_{j=1}^{N_g} p(i,j) - \mu_x \mu_y \right)$
Information Measure of Correlation	$(1 - exp[-2(HXY_2 - HXY)])^{\frac{1}{2}}$
Sum Average	$\sum_{i=2}^{2N_g} i p_{x+y}(i)$

where x and y are the coordinates (row and column) of the entry matrix, $p_{x+y}(i)$ is the probability of coordinated summing to $x + y$, μ_x, μ_y, σ_x and σ_y are the means and standard deviations of p_x and p_y which are the partial probability density functions,

$$HXY = - \sum_{i=1}^{N_g} \sum_{j=1}^{N_g} p(i,j) \log\{p(i,j)\}$$

$$HXY_2 = - \sum_{i=1}^{N_g} \sum_{j=1}^{N_g} p_x(i) p_y(j) \log\{p_x(i) p_y(j)\}$$

and HX, HY are the entropies of p_x and p_y.

Run length matrix is another way to characterize the surface of a given object or region utilizing a *gray level run*. A gray level run is a set of consecutive image points computed in any direction [16]. The matrix element (i, j) specifies the number of times that the pixel value appears in every direction. These elements correspond to the number of homogeneous runs of j voxel with gray value i [17]. From run-length method were produced 39 features. The most important run-length features identified via the interpretation of the weights of our utilized white box linear prediction model are Short Run Emphasis (SRE), Run Length Non-Uniformity Normalized (RLNUN) and Low Gray Level Run Emphasis (LGLRE) as presented in Table 2.

Table 2. Mathematic description of the most important identified features of Run Length approach.

Run-Length Features	Formula
SRE	$\frac{1}{N} \sum_{i=1}^{N_g} \sum_{j=1}^{N_r} \frac{p(i,j)}{j^2}$
RLNU	$\frac{1}{N^2} \sum_{i=1}^{N_g} \left(\sum_{j=1}^{N_r} p(i,j) \right)^2$
LGLRE	$\frac{1}{N} \sum_{i=1}^{N_g} \sum_{j=1}^{N_r} \frac{p(i,j)}{i^2}$

where Nr is the number of different run-length that occurs. Higher value of SRE indicates fine textures. RLNU measures the distribution of runs over the gray values and LGLRE is the distribution of the low gray-level runs [16]. These feature values are low when runs are equally distributed along grey levels indicating higher similarity in intensity values [17].

Statistical Values are features based on first and second order statistical analysis. The texture of an image is determined by the distribution over the pixels in calculated region. These features aim to describe specific properties of an image, such as the smoothness or irregularity, homogeneity or inhomogeneous while some extracted features are mean value, standard deviation, kurtosis, entropy, correlation and contrast.

2.2.3. Contour Features

In general, contour features aim to describe the characteristics and the information lied in the shape of objects. In our case study, tumor shape constitutes the object on every image as presented in Figure 4. For example, such features can describe if the tumor shape tends to be irregular or regular, oval or cyclic, large or small and so on. In our study, tumor size was identified to be the most significant contour feature (based on formulas described in Section 2.3.4).

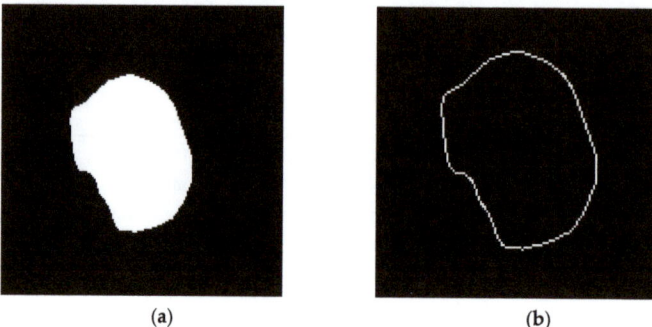

Figure 4. (**a**) Binary image, (**b**) border extraction.

This feature is described by the following formula:

$$tumor\ size = N_{in}$$

where N_{in} is the number of pixels inside the tumor object. It is worth mentioning that this is an informative feature for the final prediction model while it is also easily understandable in human terms. In general, the identification of features which are easily understandable to most humans while they are also useful for the machine learning prediction task, probably constitute some of the main research challenges and key elements in explainable machine learning domain. The identification of such useful and easily understandable features can contribute positively to this domain since the explanation of the model's decision would rely on features understandable in human terms and thus it would be able to address a much larger audience.

2.2.4. Qualitative Explanation of Extracted Features

We recall that an explainable machine learning model requires also an explainable feature representation in which the explanation output will rely on. Therefore, in the sequel it is attempted to explain in easy human understandable terms some complicated mathematically defined features of our framework. Table 3 presents a qualitative description of some of the most important identified features. For each of those features, we present two extreme example cases (high-low value comparison) in order to illustrate their main characteristics differences.

Correlation feature measures the linear relationship between two variables, which in our case, these variables are pixel coordinates. In other words, correlation measures the similarity between neighborhood sub-image's regions. In natural images, neighboring pixels tend to have similar values while a white-noise image exhibits zero (lowest value) correlation. A high correlation indicates the existence of an object, objects or some kind of structure lied in the image while a low correlation could indicate that there is no object in the image or it is not transparent enough. Regarding our case study, a correlation value can indicate how clear or not, the tumor can be seen in an image. For example, in Table 3, images on the 1st column (left) correspond to a very high correlation in contrast to images on the 2nd column (right). In the left image, a tumor (object) is clearly defined, in contrast to the right which no object can be seen at all.

Table 3. Qualitative description of some of the most important identified features.

Features	Tumor Examples		Description
	(High Value)	(Low Value)	
Correlation			Measures the linear relationship between two variables (pixels coordinates for images). In other words, measures the similarity between neighborhood sub-image's regions.
Information Measure of Correlation			Measures the amount of information that one variable contains about another. In other words, it measures how irregular is the texture of an image.
Sum Average			Provides the average of the grey values from ROI.

Information measure of correlation measures the amount of information which one variable contains about another (pixel coordinates for images). A high value can indicate that the pixel's intensities values of an image will tend to be smooth and regular while a low value that its pixel's intensities values will tend to irregular. This feature for our specific study can be defined also as "tumor's texture irregularity level".

Sum average feature aims to measure the average of the grey values from ROI. Although its mathematic definition in Table 1 seems to be a bit complicated, in practice it measures a very easily understandable in human terms feature. In particular, it aims to describe how light or dark is by average a gray image. In our case study, a high value indicates that the tumor's color tends to be white, a low value to be black, while an average value indicates that the tumor's color tends to be gray.

2.3. Machine Learning Prediction Explanations

Interpretable machine learning focuses on interpreting machine learning models' prediction mechanism in a reasonable form. More specifically, it aims to describe the mathematic or rule formula which an algorithm utilizes to make predictions, in a compact and meaningful form. An example is presented in Figure 5. Algorithm's interpretation mainly aims to present and interpret (e.g., via visualization of their decision boundaries) the model's decision function behavior. This can be very useful for machine learning developers, experts and data scientists in order to understand how a prediction model works, to identify its weaknesses and further improve its performance.

Explainable machine learning aims to explain machine learning models' predictions to human understandable terms. The definition of explainability is a very blur issue since it deals with humans and social aspects and thus explanations can be unclear and subjective [6]. Therefore, we have to define the properties of machine learning models' prediction explanations and clarify what should be considered as a good explanation. Our analysis below is based on the recent work of Christoph

Molnar in his book Interpretable machine learning [6], the popular research work of Ribeiro et al. [8] and the resent study of Robnik-Šikonja and Bohanec [9].

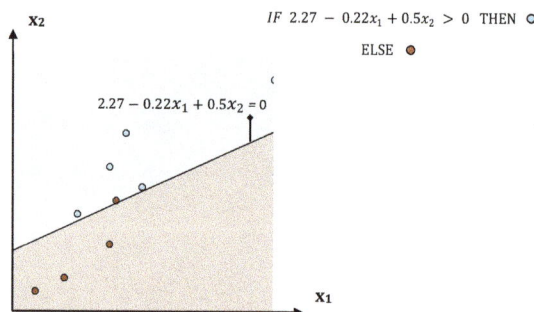

Figure 5. A visualization example presenting the decision function of a trained linear model.

2.3.1. Properties of Explanations

In general, an explanation usually has to relate in some way the features utilized by the algorithm in order to make predictions understandable to human terms. Some basic properties that explanations have, are described below.

Expressive Power is the language of the explanation output which is provided by the prediction framework. Some language examples are if-then rules, decision trees, weighted sums, finite state machines, graph diagrams, etc. This property is a very significant starting step for an explanation method since the way that this language will be defined, will determine the quality and the understandability of explanations to humans. Every machine learning algorithm has its own raw language in which makes decisions and predictions depending on its own unique computation formula and algorithm. If we just utilize the algorithm's raw output as the explanation output giving it to humans, it will be impractical, confusing and most likely not understandable at all.

For example, the raw interpretation output of a logistic regression algorithm (considered as white box model) applied on a specific dataset composed by three features could be:

$$\text{if } \frac{1}{1+e^{-(2+5x_1+7x_2-3x_3)}} > 0.5 \text{ then Output} = 1 \text{ else Output} = 0$$

which is probably not understandable and not meaningful to most humans. In contrast, decision trees models have by nature expressive power very close to human general logic since their explanation output come in an if-then-else total rule form composed by an ensemble of sub-rules which relate only one feature at a time. For example, an explanation output of a decision tree could be:

$$\text{if } \{(\text{sub-rule 1}) \text{ and } (\text{sub-rule 2}) \text{ and } (\text{sub-rule 3})\} \text{ then } (\text{Output} = 1) \text{else } (\text{Output} = 0)$$

where sub-rules 1, 2 and 3 could be $x_1 = $ "poor", $x_2 = $ "young", $x_3 > 95$ kg where $x_3 = $ "weight", respectively.

Then this is close to human reasoning and understanding as an expressive language.

Fidelity is a property, which describes how well the explanation output approximates the actual raw decision function of the prediction algorithm. For example, a decision tree model has very high fidelity since its decision function matches exactly with the utilized explanation output. In contrast, an explanation output for a black box model utilizing post-hoc methods has to approximate the original black box decision function for example with simple intrinsic models.

However, global fidelity which describes how well the explanation output approximates the complete model's decision function providing global explanations, is almost impossible to achieve in practice and thus the explanations focus on local fidelity which deals with specific data instances or local data instances and data sub-sets, providing instance and local explanations. Individual instances and local explanations are usually more significant in practice, since humans mostly care about explanations for every individual instance at a time or for instances, which belong to the same vicinity (similar instances), instead of giving a global detailed explanation for every possible instance which could lead to information overload and very confusing explanations. Nevertheless, global explanations or explanations which cover as much more instances and data sub-sets at the same time (also called representativeness of explanations), are very significant in order to ascertain trust in the model.

Stability refers to the ability of a prediction model to provide similar explanations for similar instances. This means that slight changes in the feature values of an instance will not substantially change the explanation. High stability is desirable since it can enhance the trust and reliability of model's decisions and explanations. Notice that a beneficial side effect of the stability property is that it can also diagnose possible overfitting behavior of a prediction model since lack of explanations' stability highlights also high variance of the model's decision function. Finally, it is worth mentioning that the more complicated a model's decision function is, the more unstable this model will probably be, while its function interpretation will be more difficult. This means that simple models with simple prediction function are stable models. However, this does not mean that all white box models are stable (since white boxes are usually considered simple models). A decision tree with a very large max depth will probably lead in a very complicated prediction function being probably extremely unstable just like a common complicated black box model.

Comprehensibility refers to the ability of an explanation to be short and comprehensive being understandable by most humans. This property is very significant since it defines how informative and understandable at the same time is an explanation. Comprehensibility is highly depended on the target audience. This means that different explanations may need for example, a mathematician/statistician comparing to the manager or director of a company. Therefore, this property is highly affected by the expressive power as mentioned before, since an intelligent choice and definition of the explanation's expressive power can lead to a very high comprehensibility factor with respect to the audience that the specific explanation is directed to.

Degree of importance refers to the ability of an explanation to reflect the most important features which affect the predictions. These features can describe the model's decision function in a global way, in a local way and in individual way. Global important features are the features which highly affect the decision function of the model taking into consideration all the instances trained on. Local important features are the features which highly affect the model's decision function taking into consideration local data sub-sets, while instance's important features are the features which highly affect the prediction just only for this specific individual instance. This global–local differentiation is very crucial since *"features that are globally important may not be important in the local context, and vice versa"* [8]. Therefore, an explanation for an individual prediction mostly cares for the specific features that affect this specific instance or similar to it instances, rather than describing the global important features.

2.3.2. Fundamental Property of Explanations

Nevertheless, even if an explanation possesses all of these properties, the main fundamental property than an explanation should have, is its humanistic social property which comes from the interactive dialogue between the explainer and the audience. An explanation which covers all factors for a certain prediction is not a human friendly explanation while the explanations have to be selected and come gradually via small answers based on the questions applied. More specifically, this dialogue comes up in a "questions–answers" form, where questions are in general contrastive and answers (explanations) are selected.

It was proved that humans' questions usually are contrastive and humans most of the times expect and desire selected explanations [6]. The term contrastive question means that questions are in a counterfactual form, e.g., *"Why the model predicted output 1 instead of 2?"*, *"What the prediction would be* if feature input X would be different?", "What is the minimum change required for feature input X in order the model to predict a different output result?". The term selected means that explainers usually select only one or two causes and present these as the explanation [6]. Therefore good explanations have to be able to answer contrastive questions and be selected, while this does not necessary imply that every other property described on previous section is not significant.

2.3.3. Proposed Conditions for Good Explanations

The definition and the validation of a good explanation can be considered in general extremely subjective and unclear. Therefore, taking into consideration the above analysis, we try to define three basic conditions that any prediction algorithm has to satisfy in order its prediction explanations to be considered good, stable, useful and easily understandable.

Condition A. Identification of features which highly determine the prediction result for the specific individual instance. This is probably the most significant and basic part of every explanation method since most of them mainly aim to identify these features. For example, the Grad-CAM method identifies and returns the pixels of an image which are important and determine a specific prediction for a black box model such as CNN. If the pixels' location, color level and volume can be considered as the raw initial features of every image, then such methods typically return the most significant features just like linear models would do via the interpretation of their weights on every feature variable.

Nevertheless, it is worth mentioning that by just returning the most significant pixels of an image which determined a specific prediction it does not always lead to useful explanations. If the objective is the identification of higher level representation features and properties that come out by pixels' grouping, such as shape and texture properties of an object lying in an image, which determine a prediction output, then relying only on pixels returns as explanations cannot reveal any useful information. For example, if a doctor classified a tumor image as malignant cancer and the main reason for this decision was just the tumor size and tumor's irregularity level, then pixels by itself are useless. Our proposed framework will be able to provide such type of explanations and this is the main difference comparing to other works which provide explanations based on image pixel returns.

However, explanations with pixels returns is very useful when the objective is the segmentation of an object (in our case tumor) or the identification of an object hidden in a noisy image, since the return of significant pixels would reveal if the model decided correctly utilizing the correct area of pixels or wrongly. For example, if a model classified an image as a cat, where this image actually illustrates a man hugging a dog and a cat, then explanations based on pixels returns would reveal if the model decided by cat's pixels (proper area) or another area e.g., dog's pixels where that would be obviously wrong.

Condition B. For a specific individual prediction identify some other instances such as local data sub-sets or instances that belong to the same vicinity (similar instances) which share the same prediction output and share at least one common explanation rule. This condition deals with the stability (robustness) and the representation property of model's explanations and as a result with the trust factor of a prediction model. An untruthful or unstable model, such as Deep Neural Network [18], probably will provide totally different explanations for similar instances. A very common example constitutes the adversarial attacks which aim to modify an original image in a way that the changes are almost undetectable to the human eye while the prediction function of an unstable model will probably be highly affected. In a very recent study, One pixel attack for fooling deep neural networks, 2019 [19] the authors revealed that the output of Deep Neural Networks can be easily altered by adding relatively small perturbations to the input pixel vector revealing that such models could be totally unstable and unreliable on image classification tasks.

Let assume a scenario in which an explanation method like Grad-CAM, identified for one new image (instance) the important pixels which determined a specific prediction. In order to ascertain some trust in the model, it would be very helpful if an explanation framework could also provide answers to questions like "For those identified pixels, what are their volume values in which this prediction *remains same?"* A possible answer (explanation) could be *"If the mean value of those pixels' volume is higher than 180 then the prediction will remain stable"*. In practice this means that for every new image which shares the same important identified pixels (or at least close to it) and the same rule: mean volume value > 180, then the model's prediction will remain the same. Obviously, if a method can provide meaningful explanations in a global way, this is desirable too, but generally this is almost impossible in practice and as already mentioned in previous section, humans usually care for individual explanations and explanations for local or similar instances.

Condition C. Identification of the most important features' critical values in which the prediction result will change. This condition aims to validate the explanation method's ability of answering contrastive questions based on the social humanistic property for making questions in a counterfactual form, as presented in previous section. Following the same previously defined scenario, some possible contrastive questions could be *"If those identified pixels were changing color and volume, what the prediction would be, would it be still the same? If not, what is the minimum change required for those pixel's mean volume value in order the model to predict a different output result?"* A possible answer (explanation) could be *"If their mean volume value increases by 30 then the prediction will change."*

Final Presentation form. Merge all explanation's information in a compact, selected, comprehensive and informative form, with respect to the targeted audience and application domain (significant the proper definition of expressive power). This step deals with the explanation framework's ability to create comprehensive and selected explanations which constitute some of the most significant properties of good explanations as already described in previous section. For instance, if the explanation framework was a decision tree, by default a decision tree is an example which provides information in a comprehensive and easy to read form, since one can just follow its nodes and easily verify and obtain the prediction result [7]. Nevertheless, we have to mention that even a decision tree which is naturally interpretable and explainable model, has to provide selected explanations in the case that the tree's maximum depth is very large. This means that one has to prune and select explanation rules from the global tree in order to provide selected and comprehensive individual explanations. This is a significant limitation because this procedure is not straightforward since it must define a probably subjective threshold for this pruning procedure.

2.3.4. Explanation Extraction Framework

Let assume the Logistic Regression (LR) [20] algorithm our utilized linear prediction model (it is worth mentioning that this framework theoretically can be applied on every linear interpretable prediction model). We have to note that one basic limitation of a Logistic Regression model is that it is restricted for binary classification problems and thus this limitation applies also to the proposed total prediction framework.

The prediction function of the trained LR model is given by the following formula:

$$f_{LR} = \begin{cases} 1 & F > 0.5 \\ \text{"unidentified"} & F = 0.5 \\ 0 & F < 0.5 \end{cases} \quad (1)$$

where F is defined by the following function:

$$F = \frac{1}{1 + e^{-(a_0 + \sum_{j=1}^{N} a_j x_j)}} \quad (2)$$

N is the total number of features, while if $F = 0.5$ then the prediction output f_{LR} will be *"unidentified"* meaning that the output can be either 0 or 1. In such cases, the prediction output can be chosen randomly or set by default to one value. By solving the inequality in Equation (1), the initial function can be simplified to:

$$f_{LR} = \begin{cases} 1 & G > 0 \\ \text{"unidentified"} & G = 0 \\ 0 & G < 0 \end{cases} \quad (3)$$

where G is defined by the following function:

$$G = a_0 + \sum_{j=1}^{N} a_j x_j \quad (4)$$

Let assume a new instance:

$$I_i = (x_{i1}, x_{i2}, \ldots, x_{ij}, \ldots x_{iN})$$

Verifying explanation Condition A. In linear models the absolute values of weights a_j of each feature x_j express the importance factors of its prediction function. A high weight value of a_j for feature x_j indicates that this feature is important because small changes of feature x_j multiplied by a large a_j weight value will highly affect the final output. The important features are chosen by the following formula:

$$\text{Most important features}: K = \{j : |a_j| > d_{th}\} \quad (5)$$

where d_{th} is a defined threshold which defines the minimum feature's importance factor.

Verifying explanation Condition C. For the features k identified as important: $k \in K$, we will compute their critical values in which the prediction result will change. These critical values are defined when the prediction output is in the "unidentified" region state. Based on Equations (3) and (4) the critical feature values $xcrit_k$ satisfy the following equation:

$$a_0 + \sum_{j=1}^{k-1} a_j x_{ij} + a_k xcrit_{ik} + \sum_{j=k+1}^{N} a_j x_{ij} = 0, \; \forall k \in K \quad (6)$$

and it turns out that:

$$xcrit_{ik} = -\frac{a_0 + \sum_{j=1}^{k-1} a_j x_{ij} + \sum_{j=k+1}^{N} a_j x_{ij}}{a_k}, \; \forall k \in K \quad (7)$$

Verifying explanation Condition B. If $x_k < xcrit_{ik}$ by Equation (7) it turns out that:

$$a_0 + \sum_{j=1}^{k-1} a_j x_{ij} + a_k x_k + \sum_{j=k+1}^{N} a_j x_{ij} < 0$$

while if $x_k > xcrit_{ik}$ similarly it turns out that:

$$a_0 + \sum_{j=1}^{k-1} a_j x_{ij} + a_k x_k + \sum_{j=k+1}^{N} a_j x_{ij} > 0$$

and thus by Equations (3) and (4) it turns out that:

$$y = \begin{cases} 1, & \forall x_k \geq xcrit_{ik} \text{ and } x_j = x_{ij}, \; \forall j \neq k \\ 0, & \forall x_k < xcrit_{ik} \text{ and } x_j = x_{ij}, \; \forall j \neq k \end{cases} \quad (8)$$

where y is the prediction output. For sake of simplicity we defined by default the prediction output to be 1 for the "undentifined" state.

Summarizing, the function described in Equations (3) and (4) represent the global interpretation formula of our prediction model while Equation (8) describes a local interpretation for instances similar to I_i which share the same prediction output, sharing one common explanation rule.

Final Presentation form. We have to find out a comprehensive and understandable form that will merge all information provided by conditions A, B and C while humans will be able by just following some basic rules, to easily obtain all this information. 2 main types of presentation forms are proposed for the explanation output of our prediction model: graph form since they can provide in an intelligible and compact way explanations to humans and a question–answers form since it is probably one of the most common and desirable ways that humans make explanations (Section 2.3.2). We will present it analytically in next section on our application case study scenario.

2.4. Summary of Proposed Framework

In Table 4 are summarized and described in a compact form our total proposed framework's basic steps.

Table 4. Summary of proposed framework.

Step 1. Import images $\left(X_{init}^{M \times H \times W}, y\right)$, where M is the number of images, H and W are the number of pixels corresponding to the Height and Width of every image.
Step 2. Compute Co-Occurrence, Run-length, Statistical and Contour features and extract new dataset $\left(X_{new}^{M \times N}, y\right)$, where N is the number of new extracted features.
Step 3. Train White Box Linear model LR with $\left(X^{M \times N}, y\right)$.
Step 4. Define a weight threshold d_{th} and compute most important features K.
Step 7. For every new instance $X_{new}^{1 \times N}$ and every feature $k \in K$ compute its critical values $xcrit_k$.
Step 8. Verify explanation Conditions A, B and C.
Step 9. Select and define the language of the explanation with respect to the targeted audience.
Step 10. Create the Final Presentation explanation output.

3. Results

In this section, we present our experimental results regarding to the proposed explainable prediction framework for image classification tasks, applying it on glioma prediction from MRI as a case study application scenario. In our experiments, all utilized machine learning models (Table 5) were trained using the new data representation which was created via our feature extraction framework and validated using a 10-fold cross-validation using the performance metrics: Accuracy (Acc), F_1-score (F_1), Sensitivity (sen), Specificity (spe), Positive Predictive Value (PPV), Negative Predictive Value (NPV) and the Area Under the Curve (AUC) [21]. It was considered not essential to conduct experiments based on the initial dataset (raw images) since such experiments were already performed by various CNN models based on transfer learning approach on previous works [22,23] managing to achieve around to 99% accuracy score. It is worth mentioning that since this work proposes an explainable intrinsic prediction model, obviously our goal is not to surpass the performance of these powerful black box models but manage to achieve a decent performance score with powerful explainability.

Table 5. Summary of utilized machine learning models.

WB Model	Basic Parameters	BB Model	Basic Parameters
DT_1	max depth = 3	NN_1	N.L.1 = 64, N.L.2 = 16
DT_2	max depth = 5	NN_2	N.L.1 = 128, N.L.2 = 32
DT_3	max depth = 10	NN_3	N.L.1 = 256, N.L.2 = 64
NB	No parameters	SVM_1	$C = 1$
LR_1	$C = 1$	SVM_2	$C = 500$
LR_2	$C = 500$	SVM_3	$C = 1000$
LR_3	$C = 1000$	k-NN	$k = 3$

Our experiments were performed via two phases. In the first phase, various white box (WB) models were compared while in the second phase, the best identified WB model was compared with various black box (BB) models. Table 5 depicts all the utilized machine learning models and their basic tuning parameters. All Decision Trees (DT) models were evaluated based on their max depth parameter. A high depth leads to a complex decision function while a low depth leads to a simple function but probably to biased predictions. The basic version of decision tree algorithm used in our experiments was CART algorithm since it was identified to exhibit superior performance comparing to other decision tree algorithms [24]. On Naive Bayes (NB) [20] classifier, no parameters were specified.

All Neural Networks (NNs) are fully connected networks composed by two hidden layers each and N.L.x refers to the number of Neurons in Layer x. The basic tuning parameter of a Logistic Regression (LR) constitutes the regularization parameter C, just like in Support Vector Machine (SVM) [25], where small values specify stronger regularization. All SVM models were composed by a radial basis function kernel. We have to mention that all these models' parameters were identified via exhaustive and thorough experiments in order to incur the best performance results. Finally, the k-NN [26] was implemented based on the Euclidean distance metric, while the basic tuning parameter is the number of neighbors k.

3.1. Experimental Results

Table 6 presents the performance comparison of WB models regarding the predefined performance metrics. LR_1 exhibited the best classification score (94%) while NB exhibited the worst (77%). Table 7 presents the performance comparison of the best identified WB model (LR_1) comparing to the BB models. LR_1 managed to be as accurate as the best identified BB models (NN_3 and SVM_2). This probably means that our feature extraction framework managed to filter out the noise and the complexity of the initial image representation. As a result, this framework creates a robust and simpler data representation that simple linear models can efficiently be applied on, while powerful BB models like NN are becoming unnecessary.

Table 6. Performance comparison of white box (WB) models.

WB Model	Acc	F_1	sen	spe	PPV	NPV	AUC
DT_1	0.87	0.86	0.83	0.92	0.9	0.86	0.87
DT_2	0.89	0.87	0.86	0.91	0.89	0.88	0.88
DT_3	0.87	0.86	0.86	0.88	0.87	0.88	0.87
NB	0.77	0.74	0.69	0.84	0.79	0.76	0.77
LR_1	**0.94**	**0.93**	**0.94**	**0.94**	**0.93**	**0.95**	**0.94**
LR_2	0.93	0.93	0.93	0.93	0.92	0.94	0.93
LR_3	0.93	0.93	0.93	0.93	0.92	0.94	0.93

Table 7. Performance comparison of black box (BB)–WB models.

Model	Acc	F_1	sen	spe	PPV	NPV	AUC
NN_1	0.93	0.92	0.92	0.94	0.93	0.93	0.93
NN_2	0.94	0.93	0.92	0.94	0.93	0.94	0.93
NN_3	0.94	0.93	0.92	**0.95**	**0.94**	0.93	0.94
SVM_1	0.92	0.91	0.9	0.93	0.92	0.92	0.92
SVM_2	0.93	0.93	0.92	**0.95**	**0.94**	0.93	0.93
SVM_3	0.93	0.93	0.92	0.94	0.93	0.93	0.93
k-NN	0.89	0.87	0.83	0.94	0.92	0.86	0.88
LR_1	0.94	0.93	**0.94**	0.94	0.93	**0.95**	0.94

3.2. Predictions Explanations

In the sequel, our framework's explanation output is presented for some case study predictions. The final prediction model is the LR_1. Let assume two new instances as presented in Figure 6.

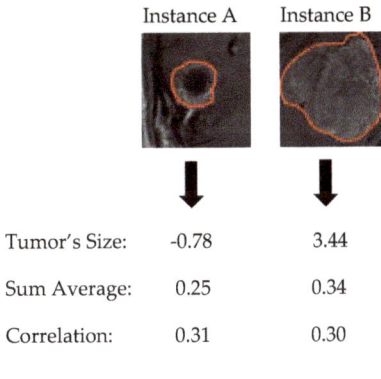

Figure 6. Two case study instances. Instance A is GLIOMA while Instance B is NON GLIOMA.

Two basic language forms are proposed for our model's explanation output, graph diagrams and questions–answers forms as presented in Figures 7 and 8, which were extracted via the formulas described in Section 2.3.4 regarding the predefined conditions A, B and C. The graph diagram provides in a compact, comprehensive and visual form, information which can easily fast extracted by just investigating every node. Each node represents one feature followed by an explanation rule in which a specific prediction output is qualified. The three displayed nodes represent the three most important identified features while the size of each node represents the importance factor of the corresponding feature.

A questions–answers form is probably one of the best ways to provide explanations since this is the main fundamental way that humans make explanations (more details in Section 2.3.2). As already mentioned before, the proper choice of the language is highly depended by the audience. Therefore, we also propose two types of questions–answers forms, Specific and Humanistic form. In specific form, the answers are extracted directly by the graph diagram without any information loss providing all details of graph's information. In humanistic form the answers are extracted via a preprocessing step aiming to simplify the explanation and convert it to a more human like explanation, by approximating the initial model's features to easier understandable abstract features (meta-features) specified by the application domain. For example, in our case the Object size can be converted to Tumor Size, the Sum Average to Tumor's Color (more details for Sum Average feature are presented in Section 2.4). Additionally, every quantitative value has to be converted to qualitative such as Small, Average, Large. For this step is essential the knowledge of a High and Low value of each feature in order to create such qualitative terms.

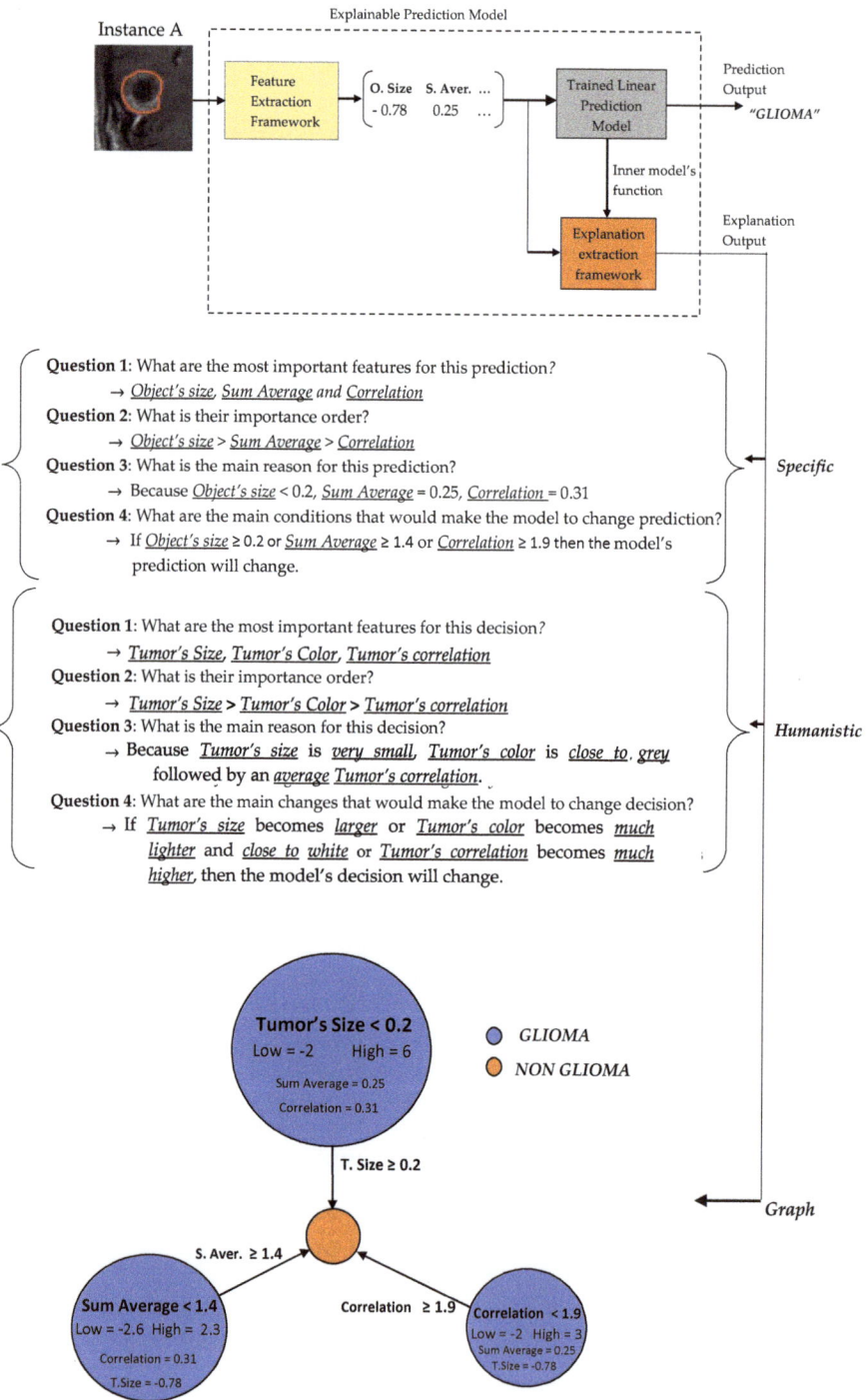

Figure 7. Explanation output for Instance A.

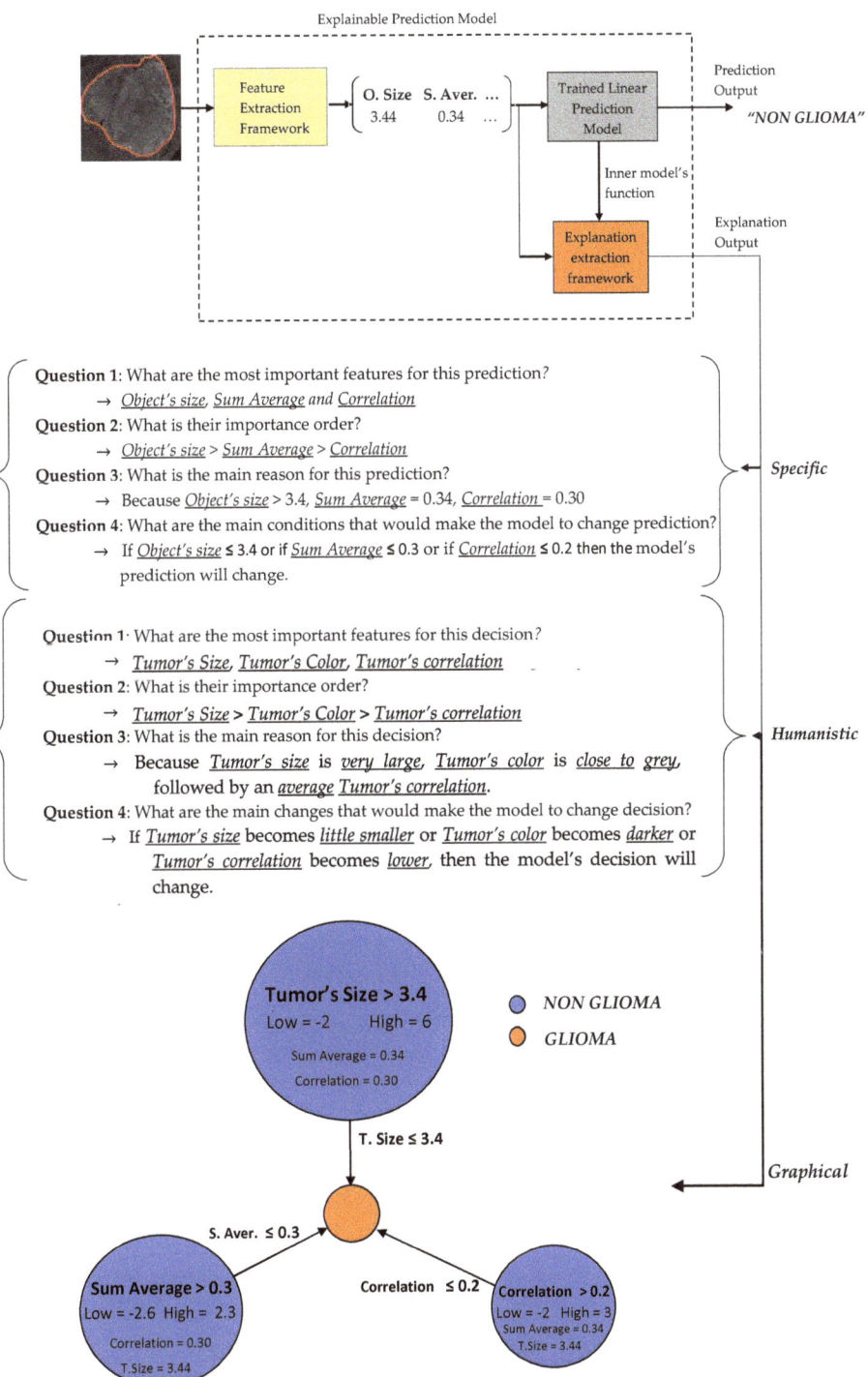

Figure 8. Explanation output for Instance A.

4. Discussion

In this study, a new prediction framework was proposed, which is able to provide accurate and explainable predictions on image classification tasks. Our experimental results indicate that our model is able to achieve a sufficient classification score comparing to state of the art CNN approaches being also intrinsic interpretable able to provide good explanations for every prediction/decision result.

One major difference comparing to other state of the art explanation frameworks for image classification tasks, is that our approach is not performing pixels based explanations. By the term pixels based (or pixel returns) we mean that the explanations are based on the visual interpretation of the most important identified pixels that determined a specific prediction. For example, if a model classified as a cat, an image which presents a cat and a dog, then meaningful pixel base explanation would probably return the cat's pixels revealing that the model classified the image utilizing the proper area of pixels. However, if the task was to recognize an owner's missing cat, then the identification of high level features which uniquely describe this cat would be essential. Such features could be cat's size, cat's color, cat's color irregularity level and cat's number of legs. In such cases, the model's prediction explanation would be useful to rely on such high level features instead of just specific pixels. If the main reason for this prediction was just that this cat has 3 legs and blue color then pixel returns probably could not reveal any useful explanation and reasoning.

As already mentioned our explanation approach is not pixel based but higher level feature based. By this term it is meant that the explanations are performed via a higher level feature representation input, in contrast to raw pixels which are the lowest level input (initial representation). Such high level features can describe the unique properties that groups of pixels possess in every image such as color of an image, color irregularity level, shape irregularity of objects lied in an image, number of objects lied in an image and so on. Obviously, these high-level feature inputs have to be understandable to humans since the model's predictions' explanations would be useless. For example, if a model classified an image as a dog because $x = 5$ without any knowledge about what the feature x means and how was calculated, then such explanation can be considered meaningless. Where instead if it was known that the feature x is the size of an object in an image or the color value of an image and so on, then we would be able to make reasoning about the model's decision and easily understand it.

Nevertheless, creating high level image features being also understandable to humans is a complex task. There is no guarantee that utilizing these features as an input for the machine model would lead to high prediction performance, as probably there are a lot of other hidden unutilized features lied in an image that are probably useful for the specific classification problem. It is hard to identify a priori such features since they are actually found out and crafted by a human sense based approach, while it could make more sense to seek the assistance of an expert with respect to the application domain. In contrast, automatic methods such as CNN models manage to automatically identify useful features in images avoiding this painful human based feature extraction process. However, these features that automatic methods manage to identify are not interpretable and explainable to humans, whereas features crafted by humans can be transparent, meaningful and understandable. This is the trade-off that we need to endure if the objective is the development of interpretable prediction models. Traditional feature extraction approaches, specialized expertise, specific knowledge domain regarding the application and the art of creating useful features for machine learning problems followed by new innovative strategies and techniques can constitute essential key elements in explainable artificial intelligent era.

5. Conclusions and Future Work

In this work, an accurate, robust and explainable prediction framework was proposed for image classification tasks proposing three types of explanations outputs with respect to the audience domain. Comparing to most approaches, our method is intrinsic interpretable providing good explanations relying on high-level feature representation inputs, extracted by images. These features aim to describe the properties that the pixels of an image possess such as its texture irregularity level, object's shape, size, etc. One basic limitation of our approach is that some of these features are probably only understandable by image analysts and specific human experts. However, we made an attempt to qualitatively explain what such features describe in simple human terms in order to make our model's explanation output more attractive and viable to a much wider audience.

Last but not least, in our experiments we utilized all features, even the least significant. We attempted to reduce the number of features in this dataset by analyzing the correlation between the features as well as their significance and by applying some feature selection techniques [27–29]. However, any attempt of removing any features was leading to decrease the overall performance of the prediction model; hence, no feature was removed. We point out the feature selection processing was not in the scope of our work since our main objective was the development and the presentation of an explainable machine learning framework for image classification tasks. Clearly, an interpretable prediction model, exhibiting even better forecasting ability, could be developed through the imposition of sophisticated feature selection techniques as a pre-processing step.

In future work, we aim to incorporate and identify features more understandable to human, being also very informative for the machine learning prediction models. In addition, it is worth investigating whether an interpretable prediction model exhibiting even better forecasting ability could be developed through the imposition of penalty functions together with the application of feature selection techniques or through additional optimized configuration of the proposed model. Finally, we also aim to develop more sophisticated algorithmic methods in order to improve the prediction performance accuracy of intrinsic white box models. Such algorithms could simplify the initial structure complexity and nonlinearity level of the initial dataset, in order to efficiently train simple white box models.

Author Contributions: Conceptualization, E.P.; methodology, E.P., M.L., I.E.L., S.K. and P.P.; validation, E.P., M.L., I.E.L., S.K. and P.P.; formal analysis, E.P., M.L., I.E.L., S.K. and P.P.; investigation, E.P., M.L., I.E.L., S.K. and P.P.; resources, E.P., M.L., I.E.L., S.K. and P.P.; data curation, E.P., M.L., I.E.L., S.K. and P.P.; writing—original draft preparation, E.P., M.L., I.E.L., S.K. and P.P.; writing—review and editing, E.P., M.L., I.E.L., S.K. and P.P.; visualization, E.P., M.L., I.E.L., S.K. and P.P.; supervision, S.K. All authors have read and agreed to the published version of the manuscript.

Funding: This research received no external funding.

Conflicts of Interest: The authors declare no conflict of interest.

References

1. Rawat, W.; Wang, Z. Deep convolutional neural networks for image classification: A comprehensive review. *Neural Comput.* **2017**, *29*, 2352–2449. [CrossRef] [PubMed]
2. Arrieta, A.B.; Díaz-Rodríguez, N.; Del Ser, J.; Bennetot, A.; Tabik, S.; Barbado, A.; García, S.; López, S.G.; Molina, D.; Benjamins, R.; et al. Explainable Artificial Intelligence (XAI): Concepts, taxonomies, opportunities and challenges toward responsible AI. *Inf. Fusion* **2020**, *58*, 82–115. [CrossRef]
3. Robnik-Šikonja, M.; Kononenko, I. Explaining classifications for individual instances. *IEEE Trans. Knowl. Data Eng.* **2008**, *20*, 589–600. [CrossRef]
4. Kuhn, M.; Johnson, K. *Applied Predictive Modeling*; Springer: New York, NY, USA, 2013; Volume 26.
5. Edwards, L.; Veale, M. Slave to the Algorithm? Why a 'Right to an Explanation' Is Probably Not the Remedy You Are Looking For. *Duke Law Technol. Rev.* **2017**, *16*, 18.
6. Molnar, C. Interpretable Machine Learning: A Guide for Making Black Box Models Explainable. Available online: https://christophm.github.io/interpretable-ml-book (accessed on 6 June 2018).
7. Pintelas, E.; Livieris, I.E.; Pintelas, P. A Grey-Box Ensemble Model Exploiting Black-Box Accuracy and White-Box Intrinsic Interpretability. *Algorithms* **2020**, *13*, 17. [CrossRef]
8. Ribeiro, M.T.; Singh, S.; Guestrin, C. "Why should I trust you?" Explaining the predictions of any classifier. In Proceedings of the 22nd ACM SIGKDD International Conference on Knowledge Discovery and Data Mining August 2016, San Francisco, CA, USA, 13–17 August 2016; pp. 1135–1144.
9. Robnik-Šikonja, M.; Bohanec, M. Perturbation-based explanations of prediction models. In *Human and Machine Learning*; Springer: Cham, Switzerland, 2018; pp. 159–175.

10. Wachter, S.; Mittelstadt, B.; Russell, C. Counterfactual Explanations without Opening the Black Box: Automated Decisions and the GPDR. *Harv. JL Tech.* **2017**, *31*, 841. [CrossRef]
11. Selvaraju, R.R.; Cogswell, M.; Das, A.; Vedantam, R.; Parikh, D.; Batra, D. Grad-cam: Visual explanations from deep networks via gradient-based localization. In Proceedings of the IEEE International Conference on Computer Vision 2017, Venice, Italy, 22–29 October 2017; pp. 618–626.
12. Goodenberger, M.L.; Jenkins, R.B. Genetics of adult glioma. *Cancer Genet.* **2012**, *205*, 613–621. [CrossRef] [PubMed]
13. Cheng, J. Brain tumor dataset. Available online: https://figshare.com/articles/brain_tumor_dataset/1512427 (accessed on 2 April 2018).
14. Haralick, R.M.; Shanmugam, K.; Dinstein, H. Texture features for Image Classification. *IEEE Trans. Syst.* **1973**, *SMC-3*, 610–621.
15. Vyas, A.; Yu, S.; Paik, J. Wavelets and Wavelet Transform. In *Multiscale Transforms with Application to Image Processing*; Springer: Singapore City, Singapore, 2018; pp. 45–92.
16. Galloway, M.M. Texture analysis using gray level run lengths. *Comput. Graph. Image Process.* **1975**, *4*, 172–179. [CrossRef]
17. Tang, X. Texture information in Run-Length Matrices. *IEEE Trans. Image Process.* **1998**, *7*, 1602–1609. [CrossRef] [PubMed]
18. Daniel, G. *Principles of Artificial Neural Networks*; World Scientific: Singapore City, Singapore, 2013; Volume 7.
19. Su, J.; Vargas, D.V.; Sakurai, K. One pixel attack for fooling deep neural networks. *IEEE Trans. Evol. Comput.* **2019**, *23*, 828–841. [CrossRef]
20. Ng, A.Y.; Jordan, M.I. On discriminative vs. generative classifiers: A comparison of logistic regression and naive bayes. In *Advances in Neural Information Processing Systems*; MIT Press: Cambridge, MA, USA, 2002; pp. 841–848.
21. Raschka, S. An overview of general performance metrics of binary classifier systems. *arXiv* **2014**, arXiv:1410.5330.
22. Deepak, S.; Ameer, P.M. Brain tumor classification using deep CNN features via transfer learning. *Comput. Biol. Med.* **2019**, *111*, 103345. [CrossRef] [PubMed]
23. Rehman, A.; Naz, S.; Razzak, M.I.; Akram, F.; Imran, M. A deep learning-based framework for automatic brain tumors classification using transfer learning. *Circuits Syst. Signal Process.* **2020**, *39*, 757–775. [CrossRef]
24. Priyam, A.; Abhijeeta, G.R.; Rathee, A.; Srivastava, S. Comparative analysis of decision tree classification algorithms. *Int. J. Curr. Eng. Technol.* **2013**, *3*, 334–337.
25. Deng, N.; Tian, Y.; Zhang, C. *Support Vector Machines: Optimization Based Theory, Algorithms, and Extensions*; Chapman and Hall/CRC: Boca Raton, FL, USA, 2012.
26. Aha, D.W. (Ed.) *Lazy Learning*; Springer Science & Business Media: Berlin, Germany, 2013.
27. Benesty, J.; Chen, J.; Huang, Y.; Cohen, I. Pearson correlation coefficient. In *Noise Reduction in Speech Processing*; Springer: Berlin/Heidelberg, Germany, 2009; pp. 1–4.
28. Hall, M.A. Correlation-based Feature Subset Selection for Machine Learning. Ph.D. Thesis, University of Waikato, Hamilton, New Zealand, 1998.
29. Kira, K.; Larry, A. Rendell: A Practical Approach to Feature Selection. In *Ninth International Workshop on Machine Learning*; Morgan Kaufmann: Burlington, MA, USA, 1992; pp. 249–256.

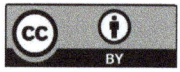

© 2020 by the authors. Licensee MDPI, Basel, Switzerland. This article is an open access article distributed under the terms and conditions of the Creative Commons Attribution (CC BY) license (http://creativecommons.org/licenses/by/4.0/).

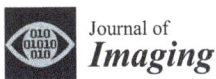

Review

A Survey of Deep Learning for Lung Disease Detection on Medical Images: State-of-the-Art, Taxonomy, Issues and Future Directions

Stefanus Tao Hwa Kieu [1], Abdullah Bade [1], Mohd Hanafi Ahmad Hijazi [2,*] and Hoshang Kolivand [3]

1. Faculty of Science and Natural Resources, Universiti Malaysia Sabah, Kota Kinabalu 88400, Sabah, Malaysia; stefanuskieu@gmail.com (S.T.H.K.); abb@ums.edu.my (A.B.)
2. Faculty of Computing and Informatics, Universiti Malaysia Sabah, Kota Kinabalu 88400, Sabah, Malaysia
3. School of Computer Science and Mathematics, Liverpool John Moores University, Liverpool L3 3AF, UK; H.Kolivand@ljmu.ac.uk
* Correspondence: hanafi@ums.edu.my

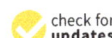

Received: 24 October 2020; Accepted: 25 November 2020; Published: 1 December 2020

Abstract: The recent developments of deep learning support the identification and classification of lung diseases in medical images. Hence, numerous work on the detection of lung disease using deep learning can be found in the literature. This paper presents a survey of deep learning for lung disease detection in medical images. There has only been one survey paper published in the last five years regarding deep learning directed at lung diseases detection. However, their survey is lacking in the presentation of taxonomy and analysis of the trend of recent work. The objectives of this paper are to present a taxonomy of the state-of-the-art deep learning based lung disease detection systems, visualise the trends of recent work on the domain and identify the remaining issues and potential future directions in this domain. Ninety-eight articles published from 2016 to 2020 were considered in this survey. The taxonomy consists of seven attributes that are common in the surveyed articles: image types, features, data augmentation, types of deep learning algorithms, transfer learning, the ensemble of classifiers and types of lung diseases. The presented taxonomy could be used by other researchers to plan their research contributions and activities. The potential future direction suggested could further improve the efficiency and increase the number of deep learning aided lung disease detection applications.

Keywords: deep learning; lung disease detection; taxonomy; medical images

1. Introduction

Lung diseases, also known as respiratory diseases, are diseases of the airways and the other structures of the lungs [1]. Examples of lung disease are pneumonia, tuberculosis and Coronavirus Disease 2019 (COVID-19). According to Forum of International Respiratory Societies [2], about 334 million people suffer from asthma, and, each year, tuberculosis kills 1.4 million people, 1.6 million people die from lung cancer, while pneumonia also kills millions of people. The COVID-19 pandemic impacted the whole world [3], infecting millions of people and burdening healthcare systems [4]. It is clear that lung diseases are one of the leading causes of death and disability in this world. Early detection plays a key role in increasing the chances of recovery and improve long-term survival rates [5,6]. Traditionally, lung disease can be detected via skin test, blood test, sputum sample test [7], chest X-ray examination and computed tomography (CT) scan examination [8]. Recently, deep learning has shown great potential when applied on medical images for disease detection, including lung disease.

Deep learning is a subfield of machine learning relating to algorithms inspired by the function and structure of the brain. Recent developments in machine learning, particularly deep learning, support the identification, quantification and classification of patterns in medical images [9]. These developments were made possible due to the ability of deep learning to learned features merely from data, instead of hand-designed features based on domain-specific knowledge. Deep learning is quickly becoming state of the art, leading to improved performance in numerous medical applications. Consequently, these advancements assist clinicians in detecting and classifying certain medical conditions efficiently [10].

Numerous works on the detection of lung disease using deep learning can be found in the literature. To the best of our knowledge, however, only one survey paper has been published in the last five years to analyse the state-of-the-art work on this topic [11]. In that paper, the history of deep learning and its applications in pulmonary imaging are presented. Major applications of deep learning techniques on several lung diseases, namely pulmonary nodule diseases, pulmonary embolism, pneumonia, and interstitial lung disease, are also described. In addition, the analysis of several common deep learning network structures used in medical image processing is presented. However, their survey is lacking in the presentation of taxonomy and analysis of the trend of recent work. A taxonomy shows relationships between previous work and categorises them based on the identified attributes that could improve reader understanding of the topic. Analysis of trend, on the other hand, provides an overview of the research direction of the topic of interest identified from the previous work. In this paper, a taxonomy of deep learning applications on lung diseases and a trend analysis on the topic are presented. The remaining issues and possible future direction are also described.

The aims of this paper are as follows: (1) produce a taxonomy of the state-of-the-art deep learning based lung disease detection systems; (2) visualise the trends of recent work on the domain; and (3) identify the remaining issues and describes potential future directions in this domain. This paper is organised as follows. Section 2 presents the methodology of conducting this survey. Section 3 describes the general processes of using deep learning to detect lung disease in medical images. Section 4 presents the taxonomy, with detailed explanations of each subtopic within the taxonomy. The analysis of trend, research gap and future directions of lung disease detection using deep learning are presented in Section 5. Section 6 describes the limitation of the survey. Section 7 concludes this paper.

2. Methodology

In this section, the methodology used to conduct the survey of recent lung disease detection using deep learning is described. Figure 1 shows the flowchart of the methodology used.

First, a suitable database, as a main source of reference, of articles was identified. The Scopus database was selected as it is one of the largest databases of scientific peer-reviewed articles. However, several significant articles, indexed by Google Scholar but not Scopus, are also included based on the number of citations that they have received. Some preprint articles on COVID-19 are also included as the disease has just recently emerged. To ensure that this survey only covers the state-of-the-art works, only articles published recently (2016–2020) are considered. However, several older but significant articles are included too. To search for all possible deep learning aided lung disease detection articles, relevant keywords were used to search for the articles. The keywords used were "deep learning", "detection", "classification", "CNN", "lung disease", "Tuberculosis", "pneumonia", "lung cancer", "COVID-19" and "Coronavirus". Studies were limited to articles written in English only. At the end of this phase, we identified 366 articles.

Second, to select only the relevant works, screening was performed. During the screening, only the title and abstract were assessed. The main selection criteria were this survey is only interested in work, whereby deep learning algorithms were applied to detect the relevant diseases. Articles considered not relevant were excluded. Based on the screening performed, only 98 articles were shortlisted.

Last, for all the articles screened, the eligibility inspection was conducted. Similar criteria, as in the screening phase, were used, whereby the full-text inspection of the articles was performed instead. All 98 screened articles passed this phase and were included in this survey. Out of the eligible articles, 90 were published in 2018 and onwards. This signifies that lung disease detection using deep learning is still a very active field. Figure 1 shows the numbers of studies identified, screened, assessed for eligibility and included in this survey.

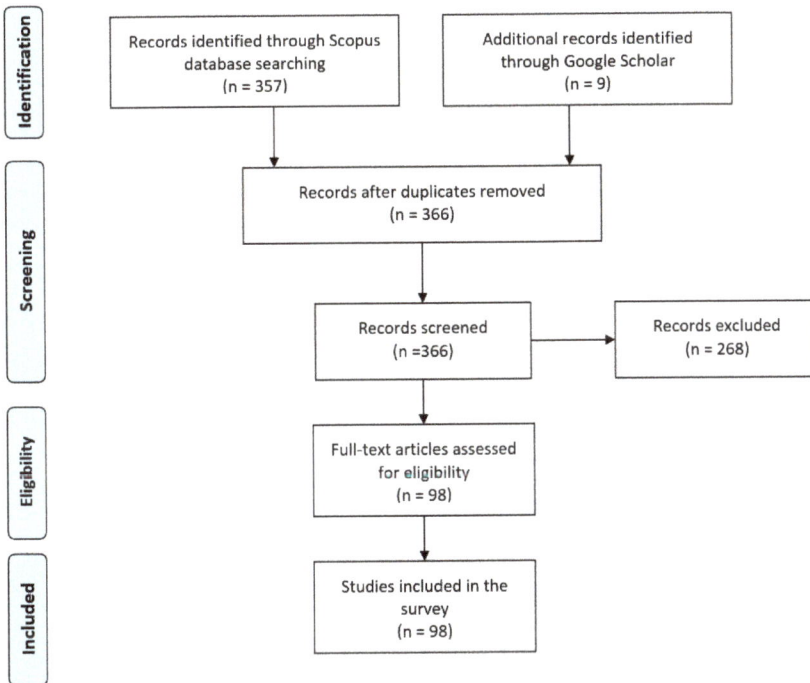

Figure 1. Flow diagram of the methodology used to conduct this survey.

3. The Basic Process to Apply Deep Learning for Lung Disease Detection

In this section, the process of how deep learning is applied to identify lung diseases from medical images is described. There are mainly three steps: image preprocessing, training and classification. Lung disease detection generally deals with classifying an image into healthy lungs or disease-infected lungs. The lung disease classifier, sometimes known as a model, is obtained via training. Training is the process in which a neural network learns to recognise a class of images. Using deep learning, it is possible to train a model that can classify images into their respective class labels. Therefore, to apply deep learning for lung disease detection, the first step is to gather images of lungs with the disease to be classified. The second step is to train the neural network until it is able to recognise the diseases. The final step is to classify new images. Here, new images unseen by the model before are shown to the model, and the model predicts the class of those images. The overview of the process is illustrated in Figure 2.

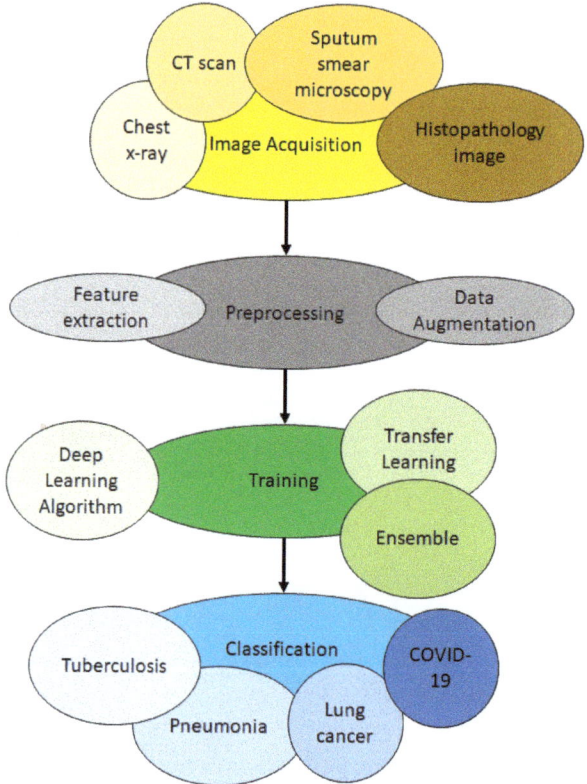

Figure 2. Overview of using deep learning for lung disease detection.

3.1. Image Acquisition Phase

The first step is to acquire images. To produce a classification model, the computer needs to learn by example. The computer needs to view many images to recognise an object. Other types of data, such as time series data and voice data, can also be used to train deep learning models. In the context of the work surveyed in this paper, the relevant data required to detect lung disease will be images. Images that could be used include chest X-ray, CT scan, sputum smear microscopy and histopathology image. The output of this step is images that will later be used to train the model.

3.2. Preprocessing Phase

The second step is preprocessing. Here, the image could be enhanced or modified to improve image quality. Contrast Limited Adaptive Histogram Equalisation (CLAHE) could be performed to increase the contrast of the images [12]. Image modification such as lung segmentation [13] and bone elimination [14] could be used to identify the region of interest (ROI), whereby the detection of the lung disease can then be performed on the ROI. Edge detection could also be used to provide an alternate data representation [15]. Data augmentation could be applied to the images to increase the amount of available data. Feature extraction could also be conducted so that the deep learning model could identify important features to identify a certain object or class. The output of this step is a set of images whereby the quality of the images is enhanced, or unwanted objects have been removed. The output of this step is images that were enhanced or modified that will later be used in training.

3.3. Training Phase

In the third step, namely training, three aspects could be considered. These aspects are the selection of deep learning algorithm, usage of transfer learning and usage of an ensemble. There are numerous deep learning algorithm, for example deep belief network (DBN), multilayer perceptron neural network (MPNN), recurrent neural network (RNN) and the aforementioned CNN. Different algorithms have different learning styles. Different types of data work better with certain algorithms. CNN works particularly well with images. Deep learning algorithm should be chosen based on the nature of the data at hand. Transfer learning refers to the transfer of knowledge from one model to another. Ensemble refers to the usage of more than one model during classification. Transfer learning and ensemble are techniques used to reduce training time, improve classification accuracy and reduce overfitting [16]. Further details concerning these two aspects could be found in Sections 4.5 and 4.6, respectively. The output of this step is models generated from the data learned.

3.4. Classification Phase

In the fourth and final step, which is classification, the trained model will predict which class an image belongs to. For example, if a model was trained to differentiate X-ray images of healthy lungs and tuberculosis-infected lungs, it should be able to correctly classify new images (images that are never seen by the model before) into healthy lungs or tuberculosis-infected lungs. The model will give a probability score for the image. The probability score represents how likely an image belongs to a certain class. At the end of this step, the image will be classified based on the probability score given to it by the model.

4. The Taxonomy of State-Of-The-Art Work on Lung Disease Detection Using Deep Learning

In this section, a taxonomy of the recent work on lung disease detection using deep learning is presented, which is the first contribution of this paper. The taxonomy is built to summarise and provide a clearer picture of the key concepts and focus of the existing work. Seven attributes were identified for inclusion in the taxonomy. These attributes were chosen as they were imminent and can be found in all the articles being surveyed. The seven attributes included in the taxonomy are image types, features, data augmentation, types of deep learning algorithms, transfer learning, the ensemble of classifiers and types of lung diseases. Sections 4.1–4.7 describe each attribute in detail, whereby the review of relevant works is provided. Section 4.8 describes the datasets used by the works surveyed. Figure 3 shows the taxonomy of state-of-the-art lung disease detection using deep learning.

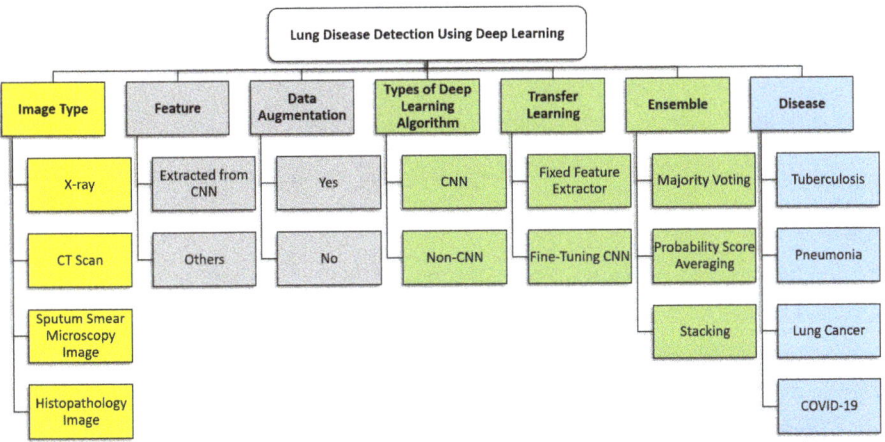

Figure 3. Taxonomy of lung disease detection using deep learning.

4.1. Image Type

In the papers surveyed, four types of images were used to train the model: chest X-ray, CT scans, sputum smear microscopy images and histopathology images. These images are described in detail in Sections 4.1.1–4.1.4. It should be noted that there are other imaging techniques exist such as positron emission tomography (PET) and magnetic resonance imaging (MRI) scans. Both PET and MRI scans could also be used to diagnose health conditions and evaluate the effectiveness of ongoing treatment. However, none of the papers surveyed used PET or MRI scans.

4.1.1. Chest X-rays

An X-ray is a diagnostic test that helps clinicians identify and treat medical problems [17]. The most widely performed medical X-ray procedure is a chest X-ray, and a chest X-ray produces images of the blood vessels, lungs, airways, heart and spine and chest bones. Traditionally, medical X-ray images were exposed to photographic films, which require processing before they can be viewed. To overcome this problem, digital X-rays are used [18]. Figure 4 shows several examples of chest X-ray with different lung conditions taken from various datasets.

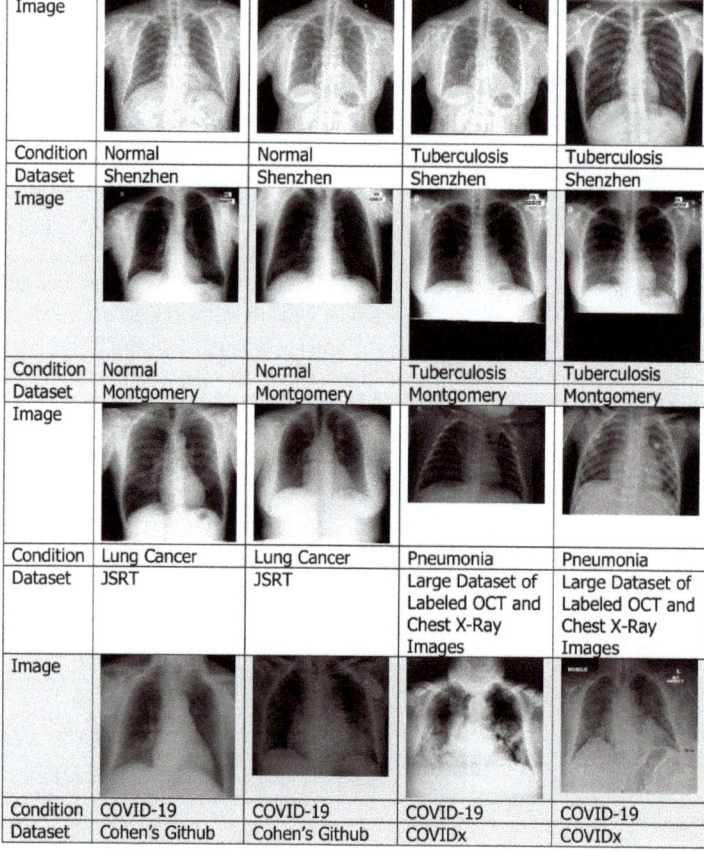

Figure 4. Examples of chest X-ray images.

Among the papers surveyed, the majority of them used chest X-rays. For example, X-rays were used for tuberculosis detection [19], pneumonia detection [20], lung cancer detection [14] and COVID-19 detection [21].

4.1.2. CT Scans

A CT scan is a form of radiography that uses computer processing to create sectional images at various planes of depth from images taken around the patient's body from different angles [22]. The image slices can be shown individually, or they can be stacked to produce a 3D image of the patient, showing the tissues, organs, skeleton and any abnormalities present [23]. CT scan images deliver more detailed information than X-rays. Figure 5 shows examples of CT scan images taken from numerous datasets. CT scans have been used to detect lung disease in numerous work found in the literature, for example for tuberculosis detection [24], lung cancer detection [25] and COVID-19 detection [26].

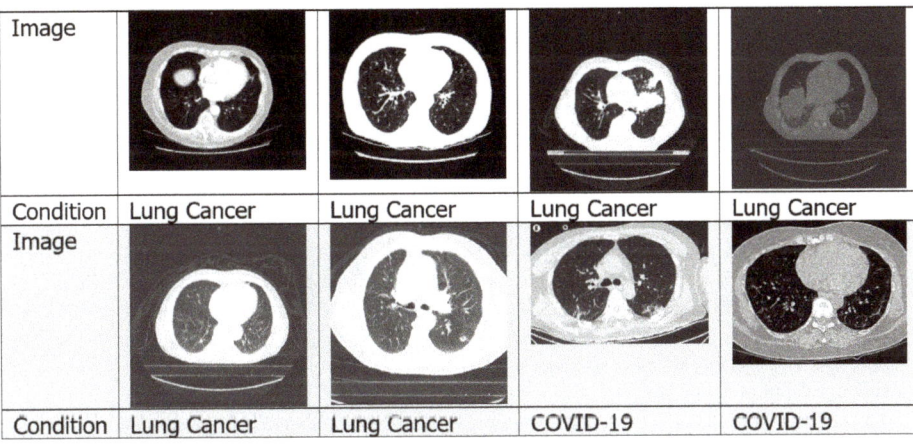

Figure 5. Examples of CT scan images.

4.1.3. Sputum Smear Microscopy Images

Sputum is a dense fluid formed in the lungs and airways leading to the lungs. To perform sputum smear examination, a very thin layer of the sputum sample is positioned on a glass slide [27]. Among the papers surveyed, only five used sputum smear microscopy image [28–32]. Figure 6 shows examples of sputum smear microscopy images.

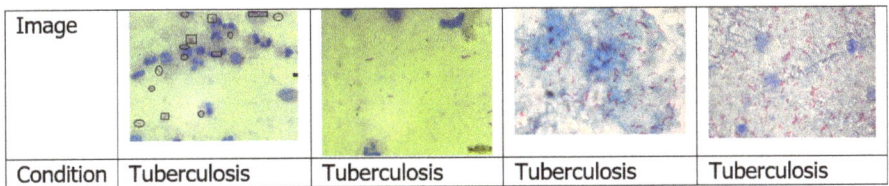

Figure 6. Examples of sputum smear microscopy images.

4.1.4. Histopathology Images

Histopathology is the study of the symptoms of a disease through microscopic examination of a biopsy or surgical specimen using glass slides. The sections are dyed with one or more stains to visualise the different components of the tissue [33]. Figure 7 shows a few examples of histopathology images. Among all the papers surveyed, only Coudray et al. [34] used histopathology images.

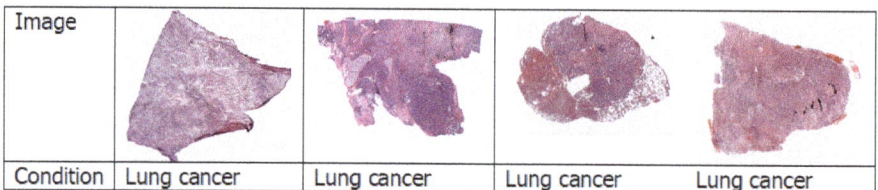

Figure 7. Examples of histopathology images.

4.2. Features

In computer vision, features are significant information extracted from images in terms of numerical values that could be used to solve specific problem [35]. Features might be in the form of specific structures in the image such as points, edges, colour, sizes, shapes or objects. Logically, the types of images affect the quality of the features.

Feature transformation is a process that creates new features using the existing features. These new features may not have the same representation as to the original features, but they may have more discriminatory power in a different space than the original space. The purpose of feature transformation is to provide a more useful feature for the machine learning algorithm for object identification. The features used in the surveyed papers include: Gabor, GIST, Local binary patterns (LBP), Tamura texture descriptor, colour and edge direction descriptor (CEDD) [36], Hu moments, colour layout descriptor (CLD) edge histogram descriptor (EHD) [37], primitive length, edge frequency, autocorrelation, shape features, size, orientation, bounding box, eccentricity, extent, centroid, scale-invariant feature transform (SIFT), regional properties area and speeded up robust features (SURF) [38]. Other feature representations in terms of histograms include pyramid histogram of oriented gradients (PHOG), histogram of oriented gradients (HOG) [39], intensity histograms (IH), shape descriptor histograms (SD), gradient magnitude histograms (GM), curvature descriptor histograms (CD) and fuzzy colour and texture histogram (FCTH). Some studies even performed lung segmentations before training their models (e.g., [13,14,36]).

From the literature, a majority of the works surveyed used features that are automatically extracted from CNN. CNN can automatically learn and extract features, discarding the need for manual feature generation [40].

4.3. Data Augmentation

In deep learning, it is very important to have a large training dataset, as the community agrees that having more images can help improve training accuracy. Even a weak algorithm with a large amount of data can be more accurate than a strong algorithm with a modest amount of data [41]. Another obstacle is imbalanced classes. When doing binary classification training, if the number of samples of one class is a lot higher than the other class, the resulting model would be biased [6]. Deep learning algorithms perform optimally when the amount of samples in each class is equal or balanced.

One way to increase the training dataset without obtaining new images is to use image augmentation. Image augmentation creates variations of the original images. This is achieved by performing different methods of processing, such as rotations, flips, translations, zooms and adding noise [42]. Figure 8 shows various examples of images after image augmentation.

Data augmentation can also help increase the amount of relevant data in the dataset. For example, consider a car dataset with two labels, X and Y. One subset of the dataset contains images of cars of label X, but all the cars are facing left. The other subset contains images of cars of label Y, but all the cars are facing right. After training, a test image of a label Y car facing left is fed into the model, and the model labels that the car as X. The prediction is wrong as the neural network search for the most obvious features that distinguish one class from another. To prevent this, a simple solution is to flip the images in the existing dataset horizontally such that they face the other side. Through augmentation, we may introduce relevant features and patterns, essentially boosting overall performance.

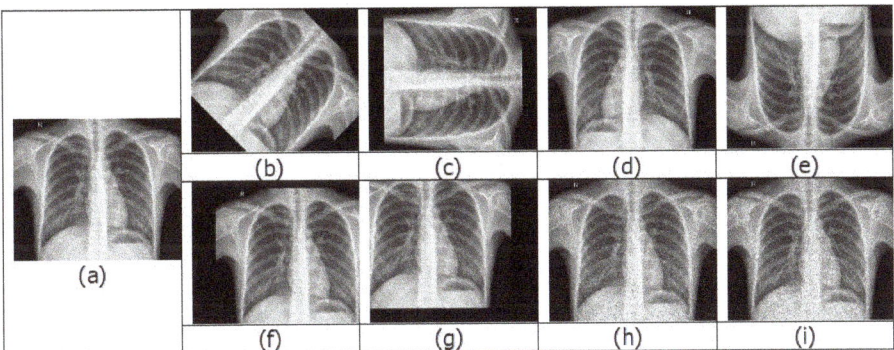

Figure 8. Examples of image augmentation: (**a**) original; (**b**) 45° rotation; (**c**) 90° rotation; (**d**) horizontal flip; (**e**) vertical flip; (**f**) positive x and y translation; (**g**) negative x and y translation; (**h**) salt and pepper noise; and (**i**) speckle noise.

Data augmentation also helps prevent overfitting. Overfitting refers to a case where a network learns a very high variance function, such as the perfect modelling of training results. Data augmentation addresses the issue of overfitting by introducing the model with more diverse data [43]. This diversity in data reduces variance and improves the generalisation of the model.

However, data augmentation cannot overcome all biases present in a small dataset [43]. Other disadvantages of data augmentation include additional training time, transformation computing costs and additional memory costs.

4.4. Types of Deep Learning Algorithm

The most common deep learning algorithm, CNN, is especially useful to find patterns in images. Similar to the neural networks of the human brain, CNNs consist of neurons with trainable biases and weights. Each neuron receives several inputs. Then, a weighted sum over the inputs is computed. The weighted sum is then passed to an activation function, and an output is produced. The difference between CNN and other neural networks is that CNN has convolution layers. Figure 9 shows an example of a CNN architecture [44]. A CNN consists of multiple layers, and the four main types of layers are convolutional layer, pooling layer and fully-connected layer. The convolutional layer performs an operation called a "convolution". Convolution is a linear operation involving the multiplication of a set of weights with the input. The set of weights is called a kernel or a filter. The input data are larger than the filter. The multiplication between a filter-sized section of the input and the filter is a dot product. The dot product is then summed, resulting in a single value. The pooling layer gradually reduces the spatial size of the representation to lessen the number of parameters and computations in the network, thus controlling overfitting. A rectified linear unit (ReLu) is added to the CNN to apply an elementwise activation function such as sigmoid to the output of the activation produced by the previous layer. More details of CNN can be found in [44,45].

CNN generally has two components when learning, which are feature extraction and classification. In the feature extraction stage, convolution is implemented on the input data using a filter or kernel. Then, a feature map is subsequently generated. In the classification stage, the CNN computes a probability of the image belongs to a particular class or label. CNN is especially useful for image classification and recognition as it automatically learns features without needing manual feature extraction [40]. CNN also can be retrained and applied to a different domain using transfer learning [46]. Transfer learning has been shown to produce better classification results [19].

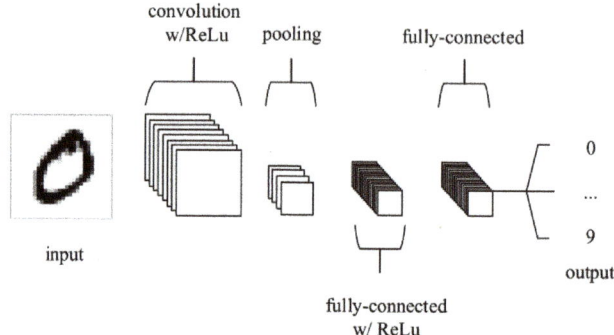

Figure 9. Example of a CNN structure.

Another deep learning algorithm is DBN. DBN can be defined as a stack of restricted Boltzmann machines (RBM) [47]. The layer of the DBN has two functions, except for the first and final layers. The layer serves as the hidden layer for the nodes that come before it, and as the input layer for the nodes that come after it. The first RBM is designed to reproduce as accurately as possible the input to train a DBN. Then, the hidden layer of the first RBM is treated as the visible layer for the second one, and the second RBM is trained using the outputs from the first RBM. This process keeps repeating until every layer of the network is trained. After this initial training, the DBN has created a model that can detect patterns in the data. DBN can be used to recognise objects in images, video sequences and motion-capture data. More details of DBN can be found in [31,48].

One more example of a deep learning algorithm used in the papers surveyed is a bag of words (BOW) model. BOW is a method to extract features from the text for use in modelling. In BOW, the number of the appearance of each word in a document is counted, then the frequency of each word was examined to identify the keywords of the document, and a frequency histogram is made. This concept is similar to the bag of visual words (BOVW), sometimes referred to as bag-of-features. In BOVW, image features are considered as the "words". Image features are unique patterns that were found in an image. The general idea of BOVW is to represent an image as a set of features, where each feature contains keypoints and descriptors. Keypoints are the most noticeable points in an image, such that, even if the image is rotated, shrunk or enlarged, its keypoints are always the same. A descriptor is the description of the keypoint. Keypoints and descriptors are used to construct vocabularies and represent each image as a frequency histogram of features. From the frequency histogram, one can find other similar images or predict the class of the image. Lopes and Valiati proposed Bag of CNN features to classify tuberculosis [19].

4.5. Transfer Learning

Transfer learning emerged as a popular method in computer vision because it allows accurate models to be built [49]. With transfer learning, a model learned from a domain can be re-used on a different domain. Transfer learning can be performed with or without a pre-trained model.

A pre-trained model is a model developed to solve a similar task. Instead of creating a model from scratch to solve a similar task, the model trained on other problem is used as a starting point. Even though a pre-trained model is trained on a task which is different from the current task, the features learned, in most cases, found to be useful for the new task. The objective of training a deep learning model is to find the correct weights for the network by numerous forward and backward iterations. By using pre-trained models that have been previously trained on large datasets, the weights and architecture obtained can be used and applied to the current problem. One of the advantages of a pre-trained model is the reduced cost of training for the new model [50]. This is because pre-trained weights were used, and the model only has to learn the weights of the last few layers.

Many CNN architectures are pre-trained on ImageNet [51]. The images were gathered from the internet and labelled by human labellers using Amazon's Mechanical Turk crowd-sourcing tool. ILSVRC uses a subset of ImageNet with approximately 1000 images in each of 1000 classes. Altogether, there are approximately 1.2 million training images, 50,000 validation images and 150,000 testing images.

Transfer learning can be used in two ways: (i) fine-tuning; or (ii) using CNN as a feature extractor. In fine-tuning, the weights of the pre-trained CNN model are preserved on some of the layers and tuned in the others [52]. Usually, the weights of the initial layers of the model are frozen while only the higher layers are retrained. This is because the features obtained from the first layers are generic (e.g., edge detectors or colour blob detectors) and applicable to other tasks. The top-level layers of the pre-trained models are retrained so that the model learned high-level features specific to the new dataset. This method is typically recommended if the training dataset is huge and very identical to the original dataset that the pre-trained model was trained on. On the other hand, CNN is used as a feature extractor. This is conducted by removing the last fully-connected layer (the one which outputs the probabilities for being in each of the 1000 classes from ImageNet) and then using the network as a fixed feature extractor for the new dataset [53]. For tasks where only a small dataset is available, it is usually recommended to take advantage of features learned by a model trained on a larger dataset in the same domain. Then, a classifier is trained from the features extracted.

There are several issues that need to be considered when using transfer learning: (i) ensuring that the pre-trained model selected has been trained on a similar dataset as the new target dataset; and (ii) using a lower learning rate for CNN weights that are being fine-tuned, because the CNN weights are expected to be relatively good, and we do not wish to distort them too quickly and too much [53].

4.6. Ensemble of Classifiers

When more than one classifier is combined to make a prediction, this is known as ensemble classification [16]. Ensemble decreases the variance of predictions, therefore making predictions that are more accurate than any individual model. From work found in the literature, the ensemble techniques used include majority voting, probability score averaging and stacking.

In majority voting, every model makes a prediction for each test instance, or, in other words, votes for a class label, and the final prediction is the label that received the most votes [54]. An alternate version of majority voting is weighted majority voting, in which the votes of certain models are deemed more important than others. For example, majority voting was used by Chouhan et al. [55].

In probability score averaging, the prediction scores of each model are added up and divided by the number of models involved [56]. An alternate version of this is weighted averaging, where the prediction score of each model is multiplied by the weight, and then their average is calculated. Examples of works which used probability score averaging are found in [15,57].

In stacking ensemble, an algorithm receives the outputs of weaker models as input and tries to learn how to best combine the input predictions to provide a better output prediction [58]. For example, stacking ensemble was used by Rajaraman et al. [12].

4.7. Type of Disease

In this section, the deep learning techniques applied for detecting tuberculosis, pneumonia, lung cancer and COVID-19 are discussed in greater detail in Sections 4.7.1–4.7.4, respectively. The first three diseases were considered as they are the most common causes of critical illness and death worldwide related to lung [2], while COVID-19 is an ongoing pandemic [3]. We also found that most of the existing work was directed at detecting these specific lung-related diseases.

4.7.1. Tuberculosis

Tuberculosis is a disease caused by Mycobacterium tuberculosis bacteria. According to the World Health Organisation, tuberculosis is among the ten most common causes of death in the world [59].

Tuberculosis infected 10 million people and killed 1.6 million in 2017. Early detection of tuberculosis is essential to increase the chances of recovery [5].

Two studies used Computer-Aided Detection for Tuberculosis (CAD4TB) for tuberculosis detection [60,61]. CAD4TB is a tool developed by Delft Imaging Systems in cooperation with the Radboud University Nijmegen and the Lung Institute in Cape Town. CAD4TB works by obtaining the patient's chest X-ray, analysing the image via CAD4TB cloud server or CAD4TB box computer, generating a heat map of the patient's lung and displaying an abnormality score from 0 to 100. Murphy et al. [60] showed that CAD4TB v6 is an accurate system, reaching the level of expert human readers. A technique for automated tuberculosis screening by combining X-ray-based computer-aided detection (CAD) and clinical information was introduced by Melendez et al. [61]. They combined automatic chest X-ray scoring by CAD with clinical information. This combination improved accuracies and specificities compared to the use of either type of information alone.

In the literature, several works use CNN to classify tuberculosis. A method that incorporated demographic information, such as age, gender and weight, to improve CNN's performance was presented by Heo et al. [62]. Results indicate that CNN, including the demographic variables, has a higher area under the receiver operating characteristic curve (AUC) score and greater sensitivity then CNN based on chest X-rays images only. A simple convolutional neural network developed for tuberculosis detection was proposed by Pasa et al. [63]. The proposed approach is found to be more efficient than previous models but retains their accuracy. This method significantly reduced the memory and computational requirement, without sacrificing the classification performance. Another CNN-based model has been presented to classify different categories of tuberculosis [64]. A CNN model is trained on the region-based global and local features to generate new features. A support vector machine (SVM) classifier was then applied for tuberculosis manifestations recognition. CNN has also been used to classify tuberculosis [65–67]. Ul Abideen et al. [68] used a Bayesian-based CNN that exploits the model uncertainty and Bayesian confidence to improve the accuracy of tuberculosis identification. In other work, a deep CNN algorithm named deep learning-based automatic detection (DLAD), was developed for tuberculosis classification that contains 27 layers with 12 residual connections [69]. DLAD shows outstanding performance in tuberculosis detection when applied on chest X-rays, obtaining results better than physicians and thoracic radiologists.

Lopes and Valiati proposed Bag of CNN features to classify tuberculosis [19] where feature extraction is performed by ResNet, VggNet and GoogLenet. Then, each chest X-ray is separated into subregions whose size is equal to the input layer of the networks. Each subregion is regarded as a "feature", while each X-ray is a "bag".

Several works that utilised transfer learning are described in this paragraph. Hwang et al. obtained an accuracy of 90.3% and AUC of 0.964 using transfer learning from ImageNet and training on a dataset of 10848 chest X-rays [70]. Pre-trained GoogLeNet and AlexNet were used to perform pulmonary tuberculosis classification by Lakhani and Sundaram [57], who concluded that higher accuracy was achieved when using the pre-trained model. Their pre-trained AlexNet achieved an AUC of 0.98 and their pre-trained GoogLeNet achieved an AUC of 0.97. Lopes and Valiati used pre-trained GoogLenet, ResNet and VggNet architectures as features extractors and the SVM classifier to classify tuberculosis [19]. They achieved AUC of 0.900–0.912. Fine-tuned ResNet-50, ResNet-101, ResNet-512, VGG16, VGG19 and AlexNet were used by Islam et al. to classify tuberculosis. These models achieved an AUC of 0.85–0.91 [71]. Instead of using networks pre-trained from ImageNet, pre-training can be performed on other datasets, such as the NIH-14 dataset [72]. This dataset contains an assortment of diseases (which does not include tuberculosis) and is from the same modality as that of the data under consideration for tuberculosis. Experiments show that the features learned from the NIH dataset are useful for identifying tuberculosis. A study performed data augmentation and then compared the performances of three different pre-trained models to classify tuberculosis [73]. The results show that suitable data augmentation methods were able to rise the accuracies of CNNs. Transfer learning was also used by Abbas and Abdelsamea [74], Karnkawinpong and Limpiyakorn [75] and Liu et al. [76]. A coarse-to-fine transfer learning was applied by Yadav et al. [77]. First, the datasets are split according to the resolution and quality of the images. Then, transfer learning is applied to the low-resolution dataset first, followed by the high-resolution dataset. In this case, the model was first trained on the low-resolution NIH dataset, and then trained on the high-resolution Shenzen and Montgomery datasets. Sahlol et al. [78] used CNN as fixed feature extractor and Artificial Ecosystem-Based Optimisation to select the optimal subset of relevant features. KNN was used as the classifier.

Several works that utilised ensemble are described in this paragraph. An ensemble method using the weighted averages of the probability scores for the AlexNet and GoogLeNet algorithms was used by Lakhani and Sundaram [57]. In [79], ensemble by weighted averages of probability scores is used. An ensemble of six CNNs was developed by Islam et al. [71]. The ensemble models were generated by calculating the simple averaging of the probability predictions given by every single model. Another ensemble classifier was created by combining the classifier from the Simple CNN Feature Extraction and a classifier from Bag of CNN features proposals [19]. Three classifiers were trained, using the features from ResNet, GoogLenet and VggNet, respectively. The Simple Features Ensemble combines all three classifiers, and the output is obtained through a simple soft-voting scheme. A stacking ensemble for tuberculosis detection was proposed by Rajaraman et al. [12]. An ensemble generated via a feature-level fusion of neural network models was also used to classify tuberculosis [80]. Three models were employed: the DenseNet, ResNet and Inception-ResNet. As such, the ensemble was called RID network. Features were extracted using the RID network, and SVM was used as a classifier. Tuberculosis classification was also executed using another ensemble of three regular architectures: ResNet, AlexNet and GoogLeNet [79]. Each architecture was trained from scratch, and different optimal hyper-parameter values were used. The sensitivity, specificity and accuracy of the ensemble were higher than when each of the regular architecture was used independently. The authors of [15,81] performed a probability score averaging ensemble of CNNs trained on features extracted from a different type of images; the enhanced chest X-ray images and the edge detected images of the chest X-ray. Rajaraman and Antani [82] studied and compared various ensemble methods that include majority voting and stacking. Results show that stacking ensemble achieved the highest classification accuracy.

Other techniques used to classify tuberculosis images include k-Nearest Neighbour (kNN), sequential minimal optimisation and simple linear regression [38]. A Multiple-Instance Learning-based approach was also attempted [83]. The advantage of this method is the lower labelling detail required during optimisation. In addition, the minimal supervision required allows easy retraining of a previously optimised system. One tuberculosis detection system uses ViDi Systems for image analysis of chest X-rays [84]. ViDi is an industrial-grade deep learning image analysis software developed by COGNEX. ViDi has shown feasible performance in the detection of tuberculosis. The authors of [36] introduced a fully automatic frontal chest screening system that is capable of detecting tuberculosis-infected lungs. This method begins with the segmentation of the lung. Then, features are extracted from the segmented images. Examples of features include shape and curvature histograms. Finally, a classifier was used to detect the disease.

For CT scans related tuberculosis detection works, a method called AECNN was proposed [85]. An AE-CNN block was formed by combining the feature extraction of CNN and the unsupervised features of AutoEncoder. The model then analyses the region of interest within the image to perform the classification of tuberculosis. A research study explores the use of CT pulmonary images to diagnose and classify tuberculosis at five levels of severity to track treatment effectiveness [24]. The tuberculosis abnormalities only occupy limited regions in the CT image, and the dataset is quite small. Therefore, depth-ResNet was proposed. Depth-ResNet is a 3D block-based ResNet combined with the injection of depth information at each layer. As an attempt to automate tuberculosis related lung deformities without sacrificing accuracy, advanced AI algorithms were studied to draw clinically actionable hypotheses [86]. This approach involves thorough image processing, subsequently performing feature extraction using TensorFlow and 3D CNN to further augment the metadata with the features extracted from the image data, and finally perform six class binary classification using the random forest. Another attempt for this problem was proposed by Zunair et al. [87]. They proposed a 16-layer 3D convolutional neural network with a slice selection. The goal is to estimate the tuberculosis severity based on the CT image. An integrated method based on optical flow and a characterisation method called Activity Description Vector (ADV) was presented to take care of the classification of chest CT scan images affected by different types of tuberculosis [88]. The important point of this technique is the interpretation of the set of cross-sectional chest images produced by CT scan, not as a volume but as a series of video images. This technique can extract movement descriptors capable of classifying tuberculosis affections by analysing deformations or movements generated in these video series. The idea of optical flow refers to the approximation of displacements of intensity patterns. In short, the ADV vector describes the activity in image series by counting for each region of the image the movements made in four directions of the 2D space.

For sputum microscopy images-related tuberculosis detection works, CNN was used for the detection and localisation of drug-sensitive tuberculosis bacilli in sputum microscopy images [29]. This method automatically localises bacilli in each view-field (a patch of the whole slide). A study found that, when training a CNN on three different image versions, namely RGB, R-G and grayscale, the best performance was achieved when using R-G images [28]. Image binarisation can also be used for preprocessing before the data were fed into a CNN [30]. Image binarisation is a segmentation method to classify the foreground and background of the microscopic sputum smear images. The segmented foreground consists of single bacilli, touching bacillus and other artefacts. A trained CNN is then given the foreground objects, and the CNN will classify the objects into bacilli and non-bacilli. Another tuberculosis detection system automatically attains all view-fields using a motorised microscopic stage [32]. After that, the data are delivered to the recognition system. A customised Inception V3 DeepNet model is used to learn from the pre-trained weights of Inception V3. Afterwards, the data were classified using SVM. DBN was also used to detect tuberculosis bacillus present in the stained microscopic images of sputum [31]. For segmentation, the Channel Area Thresholding algorithm is used. Location-oriented histogram and speed up robust feature (SURF) algorithm were used to extract the intensity-based local bacilli features. DBN is then used to classify the bacilli objects. Table 1 shows the summary of papers for tuberculosis detection using deep learning.

Table 1. Summary of papers for tuberculosis detection using deep learning.

Authors	Deep Learning Technique	Features	Dataset
[74]	CNN with transfer learning and data augmentation	Features extracted from CNN	Montgomery
[38]	K-nearest neighbour, Simple Linear Regression and Sequential Minimal Optimisation (SMO) Classification	Area, major axis, minor axis, eccentricity, mean, kurtosis, skewness and entropy	Shenzhen
[84]	ViDi	Features extracted from CNN	Unspecified
[64]	CNN	Gabor, LBP, SIFT, PHOG and Features extracted from CNN	Private dataset
[24]	CNN	Features extracted from CNN	ImageCLEF 2018 dataset
[62]	CNN with transfer learning, with demographic information	Features extracted from CNN + demographic information	Private dataset
[79]	CNN with data augmentation, and ensemble by weighted averages of probability scores	Features extracted from CNN	Montgomery, Shenzhen, Belarus, JSRT
[70]	CNN with transfer learning and data augmentation	Features extracted from CNN	Private dataset, Montgomery, Shenzhen

Table 1. *Cont.*

Authors	Deep Learning Technique	Features	Dataset
[69]	CNN	Features extracted from CNN	Private datasets, Montgomery, Shenzhen
[71]	CNN with transfer learning and ensemble by simple linear probabilities averaging	Features extracted from CNN + rule-based features	Indiana, JSRT, Shenzhen
[29]	CNN	HoG features	ZiehlNeelsen Sputum smear Microscopy image DataBase
[75]	CNN and shuffle sampling	Features extracted from CNN	Private datasets
[81]	CNN with transfer learning and ensemble by averaging	CNN extracted features from edge images	Montgomery, Shenzhen
[57]	CNN with transfer learning, data augmentation and ensemble by weighted probability scores average	Features extracted from CNN	Private dataset, Montgomery, Shenzhen, Belarus
[85]	AutoEncoder-CNN	Features extracted from CNN	Private dataset
[76]	CNN with transfer learning and shuffle sampling	Features extracted from CNN	Private dataset
[65]	End-to-end CNN	Features extracted from CNN	Montgomery, Shenzhen
[88]	Optical flow model	Activity Description Vector on optical flow of video sequences	ImageCLEF 2019 dataset
[28]	CNN	Colours	TBimages dataset
[83]	Modified maximum pattern margin support vector machine (modified miSVM)	First four moments of the intensity distributions	Private datasets
[61]	CAD4TB with clinical information	Features extracted from CNN + clinical features	Private dataset
[31]	DBN	LoH + SURF features	ZiehlNeelsen Sputum smear Microscopy image DataBase
[60]	CAD4TB	Features extracted from CNN	Private dataset
[72]	CNN with transfer learning and data augmentation	Features extracted from CNN	Montgomery, Shenzhen, NIH-14 dataset
[30]	CNN	Features extracted from CNN	TBimages dataset
[63]	CNN from scratch and data augmentation	Features extracted from CNN	Montgomery, Shenzhen, Belarus
[86]	3D CNN	Features extracted from CNN + lung volume + patient attribute metadata	ImageCLEF 2019 dataset
[12]	CNN with transfer learning and ensemble by stacking	local and global feature descriptors + features extracted from CNN	Private dataset, Montgomery, Shenzhen, India
[80]	CNN with transfer learning and feature level ensemble	Features extracted from CNN	Shenzhen
[15]	CNN with transfer learning and ensemble by averaging	CNN extracted features from edge images	Montgomery, Shenzhen
[32]	CNN with transfer learning	Features extracted from CNN	ZiehlNeelsen Sputum smear Microscopy image DataBase
[66]	CNN with data augmentation	Features extracted from CNN	Shenzhen
[73]	CNN with transfer learning and data augmentation	Features extracted from CNN	NIH-14, Montgomery, Shenzhen
[19]	CNN with transfer learning, Bag of CNN Features and ensemble by a simple soft-voting scheme	Features extracted from CNN + BOW	Private dataset, Montgomery, Shenzhen
[36]	Neural network	Shape, curvature descriptor histograms, eigenvalues of Hessian matrix	Montgomery, Shenzhen

Table 1. *Cont.*

Authors	Deep Learning Technique	Features	Dataset
[77]	CNN with transfer learning and data augmentation	Features extracted from CNN	Montgomery, Shenzhen, NIH-14
[87]	3D CNN	Features extracted from CNN	ImageCLEF 2019 dataset
[78]	CNN and Artificial Ecosystem-based Optimisation algorithm	Features extracted from CNN	Shenzhen
[67]	CNN	Features extracted from CNN	Shenzhen
[68]	Bayesian based CNN	Features extracted from CNN	Montgomery, Shenzhen
[82]	CNN with transfer learning, and ensemble by majority voting, simple averaging, weighted averaging, and stacking	Features extracted from CNN	Montgomery, Shenzhen, LDOCTCXR, 2018 RSNA pneumonia challenge dataset, Indiana dataset

4.7.2. Pneumonia

Pneumonia is a lung infection that causes pus and fluid to fill the alveoli in one or both lungs, thus making breathing difficult [89]. Symptoms include severe shortness of breath, chest pain, chills, cough, fever or fatigue. Community-acquired pneumonia is still a recurrent cause of morbidity and mortality [90]. Most of the studies used transfer learning and data augmentation. Tobias et al. [91] straightforwardly used CNN. Stephen et al. [92] trained their CNN from scratch while using rescale, rotation, width shift, height shift, shear, zoom and horizontal flip as their augmentation techniques. A pre-trained CNN was utilised by the authors of [20,55,93–97] for pneumonia detection, while the latter four also applied data augmentation on their training datasets. For data augmentation, random horizontal flipping was used by Rajpurkar et al. [96]; shifting, zooming, flipping and 40-degree angles rotation were used by Ayan and Ünver [20]; Chouhan et al. [55] used noise addition, random horizontal flip random resized crop and images intensity adjustment; and Rahman et al. [97] used rotation, scaling and translation. Hashmi et al. [98] used CNN with transfer learning, data augmentation and ensemble by weighted averaging.

In a unique study, Acharya and Satapathy [99] used Deep Siamese CNN architecture. Deep Siamese network uses the symmetric structure of the two input image for classification. Thus, the X-ray images were separated into two parts, namely the left half and the right half. Each half was then fed into the network to compare the symmetric structure together with the amount of the infection that is spread across these two regions. Training the model for both left and right parts of the X-ray images makes the classification process more robust. Elshennawy and Ibrahim [100] used CNN and Long Short-Term Memory (LSTM)-CNN for pneumonia detection. The key advantage of the LSTM is that it can model both long and short-term memory and can deal with the vanishing gradient problem by training on long strings and storing them in memory. Emhamed et al. [101] studied and compared seven different deep learning algorithms: Decision Tree, Random Forest, KNN, AdaBoost, Gradient Boost, XGBboost and CNN. Their results show CNN obtained the highest accuracy for pneumonia classification, followed by Random forest and XGBboost. Hashmi et al. [98] used CNN with transfer learning, data augmentation and ensemble by weighted averaging.

In addition, Kumar et al. [102] attempted not only pneumonia classification, but also ROI identification. Pneumonia was detected by looking at lung opacity, and Mask-RCNN based model was used to identify lung opacity that is likely to depict pneumonia. They also performed ensemble by combining confidence scores and bounding boxes. In addition to pneumonia detection, Hurt et al. [103] proposed an approach that provides a probabilistic map on the chest X-ray images to assist in the diagnosis of pneumonia. Table 2 shows the summary of papers for pneumonia detection using deep learning.

Table 2. Summary of papers for pneumonia detection using deep learning.

Reference	Deep Learning Technique	Features	Dataset
[99]	Deep Siamese based neural network	CNN extracted features from the left half and right half of the lungs	Unspecified Kaggle dataset
[20]	CNN with transfer learning and data augmentation	Features extracted from CNN	LDOCTCXR
[55]	CNN with transfer learning, data augmentation and ensemble by majority voting.	Features extracted from CNN	LDOCTCXR
[93]	CNN with transfer learning	Features extracted from CNN	LDOCTCXR
[102]	CNN with transfer learning, data augmentation and ensemble by combining confidence scores and bounding boxes.	Features extracted from CNN	Radiological Society of North America (RSNA) pneumonia dataset
[96]	CNN with transfer learning and data augmentation	Features extracted from CNN	NIH Chest X-ray Dataset
[92]	CNN from scratch and data augmentation	Features extracted from CNN	LDOCTCXR
[95]	CNN with transfer learning	Features extracted from CNN	LDOCTCXR
[91]	CNN	Features extracted from CNN	Mooney's Kaggle dataset
[100]	CNN and LSTM-CNN, with transfer learning and data augmentation	Features extracted from CNN	Mooney's Kaggle dataset
[103]	CNN with probabilistic map of pneumonia	Features extracted from CNN	2018 RSNA pneumonia challenge dataset
[101]	Decision Tree, Random Forest, K-nearest neighbour, AdaBoost, Gradient Boost, XGBboost, CNN	Multiple features	Mooney's Kaggle dataset
[98]	CNN with transfer learning, data augmentation and ensemble by weighted averaging	Features extracted from CNN	LDOCTCXR
[97]	CNN with transfer learning and data augmentation	Features extracted from CNN	Mooney's Kaggle dataset
[94]	CNN with transfer learning	Features extracted from CNN	Private dataset

4.7.3. Lung Cancer

One key characteristic of lung cancer is the presence of pulmonary nodules, solid clumps of tissue that appear in and around the lungs [104]. These nodules can be seen in CT scan images and can be malignant (cancerous) in nature or benign (not cancerous) [23].

As early as 2015, Hua et al. [105] used models of DBN and CNN to perform nodule classification in CT scans. They showed that, using deep learning, it is possible to seamlessly extract features for lung nodules classification into malignant or benign without computing the morphology and texture features. Rao et al. [25] and Kurniawan et al. [106] used CNN in a straightforward way to detect lung cancer in CT scans. Song et al. [23] compared the classification performance of CNN, deep neural network and stacked autoencoder (a multilayer sparse autoencoder of a neural network) and concluded that CNN has the highest accuracy among them. Ciompi et al. [107] used multi-stream multi-scale CNNs to classify lung nodules into six different classes: solid, non-solid, part-solid, calcified, perifissural and spiculated nodules. Specifically, they presented a multi-stream multi-scale architecture, in which CNN concurrently handles multiple triplets of 2D views of a nodule at multiple scales and then calculates the probability for the nodule in each of the six classes. Yu et al. [14] performed bone elimination and lung segmentation before training with CNN. Shakeel et al. [108] performed image denoising and enhanced the quality of the images, and then segmented the lungs by using the improved profuse clustering technique. Afterwards, a neural network is trained to detect lung cancer. The approach of Ardila et al. [13] consists of four components: lung segmentation, cancer region of interest detection model, full-volume model and cancer risk prediction model. After lung segmentation, the region of interest detection model proposes the most nodule-like regions, while the full-volume model was trained to predict cancer probability. The outputs of these two models were considered to generates the final prediction. Chen et al. [109] performed nodule enhancement and nodule segmentation before performing nodule detection.

For the works that employed transfer learning, Hosny et al. [110] and Xu et al. [111] both used CNN with data augmentation. For augmentations, both studies used flipping, translation and rotation. The authors of [112] leveraged the LUNA16 dataset to train a nodule detector and then refined that detector with the KDSB17 dataset to provide global features. Combining that and local features from a separate nodule classifier, they were able to detect lung cancer with high accuracy. The authors of [113] used transfer learning by training the model multiple times. It commenced using the more general images from the ImageNet dataset, followed by detecting nodules from chest X-rays in the ChestX-ray14 dataset, and finally detecting lung cancer nodules from the JSRT dataset. The authors of [34] is the only study surveyed to do lung cancer detection on histopathology images. Adenocarcinoma (LUAD) and squamous cell carcinoma (LUSC) are the most frequent subtypes of lung cancer, and visual examination by an experienced pathologist is needed to differentiate them. In this work, CNN was trained on histopathology slides images to automatically and accurately classify them into LUAD, LUSC or normal lung tissue. Xu et al. [114] used a CNN-long short-term memory network (LSTM) to detect lesions on chest X-ray images. Long short-term memory is an extension of RNN. This CNN-LSTM network offers probable clinical relationships between lesions to assist the model to attain better predictions. Table 3 shows the summary of papers for lung cancer detection using deep learning.

Table 3. Summary of papers for lung cancer detection using deep learning.

Reference	Deep Learning Technique	Features	Dataset
[13]	CNN	Features extracted from CNN	LUNA, LIDC, NLST
[113]	CNN with transfer learning	Features extracted from CNN	JSRT Dataset, NIH-14 dataset
[107]	Multi-stream multi-scale convolutional networks	Features extracted from CNN	MILD dataset DLCST dataset
[34]	CNN with transfer learning	Features extracted from CNN	NCI Genomic Data Commons
[110]	CNN with transfer learning and data augmentation	Features extracted from CNN	NSCLC-Radiomics, NSCLC-Radiomics-Genomics, RIDER Collections and several private datasets
[105]	CNN and DBN	Features extracted from CNN and DBN	LIDC-IDRI
[112]	CNN with transfer learning	Features extracted from CNN	Kaggle Data Science Bowl 2017 dataset, Lung Nodule Analysis 2016 (LUNA16) dataset
[25]	CNN	Features extracted from CNN	LIDC-IDRI
[108]	CNN	Features extracted from CNN	LIDC-IDRI
[23]	CNN with data augmentation	Features extracted from CNN	LIDC-IDRI database
[111]	CNN with transfer learning and data augmentation	Features extracted from CNN	Private dataset
[14]	Bone elimination and lung segmentation before training with CNN	Features extracted using CNN from bone eliminated lung images and segmented lung images	JSRT dataset
[114]	CNN-long short-term memory network	Features extracted from CNN	NIH-14 dataset

Table 3. Cont.

Reference	Deep Learning Technique	Features	Dataset
[109]	CNN with transfer learning and data augmentation	Features extracted from CNN	JSRT database
[106]	CNN with data augmentation	Features extracted from CNN	Cancer Imaging Archive

4.7.4. COVID-19

COVID-19 is an infectious disease caused by a recently discovered coronavirus [115]. Senior citizens are those at high risk to develop severe sickness, along with those that have historical medical conditions such as cardiovascular disease, chronic respiratory disease, cancer and diabetes [116].

A straightforward approach to detect COVID-19 using CNN with transfer learning and data augmentation was used by Salman et al. [21]. For transfer learning, they used InceptionV3 as a fixed feature extractor. Other works that implemented the similar approach of transfer learning for COVID-19 detection can be found in [117–122].

The authors of [123,124] performed 3-class classification using CNN with transfer learning, classifying X-ray images into normal, COVID-19 and viral pneumonia cases. Chowdhury et al. [125] utilised CNN with transfer learning and data augmentation to classify classifying X-ray images into normal, COVID-19 and viral pneumonia cases. The augmentation techniques used were rotation, scaling and translation. Wang et al. [126] trained a CNN from scratch and data augmentation to perform three-class classification. The augmentation technique used were translation, rotation, horizontal flip and intensity shift. Other work performing three-class classification can be found in [4,127–130]. Studies that employ data augmentation to increase the amount of data available can be found in [131,132]. In addition to COVID-19 detection on X-ray images, Alazab et al. [131] managed to perform prediction on the number of COVID-19 confirmations, recoveries and deaths in Jordan and Australia.

For works utilising ensemble, Ouyang et al. [133] implemented weighted averaging ensemble. Mahmud et al. [134] implemented stacking ensemble, whereby the images were classified into four categoriesL normal, COVID-19, viral pneumonia and bacterial pneumonia.

Shi et al. [135] utilised VB-Net for image segmentation and feature extraction and used a modified random decision forests method for classification. Several handcrafted features were also calculated and used to train the random forest model. More information about random forest can be found in [136].

A system that receives thoracic CT images and points out suspected COVID-19 cases was proposed by Gozes et al. [26]. The system analyses CT images at two distinct subsystems. Subsystem A performed the 3D analysis of the case volume for nodules and focal opacities, while Subsystem B performed the 2D analysis of each slice of the case to detect and localise larger-sized diffuse opacities. In Subsystem A, nodules and small opacities detection were conducted using a commercial software. Besides the detection of abnormalities, the software also provided measurements and localisation. For Subsystem B, lung segmentation was first performed, and then COVID-19 related abnormalities detection was conducted using CNN with transfer learning and data augmentation. If an image is classified as positive, a localisation map was generated using the Grad-cam technique. To provide a complete review of the case, Subsystems A and B were combined. The final outputs include per slice localisation of opacities (2D), 3D volumetric presentations of the opacities throughout the lungs and a Corona score, which is a volumetric measurement of the opacities burden.

The authors of [137] focused on location-attention classification mechanism. First, the CT images were preprocessed. Second, a 3D CNN model was employed to segment several candidate image patches. Third, an image classification model was trained and employed to categorise all image patches into one of three classes: COVID-19, Influenza-A-viral-pneumonia and irrelevant-to-infection. A location-attention mechanism was embedded in the image classification model to differentiate the structure and appearance of different infections. Finally, the overall analysis report for a single CT sample was generated using the Noisy-or Bayesian function. The results show that the proposed approach could more accurately detect COVID-19 cases than without the location-attention model. Several other studies modified the CNN for COVID-19 detection. In [138], a multi-objective differential evolution-based CNN was utilised. Sedik et al. [139] implemented CNN and LSTM with data augmentation, while Ahsan et al. [140] employed MLP-CNN based model. The authors of [141] employed capsule network-based framework with transfer learning. Table 4 shows the summary of papers for COVID-19 detection using deep learning.

Table 4. Summary of papers for COVID-19 detection using deep learning.

Authors	Deep Learning Technique	Features	Dataset
[137]	CNN with transfer learning and location-attention classification mechanism	Features extracted from CNN	Private dataset
[125]	CNN with transfer learning and data augmentation	Features extracted from CNN	SIRM database, Cohen's Github dataset, Chowdhury's Kaggle dataset
[26]	RADLogics Inc., CNN with transfer learning and data augmentation	Features extracted from RADLogics Inc and CNN	Chainz Dataset, A dataset from a hospital in Wenzhou, China, Dataset from El-Camino Hospital (CA) and Lung image database consortium (LIDC)
[123]	CNN with transfer learning	Features extracted from CNN	Cohen's Github dataset and LDOCTCXR
[21]	CNN with transfer learning and data augmentation	Features extracted from CNN	Cohen's Github dataset and unspecified Kaggle dataset
[135]	VB-Net and modified random decision forests method	96 handcrafted image features	Dataset obtained from Tongji Hospital of Huazhong University of Science and Technology, Shanghai Public Health Clinical Center of Fudan University, and China-Japan Union Hospital of Jilin University.
[126]	CNN from scratch and data augmentation	Features extracted from CNN	COVIDx Dataset
[127]	CNN with transfer learning	Features extracted from CNN	Cohen's Github dataset, Andrew's Kaggle dataset, LDOCTCXR
[117]	CNN with transfer learning	Features extracted from CNN	Cohen's Github dataset, RSNA pneumonia dataset, COVIDx
[131]	CNN with transfer learning and data augmentation	Features extracted from CNN	Sajid's Kaggle dataset
[4]	CNN with transfer learning and data augmentation	Features extracted from CNN	Cohen's Github dataset, Mooney's Kaggle dataset
[118]	CNN with transfer learning	Features extracted from CNN	COVID-CT-Dataset
[128]	CNN as feature extractor and long short-term memory (LSTM) network as classifier	Features extracted from CNN	GitHub, Radiopaedia, The Cancer Imaging Archive, SIRM, Kaggle repository, NIH dataset, Mendeley dataset
[132]	CNN with transfer learning and synthetic data generation and augmentation	Features extracted from CNN	Cohen's Github, Chowdhury's Kaggle dataset, COVID-19 Chest X-ray Dataset, Initiative
[129]	CNN with transfer learning, data augmentation and ensemble by majority voting	Features extracted from CNN	Cohen's Github, LDOCTCXR

Table 4. *Cont.*

Authors	Deep Learning Technique	Features	Dataset
[134]	CNN with transfer learning and stacking ensemble	Features extracted from CNN	Private dataset, LDOCTCXR
[130]	CNN	Features extracted from CNN	Private dataset
[138]	Multi-objective differential evolution-based CNN	Features extracted from CNN	Unspecified
[119]	CNN with transfer learning	Features extracted from CNN	Cohen's Github
[139]	CNN and ConvLSTM with data augmentation	Features extracted from CNN	Cohen's Github, COVID-CT-Dataset
[120]	CNN with transfer learning	Features extracted from CNN	Cohen's Github
[133]	CNN with ensemble by weighted averaging	Features extracted from CNN	Private hospital datasets
[121]	CNN with transfer learning	Features extracted from CNN	Cohen's Github, Mooney's Kaggle dataset, Shenzhen and Montgomery datasets
[140]	MLP-CNN based model	Features extracted from CNN	Cohen's Github
[122]	CNN with transfer learning	Features extracted from CNN	Cohen's Github, unspecified Kaggle dataset
[141]	Capsule Network-based framework with transfer learning	Features extracted from CNN	Cohen's Github, Mooney's Kaggle dataset

4.8. Dataset

The datasets used by the surveyed works are reported in this section. Tables 5–8 show the summary of datasets used for tuberculosis, pneumonia, lung cancer and COVID-19 detection, respectively. This is done to provide readers with relevant information on the datasets. Note that only public datasets are included in the tables because they are available to the public, whereas private datasets are inaccessible without permission.

According to Table 5, among the twelve datasets used for tuberculosis detection works, five of them do not contain tuberculosis medical images: JSRT dataset, Indiana dataset, NIH-14 dataset, LDOCTCXR and RSNA pneumonia dataset. JSRT dataset contains lung cancer images, while the Indiana and NIH-14 datasets contain multiple different diseases. LDOCTCXR and RSNA pneumonia datasets both contain pneumonia and normal lung images. These five datasets were used for transfer learning in several studies. Models were first trained to identify abnormalities in chest X-ray, and then they were trained to identify tuberculosis. The India, Montgomery and Shenzhen datasets contain X-ray images of tuberculosis; ImageCLEF 2018 and ImageCLEF 2019 datasets contain CT images of tuberculosis; and the Belarus dataset contains both X-ray and CT images of tuberculosis. Two of the datasets contain sputum smear microscopy images of tuberculosis: the TBimages dataset and ZiehlNeelsen Sputum smear Microscopy image DataBase.

For detection works related to pneumonia, only four public datasets are available, as shown in Table 6. All four datasets contain X-ray images only. Even though the number of datasets is low, the number of images within these datasets is high. Future studies utilising these datasets should have sufficient data.

Table 5. Summary of datasets used for tuberculosis detection.

Name	Disease	Image Type	Reference	Number of Images	Link
Belarus dataset	Tuberculosis	X-ray and CT	[142]	1299	http://tuberculosis.by
ImageCLEF 2018 dataset	Tuberculosis	CT		2287	https://www.imageclef.org/2018/tuberculosis
ImageCLEF 2019 dataset	Tuberculosis	CT	[143]	335	https://www.imageclef.org/2019/medical/tuberculosis
India	Tuberculosis	X-ray	[39]	78 tuberculosis and 78 normal	https://sourceforge.net/projects/tbxpredict/
Indiana Dataset	Multiple diseases with annotations	X-ray	[144]	7284	https://openi.nlm.nih.gov
JSRT dataset	Lung nodules and normal	X-ray and CT	[145]	154 nodule and 93 non-nodule	http://db.jsrt.or.jp/eng.php
Montgomery and Shenzhen datasets	Tuberculosis and normal	X-ray	[146]	394 tuberculosis and 384 normal	https://lhncbc.nlm.nih.gov/publication/pub9931
NIH-14 dataset	Pneumonia and 13 other diseases	X-ray	[147]	112120	https://www.kaggle.com/nih-chest-xrays/data
TBimages dataset	Tuberculosis	Sputum smear microscopy image	[148]	1320	http://www.tbimages.ufam.edu.br/
ZiehlNeelsen Sputum smear Microscopy image DataBase	Tuberculosis	Sputum smear microscopy image	[27]	620 tuberculosis and 622 normal	http://14.139.240.55/znsm/
Large Dataset of Labeled Optical Coherence Tomography (OCT) and Chest X-Ray Images (LDOCTCXR)	Pneumonia and normal	X-ray	[93]	3883 pneumonia and 1349 normal	https://data.mendeley.com/datasets/rscbjbr9sj/3
Radiological Society of North America (RSNA) pneumonia dataset	Pneumonia and normal	X-ray		5528	https://www.kaggle.com/c/rsna-pneumonia-detection-challenge/data

Table 6. Summary of datasets used for pneumonia detection.

Name	Disease	Image Type	Reference	Number of Images	Link
LDOCTCXR		X-ray	[93]	3883 pneumonia and 1349 normal	https://data.mendeley.com/datasets/rscbjbr9sj/3
NIH Chest X-ray Dataset	Pneumonia and 13 other diseases	X-ray	[147]	112,120	https://www.kaggle.com/nih-chest-xrays/data
Radiological Society of North America (RSNA) pneumonia dataset	Pneumonia and normal	X-ray		5528	https://www.kaggle.com/c/rsna-pneumonia-detection-challenge/data
Mooney's Kaggle dataset	Pneumonia and normal	X-ray		5863	https://www.kaggle.com/paultimothymooney/chest-xray-pneumonia

According to Table 7, among the ten datasets used for lung cancer detection works, only one contains histopathology images, which is the NCI Genomic Data Commons dataset. The NIH-14 dataset contains X-ray images, while the JSRT dataset contains a mix of X-ray and CT images. The rest of the datasets all contain CT images.

Table 7. Summary of datasets used for lung cancer detection.

Name	Disease	Image Type	Reference	Number of Images	Link
JSRT dataset	Lung nodules and normal lungs	X-ray and CT	[145]	154 nodule and 93 non-nodule	http://db.jsrt.or.jp/eng.php
Kaggle Data Science Bowl 2017 dataset	Lung Cancer	CT scans		601	https://www.kaggle.com/c/data-science-bowl-2017/overview
LIDC-IDRI	Lung Cancer	CT	[149]	1018	https://wiki.cancerimagingarchive.net/display/Public/LIDC-IDRI
Lung Nodule Analysis 2016 (LUNA16) dataset	Location and size of lung nodules	CT scans	[8]	888	https://luna16.grand-challenge.org/download/
NCI Genomic Data Commons	Lung Cancer	histopa-thology images	[150]	More than 575,000	https://portal.gdc.cancer.gov/
NIH-14 dataset	14 lung diseases	X-ray	[147]	112,120	https://www.kaggle.com/nih-chest-xrays/data
NLST	Lung Cancer	CT		Approximately 200,000	https://biometry.nci.nih.gov/cdas/learn/nlst/images/
NSCLC-Radiomics	Lung Cancer	CT		422	https://wiki.cancerimagingarchive.net/display/Public/NSCLC-Radiomics
NSCLC-Radiomics-Genomics	Lung Cancer	CT		89	https://wiki.cancerimagingarchive.net/display/Public/NSCLC-Radiomics-Genomics
RIDER Collections	Lung Cancer	CT		Approximately 280,000	https://wiki.cancerimagingarchive.net/display/Public/RIDER+Collections

Table 8 shows that there are thirteen public datasets related to COVID-19. With the rise of the COVID-19 pandemic, multiple datasets have been made available to the public. Many of these datasets still have a rising number of images. Therefore, the number of images within the datasets might be different from the number reported in this paper. Take note that some of the images might be contained in multiple datasets. Therefore, future studies should check for duplicate images.

Table 9 summarises the works surveyed based on the taxonomy. This allows readers to quickly refer to the articles according to their interested attributes. The analysis of the distribution of works based on the identified attributes of the taxonomy is given in the following section.

Table 8. Summary of datasets used for COVID-19 detection.

Name	Disease	Image Type	Reference	Number of Images	Link
Andrew's Kaggle dataset	COVID-19	X-ray and CT		79	https://www.kaggle.com/andrewmvd/convid19-x-rays
Chainz Dataset	COVID-19 and normal	CT		50 COVID-19, 51 normal	www.ChainZ.cn
Chowdhury's Kaggle dataset	COVID-19, normal and pneumonia	X-ray	[125]	219 COVID-19, 1341 normal and 1345 pneumonia	https://www.kaggle.com/tawsifurrahman/covid19-radiography-database
Cohen's Github dataset	COVID-19	X-ray and CT	[151]	123	https://github.com/ieee8023/covid-chestxray-dataset

Table 8. Cont.

Name	Disease	Image Type	Reference	Number of Images	Link
COVIDx Dataset	COVID-19, normal and pneumonia	X-ray	[126]	573 COVID-19, 8066 normal and 5559 pneumonia	https://github.com/lindawangg/COVID-Net/blob/master/docs/COVIDx.md
Italian Society Of Medical And Interventional Radiology (SIRM) COVID-19 Database	COVID-19	X-ray and CT		68	https://www.sirm.org/category/senza-categoria/covid-19/
LDOCTCXR	Pneumonia and normal	X-ray	[93]	3883 pneumonia and 1349 normal	https://data.mendeley.com/datasets/rscbjbr9sj/3
Lung image database consortium (LIDC)	Lung Cancer	CT	[149]	1018	https://wiki.cancerimagingarchive.net/display/Public/LIDC-IDRI
Sajid's Kaggle dataset	COVID-19 and normal	X-ray		28 normal, 70 COVID-19	https://www.kaggle.com/nabeelsajid917/covid-19-x-ray-10000-images
Mooney's Kaggle dataset	Pneumonia and normal	X-ray		5863	https://www.kaggle.com/paultimothymooney/chest-xray-pneumonia
COVID-CT Dataset	COVID-19 and normal	CT		349 COVID-19 and 463 non-COVID-19	https://github.com/UCSD-AI4H/COVID-CT
Mendeley Augmented COVID-19 X-ray Images Dataset	COVID-19 and normal	X-ray		912	https://data.mendeley.com/datasets/2fxz4px6d8/4
COVID-19 Chest X-Ray Dataset Initiative	COVID-19	X-ray		55	https://github.com/agchung/Figure1-COVID-chestxray-dataset

Table 9. Summary of the works surveyed based on the taxonomy.

Attributes	Subattributes	References
Image types	X-Ray	[4,12,14,15,19–21,24,36,38,55,57,60–85,91–103,109,113,114,117,119–129,131,132,134,139–141]
	CT Scans	[13,23,25,26,86–88,105–108,110–112,118,130,133,135,137–139]
	Sputum Smear Microscopy Images	[28–32]
	Histopathology images	[34]
Features	Extracted from CNN	[4,12–15,19–21,23–26,30,32,34,55,57,60–82,84–87,91–103,105–114,117–134,137–141]
	Others	[12,15,26,28,29,31,36,38,61,62,64,71,81,83,86,88,105,135]
Data augmentation	Yes	[4,20,21,23,26,55,57,63,66,70,73,74,77,79,92,96–98,100,102,106,109–111,114,122,125,126,128,129,131,132,139]
Types of deep learning algorithm	CNN	[4,12–15,19–21,23–26,28–30,32,34,55,57,60–69,72,74,76–82,84–86,91–103,105–114,117–134,137–141]
	Non-CNN	[19,26,31,36,38,83,88,105,135]
Transfer learning	Fixed feature extractor	[12,15,19,21,62,70,76,78,80,81,93,94,96,100,102,117,127,128,137]
	Fine-tuning CNN	[4,20,26,32,34,55,57,71–74,76,77,79,82,95,97,98,102,109–113,118–125,129,131,132,134,141]
Ensemble	Majority voting	[19,55,82,129]
	Probability score averaging	[15,57,71,79,81,82,98,102,133]
	Stacking	[12,82,134]
	Other	[80]
Disease types	Tuberculosis	[12,15,19,24,28–32,36,38,57,60–88]
	Pneumonia	[20,55,91–103]
	Lung cancer	[13,14,23,25,34,105–114]
	COVID-19	[4,21,26,117–135,137–141]

5. Analysis of Trend, Issues and Future Directions of Lung Disease Detection Using Deep Learning

In this section, the broad analysis of the existing work is presented, which is the last contribution outlined in this paper. The analysis of the trend of each attribute identified in the foregoing section is described, whereby the aim is to show the progress of the works and the direction the researchers are heading over the last five years. The shown trend could be useful to suggest the future direction of the work in this domain. Section 5.1 presents the analysis of the trend of the articles considered. The issues and potential future work to address the identified issues are described in Section 5.2.

5.1. An Analysis of the Trend of Lung Disease Detection in Recent Years

This subsection presents the analysis of lung disease detection works in recent years for each attribute of the taxonomy described in the foregoing section.

5.1.1. Trend Analysis of the Image Type Used

Figure 10a shows that the usage of X-ray images increases linearly over the years. The usage of CT images also increases over the years, with a slight dip in 2018. The sputum smear microscopy and histopathology images are combined into one as 'Others' due to the low number of previous work using them to detect lung diseases. The usage of other image types slowly increases until 2018, and then drops. This indicates that deep learning aided lung disease detection works are heading towards the direction of using X-ray images and CT images.

Figure 10b shows that the majority of the studies used X-ray images at 71%, while CT images followed second with 23%. Such observation could be due to the availability, accessibility and mobility of X-ray machines over the CT scanner. Due to the COVID-19 pandemic that has spread to all types of geographical locations, it is anticipated that the X-ray images will still be the dominant choice of medical images used to detect lung-related diseases over CT images. CT images may remain the second choice because they provide more detailed information than X-rays.

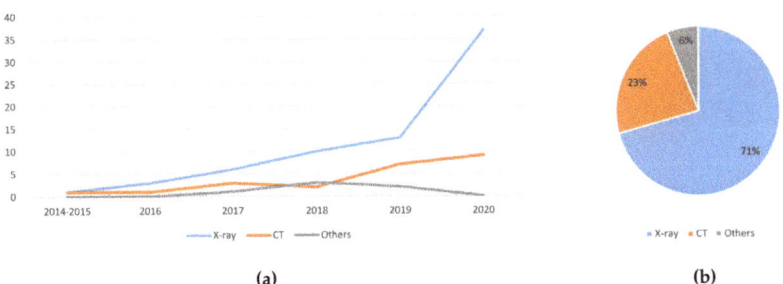

Figure 10. (a) The trend of the usage of image types in lung disease detection works in recent years; and (b) the distribution of the image type used in deep learning aided lung disease detection in recent years.

5.1.2. Trend Analysis of the Features Used

From the perspective of features used for lung disease detection in recent years, as shown in Figure 11a, the usage of CNN extracted features is steadily increasing, while the usage of other features and the combination of CNN extracted features plus other features remain low. This is because CNN allows automated feature extraction, discarding the need for manual feature generation [40]. The usage of other features was less preferred due to the fact that most recent works showed the superiority of CNN extracted features in detecting lung diseases. Figure 11b shows the distribution of work by type of features used. CNN extracted features were used in 79% of the works. The combination of CNN extracted features plus some other features were used in 13% of the recent works, while the remaining works utilised other types of features.

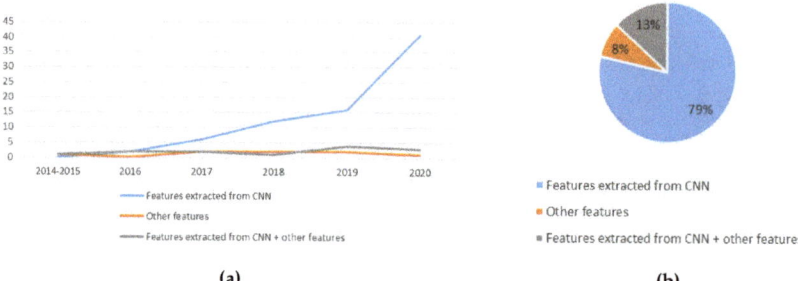

Figure 11. (a) The trend of the usage of features in lung disease detection works in recent years; and (b) the distribution of usage of data augmentation in deep learning aided lung disease detection in recent years.

5.1.3. Trend Analysis of the Usage of Data Augmentation

Figure 12a shows the trend of the usage of data augmentation. Although implementing data augmentation increased the complexity of the data pre-processing, the number of works employing data augmentation increases steadily over the years. Such trend signifies that more researchers have realised how beneficial data augmentation is to train the lung disease detection models.

Figure 12b shows the distribution of data augmentation usage in deep learning aided lung disease detection. Only about one-third of the studies used data augmentation. While it is reported that data augmentation improved the classification accuracy, the majority of works did not use data augmentation. One reason for this might be that data augmentation is not that simple to implement. As mentioned in Section 4.3, the disadvantages of data augmentation include additional memory costs, transformation computing costs and training time.

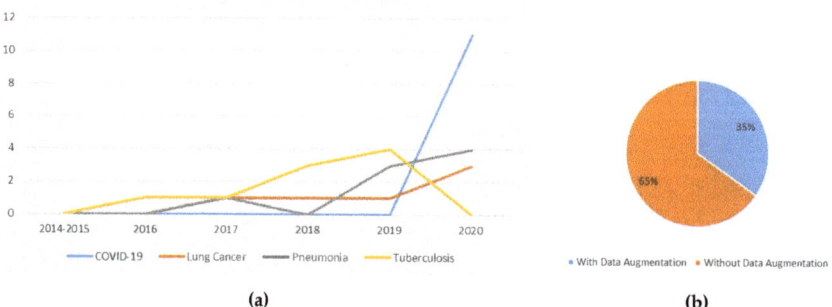

Figure 12. (a) The trend of the usage of data augmentation in lung disease detection works in recent years; and (b) the distribution of usage of data augmentation in deep learning aided lung disease detection in recent years.

5.1.4. Trend Analysis of the Types of Deep Learning Algorithm Used

Figure 13a shows the trend of the usage of deep learning algorithms in lung disease detection works in recent years. As shown in Figure 13, CNN was the most preferred deep learning algorithm for the last five years. Future works will likely follow this trend, whereby more work may prefer CNN for lung disease detection over other deep learning algorithms.

Figure 13b visualises the analysis of the usage of CNN in deep learning aided lung disease detection in recent years. The majority of the papers surveyed used CNN. This is because CNN is robust and can achieve high classification accuracy. Many of the works surveyed indicate that CNN has superior performance [74]. Other benefits of using CNN include automatic feature extraction and utilising the advantages of transfer learning, which is further analysed in the following subsection.

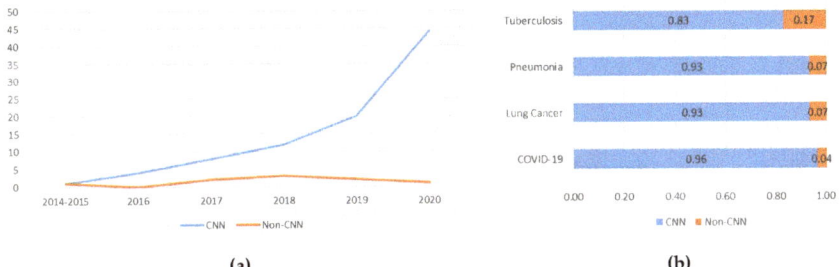

(a)   (b)

Figure 13. (a) The trend of the usage of deep learning algorithms in lung disease detection works in recent years; and (b) the distribution of the usage of CNN in deep learning aided lung disease detection in recent years.

5.1.5. Trend Analysis of the Usage Of Transfer Learning

Figure 14a shows the trend of the usage of transfer learning. As time goes on, more works employed transfer learning. With transfer learning, there is no need to define a new model. Transfer learning also allows the usage features learned while training from an old task for the new task, often increasing the classification accuracy. This could be due to the model used being more generalised as it has been trained with a greater number of images.

Figure 14b shows the usage of transfer learning among the works which used CNN. According to the figure, 57% of the recent works utilised transfer learning. Even though the number of works utilising transfer learning increased over the years, as shown in Figure 14a, the percentage of works using transfer learning is just 57%. For example, in 2020, out of 44 studies that used CNN, 28 implemented transfer learning. This suggests that works in this domain are moving towards the direction of using transfer learning, but not at a high pace. Transfer learning remains a strong approach to lung disease detection, with respect to the detection performance. Hence, the distribution of work may be skewed towards transfer learning in the near future.

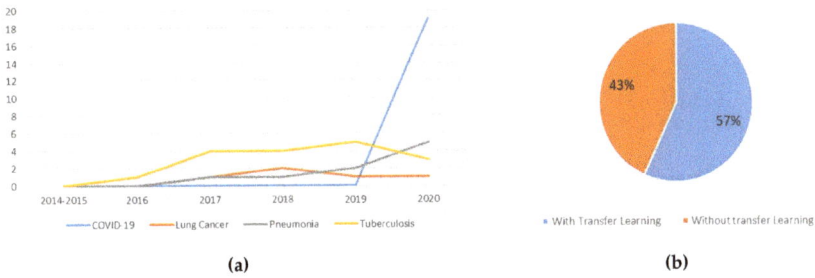

(a)   (b)

Figure 14. (a) The trend of the usage of transfer learning in lung disease detection works in recent years; and (b) the usage of transfer learning in lung disease detection works using CNN.

5.1.6. Trend Analysis of the Usage Of Ensemble

Based on Figure 15a, it seems that the ensemble was only applied on COVID-19, pneumonia and tuberculosis detection. It is observed that the usage of the ensemble is slowly growing in popularity for pneumonia and COVID-19 detection. Although less popular, the works that deployed an ensemble classifier reported better detection performance than when not using ensemble.

Figure 15b shows the distribution of the usage of the ensemble in deep learning aided lung disease detection. Only 15% of the studies used ensemble. This suggests that ensemble classifier is still less explored for lung disease detection. Only three types of ensemble techniques were found in the papers surveyed, which were majority voting, probability score averaging and stacking. The challenge to implement ensemble may be the caused of such low application. Using ensemble, the performance could only improve if the errors of the base classifiers have a low correlation. When using similar data, which may occur when the size of the datasets and the number of datasets itself are limited, the correlation of errors of the base classifiers tends to be high.

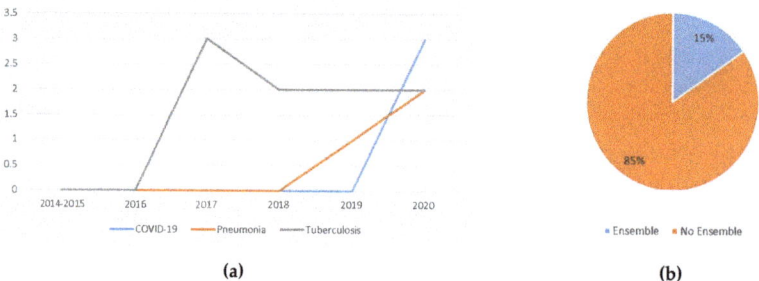

Figure 15. (**a**) The trend of the usage of ensemble classifier in lung disease detection works in recent years; and (**b**) the distribution of the usage of the ensemble in deep learning aided lung disease detection in recent years.

5.1.7. Trend Analysis of the Type Of Lung Disease Detected using Deep Learning

Based on the trend shown in Figure 16a, the total number of lung disease detection works using deep learning increased steadily over the years, with most work related to tuberculosis detection. As more lung disease medical image datasets become public, researchers have access to more data. Thus, more extensive studies were conducted. Towards 2020, the works on COVID-19 detection emerged while work conducted to detect other diseases decreased tremendously. This signifies that using deep learning to detect lung disease is still an active field of study. This also shows that much effort was directed towards easing the burden of detecting COVID-19 using the existing manual screening test, which is already anticipated.

Figure 16b shows the distribution of the diseases detected using deep learning in recent years. The majority of works were directed at tuberculosis detection, followed by COVID-19, lung cancer and pneumonia. The reason that works of tuberculosis are high is because the majority of tuberculosis-infected inhabitants were from resource-poor regions with poor healthcare infrastructure [61]. Therefore, tuberculosis detection using deep learning provides the opportunity to accelerate tuberculosis diagnosis among these communities. The reason that works of COVID-19 detection are second highest is because researchers all over the world are trying to reduce the burden of detecting COVID-19, and thus many works have been published, even though COVID-19 is a relatively new disease.

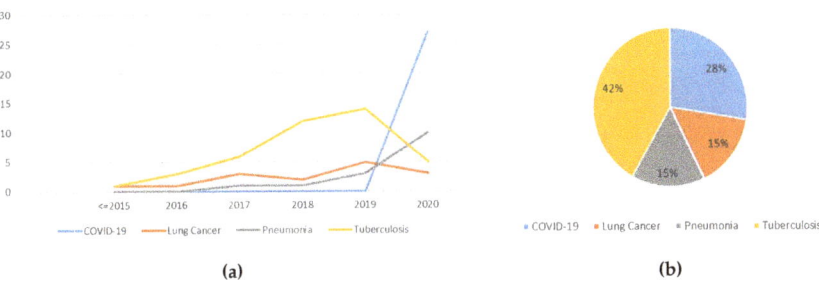

Figure 16. (a) The trend of the deep learning aided lung disease detection works in recent years; and (b) the distribution of the diseases detected using deep learning in recent years.

5.2. Issues and Future Direction of Lung Disease Detection Using Deep Learning

This subsection presents the remaining issues and corresponding future direction of lung disease detection using deep learning, which are the final contributions of this paper. The state-of-the-art lung disease detection field is suffering from several issues that can be found in the papers considered. Some of the proposed future works are designed to deal with the issues found. Details of the issues and potential future works are presented in Sections 5.2.1 and 5.2.2, respectively.

5.2.1. Issues

This section presents the issues of lung disease detection using deep learning found in the literature. Four main issues were identified: (i) data imbalance; (ii) handling of huge image size; (iii) limited available datasets; and (iv) high correlation of errors when using ensemble techniques.

(i) Data imbalance: When doing classification training, if the number of samples of one class is a lot higher than the other class, the resulting model would be biased. It is better to have the same number of images in each class. However, oftentimes that is not the case. For example, when performing a multiclass classification of COVID-19, pneumonia and normal lungs, the number of images for pneumonia far exceeds the number of images for COVID-19 [126].

(ii) Handling of huge image size: Most researchers reduced the original image size during training to reduce computational cost. It is extremely computationally expensive to train with the original image size, and it is also time-consuming to train a deeply complex model even with the aid of the most powerful GPU hardware.

(iii) Limited available datasets: Ideally, thousands of images of each class should be obtained for training. This is to produce a more accurate classifier. However, due to the limited number of datasets, the number of available training data is often less than ideal. This causes researchers to search for other alternatives to produce a good classifier.

(iv) High correlation of errors when using ensemble techniques: It requires a variety of errors for an ensemble of classifiers to perform the best. The base classifiers used should have a very low correlation. This, in turn, will ensure the errors of those classifiers also will be varied. In other words, it is expected that the base classifiers will complement each other to produce better classification results. Most of the studies surveyed only combine classifiers that were trained on similar features. This causes the correlation error of the base classifiers to be high.

5.2.2. Potential Future Works

This section presents the possible future works that should be considered to improvise the performance of lung disease detection using deep learning.

(i) Make datasets available to the public: Some researchers used private hospital datasets. To obtain larger datasets, efforts such as de-identification of confidential patients' information can be conducted to make the data public. With more data available, the produced classifiers would be more accurate. This is because, with more data comes more diversity. This decreases the generalisation error because the model becomes more general as it was trained on more examples. Medical data are hard to come by. Therefore, if the datasets were made public, more data would be available for researchers.

(ii) Usage of cloud computing: Performing training using cloud computing might overcome the problem of handling of huge image size. On a local mid-range computer, training with large images will be slow. A high-end computer might speed up the process a little, but it might still be infeasible. However, by training the deep learning model using cloud computing, we can use multiple GPUs at a reasonable cost. This allows higher computational cost training to be conducted faster and cheaper.

(iii) Usage of more variety of features: Most researchers use features automatically extracted by CNN. Some other features such as SIFT, GIST, Gabor, LBP and HOG were studied. However, many other features are still yet to be explored, for example quadtree and image histogram. Efforts can be directed to studying different types of features. This can address the issue of the high correlation of errors when using ensemble techniques. With more features comes more variation. When combining many variations, the results are often better [41]. Feature engineering allows the extraction of more information from present data. New information is extracted in terms of new features. These features might have a better ability to describe the variance in the training data, thus improving model accuracy.

(iv) Usage of the ensemble learning: Ensemble techniques show great potentials. Ensemble methods often improve detection accuracy. An ensemble of several features might provide better detection results. An ensemble of different deep learning techniques could also be considered because ensembles perform better if the errors of the base classifiers have a low correlation.

6. Limitation of the Survey

The survey presented has a limitation whereby the primary source of work considered were those indexed in the Scopus database, due to the reason described in Section 2. Exceptions were given on COVID-19 related works, as most of the articles were still at the preprint level when this survey was conducted. Concerning the publication years considered, the latest publication included were those published prior to October 2020. Therefore, the findings put forward in this survey paper did not consider contributions of works that are non-Scopus indexed and those that are published commencing October 2020 and onwards.

7. Conclusions

As time goes on, more works on lung disease detection using deep learning have been published. However, there was a lack of systematic survey available on the current state of research and application. This paper is thus produced to offer an extensive survey of lung disease detection using deep learning, specifically on tuberculosis, pneumonia, lung cancer and COVID-19, published from 2016 to September 2020. In total, 98 articles on this topic were considered in producing this survey.

To summarise and provide an organisation of the key concepts and focus of the existing work on lung disease detection using deep learning, a taxonomy of state-of-the-art deep learning aided lung disease detection was constructed based on the survey on the works considered. Analyses of the trend on recent works on this topic, based on the identified attributes from the taxonomy, are also presented. From the analyses of the distribution of works, the usage of both CNN and transfer learning is high. Concerning the trend of the surveyed work, all the identified attributes in the taxonomy observed, on average, a linear increase over the years, with an exception to the ensemble attribute. The remaining issues and future direction of lung disease detection using deep learning were subsequently established and described. Four issues of lung disease detection using deep learning were identified: data imbalance, handling of huge image size, limited available datasets and high correlation of errors when using ensemble techniques. Four potential works for lung disease detection using deep learning are suggested to resolve the identified issues: making datasets available to the public, usage of cloud computing, usage of more features and usage of the ensemble.

To conclude, investigating how deep learning was employed in lung disease detection is highly significant to ensure future research will concentrate on the right track, thereby improving the performance of disease detection systems. The presented taxonomy could be used by other researchers to plan their research contributions and activities. The potential future direction suggested could further improve the efficiency and increase the number of deep learning aided lung disease detection applications.

Author Contributions: All authors contributed to the study conceptualisation and design. Material preparation and analysis were performed by S.T.H.K. and M.H.A.H. The first draft of the manuscript was written by S.T.H.K., supervised by M.H.A.H., A.B. and H.K. All authors provided critical feedback and helped shape the manuscript. All authors have read and agreed to the published version of the manuscript.

Funding: This research was funded by Universiti Malaysia Sabah (UMS) grant number SDK0191-2020.

Conflicts of Interest: The authors declare no conflict of interest. The funders had no role in the design of the study; in the collection, analyses, or interpretation of data; in the writing of the manuscript, or in the decision to publish the results.

References

1. Bousquet, J. *Global Surveillance, Prevention and Control of Chronic Respiratory Diseases*; World Health Organization: Geneva, Switzerland, 2007; pp. 12–36.
2. Forum of International Respiratory Societies. *The Global Impact of Respiratory Disease*, 2nd ed.; European Respiratory Society, Sheffield, UK, 2017; pp. 5–42.
3. World Health Organization. *Coronavirus Disease 2019 (COVID-19) Situation Report*; Technical Report March; World Health Organization: Geneva, Switzerland, 2020.
4. Rahaman, M.M.; Li, C.; Yao, Y.; Kulwa, F.; Rahman, M.A.; Wang, Q.; Qi, S.; Kong, F.; Zhu, X.; Zhao, X. Identification of COVID-19 samples from chest X-Ray images using deep learning: A comparison of transfer learning approaches. *J. X-Ray Sci. Technol.* **2020**, *28*, 821–839. [CrossRef]
5. Yahiaoui, A.; Er, O.; Yumusak, N. A new method of automatic recognition for tuberculosis disease diagnosis using support vector machines. *Biomed. Res.* **2017**, *28*, 4208–4212.
6. Hu, Z.; Tang, J.; Wang, Z.; Zhang, K.; Zhang, L.; Sun, Q. Deep learning for image-based cancer detection and diagnosis-A survey. *Pattern Recognit.* **2018**, *83*, 134–149. [CrossRef]
7. American Thoracic Society. Diagnostic Standards and Classification of Tuberculosis in Adults and Children. *Am. J. Respir. Crit. Care Med.* **2000**, *161*, 1376–1395. [CrossRef]
8. Setio, A.A.A.; Traverso, A.; de Bel, T.; Berens, M.S.; van den Bogaard, C.; Cerello, P.; Chen, H.; Dou, Q.; Fantacci, M.E.; Geurts, B.; et al. Validation, comparison, and combination of algorithms for automatic detection of pulmonary nodules in computed tomography images: The LUNA16 challenge. *Med. Image Anal.* **2017**, *42*, 1–13. [CrossRef]
9. Shen, D.; Wu, G.; Suk, H.I. Deep Learning in Medical Image Analysis. *Annu. Rev. Biomed. Eng.* **2017**, *19*, 221–248. [CrossRef]
10. Wu, C.; Luo, C.; Xiong, N.; Zhang, W.; Kim, T.H. A Greedy Deep Learning Method for Medical Disease Analysis. *IEEE Access* **2018**, *6*, 20021–20030. [CrossRef]
11. Ma, J.; Song, Y.; Tian, X.; Hua, Y.; Zhang, R.; Wu, J. Survey on deep learning for pulmonary medical imaging. *Front. Med.* **2019**, *14*, 450–469. [CrossRef]
12. Rajaraman, S.; Candemir, S.; Xue, Z.; Alderson, P.O.; Kohli, M.; Abuya, J.; Thoma, G.R.; Antani, S.; Member, S. A novel stacked generalization of models for improved TB detection in chest radiographs. In Proceedings of the 2018 40th Annual International Conference the IEEE Engineering in Medicine and Biology Society (EMBC), Honolulu, HI, USA, 17–21 July 2018; pp. 718–721. [CrossRef]

13. Ardila, D.; Kiraly, A.P.; Bharadwaj, S.; Choi, B.; Reicher, J.J.; Peng, L.; Tse, D.; Etemadi, M.; Ye, W.; Corrado, G.; et al. End-to-end lung cancer screening with three-dimensional deep learning on low-dose chest computed tomography. *Nat. Med.* **2019**, *25*, 954–961. [CrossRef]
14. Gordienko, Y.; Gang, P.; Hui, J.; Zeng, W.; Kochura, Y.; Alienin, O.; Rokovyi, O.; Stirenko, S. Deep Learning with Lung Segmentation and Bone Shadow Exclusion Techniques for Chest X-Ray Analysis of Lung Cancer. *Adv. Intell. Syst. Comput.* **2019**, 638–647. [CrossRef]
15. Kieu, S.T.H.; Hijazi, M.H.A.; Bade, A.; Yaakob, R.; Jeffree, S. Ensemble deep learning for tuberculosis detection using chest X-Ray and canny edge detected images. *IAES Int. J. Artif. Intell.* **2019**, *8*, 429–435. [CrossRef]
16. Dietterich, T.G. Ensemble Methods in Machine Learning. *Int. Workshop Mult. Classif. Syst.* **2000**, 1–15._1. [CrossRef]
17. Webb, A. *Introduction To Biomedical Imaging*; John Wiley & Sons, Inc.: Hoboken, NJ, USA, 2003. [CrossRef]
18. Kwan-Hoong, N.; Madan M, R. X ray imaging goes digital. *Br. Med J.* **2006**, *333*, 765–766. [CrossRef]
19. Lopes, U.K.; Valiati, J.F. Pre-trained convolutional neural networks as feature extractors for tuberculosis detection. *Comput. Biol. Med.* **2017**, *89*, 135–143. [CrossRef] [PubMed]
20. Ayan, E.; Ünver, H.M. Diagnosis of Pneumonia from Chest X-Ray Images using Deep Learning. *Sci. Meet. Electr.-Electron. Biomed. Eng. Comput. Sci.* **2019**, 1–5. [CrossRef]
21. Salman, F.M.; Abu-naser, S.S.; Alajrami, E.; Abu-nasser, B.S.; Ashqar, B.A.M. COVID-19 Detection using Artificial Intelligence. *Int. J. Acad. Eng. Res.* **2020**, *4*, 18–25.
22. Herman, G.T. *Fundamentals of Computerized Tomography*; Springer: London, UK, 2009; Volume 224. [CrossRef]
23. Song, Q.Z.; Zhao, L.; Luo, X.K.; Dou, X.C. Using Deep Learning for Classification of Lung Nodules on Computed Tomography Images. *J. Healthc. Eng.* **2017**, *2017*. [CrossRef]
24. Gao, X.W.; James-reynolds, C.; Currie, E. Analysis of tuberculosis severity levels from CT pulmonary images based on enhanced residual deep learning architecture. *Neurocomputing* **2019**, *392*, 233–244. [CrossRef]
25. Rao, P.; Pereira, N.A.; Srinivasan, R. Convolutional neural networks for lung cancer screening in computed tomography (CT) scans. In Proceedings of the 2016 2nd International Conference on Contemporary Computing and Informatics, IC3I 2016, Noida, India, 14–17 December 2016; pp. 489–493. [CrossRef]
26. Gozes, O.; Frid, M.; Greenspan, H.; Patrick, D. Rapid AI Development Cycle for the Coronavirus (COVID-19) Pandemic: Initial Results for Automated Detection & Patient Monitoring using Deep Learning CT Image Analysis Article. *arXiv* **2020**, arXiv:2003.05037.
27. Shah, M.I.; Mishra, S.; Yadav, V.K.; Chauhan, A.; Sarkar, M.; Sharma, S.K.; Rout, C. Ziehl–Neelsen sputum smear microscopy image database: A resource to facilitate automated bacilli detection for tuberculosis diagnosis. *J. Med. Imaging* **2017**, *4*, 027503. [CrossRef]
28. López, Y.P.; Filho, C.F.F.C.; Aguilera, L.M.R.; Costa, M.G.F. Automatic classification of light field smear microscopy patches using Convolutional Neural Networks for identifying Mycobacterium Tuberculosis. In Proceedings of the 2017 CHILEAN Conference on Electrical, Electronics Engineering, Information and Communication Technologies (CHILECON), Pucon, Chile, 18–20 October 2017.
29. Kant, S.; Srivastava, M.M. Towards Automated Tuberculosis detection using Deep Learning. In Proceedings of the 2018 IEEE Symposium Series on Computational Intelligence (SSCI), Bengaluru, India, 18–21 November 2018; pp. 1250–1253. [CrossRef]
30. Oomman, R.; Kalmady, K.S.; Rajan, J.; Sabu, M.K. Automatic detection of tuberculosis bacilli from microscopic sputum smear images using deep learning methods. *Integr. Med. Res.* **2018**, *38*, 691–699. [CrossRef]
31. Mithra, K.S.; Emmanuel, W.R.S. Automated identification of mycobacterium bacillus from sputum images for tuberculosis diagnosis. *Signal Image Video Process.* **2019**. [CrossRef]
32. Samuel, R.D.J.; Kanna, B.R. Tuberculosis (TB) detection system using deep neural networks. *Neural Comput. Appl.* **2019**, *31*, 1533–1545. [CrossRef]
33. Gurcan, M.N.; Boucheron, L.E.; Can, A.; Madabhushi, A.; Rajpoot, N.M.; Yener, B. Histopathological Image Analysis: A Review. *IEEE Rev. Biomed. Eng.* **2009**, *2*, 147–171. [CrossRef]
34. Coudray, N.; Ocampo, P.S.; Sakellaropoulos, T.; Narula, N.; Snuderl, M.; Fenyö, D.; Moreira, A.L.; Razavian, N.; Tsirigos, A. Classification and mutation prediction from non–small cell lung cancer histopathology images using deep learning. *Nat. Med.* **2018**, *24*, 1559–1567. [CrossRef]

35. O'Mahony, N.; Campbell, S.; Carvalho, A.; Harapanahalli, S.; Hernandez, G.V.; Krpalkova, L.; Riordan, D.; Walsh, J. Deep Learning vs. Traditional Computer Vision. *Adv. Intell. Syst. Comput.* **2020**, 128–144. [CrossRef]
36. Vajda, S.; Karargyris, A.; Jaeger, S.; Santosh, K.C.; Candemir, S.; Xue, Z.; Antani, S.; Thoma, G. Feature Selection for Automatic Tuberculosis Screening in Frontal Chest Radiographs. *J. Med Syst.* **2018**, 42. [CrossRef]
37. Jaeger, S.; Karargyris, A.; Candemir, S.; Folio, L.; Siegelman, J.; Callaghan, F.; Xue, Z.; Palaniappan, K.; Singh, R.K.; Antani, S.; et al. Automatic tuberculosis screening using chest radiographs. *IEEE Trans. Med. Imaging* **2014**, *33*, 233–245. [CrossRef]
38. Antony, B.; Nizar Banu, P.K. Lung tuberculosis detection using x-ray images. *Int. J. Appl. Eng. Res.* **2017**, *12*, 15196–15201.
39. Chauhan, A.; Chauhan, D.; Rout, C. Role of gist and PHOG features in computer-aided diagnosis of tuberculosis without segmentation. *PLoS ONE* **2014**, *9*, e112980. [CrossRef]
40. Al-Ajlan, A.; Allali, A.E. CNN—MGP: Convolutional Neural Networks for Metagenomics Gene Prediction. *Interdiscip. Sci. Comput. Life Sci.* **2019**, *11*, 628–635. [CrossRef] [PubMed]
41. Domingos, P. A Few Useful Things to Know About Machine Learning. *Commun. ACM* **2012**, *55*, 78–87. [CrossRef]
42. Mikołajczyk, A.; Grochowski, M. Data augmentation for improving deep learning in image classification problem. In Proceedings of the 2018 International Interdisciplinary PhD Workshop, Swinoujscie, Poland, 9–12 May 2018; pp. 117–122. [CrossRef]
43. Shorten, C.; Khoshgoftaar, T.M. A survey on Image Data Augmentation for Deep Learning. *J. Big Data* **2019**, *6*. [CrossRef]
44. O'Shea, K.; Nash, R. An Introduction to Convolutional Neural Networks. *arXiv* **2015**, arXiv:1511.08458v2.
45. Ker, J.; Wang, L. Deep Learning Applications in Medical Image Analysis. *IEEE Access* **2018**, *6*, 9375–9389. [CrossRef]
46. Pan, S.J.; Yang, Q. A Survey on Transfer Learning. *IEEE Trans. Knowl. Data Eng.* **2010**, *22*, 1345–1359. [CrossRef]
47. Lanbouri, Z.; Achchab, S. A hybrid Deep belief network approach for Financial distress prediction. In Proceedings of the 2015 10th International Conference on Intelligent Systems: Theories and Applications (SITA), Rabat, Morocco, 20–21 October 2015; pp. 1–6. [CrossRef]
48. Hinton, G.E.; Osindero, S. A fast learning algorithm for deep belief nets. *Neural Comput.* **2006**, *18*, 1527–1554. [CrossRef]
49. Cao, X.; Wipf, D.; Wen, F.; Duan, G.; Sun, J. A practical transfer learning algorithm for face verification. In Proceedings of the IEEE International Conference on Computer Vision, Sydney, Australia, 1–8 December 2013; pp. 3208–3215. [CrossRef]
50. Wang, C.; Chen, D.; Hao, L.; Liu, X.; Zeng, Y.; Chen, J.; Zhang, G. Pulmonary Image Classification Based on Inception-v3 Transfer Learning Model. *IEEE Access* **2019**, *7*, 146533–146541. [CrossRef]
51. Krizhevsky, A.; Sutskeve, I.; Hinton, G.E. ImageNet Classification with Deep Convolutional Neural Networks. *Adv. Neural Inf. Process. Syst.* **2012**. [CrossRef]
52. Tajbakhsh, N.; Shin, J.Y.; Gurudu, S.R.; Hurst, R.T.; Kendall, C.B.; Gotway, M.B.; Liang, J. Convolutional Neural Networks for Medical Image Analysis: Full Training or Fine Tuning? *IEEE Trans. Med. Imaging* **2016**, *35*, 1299–1312. [CrossRef]
53. Nogueira, K.; Penatti, O.A.; dos Santos, J.A. Towards better exploiting convolutional neural networks for remote sensing scene classification. *Pattern Recognit.* **2017**, *61*, 539–556. [CrossRef]
54. Kabari, L.G.; Onwuka, U. Comparison of Bagging and Voting Ensemble Machine Learning Algorithm as a Classifier. *Int. J. Adv. Res. Comput. Sci. Softw. Eng.* **2019**, *9*, 1–6.
55. Chouhan, V.; Singh, S.K.; Khamparia, A.; Gupta, D.; Albuquerque, V.H.C.D. A Novel Transfer Learning Based Approach for Pneumonia Detection in Chest X-ray Images. *Appl. Sci.* **2020**, *10*, 559. [CrossRef]
56. Lincoln, W.P.; Skrzypekt, J. Synergy of Clustering Multiple Back Propagation Networks. *Adv. Neural Inf. Process. Syst.* **1990**, *2*, 650–659.
57. Lakhani, P.; Sundaram, B. Deep Learning at Chest Radiography: Automated Classification of Pulmonary Tuberculosis by Using Convolutional Neural Networks. *Radiology* **2017**, *284*, 574–582. [CrossRef]

58. Divina, F.; Gilson, A.; Goméz-Vela, F.; Torres, M.G.; Torres, J.F. Stacking Ensemble Learning for Short-Term Electricity Consumption Forecasting. *Energies* **2018**, *11*, 949. [CrossRef]
59. World Health Organisation. *Global Health TB Report*; World Health Organisation: Geneva, Switzerland, 2018; p. 277.
60. Murphy, K.; Habib, S.S.; Zaidi, S.M.A.; Khowaja, S.; Khan, A.; Melendez, J.; Scholten, E.T.; Amad, F.; Schalekamp, S.; Verhagen, M.; et al. Computer aided detection of tuberculosis on chest radiographs: An evaluation of the CAD4TB v6 system. *Sci. Rep.* **2019**, *10*, 1–11. [CrossRef]
61. Melendez, J.; Sánchez, C.I.; Philipsen, R.H.; Maduskar, P.; Dawson, R.; Theron, G.; Dheda, K.; Van Ginneken, B. An automated tuberculosis screening strategy combining X-ray-based computer-aided detection and clinical information. *Sci. Rep.* **2016**, *6*, 1–8. [CrossRef]
62. Heo, S.J.; Kim, Y.; Yun, S.; Lim, S.S.; Kim, J.; Nam, C.M.; Park, E.C.; Jung, I.; Yoon, J.H. Deep Learning Algorithms with Demographic Information Help to Detect Tuberculosis in Chest Radiographs in Annual Workers' Health Examination Data. *Int. J. Environ. Res. Public Health* **2019**, *16*, 250. [CrossRef]
63. Pasa, F.; Golkov, V.; Pfeiffer, F.; Cremers, D.; Pfeiffer, D. Efficient Deep Network Architectures for Fast Chest X-Ray Tuberculosis Screening and Visualization. *Sci. Rep.* **2019**, *9*, 2–10. [CrossRef]
64. Cao, Y.; Liu, C.; Liu, B.; Brunette, M.J.; Zhang, N.; Sun, T.; Zhang, P.; Peinado, J.; Garavito, E.S.; Garcia, L.L.; et al. Improving Tuberculosis Diagnostics Using Deep Learning and Mobile Health Technologies among Resource-Poor and Marginalized Communities. In Proceedings of the 2016 IEEE 1st International Conference on Connected Health: Applications, Systems and Engineering Technologies, CHASE, Washington, DC, USA, 27–29 June 2016; pp. 274–281. [CrossRef]
65. Liu, J.; Liu, Y.; Wang, C.; Li, A.; Meng, B. An Original Neural Network for Pulmonary Tuberculosis Diagnosis in Radiographs. In *Lecture Notes in Computer Science, Proceedings of the International Conference on Artificial Neural Networks, Rhodes, Greece, 4–7 October 2018*; Springer: Berlin/Heidelberg, Germany, 2018; pp. 158–166._16. [CrossRef]
66. Stirenko, S.; Kochura, Y.; Alienin, O. Chest X-Ray Analysis of Tuberculosis by Deep Learning with Segmentation and Augmentation. In Proceedings of the 2018 IEEE 38th International Conference on Electronics andNanotechnology (ELNANO), Kiev, Ukraine, 24–26 April 2018; pp. 422–428.
67. Andika, L.A.; Pratiwi, H.; Sulistijowati Handajani, S. Convolutional neural network modeling for classification of pulmonary tuberculosis disease. *J. Phys. Conf. Ser.* **2020**, *1490*. [CrossRef]
68. Ul Abideen, Z.; Ghafoor, M.; Munir, K.; Saqib, M.; Ullah, A.; Zia, T.; Tariq, S.A.; Ahmed, G.; Zahra, A. Uncertainty assisted robust tuberculosis identification with bayesian convolutional neural networks. *IEEE Access* **2020**, *8*, 22812–22825. [CrossRef] [PubMed]
69. Hwang, E.J.; Park, S.; Jin, K.N.; Kim, J.I.; Choi, S.Y.; Lee, J.H.; Goo, J.M.; Aum, J.; Yim, J.J.; Park, C.M. Development and Validation of a Deep Learning—based Automatic Detection Algorithm for Active Pulmonary Tuberculosis on Chest Radiographs. *Clin. Infect. Dis.* **2019**, *69*, 739–747. [CrossRef]
70. Hwang, S.; Kim, H.E.; Jeong, J.; Kim, H.J. A Novel Approach for Tuberculosis Screening Based on Deep Convolutional Neural Networks. *Med. Imaging* **2016**, *9785*, 1–8. [CrossRef]
71. Islam, M.T.; Aowal, M.A.; Minhaz, A.T.; Ashraf, K. Abnormality Detection and Localization in Chest X-Rays using Deep Convolutional Neural Networks. *arXiv* **2017**, arXiv:1705.09850v3.
72. Nguyen, Q.H.; Nguyen, B.P.; Dao, S.D.; Unnikrishnan, B.; Dhingra, R.; Ravichandran, S.R.; Satpathy, S.; Raja, P.N.; Chua, M.C.H. Deep Learning Models for Tuberculosis Detection from Chest X-ray Images. In Proceedings of the 2019 26th International Conference on Telecommunications (ICT), Hanoi, Vietnam, 8–10 April 2019; pp. 381–385. [CrossRef]
73. Kieu, T.; Ho, K.; Gwak, J.; Prakash, O. Utilizing Pretrained Deep Learning Models for Automated Pulmonary Tuberculosis Detection Using Chest Radiography. *Intell. Inf. Database Syst.* **2019**, *4*, 395–403. [CrossRef]
74. Abbas, A.; Abdelsamea, M.M. Learning Transformations for Automated Classification of Manifestation of Tuberculosis using Convolutional Neural Network. In Proceedings of the 2018 13th International Conference on Computer Engineering andSystems (ICCES), Cairo, Egypt, 18–19 December 2018; IEEE: New York, NY, USA, 2018; pp. 122–126.
75. Karnkawinpong, T.; Limpiyakorn, Y. Classification of pulmonary tuberculosis lesion with convolutional neural networks. *J. Phys. Conf. Ser.* **2018**, *1195*. [CrossRef]

76. Liu, C.; Cao, Y.; Alcantara, M.; Liu, B.; Brunette, M.; Peinado, J.; Curioso, W. TX-CNN: Detecting Tuberculosis in Chest X-Ray Images Using Convolutional Neural Network. In Proceedings of the 2017 IEEE International Conference on Image Processing (ICIP), Beijing, China, 17–20 September 2017.
77. Yadav, O.; Passi, K.; Jain, C.K. Using Deep Learning to Classify X-ray Images of Potential Tuberculosis Patients. In Proceedings of the 2018 IEEE International Conference on Bioinformatics and Biomedicine(BIBM), Madrid, Spain, 3–6 December 2018; IEEE: New York, NY, USA, 2018; pp. 2368–2375.
78. Sahlol, A.T.; Elaziz, M.A.; Jamal, A.T.; Damaševičius, R.; Hassan, O.F. A novel method for detection of tuberculosis in chest radiographs using artificial ecosystem-based optimisation of deep neural network features. *Symmetry* **2020**, *12*, 1146. [CrossRef]
79. Hooda, R.; Mittal, A.; Sofat, S. Automated TB classification using ensemble of deep architectures. *Multimed. Tools Appl.* **2019**, *78*, 31515–31532. [CrossRef]
80. Rashid, R.; Khawaja, S.G.; Akram, M.U.; Khan, A.M. Hybrid RID Network for Efficient Diagnosis of Tuberculosis from Chest X-rays. In Proceedings of the 2018 9th Cairo International Biomedical Engineering Conference(CIBEC), Cairo, Egypt, 20–22 December 2018; IEEE: New York, NY, USA, 2018; pp. 167–170.
81. Kieu, S.T.H.; Hijazi, M.H.A.; Bade, A.; Saffree Jeffree, M. Tuberculosis detection using deep learning and contrast-enhanced canny edge detected x-ray images. *IAES Int. J. Artif. Intell.* **2020**, *9*. [CrossRef]
82. Rajaraman, S.; Antani, S.K. Modality-Specific Deep Learning Model Ensembles Toward Improving TB Detection in Chest Radiographs. *IEEE Access* **2020**, *8*, 27318–27326. [CrossRef] [PubMed]
83. Melendez, J.; Ginneken, B.V.; Maduskar, P.; Philipsen, R.H.H.M.; Reither, K.; Breuninger, M.; Adetifa, I.M.O.; Maane, R.; Ayles, H.; Sánchez, C.I. A Novel Multiple-Instance Learning-Based Approach to Computer-Aided Detection of Tuberculosis on Chest X-Rays. *IEEE Trans. Med. Imaging* **2014**, *34*, 179–192. [CrossRef] [PubMed]
84. Becker, A.S.; Bluthgen, C.; van Phi, V.D.; Sekaggya-Wiltshire, C.; Castelnuovo, B.; Kambugu, A.; Fehr, J.; Frauenfelder, T. Detection of tuberculosis patterns in digital photographs of chest X-ray images using Deep Learning: Feasibility study. *Int. J. Tuberc. Lung Dis.* **2018**, *22*, 328–335. [CrossRef] [PubMed]
85. Li, L.; Huang, H.; Jin, X. AE CNN Classification of Pulmonary Tuberculosis Based on CT images. In Proceedings of the 2018 9th International Conference on Information Technology inMedicine and Education (ITME), Hangzhou, China, 19–21 October 2018; IEEE: New York, NY, USA, 2018; pp. 39–42. [CrossRef]
86. Pattnaik, A.; Kanodia, S.; Chowdhury, R.; Mohanty, S. *Predicting Tuberculosis Related Lung Deformities from CT Scan Images Using 3D CNN*; CEUR-WS: Lugano, Switzerland, 2019; pp. 9–12.
87. Zunair, H.; Rahman, A.; Mohammed, N. *Estimating Severity from CT Scans of Tuberculosis Patients using 3D Convolutional Nets and Slice Selection*; CEUR-WS: Lugano, Switzerland, 2019; pp. 9–12.
88. Llopis, F.; Fuster-Guillo, A.; Azorin-Lopez, J.; Llopis, I. *Using improved optical flow model to detect Tuberculosis*; CEUR-WS: Lugano, Switzerland, 2019; pp. 9–12.
89. Wardlaw, T.; Johansson, E.W.; Hodge, M. *Pneumonia: The Forgotten Killer of Children*; United Nations Children's Fund (UNICEF): New York, NY, USA, 2006; p. 44.
90. Wunderink, R.G.; Waterer, G. Advances in the causes and management of community acquired pneumonia in adults. *BMJ* **2017**, 1–13. [CrossRef]
91. Tobias, R.R.; De Jesus, L.C.M.; Mital, M.E.G.; Lauguico, S.C.; Guillermo, M.A.; Sybingco, E.; Bandala, A.A.; Dadios, E.P. CNN-based Deep Learning Model for Chest X-ray Health Classification Using TensorFlow. In Proceedings of the 2020 RIVF International Conference on Computing and Communication Technologies, RIVF 2020, Ho Chi Minh, Vietnam, 14–15 October 2020.
92. Stephen, O.; Sain, M.; Maduh, U.J.; Jeong, D.U. An Efficient Deep Learning Approach to Pneumonia Classification in Healthcare. *J. Healthc. Eng.* **2019**, *2019*. [CrossRef]
93. Kermany, D.S.; Goldbaum, M.; Cai, W.; Lewis, M.A. Identifying Medical Diagnoses and Treatable Diseases by Image-Based Deep Learning. *Cell* **2018**, *172*, 1122–1131.e9. [CrossRef] [PubMed]
94. Young, J.C.; Suryadibrata, A. Applicability of Various Pre-Trained Deep Convolutional Neural Networks for Pneumonia Classification based on X-Ray Images. *Int. J. Adv. Trends Comput. Sci. Eng.* **2020**, *9*, 2649–2654. [CrossRef]
95. Moujahid, H.; Cherradi, B.; Gannour, O.E.; Bahatti, L.; Terrada, O.; Hamida, S. Convolutional Neural Network Based Classification of Patients with Pneumonia using X-ray Lung Images. *Adv. Sci. Technol. Eng. Syst.* **2020**, *5*, 167–175. [CrossRef]

96. Rajpurkar, P.; Irvin, J.; Zhu, K.; Yang, B.; Mehta, H.; Duan, T.; Ding, D.; Bagul, A.; Ball, R.L.; Langlotz, C.; et al. CheXNet: Radiologist-Level Pneumonia Detection on Chest X-Rays with Deep Learning. *arXiv* **2017**, arXiv:1711.05225v3.
97. Rahman, T.; Chowdhury, M.E.H.; Khandakar, A.; Islam, K.R.; Islam, K.F.; Mahbub, Z.B.; Kadir, M.A.; Kashem, S. Transfer Learning with Deep Convolutional Neural Network (CNN) for Pneumonia Detection Using Chest X-ray. *Appl. Sci.* **2020**, *10*, 3233. [CrossRef]
98. Hashmi, M.; Katiyar, S.; Keskar, A.; Bokde, N.; Geem, Z. Efficient Pneumonia Detection in Chest Xray Images Using Deep Transfer Learning. *Diagnostics* **2020**, 1–23. [CrossRef] [PubMed]
99. Acharya, A.K.; Satapathy, R. A Deep Learning Based Approach towards the Automatic Diagnosis of Pneumonia from Chest Radio-Graphs. *Biomed. Pharmacol. J.* **2020**, *13*, 449–455. [CrossRef]
100. Elshennawy, N.M.; Ibrahim, D.M. Deep-Pneumonia Framework Using Deep Learning Models Based on Chest X-Ray Images. *Diagnostics* **2020**, *10*, 649. [CrossRef] [PubMed]
101. Emhamed, R.; Mamlook, A.; Chen, S. Investigation of the performance of Machine Learning Classifiers for Pneumonia Detection in Chest X-ray Images. In Proceedings of the 2020 IEEE International Conference on Electro Information Technology (EIT), Chicago, IL, USA, 31 July–1 August 2020; pp. 98–104.
102. Kumar, A.; Tiwari, P.; Kumar, S.; Gupta, D.; Khanna, A. Identifying pneumonia in chest X-rays: A deep learning approach. *Measurement* **2019**, *145*, 511–518. [CrossRef]
103. Hurt, B.; Yen, A.; Kligerman, S.; Hsiao, A. Augmenting Interpretation of Chest Radiographs with Deep Learning Probability Maps. *J. Thorac. Imaging* **2020**, *35*, 285–293. [CrossRef]
104. Borczuk, A.C. Benign tumors and tumorlike conditions of the lung. *Arch. Pathol. Lab. Med.* **2008**, *132*, 1133–1148.[1133:BTATCO]2.0.CO;2. [CrossRef]
105. Hua, K.L.; Hsu, C.H.; Hidayati, S.C.; Cheng, W.H.; Chen, Y.J. Computer-aided classification of lung nodules on computed tomography images via deep learning technique. *OncoTargets Ther.* **2015**, *8*, 2015–2022. [CrossRef]
106. Kurniawan, E.; Prajitno, P.; Soejoko, D.S. Computer-Aided Detection of Mediastinal Lymph Nodes using Simple Architectural Convolutional Neural Network. *J. Phys. Conf. Ser.* **2020**, *1505*. [CrossRef]
107. Ciompi, F.; Chung, K.; Van Riel, S.J.; Setio, A.A.A.; Gerke, P.K.; Jacobs, C.; Th Scholten, E.; Schaefer-Prokop, C.; Wille, M.M.; Marchianò, A.; et al. Towards automatic pulmonary nodule management in lung cancer screening with deep learning. *Sci. Rep.* **2017**, *7*, 1–11. [CrossRef]
108. Shakeel, P.M.; Burhanuddin, M.A.; Desa, M.I. Lung cancer detection from CT image using improved profuse clustering and deep learning instantaneously trained neural networks. *Meas. J. Int. Meas. Confed.* **2019**, *145*, 702–712. [CrossRef]
109. Chen, S.; Han, Y.; Lin, J.; Zhao, X.; Kong, P. Pulmonary nodule detection on chest radiographs using balanced convolutional neural network and classic candidate detection. *Artif. Intell. Med.* **2020**, *107*, 101881. [CrossRef] [PubMed]
110. Hosny, A.; Parmar, C.; Coroller, T.P.; Grossmann, P.; Zeleznik, R.; Kumar, A.; Bussink, J.; Gillies, R.J.; Mak, R.H.; Aerts, H.J. Deep learning for lung cancer prognostication: A retrospective multi-cohort radiomics study. *PLoS Med.* **2018**, *15*, 1–25. [CrossRef] [PubMed]
111. Xu, Y.; Hosny, A.; Zeleznik, R.; Parmar, C.; Coroller, T.; Franco, I.; Mak, R.H.; Aerts, H.J. Deep learning predicts lung cancer treatment response from serial medical imaging. *Clin. Cancer Res.* **2019**, *25*, 3266–3275. [CrossRef] [PubMed]
112. Kuan, K.; Ravaut, M.; Manek, G.; Chen, H.; Lin, J.; Nazir, B.; Chen, C.; Howe, T.C.; Zeng, Z.; Chandrasekhar, V. Deep Learning for Lung Cancer Detection: Tackling the Kaggle Data Science Bowl 2017 Challenge. *arXiv* **2017**, arXiv:1705.09435
113. Ausawalaithong, W.; Thirach, A.; Marukatat, S.; Wilaiprasitporn, T. Automatic Lung Cancer Prediction from Chest X-ray Images Using the Deep Learning Approach. In Proceedings of the 2018 11th Biomedical Engineering International Conference (BMEiCON), Chiang Mai, Thailand, 21–24 November 2018 .
114. Xu, S.; Guo, J.; Zhang, G.; Bie, R. Automated detection of multiple lesions on chest X-ray images: Classification using a neural network technique with association-specific contexts. *Appl. Sci.* **2020**, *10*, 1742. [CrossRef]
115. Huang, C.; Wang, Y.; Li, X.; Ren, L.; Zhao, J.; Hu, Y.; Zhang, L.; Fan, G.; Xu, J.; Gu, X. Clinical features of patients infected with 2019 novel coronavirus in Wuhan, China. *Lancet* **2020**, *395*, 497–506. [CrossRef]
116. Velavan, T.P.; Meyer, C.G. The COVID-19 epidemic. *Trop. Med. Int. Health* **2020**, *25*, 278–280. [CrossRef]

117. Shibly, K.H.; Dey, S.K.; Islam, M.T.U.; Rahman, M.M. COVID faster R–CNN: A novel framework to Diagnose Novel Coronavirus Disease (COVID-19) in X-Ray images. *Inform. Med. Unlocked* **2020**, *20*, 100405. [CrossRef]
118. Alsharman, N.; Jawarneh, I. GoogleNet CNN neural network towards chest CT-coronavirus medical image classification. *J. Comput. Sci.* **2020**, *16*, 620–625. [CrossRef]
119. Zhu, J.; Shen, B.; Abbasi, A.; Hoshmand-Kochi, M.; Li, H.; Duong, T.Q. Deep transfer learning artificial intelligence accurately stages COVID-19 lung disease severity on portable chest radiographs. *PLoS ONE* **2020**, *15*, e0236621. [CrossRef]
120. Sethi, R.; Mehrotra, M.; Sethi, D. Deep Learning based Diagnosis Recommendation for COVID-19 using Chest X-Rays Images In Proceedings of the 2020 Second International Conference on Inventive Research in Computing Applications (ICIRCA), Coimbatore, India, 15–17 July 2020.
121. Das, D.; Santosh, K.C.; Pal, U. Truncated inception net: COVID-19 outbreak screening using chest X-rays. *Phys. Eng. Sci. Med.* **2020**, *43*, 915–925. [CrossRef] [PubMed]
122. Panwar, H.; Gupta, P.K.; Siddiqui, M.K.; Morales-Menendez, R.; Singh, V. Application of deep learning for fast detection of COVID-19 in X-Rays using nCOVnet. *Chaos Solitons Fractals* **2020**, *138*, 109944. [CrossRef] [PubMed]
123. Narin, A.; Kaya, C.; Pamuk, Z. Automatic Detection of Coronavirus Disease (COVID-19) Using X-ray Images and Deep Convolutional Neural Networks. *arXiv* **2020**, arXiv:2003.10849..
124. Apostolopoulos, I.D.; Mpesiana, T.A. Covid—19: Automatic detection from X-ray images utilizing transfer learning with convolutional neural networks. *Phys. Eng. Sci. Med.* **2020**, 1–6. [CrossRef] [PubMed]
125. Chowdhury, M.E.H.; Rahman, T.; Khandakar, A.; Mazhar, R.; Kadir, M.A.; Reaz, M.B.I.; Mahbub, Z.B.; Islam, K.R.; Salman, M.; Iqbal, A.; et al. Can AI help in screening Viral and COVID-19 pneumonia? *arXiv* **2020**, arXiv:2003.13145.
126. Wang, L.; Lin, Z.Q.; Wong, A. COVID-Net: A Tailored Deep Convolutional Neural Network Design for Detection of COVID-19 Cases from Chest X-Ray Images. *Sci. Rep.* **2020**, *10*, 1–12. [CrossRef]
127. Sethy, P.K.; Behera, S.K.; Ratha, P.K.; Biswas, P. Detection of coronavirus disease (COVID-19) based on deep features and support vector machine. *Int. J. Math. Eng. Manag. Sci.* **2020**, *5*, 643–651. [CrossRef]
128. Islam, M.Z.; Islam, M.M.; Asraf, A. A combined deep CNN-LSTM network for the detection of novel coronavirus (COVID-19) using X-ray images. *Inform. Med. Unlocked* **2020**, *20*, 100412. [CrossRef]
129. Shorfuzzaman, M.; Masud, M. On the detection of covid-19 from chest x-ray images using cnn-based transfer learning. *Comput. Mater. Contin.* **2020**, *64*, 1359–1381. [CrossRef]
130. Li, L.; Qin, L.; Xu, Z.; Yin, Y.; Wang, X.; Kong, B.; Bai, J.; Lu, Y.; Fang, Z.; Song, Q.; et al. Using Artificial Intelligence to Detect COVID-19 and Community-acquired Pneumonia Based on Pulmonary CT: Evaluation of the Diagnostic Accuracy. *Radiology* **2020**, *296*, 65–71. [CrossRef]
131. Alazab, M.; Awajan, A.; Mesleh, A.; Abraham, A.; Jatana, V.; Alhyari, S. COVID-19 prediction and detection using deep learning. *Int. J. Comput. Inf. Syst. Ind. Manag. Appl.* **2020**, *12*, 168–181.
132. Waheed, A.; Goyal, M.; Gupta, D.; Khanna, A.; Al-Turjman, F.; Pinheiro, P.R. CovidGAN: Data Augmentation Using Auxiliary Classifier GAN for Improved Covid-19 Detection. *IEEE Access* **2020**, *8*, 91916–91923. [CrossRef]
133. Ouyang, X.; Huo, J.; Xia, L.; Shan, F.; Liu, J.; Mo, Z.; Yan, F.; Ding, Z.; Yang, Q.; Song, B.; et al. Dual-Sampling Attention Network for Diagnosis of COVID-19 from Community Acquired Pneumonia. *IEEE Trans. Med. Imaging* **2020**, *39*, 2595–2605. [CrossRef]
134. Mahmud, T.; Rahman, M.A.; Fattah, S.A. CovXNet: A multi-dilation convolutional neural network for automatic COVID-19 and other pneumonia detection from chest X-ray images with transferable multi-receptive feature optimization. *Comput. Biol. Med.* **2020**, *122*, 103869. [CrossRef] [PubMed]
135. Shi, F.; Xia, L.; Shan, F.; Wu, D.; Wei, Y.; Yuan, H.; Jiang, H. Large-Scale Screening of COVID-19 from Community Acquired Pneumonia using Infection Size-Aware Classification. *arXiv* **2020**, arXiv:2003.09860..
136. Breiman, L. Random forests. *Mach. Learn.* **2001**, *45*, 5–32. [CrossRef]
137. Xu, X.; Jiang, X.; Ma, C.; Du, P.; Li, X.; Ly, S.; Yu, L.; Chen, Y; Su, J.; Lang, G.; et al. A Deep Learning System to Screen Novel Coronavirus Disease 2019 Pneumonia. *Engineering* **2020**. [CrossRef]
138. Singh, D.; Kumar, V.; Kaur, M. Classification of COVID-19 patients from chest CT images using multi-objective differential evolution–based convolutional neural networks. *Eur. J. Clin. Microbiol. Infect. Dis.* **2020**, *39*, 1379–1389. [CrossRef]

139. Sedik, A.; Iliyasu, A.M.; El-Rahiem, B.A.; Abdel Samea, M.E.; Abdel-Raheem, A.; Hammad, M.; Peng, J.; Abd El-Samie, F.E.; Abd El-Latif, A.A. Deploying machine and deep learning models for efficient data-augmented detection of COVID-19 infections. *Viruses* **2020**, *12*, 769. [CrossRef]
140. Ahsan, M.M.; Alam, T.E.; Trafalis, T.; Huebner, P. Deep MLP-CNN model using mixed-data to distinguish between COVID-19 and Non-COVID-19 patients. *Symmetry* **2020**, *12*. [CrossRef]
141. Afshar, P.; Heidarian, S.; Naderkhani, F.; Oikonomou, A.; Plataniotis, K.N.; Mohammadi, A. COVID-CAPS: A capsule network-based framework for identification of COVID-19 cases from X-ray images. *Pattern Recognit. Lett.* **2020**, *138*, 638–643. [CrossRef] [PubMed]
142. Rosenthal, A.; Gabrielian, A.; Engle, E.; Hurt, D.E.; Alexandru, S.; Crudu, V.; Sergueev, E.; Kirichenko, V.; Lapitskii, V.; Snezhko, E.; et al. The TB Portals: An Open-Access, Web-Based Platform for Global Drug-Resistant-Tuberculosis Data Sharing and Analysis. *J. Clin. Microbiol.* **2017**, *55*, 3267–3282. [CrossRef] [PubMed]
143. Cid, Y.D.; Liauchuk, V.; Klimuk, D.; Tarasau, A. *Overview of ImageCLEFtuberculosis 2019—Automatic CT—Based Report Generation and Tuberculosis Severity Assessment*: CEUR-WS: Lugano, Switzerland, 2019; pp. 9–12.
144. Demner-Fushman, D.; Kohli, M.D.; Rosenman, M.B.; Shooshan, S.E.; Rodriguez, L.; Antani, S.; Thoma, G.R.; McDonald, C.J. Preparing a collection of radiology examinations for distribution and retrieval. *J. Am. Med. Inform. Assoc.* **2016**, *23*, 304–310. [CrossRef]
145. Shiraishi, J.; Katsuragawa, S.; Ikezoe, J.; Matsumoto, T.; Kobayashi, T.; Komatsu, K.I.; Matsui, M.; Fujita, H.; Kodera, Y.; Doi, K. Development of a digital image database for chest radiographs with and without a lung nodule: Receiver operating characteristic analysis of radiologists' detection of pulmonary nodules. *Am. J. Roentgenol.* **2000**, *174*, 71–74. [CrossRef] [PubMed]
146. Jaeger, S.; Candemir, S.; Antani, S.; Wáng, Y.x.J.; Lu, P.x.; Thoma, G. Two public chest X-ray datasets for computer-aided screening of pulmonary diseases. *Quant. Imaging Med. Surg.* **2014**, *4*, 475–477. [CrossRef]
147. Xiaosong, W.; Yifan, P.; Le, L.; Lu, Z.; Mohammadhadi, B.; Summers, R.M. ChestX-ray8: Hospital-scale chest X-ray database and benchmarks on weakly-supervised classification and localization of common thorax diseases. In Proceedings of the IEEE conference on computer vision and pattern recognition, Honolulu, HI, USA, 21–26 July 2017; pp. 3462–3471.
148. Costa, M.G.; Filho, C.F.; Kimura, A.; Levy, P.C.; Xavier, C.M.; Fujimoto, L.B. A sputum smear microscopy image database for automatic bacilli detection in conventional microscopy. In Proceedings of the 2014 36th Annual International Conference of the IEEE Engineering in Medicine and Biology Society, EMBC, Chicago, IL, USA, 26–30 August 2014; pp. 2841–2844. [CrossRef]
149. Armato, S.G.; McLennan, G.; Bidaut, L.; McNitt-Gray, M.F.; Meyer, C.R.; Reeves, A.P.; Zhao, B.; Aberle, D.R.; Henschke, C.I.; Hoffman, E.A.; et al. The Lung Image Database Consortium (LIDC) and Image Database Resource Initiative (IDRI): A completed reference database of lung nodules on CT scans. *Med. Phys.* **2011**, *38*, 915–931. [CrossRef]
150. Grossman, R.L.; Allison, P.; Ferrentti, V.; Varmus, H.E.; Lowy, D.R.; Kibbe, W.A.; Staudt, L.M. Toward a Shared Vision for Cancer Genomic Data. *N. Engl. J. Med.* **2016**, *375*, 1109–1112. [CrossRef]
151. Cohen, J.P.; Morrison, P.; Dao, L.; Roth, K.; Duong, T.Q.; Ghassemi, M. COVID-19 Image Data Collection: Prospective Predictions Are the Future. *arXiv* **2020**, arXiv:2006.11988..

Publisher's Note: MDPI stays neutral with regard to jurisdictional claims in published maps and institutional affiliations.

© 2020 by the authors. Licensee MDPI, Basel, Switzerland. This article is an open access article distributed under the terms and conditions of the Creative Commons Attribution (CC BY) license (http://creativecommons.org/licenses/by/4.0/).

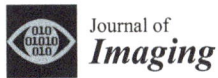

Review

Deep Learning in Selected Cancers' Image Analysis—A Survey

Taye Girma Debelee [1,2,*], Samuel Rahimeto Kebede [1,3], Friedhelm Schwenker [4] and Zemene Matewos Shewarega [1]

1. Artificial Intelligence Center, 40782 Addis Ababa, Ethiopia; samuelrahimeto@dbu.edu.et (S.R.K.); zemene.matewos@aic.et (Z.M.S.)
2. College of Electrical and Mechanical Engineering, Addis Ababa Science and Technology University, 120611 Addis Ababa, Ethiopia
3. Department of Electrical and Computer Engineering, Debreberhan University, 445 Debre Berhan, Ethiopia
4. Institute of Neural Information Processing, University of Ulm, 89081 Ulm, Germany; friedhelm.schwenker@uni-ulm.de
* Correspondence: tayegirma@gmail.com

Received: 21 July 2020; Accepted: 26 October 2020; Published: 10 November 2020

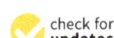

Abstract: Deep learning algorithms have become the first choice as an approach to medical image analysis, face recognition, and emotion recognition. In this survey, several deep-learning-based approaches applied to breast cancer, cervical cancer, brain tumor, colon and lung cancers are studied and reviewed. Deep learning has been applied in almost all of the imaging modalities used for cervical and breast cancers and MRIs for the brain tumor. The result of the review process indicated that deep learning methods have achieved state-of-the-art in tumor detection, segmentation, feature extraction and classification. As presented in this paper, the deep learning approaches were used in three different modes that include training from scratch, transfer learning through freezing some layers of the deep learning network and modifying the architecture to reduce the number of parameters existing in the network. Moreover, the application of deep learning to imaging devices for the detection of various cancer cases has been studied by researchers affiliated to academic and medical institutes in economically developed countries; while, the study has not had much attention in Africa despite the dramatic soar of cancer risks in the continent.

Keywords: deep learning; medical image analysis; breast cancer; brain tumor; cervical cancer; colon cancer; lung cancer

---

1. Introduction

Over the last decades, three different approaches have been practiced to deal with medical images. The first is creating awareness among the community for a regular check-up and it was not be practiced among communities. The second approach is using medical imaging technologies for screening and it is witnessed over the last decades. However, the benefits of medical imaging technology depend on the experience of the image interpreting experts or radiologists. Then, applying a computer-aided detection (CAD) approach using machine learning techniques has brought a promising result along with the imaging technologies. Machine learning techniques have evolved rapidly in recent years to solve complex problems.

The architecture of deep convolutional neural networks (DCNNs) is composed of convolutional layers, pooling layers and fully connected layers to perform feature extraction (see Figure 1), features down sampling (see Figure 2) and classification, respectively during the process of optimization [1].

In convolutional layers, local features such as colors, end-points, corners and oriented-edges are collected in the shallow layers. These local features in the shallow layers are integrated into larger structural features like circles, ellipses, specific shapes or patterns when the layer goes deeper. Afterwards, these features of structures or patterns constitute the high-level semantic representations that describe feature abstraction for each category. In pooling layers, feature down sampling is performed either using average pooling or max-pooling layers to reduce the dimensionality of the features extracted using convolutional layers [2]. On the other hand, in fully connected layers, it takes the extracted features from the convolutional layers as inputs and works as a classifier, well known as multilayer perceptron (MLP). These fully connected layers encode the spatial correspondences of those semantic features and convey the co-occurrence properties between patterns or objects.

There have been many survey papers produced on the application of deep learning on medical image analysis and few among many produced in 2017 are considered in this survey paper. Suzuki [3] in his survey paper claimed that machine learning in deep learning form has emerged in computer vision and paved the way for many researchers to work on medical image analysis using deep learning approach. The popularity of deep learning started after the AlexNet model won the competition in 2012. Suzuki has produced an interesting survey paper that aimed to address four major points: the machine learning techniques used in the computer vision field, changes observed in machine learning after the introduction of deep learning, available machine learning models in deep learning and the impact of deep learning for medical image analysis. As claimed by Litjens et al. [4], convolutional neural network-based deep learning has become a method for medical image analysis. In their survey paper, they considered papers that were related to medical image analysis, specifically for image classification, object detection, segmentation, registration and other tasks. In addition, the areas of application of deep learning were neuro, retinal, pulmonary, digital pathology, breast, cardiac, abdominal and musculoskeletal.

Dinggang Shen et al. [5] claimed that deep learning has helped many researchers in the area of computer vision to identify, classify and quantify patterns in medical images. They specifically argued that deep learning is useful in exploiting hierarchical features from data itself than feature engineering using handcrafting using human effort. Suzuki [6] in his survey paper overviewed the area of deep learning and its application in medical imaging analysis to assess what was changed before and after the introduction of deep learning in machine learning, identifying the reasons that make deep learning powerful and their applications to medical image analysis.

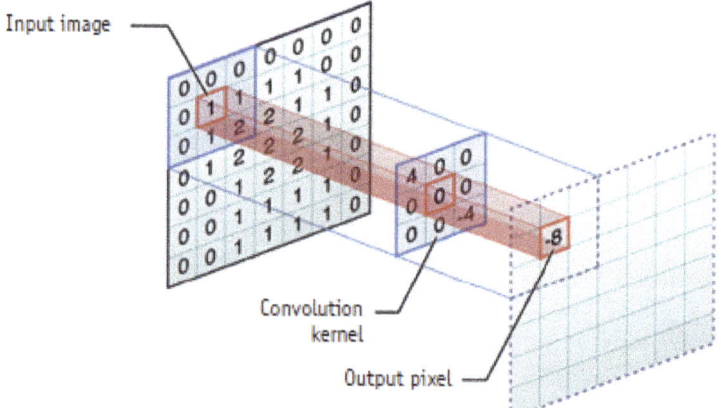

Figure 1. Example of convolution operation from [7].

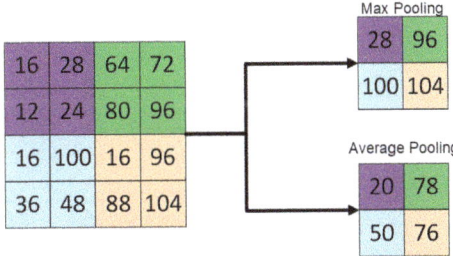

Figure 2. Example of down sampling operation using max-pooling and average-pooling.

In this survey paper, we briefly describe the breast cancer, cervical cancer, brain tumor, colon cancer and lung cancer along with their respective screening methods. Finally, we reviewed the application of deep learning for each cancer type in terms of deep learning application types like feature extraction, detection, segmentation, prediction and classification. The motivation behind selecting the cancer type for the survey was based on the cancer statistics reported in 2018 by the World Health Organization as presented in Table 1.

Table 1. World Health Organization 2018 statistical report through the global cancer observatory.

Cancer Type	New Cases (%)	Death Rate (%)
Breast Cancer	11.6	6.6
Colon Cancer	10.2	9.2
Brain Tumor	3.5	2.8
Cervical Cancer	3.2	2.5
Stomach Cancer	5.7	8.2
Liver Cancer	4.7	8.2
Lung Cancer	11.6	18.4

2. Methods

Published papers from 2016 to 2020 were considered and reviewed to (1) assess the application of deep learning for breast cancer, (2) assess the application of deep learning for cervical cancer, (3) assess the application of deep learning for a brain tumor and (4) assess the application of deep learning for colon cancer. We first defined a search criterion for the selected search databases. Our general search criteria for this survey paper are ((("colon" OR "colorectal") AND ("cancer" OR "polyp") AND ("deep learning") AND ("Image") AND ("detection" OR "classification" OR "segmentation" OR "Localization")) OR ((("breast") AND ("cancer" OR "mass") AND ("deep learning") AND ("Image") AND ("detection" OR "classification" OR "segmentation" OR "Localization")) OR ((("Brain") AND ("Tumor") AND ("deep learning") AND ("MRI") AND ("detection" OR "classification" OR "segmentation" OR "Localization")) OR (("Cervix" OR "Cervical") AND ("Deep Learning") AND ("Classification" OR "segmentation"). The searches were carried out from four databases: (1) PubMed, (2) Science Direct, (3) IEEE Xplore Digital Library and (4) Google Scholar. The search framework of the survey paper is presented in Figure 3 and the major performance metrics used to evaluate deep learning approach applied to the selected medical images are presented in Section 2.1.

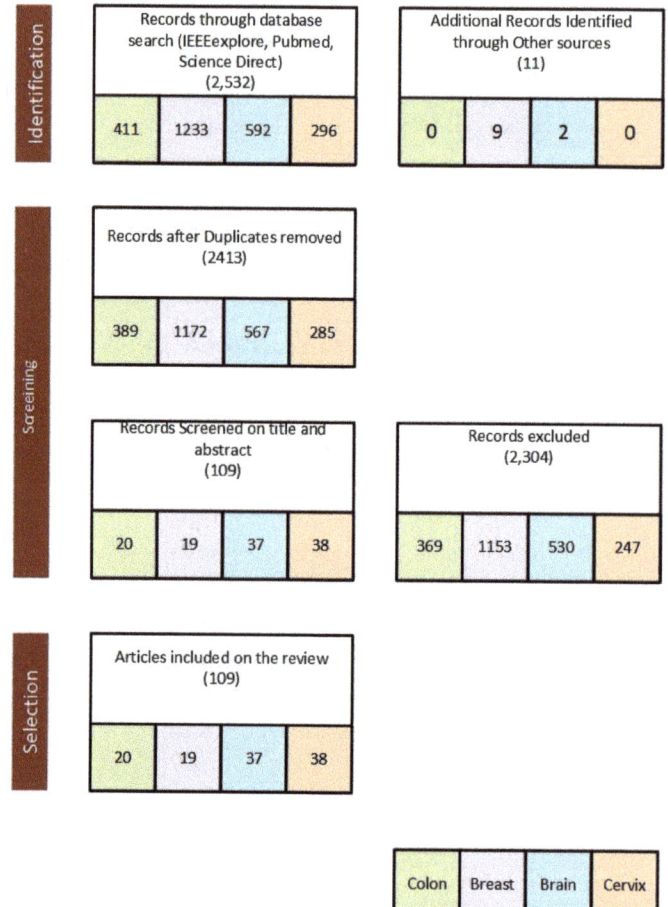

Figure 3. Search criteria framework used for IEEEexplore, PubMed, Google Scholar and Science Direct engines to select papers for review.

2.1. Segmentation and Classification Performance Metrics

Most of the performance metrics encountered in the review include area under curve (AUC), sensitivity (Sn), specificity (Sp), accuracy (Acc), precision (P), recall (R), positive predictive values (PPV), Matthews correlation coefficient (MCC), geometric mean (G-Mean), which are usually successful in describing the classification performance [8,9]. Performance measures including Dice similarity coefficient (DSC) or Zijdenbos similarity index (ZSI) or F1-score, Hausdorff distance (H) and intersection over union (IoU) are the most effective metrics for measuring system's segmentation performance [10]. Here, the true positives for the segmentation are the correctly labeled pixel while it is correctly labeled class for classification case.

3. Deep Learning in Tumor Detection, Segmentation and Classification

Region-based segmentation technique was in use in medical image analysis until the deep learning approach evolved in the field of computer vision [8]. However, Lee et al. [7] in their survey paper indicated that the existence of deep learning in the research community has become a reason to use object recognition in an image. In addition to object detection, deep learning has been applied for feature extraction, abnormality detection, cancer/tumor segmentation and classification [11].

3.1. Breast Cancer

Breast cancer occurs when there is uncontrolled growth of cells in the breast [12]. It is the most widely diagnosed type of cancer in women and the first prevalent cancer type in Ethiopia [11,13]. There are four types of breast cancer manifestation that include: mass, calcification, architectural distortion and bilateral asymmetry [11].

3.1.1. Screening Methods

As presented in Debelee et al. [11], breast cancer image analysis and breast abnormality detection start with breast cancer screening. Breast cancer screening methods include screen film mammography (SFM), digital mammography (DM), ultrasound (US), magnetic resonance imaging (MRI), digital breast tomosynthesis (DBT) and combinations of the screening methods.

3.1.2. Datasets

There are many datasets prepared for medical image analysis based on the different imaging modalities. The most common and available dataset for the breast cancer is of mammography and histopathology datasets. Some of the most common datasets are discussed in Table 2.

Table 2. Image datasets for breast cancer image analysis.

Dataset	Size	#Classes/Targets	Format	Type	Author/Repository, Year
MIAS	322	2	pgm	Mammography	Suckling, J. et al. [14]
DDSM	55,890		npy	Mammography	Scuccimarra [15]
INbreast		410	XML	Mammography	Moreira et al. [16]
Breast Cancer Wisconsin	568	3	csv	Mammography	Dua, D. and Graff, C. [17]
BreakHis	7909	2	png	Histology	Bukun [18]
BACH/ICIAR2018	400	4	tiff	Histology	G.Aresta [19]

3.1.3. Deep Learning for Detection of Breast Cancer Through Diagnostic Medical Imaging Techniques

Li Shen et al. [2] proposed a deep learning-based breast cancer detection algorithm using end-to-end training approach using mammographic images from the Digital Database for Screening Mammography (DDSM) and INbreast databases. The deep learning architectures used in their paper were ResNet-50 and VGGNet-16. The proposed approach was evaluated in terms of AUC at single model and four-model (ResNet-ResNet, ResNet-VGGNet, VGGNet-VGGNet and VGGNet-ResNet) averaging level. For the DDSM dataset, the best single model achieved a per-image AUC of 0.88, and four-model averaging improved the AUC to 0.91 with sensitivity of 86.1% and specificity of 80.1%. For INbreast database, the best single model achieved per-image AUC of 0.95, and four-model averaging achieved a better AUC value of 0.98 with sensitivity of 86.7% and specificity of 96.1%.

Wu et al. [20] proposed a DCNN architecture based on four columns of ResNet-22 to classify breast cancer screening exams using mammography. There was a total of 200,000 exams which incorporated over 1,000,000 images to train and evaluate the proposed DCNN model. The performance of their network achieved an AUC of 0.895 in predicting whether there is a cancer in the breast, when tested on the screening population and the result was compared to 14 radiologists reading results.

Alzubaidi et al. [21] transfer learning approach on their proposed 74 layer CNN. Their model was pre-trained on one same domain image dataset (erythrocytesIDB dataset, which has images of peripheral blood smears samples taken from patients with Sickle Cell Disease). They divided the original microscopy image into 12 patches and used majority voting for the classification, where the most frequent patch label is chosen to be the image label. The model achieved a patch level accuracy of 90.5% and image-level accuracy of 97.4%. The majority voting they employed seemed not a correct way since if the cells are the majority of normals and if it still has cancerous cells, the system might classify them as normal, which is not good.

Zhu et al. [22] proposed two deep learning approach to predict the occurrence of invasive cancer on MRI images. The first approach was based on transfer learning using GoogleNet pre-trained model to predict the presence of invasive cancer. As a second approach, the authors extracted features from the natural images and used SVM to predict the invasive disease. The best classification result gained in terms of AUC was 0.53 for transfer learning approach and 0.70 for extracted features.

Li et al. [23] explored the abilities of digital breast tomosynthesis (DBT) and full-field digital mammography (FFDM) in mass classification using deep neural networks equipped with or without transfer learning. They also explored an eligible combination strategy of DBT and FFDM in enhancing classification performance. They applied a 16-layer VGG network (VGG-16) and 11-layer deep convolutional neural network (DCNN) for the 2D images and extend the 11-layer DCNN to accommodate the extra dimension in 3D DBT images. The best performer from these methods, a 2D-DCNN which was trained by combining the DBT and FFDM, achieved the highest performance with average AUC, accuracy, sensitivity and specificity of 0.95, 92.13%, 83% and 93.84%, respectively on three class classification (benign, malignant, normal).

Zeiser et al. [24] explored the application of the U-Net model with different depths with or without data augmentation for the segmentation of masses on mammograms. The U-Net model trained with depth of 5 and with data augmentation was the best performer with sensitivity of 92.32%, specificity of 80.47%, accuracy of 85.95%, Dice index of 79.39% and AUC of 86.40% on the DDSM dataset.

Shen et al. [2] applied an ensemble of four best performing deep learning models which were designed based on Resnet50 and VGG16 as patch classifiers and Resnet and VGG blocks as top layer for breast cancer classification. The ensemble of these classifiers achieved the best AUC of 0.91 (sensitivity: 86.1%, specificity: 80.1%) on the detection of benign and malignant masses and classifications on the DDSM dataset.

Zhang et al. [25] used U-net architecture for the segmentation and extraction of fat tissue, fibroglandular tissue (FGT) inside the breast, and all nonbreast tissues outside the breast in breast MRI. They achieved mean DSC of 0.95 for breast and 0.91 for FGT; and mean accuracy of 0.98 for breast and 0.97 for FGT.

Zhou et al. [26] applied 3D deep convolutional neural network (CNN) based on 3D DenseNet [27] architecture with 37 layers for diagnosing breast cancer and localizing the lesions at dynamic contrast enhanced (DCE) MRI data in a weakly supervised manner. The proposed algorithm performance for breast cancer diagnosis showed 83.7% accuracy, 90.8% sensitivity, 69.3% specificity, 0.859 AUC and 0.501 Dice distance.

Summary of the performance of the above reviewed work can be summarized in Table 3.

3.1.4. Deep Learning for Breast Histopathology Image Analysis

Breast histopathology helps to confirm the presence of cancerous sales detected by other imaging modalities. Since histology slides may contain millions of cells and identifying the cancerous sales from the slides is time consuming and tedious job. Hence there are many varieties of research done in this area.

Table 3. Summary of scientific papers on detection of breast cancer using diagnostic medical imaging techniques.

Author and Citation	Dataset	AUC	Sn (%)	Sp (%)	Acc (%)	Target
	Siemens and Hologic	0.933	-	-	-	Detection
Wu et al. [20]	Personal	0.895	-	-	-	Classification/Prediction
Shen et al. [2] (Single-Model)	DDSM	0.88	-	-	-	Detection
	INbreast	0.95	-	-	-	Detection
Shen et al. [2] (Four-Models Average)	DDSM	0.91	86.1	80.1	-	Detection
	INbreast	0.98	86.7	96.1	-	Detection
Zhu et al. [22] (Transfer learning)	-		0.53	-	-	Prediction
Zhu et al. [22] (SVM)	-		0.7	-	-	Prediction
Li et al. [23]	-		0.95	83	93.84	92.13	Classification
Zeiser et al. [24]	DDSM	0.86	92.32	80.47	85.95	Segmentation
Zhang et al. [28]	-	-	-	-	97.5	Detection
Zhou et al. [26]	-	0.86	90.8	69.3	83.7	Classification

Sheikh et al. [29] proposed a multi-scale input and multi-feature CNN network for the classification of histopathological images. They concatenate four scales (1 ×, 0.5 ×, 0.33 × and 0.25 ×) of the original normalized image to accommodate the scale variant property of the cells and used it as an input to the CNN network. They trained their proposed model on ICIAR2018 and BreakHits datasets. The model achieved a satisfactory max accuracy of 0.83 for the ICIAR2018 dataset and 0.98 for the BreakHis dataset for binary classification. For the multiclass classification, the proposed model's accuracy was rather unsatisfactory reaching as low as 60% for the ICIAR2018 dataset.

Li et al. [30] modified the Densenet-121 architecture by removing the pooling layers of the 4th Dense-block and feeding the extracted feature maps from each Dense-block to the squeeze-and-excitation (SENet) module for breast histopathology images. The used SENet for receiving more channel-wise information. After concatenating each SENet output, they used a fully-connected layer for the classification purpose. They used a pre-trained Densenet model for their architecture using the transfer-learning approach. Using the publicly available BreakHis dataset, their algorithm achieved an average accuracy of 88% over different magnification levels for binary classification.

Yan et al. [31] used the transfer-learning approach by using Google's Inception-V3 model as patch-wise feature extraction and image-wise long short-term memory (LSTM) for classifying breast histopathological images into four classes, namely normal, benign, in situ and invasive. They fine-tuned the Inception-V3 model. Their proposed model achieved an average accuracy of 91% on the ICIAR2018 dataset.

Sharma et al. [32] studied the use of pre-trained deep learning networks as feature extractor from breast cancer histopathology images. They used transfer learning on the pre-existing networks (VGG16, VGG19 and ResNet50) for using them as feature extractor. The extracted features were then classified using SVM classifier. The VGG16 network with linear SVM achieved the highest accuracy (93.97% for 40 ×, 92.92% for 100 ×, 91.23% for 200 × and 91.79% for 400 × magnifications).

Vang et al. [33] proposed ensemble classifier and reinforcement backed deep learning approach using inception-V3 for multiclass (normal, benign, in situ and invasive) classification. The ensemble fusion approach for image level prediction involved majority voting, gradient boosting machine (GBM) and logistic regression. Their approach performed low in terms of sensitivity for the two classes (benign and normal). The sensitivity of the normal and benign predicted classes was improved by adding a dual path network (DPN) to use it as feature extractor. However, the extracted features were further sent to the next layer of ensemble prediction fusion using GBM, logistic regression and support vector machine (SVM) to refine predictions. This approach was evaluated in terms of accuracy and scored an accuracy of 87.5%.

Alzubaidi et al. [21] transfer learning approach onto their proposed 74 layer CNN. They pre-trained their model on one same domain image dataset (erythrocytesIDB dataset, which has images of peripheral blood smears samples taken from patients with Sickle Cell Disease). They divided the original microscopy image into 12 patches and used majority voting for the classification, where the most frequent patch label is chosen to be the image label. The model training was don on the ICIAR 2018 dataset. The model achieved patch level accuracy of 90.5% and image level accuracy of 97.4%. The majority voting they employed seemed not a correct way since if the cells are majority of normal and if it still has cancerous cells the system might classify them as normal, which is not good.

The summary of papers explored in classification of breast histological slides can be summarized in Table 4. From the literature reviews the algorithm proposed by Yan et al. [31] seems the best method for histopathological breast cancer detection.

Table 4. Summary of scientific papers on classification of breast cancer using histopathological images.

Author and Citation	Dataset	Acc	Sn (%)	Sp (%)
	Siemens and Hologic	0.933	-	-
Vang et al. [33]	ICIAR2018 (H & E)	87.5	-	-
Sharma and Mehra [32]	BreakHis	93.97	-	-
Sheikh et al. [29]	ICIAR2018 and BreakHis	83 98	-	-
Li et al. [30]	ICIAR2018	88	-	-
Yan et al. [31]	ICIAR2018	91	-	-
Alzubaidi et al. [21]	ICIAR 2018	97.4	-	-

3.1.5. Summary

As presented in Tables 5 and 6, the deep learning architecture involved in the recently published, from 2016 to 2020, breast cancer we considered in this survey paper were ResNet, VGGNet, AlexNet, Inception V3, U-Net and DenseNet.

Table 5. Summary of breast cancer scientific papers in terms of convolutional neurla network (CNN) architecture and type of environment used in the selected papers.

Authors	Network	Pre-Training	Transfer Learning	Environment
Wu et al. [20]	ResNet-22	Yes	No	TensorFlow
Shen et al. [2]	ResNet-50, VGGNet-16	Yes	Yes	-
Vang et al. [33]	Inception V3	Yes	No	TensorFlow
Zhu et al. [22]	GoogleNet	Yes	Yes	Caffe
Li et al. [23]	VGGNet-16	Yes	Yes	-
Sharma and Mehra [32]	VGGNet-16, VGGNet-19, ResNet50	Yes	Yes	Keras, TensorFlow
Zeiser et al. [24]	U-net	No	No	-
Zhang et al. [28]	U-net	No	No	TensorFlow
Zhou et al. [26]	3D DensNet	No	No	-
Sheikh et al. [29]	MSI-MFNet	No	No	Keras
Li et al. [30]	IDSNet	Yes	Yes	Tensorflow
Yan et al. [31]	Inception-V3	Yes	Yes	Tensorflow
Alzubaidi et al. [21]	ResNet	Yes	Yes	-

Table 6. Summary of breast cancer scientific papers in terms of publication year, name of journal/conference for the selected papers and its impact factor with year of impact factor.

Authors	Publication Year	Journal/Conf.	Impact Factor	Year of Impact Factor
Wu et al. [20]	2020	ITMI	6.85	2020
Shen et al. [2]	2019	Scientific Reports	3.998	2019
Vang et al. [33]	2018	CBM	5.4	2019
Zhu et al. [22]	2019	CBM	3.434	2020
Li et al. [23]	2019	European Radiology	4.101	2019
Sharma and Mehra [32]	2020	Journal of Digital Imaging	2.99	2018
Zeiser et al. [24]	2020	Journal of Digital Imaging	2.99	2018
Zhang et al. [28]	2018	Academic Radiology	2.50	2020
Dembrower et al. [34]	2020	Radiology	7.608	2018
Zhou et al. [26]	2019	Journal of Magnetic Resonance Imaging	2.112	2018
Sheikh et al. [29]	2020	MDPI, Cancers	6.126	2019
Li et al. [30]	2020	Plos One	2.74	2019
Yan et al. [31]	2020	Elsevier, Methods	3.812	2019
Alzubaidi et al. [21]	2020	MDPI, electronics	2.412	2019

As indicated in Table 7, the result of almost all papers in this survey paper were not compared with the domain specialists and performance of the traditional machine learning algorithms.

Table 7. Summary of breast cancer scientific papers in terms of comparison to specialists and/or traditional techniques.

Author and Citation	Comparison to Specialists	Comparison to Traditional Technique (Yes/No)
Hagos et al. [35]	No	No
Wu et al. [20]	Yes	No
Shen et al. [2]	No	No
Vang et al. [33]	No	No
Zhu et al. [22]	No	No
Li et al. [23]	No	No
Sharma and Mehra [32]	No	Yes
Zeiser et al. [24]	No	Yes
Zhang et al. [28]	No	No
Zhou et al. [26]	Yes	Yes
Sheikh et al. [29]	No	Yes
Li et al. [30]	No	Yes
Yan et al. [31]	No	Yes
Alzubaidi et al. [21]	No	yes

3.2. Cervical Cancer

Cervical cancer is one of the most common cancers among women worldwide, especially in developing nations, and it has a relatively high incidence and mortality rates [36]. Cervical cancer usually develops slowly over time. When cervical cancer begins in the cervix, cervical cells go through changes called dysplasia, in which cells that are not normal begin to appear in the cervical tissue. In its later stage, cancer cells start to multiply and proliferate more deeply into the cervix and to surrounding areas. Fortunately, cervical cancer is mostly preventable with active screening and detection techniques.

For example, preventive screening and early detection can decrease the morbidity of cervical cancer by about 70% in the United States [37].

3.2.1. Screening Methods

Nowadays, there are a few frequently-used cervical cancer screening techniques, such as high-risk human papillomavirus (HPV) testing, Pap smear cytology testing, colposcopy and visual inspection of the cervix with acetic acid (VIA), each of which has its advantages and disadvantages.

- **Bimanual pelvic examination.** This is a visual and physical inspection by the physician. It consists of both visual inspections using a device called a speculum and physical inspection by using fingers. This test is not enough on its own and the Pap test is usually performed next.
- **Cervical cytopathology** Papanicolaou Smear (Pap smear) or liquid-based cytology is a process of gently scraping cervical cells and inspection of those cells under a microscope. It can also be analyzed digitally using computers.
- **HPV typing test.** Cervical cancer usually occurs from persistent infection of the cervix with some carcinogenic types of human papillomavirus (HPV) such as HPV16 and HPV18 [38]. It is usually performed along with a Pap test or after Pap test results show abnormal changes to the cervix. The occurrence of HPV does not confirm cancer.
- **Colposcopy.** Colposcopy is a visual inspection of the cervix using a special instrument called a colposcope. The device magnifies the cervix area under inspection like a microscope. It can be used for pregnant women.

Other types of tests were also used for cervical cancer screening such as X-ray, CT scan, MRI and PET scan but they are more expensive and used to detect advanced stages of cancer.

Cervical cytology (Pap test) is the most common test used to look for early changes in cells that can lead to cervical cancer [39]. It has been widely used for the screening of cervical cancer in developed countries and is effective in reducing the number of deaths. It is still unavailable for population-wide screening in the developing countries. This is because screening using cervical cytology is difficult, tedious, time-consuming, expensive and subjected to errors because each slide contains around three million cells with large shape and appearance variation between cells, the poor contrast of cytoplasm boundaries and the overlap between cells [40]. In developed countries like the United Kingdom, cervical cancer screening is performed every 3 years for women aged 25 to 49 years and every 5 years aged 50 to 64 years [41]. Over the past few decades, many types of research were performed in developing a computer-assisted cervical cancer screening method. Most of these researches tried to automatically identify the various stages of cancer or abnormality types by classifying cells on the Pap-smear slides. Most of these classifications consist of cell or nuclei segmentation, feature extraction and classification steps [42].

3.2.2. Datasets for Cervical Cancer

Most of the research regarding the detection and segmentation of cervical cancer used the Herlev dataset. The pap-smear benchmark database provides data for comparing classification methods. The data consists of 917 images of pap-smear cells, classified carefully by cyto-technicians and doctors [43]. The dataset is distributed unevenly into seven classes, namely superficial squamous, squamous intermediate, columnar, moderate dysplasia, moderate dysplasia, severe dysplasia and carcinoma in situ. Each image in the Herlev dataset contains only a single cell. Each slide contains many cells and cells might also overlap. Hussien [44] prepared a more realistic dataset for the classification of cervical cells. Summary of the publicly available datasets for classification and segmentation of cervical cells and cervix is given in Table 8.

Table 8. Image datasets for cervical cancer.

Dataset	Size	#Classes/Targets	Format	Type	Author, Year
Herlev	917	187	Bit Map(BMP)	Histology	Dr J. Jantzen [43]
DANS-KNAW	963	4	jpg	Histology	Hussien [44]
CRIC	400	6	png and csv	Histology	M.T. Rezende et al. [45]
Zenodo	962	4	jpg	Histology	Franco et al. [46]
ALTS	938	2	jpg	Colposcopy	Alts Group [47]
MobileODT	1448	3	jpg	Colposcopy	MobileODT [48]

3.2.3. Deep Learning for Segmentation of Cervical Cells

Traditional cytological criteria for classifying cervical cell abnormalities are based on the changes in the nucleus to cytoplasm ratio, nuclear size, irregularity of nuclear shape and membrane. In normal cells, the cytoplasm appears much larger than the nucleus with the regular shaped nuclei. Therefore numerous works are focusing on the segmentation of cell or cell components (nuclei, cytoplasm) [41]. Deep learning has been applied for the segmentation of cervical cell nuclei and the whole cell itself. The successful segmentation of each cervical cell from the slides gives a better performance for cancerous cells. Nuclei detection is only maybe helpful and is easier than segmentation of the whole cell and may be enough for the detection of cancer or help for the segmentation of the whole cell.

Song et al. [49] tried to improve cervical cell segmentation by using learning-based segmentation when overlapping cells are encountered. They include high-level shape information to guide the segmentation algorithm which is done by the convolutional neural network algorithm. They evaluated their algorithm in nuclei detection and cervical cell segmentation. By using the datasets ISBI 2015 challenge dataset, and SZU dataset they achieved a Dice similarity coefficient (DSC) of 0.95 and 0.89, respectively.

Zhao et al. [50] proposed an algorithm called Progressive Growing of U-net + (PGU-net +) for Automated Cervical Nuclei Segmentation, which tried to modify the original U-net algorithm [51], which augmented the limited medical dataset for use of deep learning. They claimed these augmentations mix the information of different scales that affect each other; hence, it limits the segmentation accuracy of the model. they proposed a progressive growing U-net (PGU-net +) model, which extracts image features at each scale independently and passing residual information with the next scale. They achieved a segmentation accuracy of 0.925 on the Herlev dataset, with precision 0.901 ± 0.13, recall 0.968 ± 0.04 and ZSI of 0.925 ± 0.09.

Sompawong et al. [52] applied a pre-trained Mask R-CNN for cervical cancer nuclei detection, segmentation and classification into normal and abnormal ones. They used liquid-based histological slides obtained from Thammasat University (TU) Hospital and obtained mean average precision (mAP) of 57.8%, the accuracy of 91.7%, the sensitivity of 91.7% and specificity of 91.7% per image. They used DeepPap as a benchmark to evaluate their algorithm. Since DeepPap used the Herlev dataset (containing images of single cells) for training and testing. It needs to be modified and retrained on the TU dataset. They showed the proposed algorithm performs better than the modified DeepPap on the TU dataset. They did not evaluate the Mask R-CNN algorithm on the Herlev dataset.

Liu et al. [53] proposed a cervical nucleus segmentation method in which pixel-level prior information was utilized to provide the supervisory information for the training of a mask regional convolutional neural network (Mask R-CNN). They added a local fully-connected conditional random field (LFCCRF) to refine the segmentation. Using the Herlev Pap smear dataset, the proposed method achieved 0.96 in both precision and recall and 0.95 in the Zijdenbos similarity index.

Liang et al. [42] used a comparison based detection which combines the decision of two CNN architectures. First reference, samples were obtained by using the ResNet50 with Feature Pyramid Network (FPN) architecture from each cell image from the dataset. At the same time features from the whole slide image, which contains many cells, were extracted through ResNet50 with FPN and region proposal network (RPN). They replaced the original parameter classifier from their baseline network, Faster R-CNN with FPN with their comparison classifier. Their proposed algorithm can detect 11 different cell types from the whole slide. The performance of the proposed algorithm achieved mean average precision (mAP) of 26.3% and average recall (AR) of 35.7%. They argue these performance measurements do not reflect how good the algorithm was since the proposed algorithm groups multiple neighboring cells with the same category into one result.

Kurnianingsih et al. [54] used deep learning methods to segment cervical cells and classify them. For the segmentation purpose, transfer learning was applied on Mask R-CNN weights trained using the COCO dataset. The pre-trained model was trained to segment cervical cell area consisting of both nuclei and cytoplasm. In the segmentation phase, when Mask R-CNN is applied to the whole cell, it outperforms the previous segmentation method in precision (0.92 ± 0.06), recall (0.91 ± 0.05) and ZSI (0.91 ± 0.04).

Deep learning-based segmentation into nuclei segmentation and cell segmentation can be summarized (see Tables 9 and 10).

Table 9. Summary of selected papers on nuclei segmentation.

Authors	Method	Dataset	Acc	P	R	F1	Sp	Sn	ZSI
Zhao et al. [50]	Progressive Growing of U-net+(PGU-net+)	Herlev	0.925	0.901	0.968				0.925
Liu et al. [53]	Mask-RCNN with LFCCRF	Herlev		0.96	0.96				0.95
Sompawong et al. [52]	Mask-RCNN	TU	89.8%				94.3%	72.5%	

Table 10. Summary of selected papers on cervical cell segmentation.

Authors	Method	Dataset	Acc	P	R	ZSI	DSC
Kurnianingsih et al. [54]	Mask R-CNN	Herlev		0.92	0.91	0.91	
Song et al. [49]	CNN with Shape information	Herlev					0.92
Liang et al. [42]	comparison based Faster R-CNN	local		26.3	35.7		

3.2.4. Deep Learning for Cervical Cell Classification

Zhang et al. [55] tried to directly classify cervical cells—without prior segmentation—based on deep features, using convolutional neural networks (ConvNets). In their algorithm (DeepPap), a pre-trained ConvNets was trained on a cervical cell dataset consisting of adaptively re-sampled image patches coarsely centered on the nuclei. Then they applied aggregation to average the prediction scores of a similar set of image patches. The proposed algorithm achieved classification accuracy (98.3%), area under the curve (AUC) (0.99) values and specificity (98.3%) on the Herlev dataset.

Hyeon et al. [56] proposed a CNN-based pre-trained model, VGGNet-16 for feature extraction, and use different classifiers namely: logistic regression, random forests, AdaBoost and SVM for classification of the pap-test images into normal and abnormal. From these classifiers, the highest scoring one is the SVM classifier with an F1-score of 0.7817 on a dataset collected locally.

LIN et al. [57] applied the transfer learning approach to fine-tune different CNN models (AlexNet, GoogLeNet, ResNet and DenseNet) which were pre-trained on ImageNet dataset [58]. The pre-trained models were fine-tuned on the Herlev cervical dataset with additional cytoplasm and nucleus morphological masks. They achieved classification accuracies of 94.5%, 71.3% and 64.5%, for two-class (abnormal versus normal), four-class (normal, low-grade squamous intraepithelial lesion (LSIL), high-grade squamous intraepithelial lesion (HSIL) and carcinoma-in-situ (CIS) [59]) and seven-class ("World Health Organization classification system") classification tasks, respectively.

Chen et al. [60] tried to combine features extracted from different types of tests. They proposed a Faster R-CNN, which is based on Faster R-CNN for fusing acetic and iodine images of the cervix.

They fuse non-image features extracted from the cervix transformation zone type, pap test, HPV test and age after they non-linearly compression of the fused image features to 29D by using one fully connected (FC) layer. They did not mention which classifier they used for normal–abnormal classification but achieved an accuracy of 87.4% (88.6% sensitivity and 86.1% specificity) on a locally collected dataset.

Kurnianingsih et al. [54] trained a compact VGG network based on their Mask R-CNN based segmentation algorithm. For the classification, a compact VGG Net classifier yields a sensitivity score of more than 96% with a low standard deviation ($\pm$ 2.8%) for the binary classification problem and yields a higher result of more than 95% with low standard deviation (maximum 4.2%) for the 7-class problem.

Performance comparison of different pre-trained deep learning models on Pap smear classification was done by Promworn et al. [61]. They compared the performance of CNN models namely resnet101, densenet161, AlexNet, vgg19_bn and squeeznet1_1, which are the top five models based on accuracy in ImageNet. The models are retrained on the Herlev dataset. Based on accuracy, densenet161 was the best performer on both binary classification (94.38%) and multiclass classification (68.54). Based on sensitivity, AlexNet and resnet have achieved 100% on binary classification. Whereas densenet161 was the best performer on multiclass classification with 68.18%. Again, based on specificity, densenet161 was superior with values 82.61% for binary and 69.57% for multiclass classification.

Yutao Ma et al. [62] developed a CADx system by using a convolutional neural network (CNN) for feature extraction and support vector machines (SVM) for classifying the optical coherence microscopy (OCM) images into five classes namely normal, ectropion, low-grade and high-grade squamous intraepithelial lesions (LSIL and HSIL) and cancer. They also used HPV test results for the classification in conjunction with features extracted from the OCM images by the CNN. An 88.3 $\pm$ 4.9% classification accuracy was achieved for all five classes. In the binary classification task (low-risk (normal, ectropion and LSIL) vs. high-risk (HSIL and cancer)), the CADx method achieved an area under the curve (AUC) value of 0.959 with 86.7 $\pm$ 11.4% sensitivity and 93.5 $\pm$ 3.8% specificity.

Ahmed et al. [63] proposed transfer learning-based approaches for the classification of cervical cells. They explored six different methods for the classification of cervical cells by combining three pre-trained models as features, shallow CNN, which consisted of only two convolutional layers and two max-pooling layers, VGG-16 Net and CaffeNet as a feature extraction technique and two classifiers, extreme learning machine (ELM) and auto encoder (AE) for the classification purpose. They used the Herlev dataset for training and testing their system. The best performer from these combinations is the CaffeNet+ELM which achieved a binary classification accuracy of 99.7 and 97.2 for the 7 class classification.

Dong et al. [64] used artificially extracted features such as color, texture and morphology along with the Inception-V3 model for the classification of cervical cells. They used features extracted manually since the features extracted from the CNN architecture since the knowledge of cervical cells is lacking there. Nine artificial features were combined with features extracted from the Inception-V3 architecture joined on the fully connected layer and used the Softmax function for the classification. They keep the aspect ratio of the cells when resizing for the Inception-V3 network will harm the morphological features. The proposed algorithm achieved an overall accuracy of 98.2%, the sensitivity of 99.4% and specificity of 96.73% for normal abnormal classification on the Herlev dataset.

Martinez-Mias et al. [65] tried to improve and make it realistic the cervical classification from PAP smears using a cell merger approach. They used CNN for PAP smear image classification, and optimize and integrate the cell fusion approach since most PAP smear slides contain overlapping cells. They used a local PAP smear dataset collected from ten patients and labeled using biopsy results. Hence, it was used as a gold standard. They trained the CaffeNet model using data prepared using a cell merger to reflect the reality of the PAP smear examination. For classifying the cervical cells into four classes the CaffeNet with the cell merger dataset achieved an average accuracy of just 55.6% with the performance as low as just 16.7% for LSIL class. For the normal/abnormal classification, their proposed algorithm achieved an accuracy, sensitivity and specificity of 88.8%, 0.92 and 0.83, respectively. This performance is satisfactory considering the classification was done on overlapping cell regions.

Xiang et al. [66] used YOLOv3 as a cell detector and Inception-V3-based classifier for cervical cell classification into ten classes that could be present on the slide namely, normal cells (NORMAL), atypical squamous cells-undetermined significance (ASC-US), atypical squamous cells-cannot exclude HSIL(ASC-H), low-grade squamous intraepithelial lesion (LSIL), high-grade squamous intraepithelial lesion (HSIL), atypical glandular cells (AGC), adenocarcinoma (ADE), vaginalis trichomoniasis (VAG), monilia (MON) and dysbacteriosis (DYS). The model achieves 97.5% sensitivity (Sens) and 67.8% specificity (Spec) on cervical cell image-level screening.

The cervical cell classification algorithms can be categorized into two categories, binary and multiclass. In the binary classification cervical cells are classified into normal and abnormal cells (see Table 11). Multiclass classification describing the severity of the cancer including the normal ones (see Table 12).

Table 11. Summary of selected papers on cervical cell binary classification.

Authors	Method	Dataset	Acc(%)	Sn(%)	Sp(%)	AUC	F1	P	R
Zhang et al. [55]	DeepPap	Herlev	98.3	-	98.3	0.99	-	-	-
Hyeon et al. [56]	VGG16	SVM	local	-	-	-	0.78	0.78	0.78
Lin et al. [57]	GoogleNet5C	Herlev	94.5	-	-	-	-	-	-
Chen et al. [60]	Mask R-CNN 7 class	local-	87.4	88.6	86.1	-	-	-	-
Kurnianingsih et al. [54]	Mask R-CNN	Herlev	98.1	96.7	98.6	96.5	-	-	-
Promworn et al. [61]	densenet161	Herlev	94.38	100	-	-	-	-	-
Yutao Ma et al. [62]	CNN and SVM	OCM image	-	86.7	93.5	0.96	-	-	-
Ahmed et al. [63]	CaffNet+ELM	Herlev	99.5	-	-	-	-	-	-
Dong et al. [64]	Inception-V3	Herlev	98.23	99.4	96.7	-	-	-	-
Martinez-Mias et al. [65]	CaffeNet	Local	88.8	92	83	-	-	-	-

Table 12. Summary of selected papers on cervical cell multiclass classification.

Authors	Method	Dataset	Acc	Sn	Sp	Others
	regressor 7 classes					
Yutao Ma et al. [62]	CNN and SVM 5 classes	OCM image	88.3			
Lin et al. [57]	GoogleNet5C 4 classes	Herlev Dataset	71.3			
Lin et al. [57]	GoogleNet5C seven classes	Herlev Dataset	64.5			
Kurnianingsih et al. [54]	Mask R-CNN 7 class	Herlev	95.9	96.2	99.3	
Promworn et al. [61]	densenet161 7 classes	Herlev dataset	68.54	68.18	69.57	
Ahmed et al. [63]	CaffNet+ELM	Herlev	91.2	-	-	-
Martinez-Mias et al. [65]	CaffeNet	Local	55.6	-	-	-
Xiang et al. [66]	YOLOv3+InceptionV3	local	89.3	97.5	67.8	-

3.2.5. Deep Learning for Cervix Classification

Colposcopic images are also used for cervical cancer detection using deep learning methods. A colposcopy helps to observe the cervix at up to ×10 magnification [67]. Cervical intraepithelial lesions are easily recognized when treated with acetic acid solutions using colposcopy.

Cervix type classification from smartphone camera was tried in [68] using capsule networks which achieves an accuracy of 94%. A more advanced approach called CervixNet [69] which is designed based on a novel hierarchical convolutional mixture of experts (HCME) method achieved an accuracy of 96.77%.

M. Arora et al. [70] used the transfer learning approach from a pre-trained CNN, Inception V3 model [71] by modifying the output layer. The output layer was replaced by a pooling layer and a fully connected layer for the classification of the cervix based on its image. A cervical image dataset from Kaggle was used here, which has three types of cervix based on the location of the transformation layer. The type of cervix will help the physician whether further tests are needed or not. They obtained an average accuracy of just 54.54%.

Guo et al. [72] explored the application of two versions of regions with convolutional neural networks (R-CNN), Mask R-CNN and Mask^X R-CNN, on three different dataset for cervix classification for automatic segmentation of cervix region. Mask R-CNN is effective on datasets with annotations having the exact boundaries. The Mask^X R-CNN can also trained the bounding box annotation. The highest performance was achieved using Mask R-CNN with Dice and IoU of 0.947 and 0.901, respectively. Mask^X R-CNN also achieved a very good performance with Dice and IoU of 0.92 and 0.86 respectively. These colposcopy images suffer from presense of many distractors such as pubic hair, intra-uterine devices (IUDs), the speculum and even parts of human hand. The main problem in cervix classification from cervix photos is the presence of out of focus images [73].

Guo et al. [74] used an ensemble of three deep learning architectures, RetinaNet, Deep SVDD and a customized CNN for the detection of cervix on smartphone captured images. They achieved an average accuracy and F1-score of 91.6% and 0.890, respectively.

3.2.6. Summary

Screening through a Pap test for cervical cancer can take days for the final analysis to complete since the pathologist needs to go through millions of cells. A deep learning-based system can detect those cells in minutes if it is accurate enough to be trusted. One of the main challenges of deep learning methods is the presence of other types of cells and other materials present in the image and the overlapping between two adjacent cervical cells. To solve these problems, a large and carefully annotated dataset needs to be built for the algorithms to learn. Building this many datasets for medical images is very difficult. The most commonly used dataset for cervical cancer screening is the Herlev dataset as shown in Table 10.

Deep learning has been applied for cervical cancer screening in many of its screening methods. Most of the successful deep learning-based cervical cancer detection methods were based on a dataset using pap smear histology images. Colposcopic images are also taking more attention since they are easy to take and not invasive. Their accuracies on the detection of cervical cancers is not as good as that of the histology images. Cervical cancer detection using the deep learning methods based on the colposcopic images are becoming common since a large dataset can be collected and annotated easily. Colposcopic screening could be applied for mass screening purposes with the aid of deep learning, since taking samples are easy. As we can see from Tables 9–12, the Herlev dataset is the most used dataset for cervical cell classification and segmentation works. Most of the coloscopic datasets used for cervix classifications are locally collected. We can also see that the deep learning methods for nuclei segmentation are more accurate than that of cell segmentations since cell boundaries might overlap between adjacent cells. For the classification case, binary classifiers are more accurate than that of multiclass classifiers which can detect the type of abnormalities in the cells.

From Tables 11–13, we can see those deep learning methods with pre-trained networks and those with transfer learning mechanisms are more accurate than networks trained from scratch with TensorFlow the widely used software.

Most of the reviewed papers on the application of deep learning on cervical cancer screening were published in 2019 with an average impact factor of 3.4 (see Table 14). And, as shown in Table 15, only one of the papers compares the algorithm performance with that of the specialist.

Table 13. Summary of cervical cancer scientific papers in terms of CNN architecture, and type of environment used in the selected papers.

Author and Citation	Network	Pre-Training	Transfer Learning	Environment
Zhao et al. [50]	U-Net	No	No	-
Liu Y. et al. [53]	Mask-RCNN	Yes	No	Tensorflow
Sompawong et al. [52]	Mask-RCNN	Yes	Yes	-
Kurnianingsih et al. [54]	Mask-RCNN and VGGNet	Yes	Yes	-
Song et al. [49]	CNN-Custom	No	No	-
Lianget al. [42]	ResNet50	Yes	Yes	Tensorflow
Zhang et al. [55]	ConvNet	Yes	Yes	Caffe
Hyeon et al. [56]	CNN	Yes	Yes	-
Yutao Ma et al. [62]	VGG-16	Yes	Yes	Tensorflow
Lin et al. [57]	GoogLeNet	Yes	Yes	Caffe
Promworn et al. [61]	DenseNet161	No	No	PytTorch
Wimpy and Suyanto [68]	Capsule Network	Yes	No	Tensorflow
Gorantla et al. [69]	ResNet101	yes	Yes	-
Arora et al. [70]	CNN-Custom	No	No	-
Ahmed et al. [63]	CaffeNet	yes	yes	Caffe
Martinez-Mias et al. [65]	CaffeNet	yes	yes	Caffe

Table 14. Summary of cervical cancer scientific papers in terms of article publication year, name of the journal for the selected papers and its impact factor with year of impact factor.

Author and Citation	Publication Year	Journal/Conference	Impact Factor	Impact Assigned Year
Zhao et al. [50]	2019	MMMI 2019	-	-
Liu Y. et al. [53]	2018	IEEE Access	4.098	2018
Sompawong et al. [52]	2019	Conference ACEMBS	0.54	2019
Kurnianingsih et al. [54]	2019	IEEE Access	4.098	2018
Song et al. [49]	2016	Conference ISBI	1.51	2019
Liang et al. [42]	2019	Neurocomputing	3.317	2016
Zhang et al. [55]	2017	JBHI	5.223	2020
Hyeon etal. [56]	2017	Conference ICMDM	-	-
Yutao Ma et al. [62]	2019	IEEE Transaction on Biomedical Engineering	4.78	2019
Lin et al. [57]	2019	IEEE Access	4.098	2018
Promworn et al. [61]	2019	Conference ICNEMS	0.312	2019
Wimpy and S. Suyanto [68]	2019	Conference ISRITI	-	-
Gorantla et al. [69]	2019	BIBE	0.392	2012
Arora et al. [70]	2018	Conference ICSCCC	0.91	2019
Ahmed et al. [63]	2019	Future Generation computer systems	6.125	2019
Dong et al. [64]	2020	ASCJ	5.5	2020
Martinez-Mias et al. [65]	2020	ESWA	5.45	2020

Table 15. Summary of cervical cancer scientific papers in terms of comparison to specialists and/or traditional techniques.

Author and Citation	Comparison to Specialists	Comparison to Traditional Technique (Yes/No)
Zhao et al. [50]	No	Yes
Liu Y. et al. [53]	No	Yes
Sompawong et al. [52]	No	Yes
Kurnianingsih et al. [54]	No	Yes
Song et al. [49]	No	Yes
Liang et al. [42]	No	Yes
Zhang et al. [55]	Yes	No
Hyeon et al. [56]	No	No
Yutao Ma et al. [62]	Yes	No
Lin et al. [57]	No	Yes
Promworn et al. [61]	No	Yes
Wimpy and S. Suyanto [68]	No	Yes
Gorantla et al. [69]	No	Yes
Arora et al. [70]	No	No
Ahmed et al. [63]	No	Yes
Dong et al. [64]	No	Yes
Martinez-Mias et al. [65]	No	No

3.3. Brain Tumor

Brain tumor is a group of abnormal cells around or inside the brain due to the uncontrolled division of cells with a serious effect of deterring the normal functionality of the brain activity and destroying the healthy cells[75].

Brain tumor is classified into benign or low-grade (grade I and II) and malignant or high-grade (grade III and IV). Benign is a non-cancerous tumor that does not exhibit any progression and cannot spread to other parts of the body; it started in the brain with a very low growth rate. On the other hand, a malignant tumor is cancerous with an attribute of growing rapidly and spreading to other parts of the body. Malignant tumors can further be categorized as primary and secondary. Primary malignant tumor originates in the brain itself; whereas, the secondary type begins from somewhere else in the body and spreads to the brain. Cancerous cells that spread to the brain commonly originate from the lung, kidney, breast, skin and colon. A metastatic brain tumor is another expression for this type of brain tumor. Glioblastoma multiform (GBM) is the most common type of primary brain tumor that grows fast from glial cells. An intense clinical treatment plan is required for high-grade gliomas (HGG) as they have a higher spreading rate than the low-grade gliomas (LCG) [76]. It is evidenced that patients with GBMs decease in less than a year. Early detection helps a therapeutic plan of patients and improves the overall survival rate [77]. The most prevalent brain cancer is high-grade glioma with 85% of new cases of malignant primary tumor diagnosed every year [78].

3.3.1. Screening Methods

Magnetic resonance imaging is the most common brain tumor diagnosis and has a great role in treatment planning strategies [79]. These images have an important contribution towards an automatic medical image analysis field as they provide quite a lot of information about the brain structure and abnormalities [80].

This is the reason why MRI images have a great impact on the automatic medical image analysis field. There are various steps taken in the course of brain tumor treatment. The first step is determining if the tumor does exist in the brain or not. Then, the infected region in the brain tissues must be extracted from an MRI image in a process called segmentation [81]. Segmentation is not an easy task as MRI images may not help human readers easily discern regions of concern for various technical reasons. However, segmentation is a very important task in properly conducting the diagnosis, treatment and appraisal of treatment outcomes. A great number of automatic segmentation methods with varying degrees of accuracy have been developed as applications of the computational science for utilization of imaging devices advance.

There are different modalities of the MRI including T1-weighted (T1), T2-weighted contrast-enhanced (T1c), T2-weighted (T2) and T2-weighted fluid attenuated inversion recovery (FLAIR) for segmenting the brain tumor [82]. Moreover, features of the MRI like textures, local histograms and structure tensor eigenvalues have been used in brain tumor segmentation [83]. Deep learning-based methods have become state-of-the-art as they score superior performance in image analysis fields [84].

3.3.2. Datasets

Most of the researchers have applied publicly available brain tumor image datasets to test their methods. Summary of publicly available datasets for brain tumor segmentation and classification is summarized in Table 16.

Table 16. Image datasets for brain tumor (N—normal, AB—abnormal).

Dataset	Size	#Classes	Format/Targets	Type	Author, Year
LBPA40	288	2	html	MRI	Shattuck et al. [85]
BRATS 2015	43,708	2	.mha	MRI	Menze et al. [86]
BRATS2013	1799	2	.mha	MRI	Menze et al. [86]
RIDER_NEURO_MRI	29	2	.tcia	MRI	Barboriak et al. [87]
SUH	49	2	-	MRI	Fabelo et al. [88]
HMS	66	2	.gif	MRI	Keith A. Johnson
FBT	3064	2	.mat	MRI	C. Jun [89]
NHTM	3064	2	.png	MRI	C. Jun [89]
GCE	150	2	.png	MRI	Jun Cheng [90]

3.3.3. Deep Learning in Brain Tumor Segmentation

Alkassar et al. [91] proposed transfer learning and fully convolution network (FCN) to achieve robust tumor segmentation using VGG-16 networks. The proposed method achieved a global accuracy of 0.97785 and a 0.89 Dice score in terms of whole tumor segmentation on MRI images from the BRATS2015 dataset.

Amiri et al. [92] proposed a simple and reliable brain segmentation method in MRI images through recursively and deeply transferring a learned random forest (RF) to guide an SVM classifier for segmenting tumor lesions while capturing the complex characteristics of brain tumor appearance. They tested this method on 20 patients with high-grade gliomas from the Brain Tumor Image Segmentation Challenge (BRATS) dataset. Their method outperforms both SVM and RF with a high statistical significance using paired t-test; i.e., a mean Dice index of 72% compared to SVM (59%) and RF (63%).

Chahal et al. [93] proposed a novel approach using deep learning which utilizes both global and local brain image datasets for precise segmentation. Their proposed deep learning model combines two-pathway and cascade architectures to analyze and implement brain segmentation. The results are evaluated over Input Cascade and the outcomes showed better performance—that is, a metrics of Dice score for high grade and low-grade image with values 0.943 and 0.950, respectively—than existing MFC cascade.

Ding et al. [94] proposed deep residual dilate network with middle supervision (RDM-Net) which combines the residual network with dilated convolution. By evaluating their framework on the BRATS 2015 challenge, their framework proved to achieve better performance than other state-of-the-art methods incomplete tumor (Dice score of 0.86) and core tumor segmentation (Dice score of 0.78). However, the Dice score for enhancing tumors only achieves 0.63 which is not as good as the other counterpart methods. The reason for this could be the focus on the 2D slices segmentation by the proposed framework which pays less attention to the context information within slices by comparing with 3D segmentation. The loss of context information may lead to worse performance on the enhancing tumor segmentation.

Mallick et al. [95] have used a deep wavelet autoencoder (DWA) for an image compression technique which blends the basic feature reduction property of autoencoder along with image decomposition property of wavelet transform for further classification task by using DNN. The performance of the DWA-DNN classifier was compared with other existing classifiers like autoencoder-DNN or DNN and the proposed method surpasses them all with an overall accuracy of 96% where that of AE-DNN is 93% and DNN is 91%.

Ramirez et al. [96] proposed a new variational model for saliency detection in images and its application to brain tumor segmentation. The model works by incorporating a saliency term to a classical total variation-based restoration functional and hence discriminates what is relevant (salient) from the background. They have, therefore, introduced a deep learning framework for using available knowledge from a specific application to optimize the parameters of the energy functional. The proposed framework achieved a Dice score of 0.857, precision 0.845 and recall 0.882.

Sajid et al. [97] proposed a deep learning-based method that uses different modalities of MRI for the segmentation of brain tumors. The proposed hybrid convolutional neural network architecture uses a patch-based approach and deals with the over-fitting problems by utilizing dropout regularize alongside batch normalization, whereas the data imbalance problem is dealt with by using a two-phase training procedure. The proposed method contains a preprocessing step, in which images are normalized and bias field corrected, a feed-forward pass through a CNN and a post-processing step as a means of removing remnant false positives in the skull portion. The proposed method is validated on the BRATS 2013 dataset, where it achieves scores of 0.86, 0.86 and 0.91 in terms of Dice score, sensitivity and specificity for whole tumor region, improving results compared to existing state-of-the-art techniques.

Wang et al. [98] proposed an automatic method named residual and pyramid pool network (WRN-PPNet) to segment brain tumor by first obtaining 2D slices from 3D MRI brain tumor images and then normalizing the 2D slices and putting them in the model. The model will output the tumor segmentation results. The experimental results show that the proposed method is simple and robust compared to the other state-of-the-art methods with an average Dice, sensitivity and PPV values on randomly selected datasets 0.94, 0.92 and 0.97, respectively.

Zhao et al. [99] proposed a new method for brain segmentation which is an integration of fully convolutional neural networks (FCNNs) and conditional random fields (CRFs) in a unified framework. The result helps to obtain segmentation results with the appearance and spatial consistency. The following steps are taken to for training the deep learning model using 2D image patches and image slices: (1) training FCNNs using image patches; (2) training CRFs as recurrent neural networks (CTF-RNN) using image slices with parameters of FCNNs fixed; and (3) fine-tuning the FCNNs and the CRF-RNN using image slices. In the model, 3 segmentation models are particularly trained using 2D image patches and slices obtained in axial, coronal, and sagittal views respectively are combined to segment brain tumors using a voting-based fusion strategy. The method used BRTS 2013, BRATS 2015 and BRATS 2016 with an experimental result of a competitive score. The method achieved a promising performance on the BRATS 2013 and BRATS 2015 testing dataset. The method could also achieve competitive performance with only 3 imaging modalities (FLAIR, T1c and T2) rather than 4(FLAIR, T1, T1c and T2). In BRATS 2016, the method ranked first on its multi-temporal evaluation.

Kuzina et al. [100] proposed a knowledge transfer method between diseases via the generative Bayesian prior network to mitigate the common challenge of obtaining large image datasets for automatic segmentation. They have applied deep weight prior; hence the name UNet-DWP for their method, to incorporate information about the structure of previously learned convolutional filters during the training of a new model. A comparison between a pre-trained approach and random initialization to this approach proves that this method yields the best results in terms of the Dice similarity coefficient metric on a small subset of the BRATS2018 dataset. The performance of the model was rated by taking subsets containing 5, 10, 15 or 20 randomly selected images from the dataset and comparing them with the fixed test sample size of 50 images. They have also used a blend of binary cross-entropy and Dice losses to train U-Net in the non-Bayesian setting. The results indicate that the model outperforms both pre-trained and randomly initialized U-Nets for all the training sizes.

Zeineldin et al. [101] proposed a new generic deep learning architecture named DeepSeg to address the challenge of distinguishing tumor boundaries from healthy cells in the brain tumor diagnosis. This method helps to wholly automate detection and segmentation of the brain lesion using FLAIR MRI data. The developed system is a decoupling framework interacting encoding and decoding relationship where the encoder part performs spatial information using a convolutional neural network and the decoder provides the full-resolution probability map from the resulting semantic map. The study has employed different CNN models such as residual neural network (ResNet), dense convolutional network (DenseNet) and NASNet using modified U-Net architecture. The proposed architecture has been tested on MRI datasets of brain tumor segmentation (BRATS2019) challenge which includes s336 cases as training data and 125 cases for validation data yielding Dice and Hausdorff distance scored of about 0.81 to 0.84 and 9.8 to 19.7, respectively. The proposed DeepSeg is open source and freely available at https://github.com/razeineldin/DeepSeg/.

Fabelo et al. [102] suggested a deep learning-based hyperspectral image (HSI) processing modality to be used as a reliable support in real-time neurosurgical procedure for carrying out accurate resection of the tumor without affecting much of the normal brain tissue. The study employed a number of deep learning techniques for the detection of brain tumors using HSI. The HS image database was obtained during the course of operation and the system employed a highly sophisticated and specialized visible and near-infrared (VNIR) push broom camera. Classification methods with 2D-CNN and pixel-wise classification with 1D-DNN have been found to yield a very good result. Despite the challenge in obtaining sufficient number of training samples and the anomalies incurred due to brain movement during scanning, the overall average accuracy for the proposed method was 80%. The method has also achieved a very high specificity for both binary and multiclass classification schemes with values of 100% and 90%, respectively.

The summary of researches on deep learning methods for brain tumor segmentation is presented in Table 17.

3.3.4. Deep Learning in Brain Tumor Classification

Like in the segmentation, deep learning-based methods have performed fairly well in image classification of brain tumors. Yet, variation in the shape, size, location and contrast of tumor tissue cells is the major factor that impacts the accurate classification of brain tumors from MRI images [103].

Deep learning techniques involving different enhancement methods are used to classify different types of brain tumors—glioma, meningioma and pituitary. The classification is further categorized into axial, coronal and sagittal planes that are used by various algorithms to minimize the error rate of neural networks in identifying the brain tumor [104].

Mohsen et al. [80] employed a DNN classifier where a 7-fold cross-validation technique was applied for building and training the DNN of 7-hidden layers structure for classifying a dataset of brain MRIs into four classes, i.e., normal, glioblastoma, sarcoma and metastatic bronchogenic carcinoma.

They have combined the classifier with the discrete wavelet transform (DWT)—a powerful feature extraction tool—and principal components analysis (PCA). They achieved a classification rate of 96.97%, recall 0.97, precision 0.97, F-measure 0.97 and AUC (ROC) 0.984.

Table 17. Summary of selected papers on brain tumor segmentation.

Authors	Method Learning	Dataset	Acc.	P	R	F	Sp	Sn	Dice	PPV
Alkassar et al. [91]	DNN+FCN+VGG-16	BRATS2015	0.98						0.89	
Amiri et al. [92]	RF-SVM	BRATS							0.72	
Chahal et al. [93]	CNN	BRATS2013			0.96				0.93	0.95
Ding et al. [94]	RDM-Net	BRATS2015							0.86	
Mallick et al. [95]	DWA-DNN	RIDER_NEURO_MRI	0.93				0.93	0.92	0.94	
Ramirez et al. [96]	CNN+TVS	Flair-MRI Brats2015		0.84	0.88				0.86	
Sajid et al.[97]	hybrid CNN	BRATS 2013					0.91	0.86	0.86	
Wang et al. [98]	WRN-PPNet	BRATS2015						0.92	0.94	0.97
Zhao et al. [99]	FCNNs and CRF-RNN	BRATS 2013–16						0.82	0.84	0.89
Kuzina et al. [100]	UNet-DWP	BRATS2018							0.76	
Zeineldin et al. [101]	DeepSeg	BRATS 2019							0.81–0.84	
Fabelo et al. [102]	HSI+2D-CNN	SUH	80					80–100		

Alqudah et al. [105] used a convolutional neural network (CNN) for classifying a dataset of 3064 T1 weighted contrast-enhanced brain MR images for grading the brain tumors into three classes called glioma, meningioma and pituitary. The research has used T1-weighted contrast-enhanced brain MR images for classifying brain tumor grades. They have used a free online available dataset at [90] which contains images having the above-mentioned attributes. A total of 18 layers in the proposed CNN architecture would enable the classifier to rate the brain tumor effectively. In their work they proved that the proposed CNN classifier is a powerful tool with an accuracy of 98.93% and sensitivity 98.18% for cropped lesions; for the uncropped lesions, they have obtained an accuracy of 99% and 98.52% sensitivity; for segmented lesion images, the result is 97.62 accuracy and 97.40% sensitivity.

Ucuzal et al. [106] developed a deep learning free web-based software that can be utilized in the detection and diagnosis of the three types of brain tumors (glioma/meningioma/pituitary) on T1-weighted magnetic resonance imaging. In the research, 3064 T1-weighted MR image scans for the three types of brain tumors have been used. Out of which, 2599 instances were used in the training phase; whereas, the remaining 465 were used in the testing phase. A python programming language library called Auto Keras was used in image pre-processing (image rotation, changing width and length, truncating images, rescaling, etc). Furthermore, a Bayesian optimization technique was used to tune the hyperparameters of the model. With this, they have verified that all the calculated performance metrics—i.e., accuracy, precision, sensitivity, specificity, F1-score, MCC, G-Mean of the experimental results are higher than 98% for classifying the types of brain tumors on the testing dataset obtained from Nanfang Hospital and Tianjin Medical University General Hospital which is an open-source dataset downloaded from [107]. This data set consists of 3064 T1-weighted contrast-enhanced MR images from 233 patients: 708 meningiomas, 1426 glioma and 930 pituitary tumors. The developed web-based software can be publicly available at [108].

Selvy et al. [109] developed a model that makes use of an image processing technique and artificial neural network for successful detection of the brain tumor. To enhance the contrast of the original image in its analysis and manipulation, they have used histogram equalization (HE) technique where gray level co-occurrence matrix (GLCM) would be used on the feature extraction. A probabilistic neural network (PNN) classifier is applied to the obtained feature to accurately determine tumor location in brain MRI images. The PNN classifier has produced an accuracy of 90.9%, specificity of 100% and sensitivity 85.75%.

Sultan et al. [110] proposed a deep learning (DL) model to classify different brain tumor types. The model which bases a convolutional neural network has employed two publicly available datasets acquired from Nanfang Hospital and General Hospital, Tianjing Medical University, China from 2005 to 2010. The two datasets entail 233 and 73 patients with a total of 3064 and 516 images on T1-weighted contrast-enhanced images, respectively. The overall accuracy of the proposed network is 96.13% for the first and 98.7% for the second dataset. The result inferred that the model has the ability to perform brain tumor multi-classification. The network training and performance computations are finally presented. The system parameters used to train the neural network structure are Intel i7-7700HQ CPU (2.8 GHz), NVIDIA GTX 1060 (6 GB) GPU, 16GB RAM, Matlab 2018b and Python 3. The network is constructed from 16 layers where the input layer holds the pre-processed images passing through the convolution layers and their activation functions (3 convolution, 3 ReLU, normalization and 3 max-pooling layers). Additionally, two dropout layers are used to prevent overfitting followed by a fully connected layer and a softmax layer to predict the output and finally a classification layer that produces the predicted class. Although the dataset is relatively not big (due to the variety of imaging views), data augmentation helped well to show better results and hence, overcome this problem.

Badža and Barjaktarovic [111] presented a new CNN architecture for Brain Tumor Image Segmentation and classification for three tumor types. The study has employed an image database that contains 3064 T1-weighted contrast-enhanced MRI images acquired from Nanfang Hospital and General Hospital, Tianjin Medical University, China from 2005 to 2010. The input layer of the proposed network was represented by MRI images of the database after being normalized to 256 × 256 pixels. The network architecture having consisted of input, two main blocks, classification block and output was employed to perform tumor classification. The blocks consist of the rectified linear unit (ReLU) activation layer, the dropout layer and the max-pooling layer engaged in fine-tuning and resizing the images. A CNN developed in Matlab R2018a (The MathWorks) was employed for the tumor classification. The evaluation of the network was assessed using four approaches: combinations of two 10-fold cross-validation methods and the two databases mentioned above. The generalization capability of the network was tested with one of the 10-fold methods, subject-wise cross-validation, and the improvement was tested by using an augmented image database. The best result for the 10-fold cross-validation method was obtained for the record-wise cross-validation for the augmented data set, and, in that case, the accuracy was 96.56%. With good generalization capability and good execution speed, the new developed CNN architecture could be used as an effective decision-support tool for radiologists in medical diagnostics.

The summary of the papers reviewed is presented in Table 18.

Table 18. Summary of selected papers on brain tumor classification.

Authors	Method	Dataset	Acc.	P	R	F	Sp	Sn	MCC	G-Mean
Mohsen et al. [80]	DWT-DNN	Harvard		0.97	0.97	0.97				
Alqudah et al. [105]	CNN	Online	98.40	98.19			99.19	98.18		
Ucuzal et al. [106]	CNN Multiclass	NHTM	99.74	99.58			99.59	99.81	99.60	99.39	99.70
Selvy et al. [109]	PNN	GCE	90				100	85.75		
Sultan et al. [110]	CNN	NHTM	96.13–98.7							
Badža and Barjaktarovic [111]	CNN	NHTM	96.56							

3.3.5. Summary

As shown in Table 19, papers from 2016, 2018, 2019, and 2020 were reviewed here. Unlike other cancer type papers, reviewed papers on brain tumors consist of a significant number of papers that compared the performance of their model with that of the domain expert(see Table 20).

As indicated in Tables 17 and 18, Brain Tumor Image Segmentation Challenge (BRATS) of various versions is the most widely used dataset among the researchers and appeared in ten out of the seventeen papers reviewed.

From Table 21 it was found that a Tensor flow-based framework run by a high-speed core processor or a GPU was widely used, seven out of seventeen, followed by PyTorch, two out of seventeen, to implement the experiments and conducting the deep learning training. However, the rest of the papers have not explicitly indicated which software platform they have applied. On the other hand, VGGNet is the most frequently applied network to achieve robust tumor segmentation 52.9% of the papers have made a comparison with domain experts; on the other hand, 94.1% of the paper has made a comparison with the traditional method.

Table 19. Summary of brain tumor scientific papers in terms of article publication year, name of journal for the selected papers and its impact factor with year of impact factor.

Author and Citation	Publication Year	Journal	Impact Factor	Impact Assigned Year
Alkassar et al. [91]	2019	ICECCPCE19 Conference	0.627	2019
Amiri et al. [92]	2016	ATSIP 2016 Conference	0.17	2019
Chahal et al. [93]	2019	RDCAPE Conference	-	-
Ding et al. [94]	2019	IEEE Access	3.745	2019
Mallick et al. [95]	2019	IEEE Access	3.745	2019
Ramirez et al. [96]	2018	ISBI Conference	1.51	2019
Sajid et al.[97]	2019	Arabian Journal for Science and Engineering	0.33	2019
Wang et al. [98]	2019	IJCNN Conference	0.37	2019
Zhao et al. [99]	2018	Medical Image Analysis	3.88	2019
Kuzina et al. [100]	2019	Frontiers in Neuroscince	3.7	2020
Mohsen et al. [80]	2018	Future Computing and Informatics	3.88	2019
Alqudah et al. [105]	2019	IJATCSE	0.2	2019
Ucuzal et al. [106]	2019	ISMSIT	0.84	2019
Zeineldin et al. [101]	2020	IJCARS	1.961	2017
Fabelo et al. [102]	2019	MDPI	3.275	2019
Selvy et al. [109]	2019	IJSRCSEIT	1.638	2016
Sultan et al. [110]	2019	IEEE Access	3.745	2019
Badža and Barjaktarovic [111]	2020	MDPI	2.474	2019

Table 20. Summary of brain tumor scientific papers in terms of comparison to specialists and/or traditional techniques.

Author and Citation	Comparison to Specialists (Yes/No)	Comparison to Traditional Technique (Yes/No)
Alkassar et al. [91]	Yes	Yes
Amiri et al. [92]	No	Yes
Chahal et al. [93]	No	Yes
Ding et al. [94]	No	Yes
Mallick et al. [95]	No	Yes
Ramirez et al. [96]	Yes	Yes
Sajid et al.[97]	No	Yes
Wang et al. [98]	Yes	Yes
Zhao et al. [99]	Yes	Yes
Kuzina et al. [100]	No	Yes
Mohsen et al. [80]	No	Yes
Alqudah et al. [105]	No	Yes
Ucuzal et al. [106]	Yes	No
Zeineldin et al. [101]	Yes	Yes
Fabelo et al. [102]	Yes	Yes
Selvy et al. [109]	No	No
Sultan et al. [110]	Yes	Yes
Badža and Barjaktarovic [111]	No	Yes

Table 21. Summary of brain tumor scientific papers in terms of CNN architecture, and type of environment used in the selected papers.

Author and Citation	Network	Pre-Training	Transfer Learning	Environment
Alkassar et al. [91]	VGGNet-16	Yes	Yes	
Amiri et al. [92]	RF+SVM	Yes	Yes	
Chahal et al. [93]	CNN	Yes	Yes	
Ding et al. [94]	RDM-Net	Yes	Yes	
Mallick et al. [95]	DWA-DNN	Yes	Yes	Tensor flow
Ramirez et al. [96]	CNN+TVS	Yes	Yes	Tensor flow
Sajid et al. [97]	hybrid CNN	Yes	Yes	Tensor Flow
Wang et al. [98]	WRN-PPNet	Yes	Yes	Tensor flow
Zhao et al. [99]	FCNNs and CRF-RNN	Yes	Yes	Tensor flow
Kuzina et al. [100]	UNet-DWP	Yes	Yes	
Mohsen et al. [80]	DWT-DNN	Yes	Yes	
Alqudah et al. [105]	VGGNet-19	Yes	Yes	
Ucuzal et al. [106]	UNet-DWP	Yes	Yes	Tensor flow and Keras
Zeineldin et al. [101]	ResNet+DenseNet+NasNet	Yes	Yes	Keras, Tensor Flow
Fabelo et al. [102]	UNet	Yes	Yes	Tensor Flow
Selvy et al. [109]	GLCM+PNN	Yes	Yes	
Sultan et al. [110]	CNN	Yes	Yes	Matlab 2018b and Python
Badža and Barjaktarovic [111]	CNN	Yes	Yes	Matlab 2018b

3.4. Colorectal Cancer (CRC)

Worldwide in 2018, more than 1,849,518 (which accounts for 10.2% of overall cancer cases) new cases of colorectal cancer (CRC) are diagnosed and nearly 880,792 people died which is 9.2% of all cancer-related deaths [112]. It is the third most common cancer worldwide and the second most deadly [112]. Since colorectal cancer takes a long time before it becomes invasive, it is often curable if found early. Hence, casual screening for colorectal cancer can substantially reduce its mortality. Approximately 95% of all colorectal cancers are adenocarcinomas [113]. Colorectal adenocarcinomas develop in the lining of the colon or rectum and are characterized by glandular formation.

3.4.1. Screening Methods

There are three common screening methods for colorectal cancer: fecal occult blood test (FOBt), flexible sigmoidoscopy (FS) and total colonoscopy (TC) [114]. FOBt reveals traces of blood in stool samples which is an early sign of colorectal cancer. FS involves visual inspection of the distal bowel for polyps and cancers. TC visualizes the entire bowel and therefore is a more invasive examination. The advancement of whole slide imaging (WSI) scanners has opened new opportunities in automating pathology image analysis by digitizing the slides [115]. Histological examination of the glands, most frequently with the hematoxylin & eosin (H & E) stain, is routine practice for assessing the differentiation of cancer within colorectal adenocarcinoma [113]. Pathologists use the degree of glandular formation as an important factor in deciding the grade of the tumor. Accurate segmentation of structures of the glandular formations such as glands and nuclei have crucial importance, because their morphological properties can assist the pathologist in screening the malignancy [113].

3.4.2. Datasets

In Table 22, we present some of the publicly available and widely used datasets for colorectal cancer detection and segmentation.

Table 22. Publicly available datasets for colorectal cancer (CRC), UMCM—University Medical Center Mannheim, CVC—computer vision center.

Dataset	Size	#Classes/Targets	Format	Type	Author, Year
CVC-EndoSceneStill	912	4	bmp	Colonoscopy	Vázquez et al. [116], 2017
CVC-ColonDB	300	4	bmp	Colonoscopy	J. Bernal et al. [117], 2012
CVC-ClinicDB	612	4	tiff	Colonoscopy	J. Bernal et al. [118], 2015
UMCM	500	8	mat	histology	Kather et al. [119], 2016

3.4.3. Deep Learning for Cell Detection and Classification on Histological Slides

Kainz et al. [120] applied deep learning methods to segment and classify colon glands into benign and malignant types for GlaS@MICCAI2015 challenge. They first pre-processed the stained RGB by taking the Red channel and ignoring the others. Then contrast enhancement was performed using contrast limited adaptive histogram equalization (CLAHE) technique. Two CNN classifiers were trained: Object-Net, Separator-Net. Object-Net is for the detection of benign and malignant glands from their respective backgrounds. Separator-Net is for classifying gland-separating structures since the Object-Net architecture segment two neighboring glands as one. These to classifiers are then regularized using a figure-ground segmentation based on weighted total variation to produce the final segmentation result. They have achieved 96% average accuracy on the two tests provided by the challenge.

Sirinukunwattana et al. [121] proposed a spatially constrained convolutional neural network (SC-CNN) that includes parameter estimation layer and spatially constrained layer for spatial regression to predict the probability of a pixel being the center of a nucleus in hematoxylin and eosin (H & E) stained histopathology images. For classifying the detected nuclei they combine neighboring ensemble predictor (NEP) with a standard softmax CNN (s-CNN). For the nuclei detection using SC-CNN, they achieved 0.77 precision, 0.82 recall, and 0.8 F1-score. The NEP&s-CNN classifier achieved an F1-score of 0.784 and the overall nuclei detection and classification (SC-CNN+NEP&s-CNN) achieved an F1-score of 0.69.

Graham et al. [113] used a fully convolutional neural network that counters the loss of information caused by the max-pooling layer by introducing original down-sampled image into the residual unit using the minimal information loss (MIL) units. They applied atrous spatial pyramid pooling for multi-level aggregation and preserving the resolution. They achieved an F1-score of 0.92 for gland segmentation using the GlaS challenge dataset.

Chamanzar et al. [122] develop a deep learning method that can detect and segment a single cell using only point labeled dataset. They combined Voronoi transformation, Local pixel clustering and Repel encoding methods with U net with Resnet encoder by feeding them to a multi-task scheduler for training the system. They achieved an accuracy of 93% for cell segmentation and 94.1% for detection of adenocarcinoma.

Sari et al. [123] proposed a novel approach for feature extraction, which defines the features by considering only the salient subregions of the image. The salient subregions were detected by the detection of nuclear and non-nuclear pixels using an algorithm presented in [124]. Then a deep belief network of restricted Boltzmann machines (RBMs) re-characterizes these regions and extract features. These features are clustered using the k-means clustering algorithm and SVM classifier for categorizing those regions. They achieved an average precision, recall, and F1-score of 82.3%, 89.9% and 85.1, respectively at the detection of colon adenocarcinoma.

Shapcott et al. [125] proposed a deep learning-based cell identification on histological images of the colon with a systematic random sampling of the WSI slides. Their proposed system consists of two CNNs in series in which the first one detects cells on the WSI slide while the second one classifies those cells into epithelial, inflammatory, a fibroblast or "other". The training was performed on a local dataset and Evaluated using the "The Cancer Genome Atlas (TCGA)" dataset. Using five patients' slides, they achieved an average accuracy of 65% in the detection of cells and 76% in the classification.

Tang et al. [126] proposed Segnet based gland segmentation on the histology image of the colon. Augmented MICCAI2015 challenge dataset was used to train the SegNet network which is a CNN with encode-decoder architecture for pixel-wise segmentation. SegNet achieved an average Dice similarity index of 0.872 and Hausdorff distance of 104.61.

Vuong et al. [127] proposed an algorithm based on DenseNet121 that can perform both classification and regression tasks on WSI images, for improving the overall performance of the system. They designed this multi-task deep learning model by adding two fully connected layers, one for classification and one for regression, after the DenseNet121 network. The classifier classifies the tissue image into four distinctive pathologies and the regressor considers these four pathological categories as continuous values. They achieved 85.1% accuracy in classifying colon tissues into four categories.

Sabol et al. [128] proposed a semantically explainable fuzzy classifier called cumulative fuzzy class membership criterion (CFCMC) for classifying WSI of colorectal cancer tissue into eight different tissue types. They compared many CNN architectures as feature extraction for the CFCMC classifier with the Xception architecture performance being the best feature extractor for the CFCMC. The explainability of the system is its ability to provide a degree of confidence for each of its predictions. The proposed method achieved an accuracy of 92.78% for the classification of the different tissue samples. The explainability was evaluated by pathologists based on its objectivity, level of details, reliability and quality. Based on these measures, they confirmed that the explainability of the system is better than the traditional CNN architectures.

3.4.4. Deep Learning for Classification of Polyps on Endoscopic Images

Colorectal polyps are abnormalities in the colon tissues that can develop into colorectal cancer. The survival rate for patients is higher when the disease is detected at an early stage and polyps can be removed before they develop into malignant tumors. These tests are usually performed using endoscopic analysis of the colon. During this study, the endoscopist explores the colon cavity looking for abnormal growths of tissue, polyps. However, polyp detection is a challenging problem given its high variation in appearance, size, shape and in many cases its high similarity with the surrounding tissue.

The application of CTs for the screening of colorectal cancer suffers from false positives due to the similarity between polyps and colorectal tubes on the CT image. Approaches in [129] can help to distinguish between colorectal tubes and polyps in CT scans of the colon area using a three dimensional massive-training artificial neural network (3D-MTANN). The proposed model manages to reduce false positives by 33% while keeping a sensitivity of 96%.

Ornela Bardhi et al. [130] used CNNs with auto-encoders for the automatic detection of colon polyp. They used the SegNet architecture from the TensorFlow to build the model and train it from scratch using three datasets: CVC-ColonDB, CVC-ClinicDB and ETIS-LaribPolypDB. They achieved a maximum accuracy of 96.7% on the EITS dataset for the detection of colon polyps.

Bour et al. [131] trained different architectures: ResNet50, ResNet101, Xception, VGG19 and Inception V3 for classification of polyps. ResNet50 achieved the highest accuracy of 87.1 % with precision 87.1%, recall 87.1%, F1-score 87.1% and specificity 93%.

Liu et al. [132] used a deep learning network, faster_rcnn_inception_resnet_v2 model for localization and classification of endoscopic images of the colon. They achieved 90.645% mean average precision and 0.5 for the intersection over union (IoU).

Ozawa et al. [133] used deep convolutional neural network (CNN) architecture called single shot multibox detector (SSD) for the detection of colorectal polyps. All layers were fine-tuned using stochastic gradient descent with a global learning rate of 0.0001. The trained SSD detected the trained CNN detected 1246 colorectal polyps from a dataset collected at Tada Tomohiro Institute of Gastroenterology and Proctology with a sensitivity of 92% and a positive predictive value (PPV) of 86%.

Nadimi et al. [134] used a modified version of ZF-net, a CNN architecture proposed by Matthew D. Zeiler and Rob Fergus [135], as the basis for a Faster R-CNN to localize regions of images containing colorectal polyps. They trained their architectures using a locally collected dataset labeled as colorectal polyps (N = 4800) and normal mucosa (N = 6500). The proposed architecture achieved an accuracy, sensitivity and specificity of 98.0%, 98.1% and 96.3%, respectively. The proposed approach produces the bounding box annotation of the polyp.

3.4.5. Summary

The most common colorectal cancer screening methods use endoscopic images to find abnormal colon tissues, polyps and locating cancerous cells or glands on WSI images. Hence most of the application of deep learning for detecting colorectal cancer is either finding adenocarcinoma on WSI or detection of polyps on colonoscopic images. Most of the research shows promising results in both polyp detection and adenocarcinoma or glands detection as seen in Tables 23 and 24.

Table 23. Summary of selected papers on detection and classification for colorectal cancer histological slides.

Authors	Method	Dataset	Acc	P	R	F1	DSC	H
Kainz et al. [120]	Separator-Net and Object-Net	MICCAI2015	96	59	74	62	-	-
Graham et al. [113]	MILD-Net	GlaS+	-	-	-	87	88	142
Chamanzar et al. [122]	WSMTL	local	93	-	-	79.1	78.4	-
Sari et al. [123]	DeepFeature	local	-	82.3	89.9	85.1	-	-
Shapcott et al. [125]	CNNs	local and TCGA	65	-	-	-	-	-
Sirinukunwattana et al. [121]	SC-CNN+NEP & s-CNN	MICCAI2015	-	-	-	-	69	-
Tang et al. [126]	Segnet	MICCAI2015	-	-	-	-	87.2	104.61
Vuong et al. [127]	Multitask DensNet121	local	85.1	-	-	-	-	-
Sabol et al. [128]	CFSCMC	UMCM	92.78	-	-	-	-	-

The main challenge for the analysis of colposcopic images is most of the dataset suffers from out of focus problems. Detection of polyps from endoscopic images presents a big opportunity for deep learning methods to shine since most of the physicians may miss smaller polyps. Still, challenges are there due to low-quality samples and the operator might miss some areas.

Papers who used pre-trained models and applied transfer learning approaches discuss their findings in detail and are from reputable journals (see Tables 25 and 26). From Table 27, only two of the papers measure the performance of their proposed model against expert physicians.

Table 24. Summary of selected papers on colorectal cancer polyp detection.

Authors	Method	Dataset	Acc	P	R	F1	Sp	Sn	PPV
Ornela Bardhi et al. [130]	SegNet	EITs	96.7	-	-	-	-	-	-
Bour et al. [131]	Resnet50	local	87.1	87.1	87.1	87.1	93	-	-
Liu et al. [132]	faster_rcnn_inception_resnet_v2	local	90.6	-	-	-	-	-	-
Ozawa et al. [133]	SSD	local	-	-	-	-	-	92	86
Nadimi et al. [134]	mZF-net+ResNet	local	98	-	-	-	98.1	96	-

Table 25. Summary of colorectal cancer in terms of article publication year, name of journal for the selected papers and its impact factor with year impact factor has been assigned.

Author and Citation	Publication Year	Journal/Conference	Impact Factor	Impact Assigned Year
Kainz et al. [120]	2017	PeerJ	2.38	2019
Graham et al. [113]	2018	Medical Image Analysis	8.79	2018
Chamanzar et al. [122]	2020	ISBI conference	2.283	2019
Sari et al. [123]	2019	IEEE Transactions on Medical Imaging	9.71	2019
Shapcott et al. [125]	2019	Frontiers in bioengineering and biotechnology	3.644	2020
Sirinukunwattana et al. [121]	2016	IEEE transactions on medical imaging	9.71	2019
Tang et al. [126]	2018	Conference YAC	1.461	2019
Vuong et al. [127]	2020	Conference ICEIC	0.76	2019
Ornela Bardhi et al. [130]	2017	Conference ISSPIT	1.393	2019
Bour et al. [131]	2017	Conference ISSPIT	1.393	2019
Liu et al. [132]	2019	Conference ISNE	0.152	2019
Ozawa et al. [133]	2020	Therapeutic advances in gastroenterology	4.08	2020
Nadimi et al. [134]	2020	CEE	2.663	2020
Sabol et al. [128]	2020	YJBIN	3.526	2020

Table 26. Summary of colorectal cancer in terms of CNN architecture and type of environment used in the selected papers.

Author and Citation	Network	Pre-Training	Transfer Learning	Environment
Kainz et al. [120]	Object-Net and SeparatorNet—custom	No	No	Matlab
Graham et al. [113]	MILD-Net—custom	No	No	Tensorflow
Chamanzar et al. [122]	U-net and Resnet	Yes	Yes	PyTorch
Sari et al. [123]	DeepBelief	Yes	Yes	-
Shapcott et al. [125]	-	No	No	Tensorflow
Sirinukunwattana et al. [121]	-	No	No	Matlab
Tang et al. [126]	SegNet	No	No	Caffe
Vuong et al. [127]	DensNet121	No	No	PyTorch
Ornela Bardhi et al. [130]	SegNet	No	No	Tensorflow
Bour et al. [131]	ResNet50	Yes	Yes	Tensorflow
Liu et al. [132]	faster_rcnn_inception_resnet_v2	No	No	Tensorflow
Ozawa et al. [133]	Single Shot MultiBox Detector (SSD)	No	No	Caffe
Nadimi et al. [134]	mZF-Net+ResNet	Yes	Yes	Matlab 2018a
Sabol et al. [128]	Xception+CFCMC	Yes	Yes	-

Table 27. Summary of colorectal cancer papers in terms of comparison to specialists and/or traditional techniques.

Author and Citation	Comparison to Specialists	Comparison to Traditional Technique (Yes/No)
Kainz et al. [120]	No	No
Graham et al. [113]	No	Yes
Chamanzar et al. [122]	No	Yes
Sari et al. [123]	No	No
Shapcott et al. [125]	No	No
Sirinukunwattana et al. [121]	No	Yes
Tang et al. [126]	No	Yes
Vuong et al. [127]	No	No
Ornela Bardhi et al. [130]	No	No
Bour et al. [131]	Yes (Approval)	No
Liu et al. [132]	No	Yes
Ozawa et al. [133]	No	No
Nadimi et al. [134]	No	No
Sabol et al. [128]	Yes	Yes

3.5. Lung Cancer

Lung cancer is the deadliest cancer worldwide with the highest incidence rate [112]. The death rate is so high because the majority of the cases are discovered at an advanced stage, where curative treatment is no longer feasible. Hence, screening for early detection is significant enough for decreasing mortality.

3.5.1. Screening Methods

The recommended screening test for lung cancer is low-dose computed tomography (LDCT), which uses a low dose of X-ray radiation to get detailed images of the lungs. Physicians will study different slices of the LDCT to determine the presence of an abnormal area called lung nodule (or mass) [136]. Other approaches also exist like chest X-ray(the usual X-ray image), sputum cytology (microscopic analysis of mucus from the lungs). According to a study performed in [136], these approaches do not seem to decrease the mortality rate.

3.5.2. Datasets

In Table 28, some of the publicly available and widely used datasets for lung cancer detection and segmentation are listed.

Table 28. Publicly available datasets for CRC, UMCM—University Medical Center Mannheim, CVC—computer vision center.

Dataset	Size	#Classes/Targets	Format	Type	Author, Year
UCI ML repository	32	3		CSV	Hong and Yang [137], 1991
SPIE-AAPM-NCI	22489	2	dicom	CT	Armato et al. [138], 2015
Lung Nodule Malignancy	6690	2	hdf5	CT	Scott Mader [139], 2017
LUNA2016	888	2	mhd.zip	CT	Consortium for Open Medical Image Computing [119], 2016

3.5.3. Deep Learning for Lung Nodules Detection

Before the introduction of convolution-based deep learning methods, Suzuki [140] uses massive training artificial neural networks (MTANN) for the detection and decreasing false positives in lobules detection using extracted subregions from LDCT images. MTANNs are designed based on the concepts of artificial neural network filters, where MTANN will classify each subregion (kernel) independently. Hence, the convolution process is external. They used Multiple MTANNs in parallel to distinguish between nodules and non-nodules by training each MTANN with the same nodules but different types of non-nodules. multi-MTANN was applied to differentiate between benign and malignant nodules from LDCT images in [141].

Tajbakhsh and Suzuki [142] compared the performances of the two widely studied deep learning models, CNNs and MTANNs, for the detection and classification of lung nodules. The proposed MTANN-based architecture outperforms the best performing CNN (AlexNet in their experiment) insensitivity and false-positive rates achieving 100% sensitivity and 2.7 false positives per patient. In the classifications of the nodules into benign and malignant the MTANNs achieved an AUC of 0.88.

Gu et al. [143] proposed a novel CAD system for the detection of lung nodules using a 3D-CNN. They implemented a multiscale approach for making the system more efficient at the detection of various sizes of nodules. The proposed CAD system considers the preprocessing step, which is usually essential in building a standalone CAD system. It has a volume segmentation step for generating ROI cubes for the 3D-CNN to classify them. After the classification, DBSCAN was used to merge neighboring regions into one since they might be different parts of the same nodule. Using the LUNA16 dataset, they found out that small scale cubes are efficient in the detection of smaller nodules (92% sensitivity and four false positives per patient), but larger ones have lower sensitivity (88%), but with an average of one false positive per patient.

Sahu et al. [144] proposed a multiple view sampling-based multi-section CNN model for nodule classification and malignancy estimation from CT scans. Their proposed model is computationally lighter than the widely used and relatively efficient 3D-CNNs. They used sample slices extracted at different orientations, with spherical sampling performing the best, and a pre-trained MobileNet network to build their system. On the classification task, the proposed model achieved a sensitivity of 96% and AUC of 98% on the LUNA2016 dataset. They measure the severity of malignancy by training the logistic regression model to estimate the class probability of malignancy. It achieved an accuracy of 93.79% on malignancy estimation. Since it is a lightweight model, the model can work on smaller devices such as smart-phones, tablets, etc.

Ozdemir et al. [145] proposed an efficient end-to-end CAD system by coupling nodule detection with malignancy ranking step. They called the nodule detection system as CAD_e (detection) whose output is an input for malignancy ranking step, CAD_x (diagnosis) step in the complete CAD system. Training and evaluation were performed on the LUNA16 and Kaggle Bowl datasets [146]. The proposed model includes model uncertainty in its decision, making it relatively trustworthy in a real-world application. The proposed CAD_e system achieved a sensitivity of 96.5%+ and 19.7 false positives per patient without using false positive reduction techniques. The CAD_x system also achieves an AUC of 98%. The combination of the two systems was further tuned to build the full CAD system.

Bansal et al. [147] proposed Deep3DSCan for lung cancer segmentation and classification. They used a deep 3D segmentation algorithm to extract a 3D volume of interest from CTs. A combination of features extracted using a deep fine-tuned residual network and morphological features were used to train the ResNet based model. Training and testing used the publicly available LUNA16 dataset. The proposed architecture achieved an accuracy of 88% in segmentation and classification tasks with an F1-score of 0.88.

3.5.4. Summary

Many of the papers discussed here studied the detection and classification of lung nodules from the LDCT images. The end-to-end papers covered in these reviews ([142,145,147]) can help to build an effective CAD system to assist the radiologist.Bansal et al. [147] seems to work better than the other works reviewed here since its performance covers both the detection and classification tasks (see Table 29). We must also consider MTANN-based papers since they deliver a satisfactory result with smaller data sizes. Papers reviewed here can be summarized in Tables 30 and 31. Here we did not consider to create a table for domain expert approval since none was participated in the papers we reviewed.

Table 29. Summary of selected papers on lung cancer detection and classification.

Authors	Method	Dataset	Acc	FPR	Sp	Sn	AUC
Tajbakhsh and Suzuki [142]	MTANN, detection	local	-	2.7	-	100	-
Tajbakhsh and Suzuki [142]	MTANN, classification	local	-	-	-	-	0.88
Gu et al. [143]	3D-CNN, detection	LUNA16	-	2.5	-	90	-
Sahu et al. [144]	multi-section MobileNet	LUNA16	93.8	-	-	96	0.98
Ozdemir et al. [145]	V-Net, classification	LUNA16	-	19	-	96.5	0.98
Bansal et al. [147]	ResNet	LUNA16	88	-	89.7	87	0.88

Table 30. Summary of lung cancer in terms of article publication year, name of journal for the selected papers and its impact factor with the year impact factor has been assigned.

Author and Citation	Publication Year	Journal/Conference	Impact Factor	Impact Assigned Year
Tajbakhsh and Suzuki [142]	2017	Pattern Recognition	7.196	2019
Gu et al. [143]	2018	CBM	3.43	2019
Sahu et al. [144]	2019	IEEE-JBHI	5.180	2020
Ozdemir et al. [145]	2020	IEEE Transactions on Medical Imaging	9.71	2020
Bansal et al. [147]	2020	IET Image Processing	2.61	2020

Table 31. Summary of Colorectal cancer in terms of CNN architecture and type of environment used in the selected papers.

Author and Citation	Network	Pre-Training	Transfer Learning	Environment
Tajbakhsh and Suzuki [142]	MTANN	-	-	Caffe
Gu et al. [143]	3D-CNN	-	-	Keras
Sahu et al. [144]	Mobile-Net	Yes	Yes	Keras
Ozdemir et al. [145]	Vnet	-	-	-
Bansal et al. [147]	Resnet	-	-	Pythorch

3.5.5. Deep Learning for Other Cancer Detection and Segmentation

In this sub-section, we included the application of deep learning on skin, liver and stomach cancer detection. Melanoma is skin cancer which is the deadliest cancer in its nature. In a normal diagnosis distinguishing melanoma lesions from nonmelanoma, lesions are very challenging [148]. For such difficulties, researchers have introduced an automatic skin cancer diagnosis system for detection and segmentation. As a result of uneasy visual characteristics of skin lesion that include inhomogeneous features and fuzzy boundaries. To overcome the challenges, Adegun and Viriri [148] proposed a deep learning-based automatic melanoma lesion detection and segmentation algorithm. They evaluated their approach in terms of Dice coefficient and accuracy 92% and 95% on ISIC 2017 dataset and accuracy and Dice coefficient of 95% and 93% on PH2 datasets.

Another deadly cancer with high morbidity is liver cancer. There are no widely recommended methods for early detection of liver cancer. For patients at higher risk, an imaging test such as CT, MRI, ultrasound and angiography can be used to test for liver cancer. If the physician believes in the need, a biopsy may be used to confirm the diagnosis. Hence, deep learning methods have been proposed in assisting physicians in the diagnosis of liver cancers, including hepatocellular carcinoma (HCC), liver metastasis, cysts, hemangioma and other masses [149]. A custom CNN for classifying HCC in liver cancer from MRI images, which achieved 92% sensitivity (Sn), 98% specificity (Sp) and 92% accuracy was proposed in [150]. In [151], VGGNet was used to develop a CAD system that identifies four types of liver cancers, cysts, hemangiomas, HCC and metastatic liver cancer from ultrasound images. The developed CAD system achieved an average accuracy of 88%. A hybridized fully convolutional neural network (HFCNN) was applied in the detection of liver cancer from abdominal CT images in [64]. HFCNN accurately segments 94.7% of the tumor volume.

Stomach (gastric) cancer is also another common cancer with the fourth-highest incidence rate and the third-highest mortality rate in the world [112]. The most common screening methods for stomach cancer are UGI series, serum pepsinogen (PG) testing, Hpylori serology and endoscopy [152]. Endoscopy is the most accurate of these methods, but it is highly invasive [152]. Some popular deep learning architectures, the inception, ResNet and VGGNet that were pre-trained on ImageNet were applied using transfer learning methods has been applied to identify benign ulcer and cancer from gastrointestinal endoscopic color images in [153]. The ResNet model achieved the highest performance with normal versus abnormal accuracies of 90% and ulcer versus cancer accuracy of 77%. A pre-trained Inception-Resnet-v2 model was trained and compared with endoscopists in classifying classification of gastric neoplasms in [154]. The Inception-Resnet-v2 model performance was lower in five-class (advanced gastric cancer, early gastric cancer, high-grade dysplasia, low-grade dysplasia and no neoplasm) classification, i.e., 76.4% vs. 87.6%. The Inception-Resnet-v2 model performance is comparable with endoscopist in the differentiation of gastric cancer and neoplasm (accuracy 76.0% vs. 82.0%).

4. Conclusions

The paper review indicates that deep learning methods have achieved state-of-the-art breast cancer, cervical cancer, brain tumor. colon cancer and lung cancer detection, feature extraction, classification and segmentation. In this article, a good number of deep learning-based methods for breast cancer, cervical cancer, brain tumor and colon cancer image analysis are studied. The developed and implemented methods employed a CNN approach combined with other techniques to mitigate the existing challenge arising from a large dataset demand for such systems to learn. Problems related to noise and corrupted images have been properly addressed in some of the works as they suggest utilizing normal images and limited dataset size in modes that encompass a combination of two or more architectures to discern breast, cervical, brain and colon abnormalities.

The use of enhanced activation functions have also been recommended to improve the overall performance of deep learning-based systems in medical image analysis. Moreover, many researchers have added multiple layers in the CNN architecture to increase the performance of the system. Some researchers worked on designing unique architectures for specific task properties instead of using CNN as it is. Subsequently, most of the methods are proved to produce a successful performance in terms of specificity, sensitivity and Dice score when tested on renowned datasets and BRATS challenges. The lack of sufficient datasets can be considered a challenge for many of the deep learning-based researches. All of the reviewed papers have not used different medical images other than MRI for brain and in most cases mammograms for breast.

Author Contributions: Conceptualization, T.G.D. and S.R.K.; Methodology, T.G.D., S.R.K. and F.S.; Validation, F.S., and T.G.D.; Writing—original draft preparation, T.G.D., S.R.K. and Z.M.S.; Writing—review and editing, S.R.K., Z.M.S.and T.G.D. All authors have read and agreed to the published version of the manuscript.

Funding: This research received funding from Artificial Intelligence Center and University of Ulm.

Conflicts of Interest: The authors declare no conflict of interest.

References

1. Afework, Y.K.; Debelee, T.G. Detection of Bacterial Wilt on Enset Crop Using Deep Learning Approach. *Int. J. Eng. Res. Afr.* **2020**, *51*, 1–17.
2. Shen, L.; Margolies, L.R.; Rothstein, J.H.; Fluder, E.; McBride, R.; Sieh, W. Deep Learning to Improve Breast Cancer Detection on Screening Mammography. *Sci. Rep.* **2019**, *9*. [CrossRef] [PubMed]
3. Suzuki, K. Survey of Deep Learning Applications to Medical Image Analysis. *Med. Imaging Technol.* **2017**, *35*, 212–226.
4. Litjens, G.; Kooi, T.; Bejnordi, B.E.; Setio, A.A.A.; Ciompi, F.; Ghafoorian, M.; van der Laak, J.A.W.M.; van Ginneken, B.; Sánchez, C.I. A survey on deep learning in medical image analysis. *Med. Image Anal.* **2017**, *42*, 60–88. [CrossRef] [PubMed]
5. Shen, D.; Wu, G.; Suk, H.I. Deep Learning in Medical Image Analysis. *Annu. Rev. Biomed. Eng.* **2017**, *19*, 221–248. [CrossRef] [PubMed]
6. Suzuki, K. Overview of deep learning in medical imaging. *Radiol. Phys. Technol.* **2017**, *10*, 257–273. [CrossRef] [PubMed]
7. Lee, J.; Jun, S.; Cho, Y.; Lee, H.; Kim, G.B.; Seo, J.B.; Kim, N. Deep Learning in Medical Imaging: General Overview. *Korean J. Radiol.* **2017**, *18*, 570–584. [CrossRef]
8. Debelee, T.G.; Schwenker1, F.; Rahimeto, S.; Yohannes, D. Evaluation of modified adaptive k-means segmentation algorithm. *Comput. Vis. Media* **2019**. [CrossRef]

9. Kebede, S.R.; Debelee, T.G.; Schwenker, F.; Yohannes, D. Classifier Based Breast Cancer Segmentation. *J. Biomim. Biomater. Biomed. Eng.* **2020**, *47*, 1–21.
10. Rahimeto, S.; Debelee, T.; Yohannes, D.; Schwenker, F. Automatic pectoral muscle removal in mammograms. *Evol. Syst.* **2019**. [CrossRef]
11. Debelee, T.G.; Schwenker, F.; Ibenthal, A.; Yohannes, D. Survey of deep learning in breast cancer image analysis. *Evol. Syst.* **2019**. [CrossRef]
12. Debelee, T.G.; Gebreselasie, A.; Schwenker, F.; Amirian, M.; Yohannes, D. Classification of Mammograms Using Texture and CNN Based Extracted Features. *J. Biomim. Biomater. Biomed. Eng.* **2019**, *42*, 79–97. [CrossRef]
13. Debelee, T.G.; Amirian, M.; Ibenthal, A.; Palm, G.; Schwenker, F. Classification of Mammograms Using Convolutional Neural Network Based Feature Extraction. *LNICST* **2018**, *244*, 89–98.
14. Suckling, J.; Parker, J.; Dance, D.; Astley, S.; Hutt, I.; Boggis, C.; Ricketts, I. *Mammographic Image Analysis Society (MIAS) Database v1.21 [Dataset]*; Dataset; Digital Mammogram Database Exerpta Medica: Dordrecht, The Netherland, 2015.
15. Scuccimarra, E.A. *DDSM Mammography [Dataset]*; Dataset; Digital Mammogram Database Exerpta Medica: Dordrecht, The Netherland, 2018.
16. Moreira, I.C.; Amaral, I.; Domingues, I.; Cardoso, A.; Cardoso, M.J.; Cardoso, J.S. INbreast. *Acad. Radiol.* **2012**, *19*, 236–248. [CrossRef]
17. Dua, D.; Graff, C. *UCI Machine Learning Repository*; University of California, Irvine, School of Information and Computer Sciences: Newport Beach, CA, USA, 2017.
18. Bukun. *Breast Cancer Histopathological Database (BreakHis)*; Dataset; P and D Laboratory—Pathological Anatomy and Cytopathology: Parana, Brazil, 2019.
19. Aresta, G.; Araújo, T.; Kwok, S.; Chennamsetty, S.S.; Safwan, M.; Alex, V.; Marami, B.; Prastawa, M.; Chan, M.; Donovan, M.; et al. BACH: Grand challenge on breast cancer histology images. *Med. Image Anal.* **2019**, *56*, 122–139. [CrossRef]
20. Wu, N.; Phang, J.; Park, J.; Shen, Y.; Huang, Z.; Zorin, M.; Jastrzebski, S.; Fevry, T.; Katsnelson, J.; Kim, E.; et al. Deep Neural Networks Improve Radiologists' Performance in Breast Cancer Screening. *IEEE Trans. Med. Imaging* **2020**, *39*, 1184–1194. [CrossRef]
21. Alzubaidi, L.; Al-Shamma, O.; Fadhel, M.A.; Farhan, L.; Zhang, J.; Duan, Y. Optimizing the Performance of Breast Cancer Classification by Employing the Same Domain Transfer Learning from Hybrid Deep Convolutional Neural Network Model. *Electronics* **2020**, *9*, 445. [CrossRef]
22. Zhu, Z.; Harowicz, M.; Zhang, J.; Saha, A.; Grimm, L.J.; Hwang, E.S.; Mazurowski, M.A. Deep learning analysis of breast MRIs for prediction of occult invasive disease in ductal carcinoma in situ. *Comput. Biol. Med.* **2019**, *115*, 103498. [CrossRef]
23. Li, X.; Qin, G.; He, Q.; Sun, L.; Zeng, H.; He, Z.; Chen, W.; Zhen, X.; Zhou, L. Digital breast tomosynthesis versus digital mammography: Integration of image modalities enhances deep learning-based breast mass classification. *Eur. Radiol.* **2019**, *30*, 778–788. [CrossRef]
24. Zeiser, F.A.; da Costa, C.A.; Zonta, T.; Marques, N.M.C.; Roehe, A.V.; Moreno, M.; da Rosa Righi, R. Segmentation of Masses on Mammograms Using Data Augmentation and Deep Learning. *J. Digit. Imaging* **2020**. [CrossRef]
25. Zhang, Y.; Chen, J.H.; Chang, K.T.; Park, V.Y.; Kim, M.J.; Chan, S.; Chang, P.; Chow, D.; Luk, A.; Kwong, T.; et al. Automatic Breast and Fibroglandular Tissue Segmentation in Breast MRI Using Deep Learning by a Fully-Convolutional Residual Neural Network U-Net. *Acad. Radiol.* **2019**, *26*, 1526–1535. [CrossRef]
26. Zhou, J.; Luo, L.Y.; Dou, Q.; Chen, H.; Chen, C.; Li, G.J.; Jiang, Z.F.; Heng, P.A. Weakly supervised 3D deep learning for breast cancer classification and localization of the lesions in MR images. *J. Magn. Reson. Imaging* **2019**, *50*, 1144–1151. [CrossRef]
27. Huang, G.; Liu, Z.; Maaten, L.V.D.; Weinberger, K.Q. Densely Connected Convolutional Networks. In Proceedings of the 2017 IEEE Conference on Computer Vision and Pattern Recognition (CVPR), Honolulu, HI, USA, 21–26 July 2017. [CrossRef]
28. Zhang, J.; Saha, A.; Soher, B.J.; Mazurowski, M.A. Automatic deep learning-based normalization of breast dynamic contrast-enhanced magnetic resonance images. *arXiv* **2018**, arXiv:1807.02152v1.

29. Sheikh, T.S.; Lee, Y.; Cho, M. Histopathological Classification of Breast Cancer Images Using a Multi-Scale Input and Multi-Feature Network. *Cancers* **2020**, *12*, 2031. [CrossRef] [PubMed]
30. Li, X.; Shen, X.; Zhou, Y.; Wang, X.; Li, T.Q. Classification of breast cancer histopathological images using interleaved DenseNet with SENet (IDSNet). *PLoS ONE* **2020**, *15*, e0232127. [CrossRef]
31. Yan, R.; Ren, F.; Wang, Z.; Wang, L.; Zhang, T.; Liu, Y.; Rao, X.; Zheng, C.; Zhang, F. Breast cancer histopathological image classification using a hybrid deep neural network. *Methods* **2020**, *173*, 52–60. [CrossRef]
32. Sharma, S.; Mehra, R. Conventional Machine Learning and Deep Learning Approach for Multi-Classification of Breast Cancer Histopathology Images—a Comparative Insight. *J. Digit. Imaging* **2020**, *33*, 632–654. [CrossRef]
33. Vang, Y.S.; Chen, Z.; Xie, X. Deep Learning Framework for Multi-class Breast Cancer Histology Image Classification. In *Lecture Notes in Computer Science*; Springer International Publishing: Berlin/Heidelberg, Germany, 2018; pp. 914–922. [CrossRef]
34. Dembrower, K.; Liu, Y.; Azizpour, H.; Eklund, M.; Smith, K.; Lindholm, P.; Strand, F. Comparison of a Deep Learning Risk Score and Standard Mammographic Density Score for Breast Cancer Risk Prediction. *Radiology* **2020**, *294*, 265–272. [CrossRef]
35. Hagos, Y.B.; Merida, A.G.; Teuwen, J. Improving Breast Cancer Detection using Symmetry Information with Deep Learning. *arXiv* **2018**, arXiv:1808.08273v1.
36. Ferlay, J.; Shin, H.R.; Bray, F.; Forman, D.; Mathers, C.; Parkin, D.M. Estimates of worldwide burden of cancer in 2008: GLOBOCAN 2008. *Int. J. Cancer* **2010**, *127*, 2893–2917. [CrossRef]
37. Wingo, P.A.; Cardinez, C.J.; Landis, S.H.; Greenlee, R.T.; Ries, L.A.G.; Anderson, R.N.; Thun, M.J. Long-term trends in cancer mortality in the United States, 1930–1998. *Cancer* **2003**, *97*, 3133–3275. [CrossRef] [PubMed]
38. Schiffman, M.; Doorbar, J.; Wentzensen, N.; De Sanjosé, S.; Fakhry, C.; Monk, B.J.; Stanley, M.A.; Franceschi, S. Carcinogenic human papillomavirus infection. *Nat. Rev. Dis. Prim.* **2016**, *2*, 1–20. [CrossRef]
39. Patten, J. (Ed.) *Comprehensive Cervical Cancer Control: A Guide to Essential Practice*; World Health Organization: Geneva, Switzerland, 2014.
40. GençTav, A.; Aksoy, S.; ÖNder, S. Unsupervised segmentation andclassification of cervical cell images. *Pattern Recognit.* **2012**, *45*, 4151–4168. [CrossRef]
41. Tang, G.Y.; Parekh, J. Methods of Screening for Cervical Cancer. *JAMA* **2018**, *320*, 1938. [CrossRef]
42. Liang, Y.; Tang, Z.; Yan, M.; Chen, J.; Liu, Q.; Xiang, Y. Comparison-Based Convolutional Neural Networks for Cervical Cell/ClumpsDetection in the Limited Data Scenario. *arXiv* **2019**, arXiv:1810.05952.
43. Jantzen, J.; Norup, J.; Dounias, G.; Bjerregaard, B. Pap-smear benchmark data for pattern classification. In Proceedings of the Nature Inspired Smart Information Systems (NiSIS 2005), Albufeira, Portugal, 3–5 October 2005.
44. Hussain, E. Liquid based cytology pap smear images for multi-class diagnosis of cervical cancer. *Data Brief* **2019**. [CrossRef]
45. Rezende, M.T.; Tobias, A.H.G.; Silva, R.; Oliveira, P.; Medeiros, F.S.D.; Ushizima, D.; Carneiro, C.M.; Bianchi, A.G.C. CRIC Cervix Cell Classification. 2020. Available online: https://figshare.com/collections/CRIC_Cervix_Cell_Classification/4960286 (accessed on 11 August 2020). [CrossRef]
46. Franco, R.A.S.; Carvalho, M.A.G.; Coelho, G.P.; Martins, P.; Enciso, J.L. Dataset of Cervical Cell Images for the Study of Changes Associated with Malignancy in Conventional Pap Test. *ZENODO* **2018**. [CrossRef]
47. Group, A. Human Papillomavirus Testing for Triage of Women With Cytologic Evidence of Low-Grade Squamous Intraepithelial Lesions: Baseline Data From a Randomized Trial. *J. Natl. Cancer Inst.* **2000**, *92*, 397–402. [CrossRef] [PubMed]
48. MobileODT. Intel & Mobile ODT Cervical Cancer Screening. 2017. Available online: https://www.kaggle.com/c/intel-mobileodt-cervical-cancer-screening (accessed on 14 August 2020).
49. Song, Y.; Cheng, J.Z.; Ni, D.; Chen, S.; Lei, B.; Wang, T. Segmenting overlapping cervical cell in Pap smear images. In Proceedings of the 2016 IEEE 13th International Symposium on Biomedical Imaging (ISBI), Prague, Czech Republic, 13–16 April 2016. [CrossRef]
50. Zhao, J.; Dai, L.; Zhang, M.; Yu, F.; Li, M.; Li, H.; Wang, W.; Zhang, L. PGU-net+: Progressive Growing of U-net+ for Automated Cervical Nuclei Segmentation. In *Multiscale Multimodal Medical Imaging*; Springer International Publishing: Berlin/Heidelberg, Germany, 2019; pp. 51–58. [CrossRef]

51. Ronneberger, O.; Fischer, P.; Brox, T. U-Net: Convolutional Networks for Biomedical Image Segmentation. In *Lecture Notes in Computer Science*; Springer International Publishing: Berlin/Heidelberg, Germany, 2015; pp. 234–241. [CrossRef]
52. Sompawong, N.; Mopan, J.; Pooprasert, P.; Himakhun, W.; Suwannarurk, K.; Ngamvirojcharoen, J.; Vachiramon, T.; Tantibundhit, C. Automated Pap Smear Cervical Cancer Screening Using Deep Learning. In Proceedings of the 2019 41st Annual International Conference of the IEEE Engineering in Medicine and Biology Society (EMBC), Berlin, Germany, 23–27 July 2019. [CrossRef]
53. Liu, Y.; Zhang, P.; Song, Q.; Li, A.; Zhang, P.; Gui, Z. Automatic Segmentation of Cervical Nuclei Based on Deep Learning and a Conditional Random Field. *IEEE Access* **2018**, *6*, 53709–53721. [CrossRef]
54. Kurnianingsih, A.K.H.S.; Nugroho, L.E.; Widyawan; Lazuardi, L.; Prabuwono, A.S.; Mantoro, T. Segmentation and Classification of Cervical Cells Using Deep Learning. *IEEE Access* **2019**, *7*, 116925–116941. [CrossRef]
55. Zhang, L.; Lu, L.; Nogues, I.; Summers, R.M.; Liu, S.; Yao, J. DeepPap: Deep Convolutional Networks for Cervical Cell Classification. *IEEE J. Biomed. Health Inform.* **2017**, *21*, 1633–1643. [CrossRef]
56. Hyeon, J.; Choi, H.J.; Lee, K.N.; Lee, B.D. Automating Papanicolaou Test Using Deep Convolutional Activation Feature. In Proceedings of the 2017 18th IEEE International Conference on Mobile Data Management (MDM), Daejeon, Korea, 29 May–1 June 2017. [CrossRef]
57. Lin, H.; Hu, Y.; Chen, S.; Yao, J.; Zhang, L. Fine-Grained Classification of Cervical Cells Using Morphological and Appearance Based Convolutional Neural Networks. *IEEE Access* **2019**, *7*, 71541–71549. [CrossRef]
58. Deng, J.; Dong, W.; Socher, R.; Li, L.J.; Li, K.; Fei-Fei, L. Imagenet: A large-scale hierarchical image database. In Proceedings of the 2009 IEEE Conference on Computer Vision and Pattern Recognition, Miami, FL, USA, 20–25 June 2009; pp. 248–255.
59. Nayar, R.; Wilbur, D.C. The Pap test and Bethesda 2014. *Cancer Cytopathol.* **2015**, *123*, 271–281. [CrossRef]
60. Chen, T.; Ma, X.; Ying, X.; Wang, W.; Yuan, C.; Lu, W.; Chen, D.Z.; Wu, J. Multi-Modal Fusion Learning For Cervical Dysplasia Diagnosis. In Proceedings of the 2019 IEEE 16th International Symposium on Biomedical Imaging (ISBI 2019), Venice, Italy, 8–11 April 2019. [CrossRef]
61. Promworn, Y.; Pattanasak, S.; Pintavirooj, C.; Piyawattanametha, W. Comparisons of PAP-Smear Classification with Deep Learning Models. In Proceedings of the 14th annual IEEE International Conference on Nano/Micro Engineering and Molecular Systems, Bangkok, Thailand, 11–14 April 2019.
62. Ma, Y.; Xu, T.; Huang, X.; Wang, X.; Li, C.; Jerwick, J.; Ning, Y.; Zeng, X.; Wang, B.; Wang, Y.; et al. Computer-Aided Diagnosis of Label-Free 3-D Optical Coherence Microscopy Images of Human Cervical Tissue. *IEEE Trans. Biomed. Eng.* **2019**, *66*, 2447–2456. [CrossRef] [PubMed]
63. Ghoneim, A.; Muhammad, G.; Hossain, M.S. Cervical cancer classification using convolutional neural networks and extreme learning machines. *Future Gener. Comput. Syst.* **2020**, *102*, 643–649. [CrossRef]
64. Dong, N.; Zhao, L.; Wu, C.; Chang, J. Inception v3 based cervical cell classification combined with artificially extracted features. *Appl. Soft Comput.* **2020**, *93*, 106311. [CrossRef]
65. Martínez-Más, J.; Bueno-Crespo, A.; Martínez-España, R.; Remezal-Solano, M.; Ortiz-González, A.; Ortiz-Reina, S.; Martínez-Cendán, J.P. Classifying Papanicolaou cervical smears through a cell merger approach by deep learning technique. *Expert Syst. Appl.* **2020**, *160*, 113707. [CrossRef]
66. Xiang, Y.; Sun, W.; Pan, C.; Yan, M.; Yin, Z.; Liang, Y. A novel automation-assisted cervical cancer reading method based on convolutional neural network. *Biocybern. Biomed. Eng.* **2020**, *40*, 611–623. [CrossRef]
67. Garcia-Arteaga, J.; Kybic, J.; Li, W. Automatic colposcopyvideo tissue classification using higher order entropy-basedimage registration. *Comput. Biol. Med.* **2011**, *41*, 960–970. [CrossRef]
68. Wimpy, B.; Suyanto, S. Classification of Cervical and Type Image and Using and Capsule Networks. In Proceedings of the 2019 International Seminar on Research of Information Technology and Intelligent Systems (ISRITI), Yogyakarta, Indonesia, 5–6 December 2019.
69. Gorantla, R.; Singh, R.K.; Pandey, R.; Jain, M. Cervical Cancer Diagnosis using CervixNet—A Deep Learning Approach. In Proceedings of the 2019 IEEE 19th International Conference on Bioinformatics and Bioengineering (BIBE), Athens, Greece, 28–30 October 2019. [CrossRef]
70. Arora, M.; Dhawan, S.; Singh, K. Deep Neural Network for Transformation Zone Classification. In Proceedings of the 2018 First International Conference on Secure Cyber Computing and Communication (ICSCCC), Jalandhar, India, 15–17 December 2018.

71. Tang, J. *Intelligent Mobile Projects with TensorFlow: Build 10+ Artificial Intelligence Apps Using TensorFlow Mobile and Lite for iOS, Android, and Raspberry Pi*; Packt Publishing: Birmingham, UK, 2018.
72. Guo, P.; Xue, Z.; Long, L.R.; Antani, S. Cross-Dataset Evaluation of Deep Learning Networks for Uterine Cervix Segmentation. *Diagnostics* **2020**, *10*, 44. [CrossRef]
73. Guo, P.; Singh, S.; Xue, Z.; Long, R.; Antani, S. Deep Learning for Assessing Image Focus for Automated Cervical Cancer Screening. In Proceedings of the 2019 IEEE EMBS International Conference on Biomedical & Health Informatics (BHI), Chicago, IL, USA, 19–22 May 2019. [CrossRef]
74. Guo, P.; Xue, Z.; Mtema, Z.; Yeates, K.; Ginsburg, O.; Demarco, M.; Long, L.R.; Schiffman, M.; Antani, S. Ensemble Deep Learning for Cervix Image Selection toward Improving Reliability in Automated Cervical Precancer Screening. *Diagnostics* **2020**, *10*, 451. [CrossRef]
75. Sharma, M.; Mukharjee, S. Brain Tumor Segmentation Using Genetic Algorithm and Artificial Neural Network Fuzzy Inference System (ANFIS). In *Advances in Computing and Information Technology*; Springer: Berlin/Heidelberg, Germany, 2013; pp. 329–339. [CrossRef]
76. Hanif, F.; Muzaffar, K.; Perveen, K.; Malhi, S.M.; Simjee, S.U. Glioblastoma Multiforme: A Review of its Epidemiology and Pathogenesis through Clinical Presentation and Treatment. *Asian Pac. J. Cancer Prev. APJCP* **2017**, *18*, 3–9. [CrossRef]
77. Rees, J.H. Diagnosis and treatment in neuro-oncology: An oncological perspective. *Br. J. Radiol.* **2011**, *84*, S82–S89. [CrossRef]
78. Rasmussen, B.K.; Hansen, S.; Laursen, R.J.; Kosteljanetz, M.; Schultz, H.; Nørgård, B.M.; Guldberg, R.; Gradel, K.O. Epidemiology of glioma: Clinical characteristics, symptoms, and predictors of glioma patients grade I–IV in the the Danish Neuro-Oncology Registry. *J. Neuro Oncol.* **2017**, *135*, 571–579. [CrossRef]
79. Kalpathy-Cramer, J.; Gerstner, E.R.; Emblem, K.E.; Andronesi, O.; Rosen, B. Advanced magnetic resonance imaging of the physical processes in human glioblastoma. *Cancer Res.* **2014**, *74*, 4622–4637. [CrossRef] [PubMed]
80. Mohsen, H.; El-Dahshan, E.S.A.; El-Horbaty, E.S.M.; Salem, A.B.M. Classification using deep learning neural networks for brain tumors. *Future Comput. Inform. J.* **2018**, *3*, 68–71. [CrossRef]
81. Bahadure, N.B.; Ray, A.K.; Thethi, H.P. Image Analysis for MRI Based Brain Tumor Detection and Feature Extraction Using Biologically Inspired BWT and SVM. *Int. J. Biomed. Imaging* **2017**, *2017*, 1–12. [CrossRef] [PubMed]
82. Srinivas, B.; Rao, G.S. Segmentation of Multi-Modal MRI Brain Tumor Sub-Regions Using Deep Learning. *J. Electr. Eng. Technol.* **2020**, *15*, 1899–1909. [CrossRef]
83. Nadeem, M.W.; Ghamdi, M.A.A.; Hussain, M.; Khan, M.A.; Khan, K.M.; Almotiri, S.H.; Butt, S.A. Brain Tumor Analysis Empowered with Deep Learning: A Review, Taxonomy, and Future Challenges. *Brain Sci.* **2020**, *10*, 118. [CrossRef] [PubMed]
84. Akkus, Z.; Galimzianova, A.; Hoogi, A.; Rubin, D.L.; Erickson, B.J. Deep Learning for Brain MRI Segmentation: State of the Art and Future Directions. *J. Digit. Imaging* **2017**, *30*, 449–459. [CrossRef]
85. Shattuck, D.W.; Prasad, G.; Mirza, M.; Narr, K.L.; Toga, A.W. Online resource for validation of brain segmentation methods. *NeuroImage* **2009**, *45*, 431–439. [CrossRef] [PubMed]
86. Menze, B.H.; Jakab, A.; Bauer, S.; Kalpathy-Cramer, J.; Farahani, K.; Kirby, J.; Burren, Y.; Porz, N.; Slotboom, J.; Wiest, R.; et al. The Multimodal Brain Tumor Image Segmentation Benchmark (BRATS). *IEEE Trans. Med. Imaging* **2015**, *34*, 1993–2024. [CrossRef]
87. Barboriak, D. Data From RIDER_NEURO_MRI. 2015. Available online: https://wiki.cancerimagingarchive.net/display/Public/RIDER+NEURO+MRI (accessed on 15 August 2020). [CrossRef]
88. Fabelo, H.; Ortega, S.; Szolna, A.; Bulters, D.; Pineiro, J.F.; Kabwama, S.; J-O'Shanahan, A.; Bulstrode, H.; Bisshopp, S.; Kiran, B.R.; et al. In-Vivo Hyperspectral Human Brain Image Database for Brain Cancer Detection. *IEEE Access* **2019**, *7*, 39098–39116. [CrossRef]
89. Cheng, J.; Huang, W.; Cao, S.; Yang, R.; Yang, W.; Yun, Z.; Wang, Z.; Feng, Q. Enhanced Performance of Brain Tumor Classification via Tumor Region Augmentation and Partition. *PLoS ONE* **2015**, *10*, e0140381. [CrossRef]
90. Cheng, J. Brain Tumor Dataset. 2017. Available online: https://doi.org/10.6084/m9.figshare.1512427.v5 (accessed on 26 October 2020).

91. Alkassar, S.; Abdullah, M.A.M.; Jebur, B.A. Automatic Brain Tumour Segmentation using fully Convolution Network and Transfer Learning. In Proceedings of the 2019 2nd International Conference on Electrical, Communication, Computer, Power and Control Engineering (ICECCPCE), Mosul, Iraq, 13–14 February 2019. [CrossRef]
92. Amiri, S.; Rekik, I.; Mahjoub, M.A. Deep random forest-based learning transfer to SVM for brain tumor segmentation. In Proceedings of the 2016 2nd International Conference on Advanced Technologies for Signal and Image Processing (ATSIP), Monastir, Tunisia, 21–23 March 2016. [CrossRef]
93. Chahal, E.S.; Haritosh, A.; Gupta, A.; Gupta, K.; Sinha, A. Deep Learning Model for Brain Tumor Segmentation & Analysis. In Proceedings of the 2019 3rd International Conference on Recent Developments in Control, Automation & Power Engineering (RDCAPE), Noida, India, 10–11 October 2019. [CrossRef]
94. Ding, Y.; Li, C.; Yang, Q.; Qin, Z.; Qin, Z. How to Improve the Deep Residual Network to Segment Multi-Modal Brain Tumor Images. *IEEE Access* **2019**, *7*, 152821–152831. [CrossRef]
95. Mallick, P.K.; Ryu, S.H.; Satapathy, S.K.; Mishra, S.; Nguyen, G.N.; Tiwari, P. Brain MRI Image Classification for Cancer Detection Using Deep Wavelet Autoencoder-Based Deep Neural Network. *IEEE Access* **2019**, *7*, 46278–46287. [CrossRef]
96. Ramirez, I.; Martin, A.; Schiavi, E. Optimization of a variational model using deep learning: An application to brain tumor segmentation. In Proceedings of the 2018 IEEE 15th International Symposium on Biomedical Imaging (ISBI 2018), Washington, DC, USA, 4–7 April 2018. [CrossRef]
97. Sajid, S.; Hussain, S.; Sarwar, A. Brain Tumor Detection and Segmentation in MR Images Using Deep Learning. *Arab. J. Sci. Eng.* **2019**, *44*, 9249–9261. [CrossRef]
98. Wang, Y.; Li, C.; Zhu, T.; Yu, C. A Deep Learning Algorithm for Fully Automatic Brain Tumor Segmentation. In Proceedings of the 2019 International Joint Conference on Neural Networks (IJCNN), Budapest, Hungary, 14–19 July 2019. [CrossRef]
99. Zhao, X.; Wu, Y.; Song, G.; Li, Z.; Zhang, Y.; Fan, Y. A deep learning model integrating FCNNs and CRFs for brain tumor segmentation. *Med. Image Anal.* **2018**, *43*, 98–111. [CrossRef] [PubMed]
100. Kuzina, A.; Egorov, E.; Burnaev, E. Bayesian Generative Models for Knowledge Transfer in MRI Semantic Segmentation Problems. *Front. Neurosci.* **2019**, *13*. [CrossRef] [PubMed]
101. Zeineldin, R.A.; Karar, M.E.; Coburger, J.; Wirtz, C.R.; Burgert, O. DeepSeg: Deep neural network framework for automatic brain tumor segmentation using magnetic resonance FLAIR images. *Int. J. Comput. Assist. Radiol. Surg.* **2020**, *15*, 909–920. [CrossRef]
102. Fabelo, H.; Halicek, M.; Ortega, S.; Shahedi, M.; Szolna, A.; Piñeiro, J.; Sosa, C.; O'Shanahan, A.; Bisshopp, S.; Espino, C.; et al. Deep Learning-Based Framework for In Vivo Identification of Glioblastoma Tumor using Hyperspectral Images of Human Brain. *Sensors* **2019**, *19*, 920. [CrossRef]
103. Shree, N.V.; Kumar, T.N.R. Identification and classification of brain tumor MRI images with feature extraction using DWT and probabilistic neural network. *Brain Inform.* **2018**, *5*, 23–30. [CrossRef]
104. Tandel, G.S.; Biswas, M.; Kakde, O.G.; Tiwari, A.; Suri, H.S.; Turk, M.; Laird, J.; Asare, C.; Ankrah, A.A.; Khanna, N.N.; et al. A Review on a Deep Learning Perspective in Brain Cancer Classification. *Cancers* **2019**, *11*, 111. [CrossRef] [PubMed]
105. Alqudah, A.M. Brain Tumor Classification Using Deep Learning Technique—A Comparison between Cropped, Uncropped, and Segmented Lesion Images with Different Sizes. *Int. J. Adv. Trends Comput. Sci. Eng.* **2019**, *8*, 3684–3691. [CrossRef]
106. Ucuzal, H.; Yasar, S.; Colak, C. Classification of brain tumor types by deep learning with convolutional neural network on magnetic resonance images using a developed web-based interface. In Proceedings of the 2019 3rd International Symposium on Multidisciplinary Studies and Innovative Technologies (ISMSIT), Ankara Turkey, 11–13 October 2019. [CrossRef]
107. Bazin, P. Example MP2RAGEME Data Set. 2019. Available online: https://uvaauas.figshare.com/articles/Example_MP2RAGEME_data_set/7938326 (accessed on 15 August 2020). [CrossRef]
108. Tetik, B.; Ucuzal, H.; Yasar, S.; Colak, C. Brain Tumor Classification Software[Web-Based Software]. Available online: http://biostatapps.inonu.edu.tr/BTSY (accessed on 17 August 2020)
109. Selvy, P.T.; Dharani, V.P.; Indhuja, A. Brain Tumour Detection Using Deep Learning Techniques. *Int. J. Sci. Res. Comput. Sci. Eng. Inf. Technol.* **2019**, 169–175. [CrossRef]
110. Sultan, H.H.; Salem, N.M.; Al-Atabany, W. Multi-Classification of Brain Tumor Images Using Deep Neural Network. *IEEE Access* **2019**, *7*, 69215–69225. [CrossRef]

111. Badža, M.M.; Barjaktarović, M.Č. Classification of Brain Tumors from MRI Images Using a Convolutional Neural Network. *Appl. Sci.* **2020**, *10*, 1999. [CrossRef]
112. WHO. Global Cancer Observatory (GCO). 2018. Available online: https://gco.iarc.fr/ (accessed on 1 July 2020).
113. Graham, S.; Chen, H.; Gamper, J.; Dou, Q.; Heng, P.A.; Snead, D.; Tsang, Y.W.; Rajpoot, N. MILD-Net: Minimal Information Loss Dilated Network for Gland Instance Segmentation in Colon Histology Images. *Med. Image Anal.* **2018**. [CrossRef]
114. Benson, V.S.; Patnick, J.; Davies, A.K.; Nadel, M.R.; Smith, R.A.; Atkin, W.S. Colorectal cancer screening: A comparison of 35 initiatives in 17 countries. *Int. J. Cancer* **2007**, *122*, 1357–1367. [CrossRef] [PubMed]
115. Rony, J.; Belharbi, S.; Dolz, J.; Ayed, I.B.; McCaffrey, L.; Granger, E. Deep weakly-supervised learning methods for classification and localization in histology images: A survey. *arXiv* **2019**, arXiv:1909.03354v3.
116. Vázquez, D.; Bernal, J.; Sánchez, F.J.; Fernández-Esparrach, G.; López, A.M.; Romero, A.; Drozdzal, M.; Courville, A. A Benchmark for Endoluminal Scene Segmentation of Colonoscopy Images. *J. Healthc. Eng.* **2017**, *2017*, 1–9. [CrossRef] [PubMed]
117. Bernal, J.; Sánchez, J.; Vilariño, F. Towards automatic polyp detection with a polyp appearance model. *Pattern Recognit.* **2012**, *45*, 3166–3182. [CrossRef]
118. Bernal, J.; Sánchez, F.J.; Fernández-Esparrach, G.; Gil, D.; Rodríguez, C.; Vilariño, F. WM-DOVA maps for accurate polyp highlighting in colonoscopy: Validation vs. saliency maps from physicians. *Comput. Med. Imaging Graph.* **2015**, *43*, 99–111. [CrossRef]
119. Kather, J.N.; Weis, C.A.; Bianconi, F.; Melchers, S.M.; Schad, L.R.; Gaiser, T.; Marx, A.; Zöllner, F.G. Multi-class texture analysis in colorectal cancer histology. *Sci. Rep.* **2016**, *6*. [CrossRef]
120. Kainz, P.; Pfeiffer, M.; Urschler, M. Segmentation and classification of colon glands with deep convolutional neural networks and total variation regularization. *PeerJ* **2017**, *5*, e3874. [CrossRef]
121. Sirinukunwattana, K.; Ahmed Raza, S.E.; Tsang, Y.W.; Snead, D.R.J.; Cree, I.A.; Rajpoot, N.M. Locality Sensitive Deep Learning for Detection and Classification of Nuclei in Routine Colon Cancer Histology Images. *IEEE Trans. Med. Imaging* **2016**, *35*, 1196–1206. [CrossRef]
122. Chamanzar, A.; Nie, Y. Weakly Supervised Multi-Task Learning for Cell Detection and Segmentation. In Proceedings of the 2020 IEEE 17th International Symposium on Biomedical Imaging (ISBI), Iowa City, IA, USA, 4 April 2020. [CrossRef]
123. Sari, C.T.; Gunduz-Demir, C. Unsupervised Feature Extraction via Deep Learning for Histopathological Classification of Colon Tissue Images. *IEEE Trans. Med. Imaging* **2019**, *38*, 1139–1149. [CrossRef] [PubMed]
124. Ozdemir, E.; Gunduz-Demir, C. A Hybrid Classification Model for Digital Pathology Using Structural and Statistical Pattern Recognition. *IEEE Trans. Med. Imaging* **2013**, *32*, 474–483. [CrossRef]
125. Shapcott, M.; Hewitt, K.J.; Rajpoot, N. Deep Learning With Sampling in Colon Cancer Histology. *Front. Bioeng. Biotechnol.* **2019**, *7*, 52. [CrossRef]
126. Tang, J.; Li, J.; Xu, X. Segnet-based gland segmentation from colon cancer histology images. In Proceedings of the 2018 33rd Youth Academic Annual Conference of Chinese Association of Automation (YAC), Nanjing, China, 18 May 2018. [CrossRef]
127. Vuong, T.L.T.; Lee, D.; Kwak, J.T.; Kim, K. Multi-task Deep Learning for Colon Cancer Grading. In Proceedings of the 2020 International Conference on Electronics, Information, and Communication (ICEIC), Fukuoka, Kapan, 5–7 September 2020. [CrossRef]
128. Sabol, P.; Sinčák, P.; Hartono, P.; Kočan, P.; Benetinová, Z.; Blichárová, A.; Verbóová, Ľ.; Štammová, E.; Sabolová-Fabianová, A.; Jašková, A. Explainable classifier for improving the accountability in decision-making for colorectal cancer diagnosis from histopathological images. *J. Biomed. Inform.* **2020**, *109*, 103523. [CrossRef]
129. Suzuki, K.; Yoshida, H.; Näppi, J.; Dachman, A.H. Massive-training artificial neural network (MTANN) for reduction of false positives in computer-aided detection of polyps: Suppression of rectal tubes. *Med. Phys.* **2006**, *33*, 3814–3824. [CrossRef] [PubMed]
130. Bardhi, O.; Sierra-Sosa, D.; Garcia-Zapirain, B.; Elmaghraby, A. Automatic colon polyp detection using Convolutional encoder-decoder model. In Proceedings of the 2017 IEEE International Symposium on Signal Processing and Information Technology (ISSPIT), Bilbao, Spain, 18–20 December 2017. [CrossRef]

131. Bour, A.; Castillo-Olea, C.; Garcia-Zapirain, B.; Zahia, S. Automatic colon polyp classification using Convolutional Neural Network: A Case Study at Basque Country. In Proceedings of the 2019 IEEE International Symposium on Signal Processing and Information Technology (ISSPIT), Ajman, UAE, 10–12 December 2019. [CrossRef]
132. Liu, X.; Li, Y.; Yao, J.; Chen, B.; Song, J.; Yang, X. Classification of Polyps and Adenomas Using Deep Learning Model in Screening Colonoscopy. In Proceedings of the 2019 8th International Symposium on Next Generation Electronics (ISNE), Zhengzhou, China, 9–10 October 2019. [CrossRef]
133. Ozawa, T.; Ishihara, S.; Fujishiro, M.; Kumagai, Y.; Shichijo, S.; Tada, T. Automated endoscopic detection and classification of colorectal polyps using convolutional neural networks. *Ther. Adv. Gastroenterol.* **2020**, *13*, 1756284820910659. [CrossRef]
134. Nadimi, E.S.; Buijs, M.M.; Herp, J.; Kroijer, R.; Kobaek-Larsen, M.; Nielsen, E.; Pedersen, C.D.; Blanes-Vidal, V.; Baatrup, G. Application of deep learning for autonomous detection and localization of colorectal polyps in wireless colon capsule endoscopy. *Comput. Electr. Eng.* **2020**, *81*, 106531. [CrossRef]
135. Zeiler, M.D.; Fergus, R. Visualizing and Understanding Convolutional Networks. In *Computer Vision—ECCV 2014*; Springer International Publishing: Berlin/Heidelberg, Germany, 2014; pp. 818–833. [CrossRef]
136. Lung Cancer Screening (PDQ®): Patient Version. 2020. Available online: https://www.cancer.gov/types/lung/hp/lung-screening-pdq (accessed on 11 October 2020).
137. Hong, Z.Q.; Yang, J.Y. Optimal discriminant plane for a small number of samples and design method of classifier on the plane. *Pattern Recognit.* **1991**, *24*, 317–324. [CrossRef]
138. Armato, S.G., III; Hadjiiski, L.; Tourassi, G.D.; Drukker, K.; Giger, M.L.; Li, F.; Redmond, G.; Farahani, K.; Kirby, J.S.; Clarke, L.P. SPIE-AAPM-NCI Lung Nodule Classification Challenge Dataset. *Cancer Imaging Arch.* **2015**. [CrossRef]
139. Mader, S. Lung Nodule Malignancy. Data available at Kaggle. 2017. Available online: https://www.kaggle.com/kmader/lungnodemalignancy (accessed on 14 August 2020).
140. Suzuki, K.; Armato, S.G.; Li, F.; Sone, S.; Doi, K. Massive training artificial neural network (MTANN) for reduction of false positives in computerized detection of lung nodules in low-dose computed tomography. *Med. Phys.* **2003**, *30*, 1602–1617. [CrossRef]
141. Suzuki, K.; Li, F.; Sone, S.; Doi, K. Computer-aided diagnostic scheme for distinction between benign and malignant nodules in thoracic low-dose CT by use of massive training artificial neural network. *IEEE Trans. Med. Imaging* **2005**, *24*, 1138–1150. [CrossRef]
142. Tajbakhsh, N.; Suzuki, K. Comparing two classes of end-to-end machine-learning models in lung nodule detection and classification: MTANNs vs. CNNs. *Pattern Recognit.* **2017**, *63*, 476–486. [CrossRef]
143. Gu, Y.; Lu, X.; Yang, L.; Zhang, B.; Yu, D.; Zhao, Y.; Gao, L.; Wu, L.; Zhou, T. Automatic lung nodule detection using a 3D deep convolutional neural network combined with a multi-scale prediction strategy in chest CTs. *Comput. Biol. Med.* **2018**, *103*, 220–231. [CrossRef]
144. Sahu, P.; Yu, D.; Dasari, M.; Hou, F.; Qin, H. A Lightweight Multi-Section CNN for Lung Nodule Classification and Malignancy Estimation. *IEEE J. Biomed. Health Inform.* **2019**, *23*, 960–968. [CrossRef] [PubMed]
145. Ozdemir, O.; Russell, R.L.; Berlin, A.A. A 3D Probabilistic Deep Learning System for Detection and Diagnosis of Lung Cancer Using Low-Dose CT Scans. *IEEE Trans. Med. Imaging* **2020**, *39*, 1419–1429. [CrossRef] [PubMed]
146. Hamilton, B.A. Data Science Bowl 2017. Data Available at Kaggle. 2017. Available online: https://www.kaggle.com/c/data-science-bowl-2017 (accessed on 1 August 2020).
147. Bansal, G.; Chamola, V.; Narang, P.; Kumar, S.; Raman, S. Deep3DSCan: Deep residual network and morphological descriptor based framework for lung cancer classification and 3D segmentation. *IET Image Process.* **2020**, *14*, 1240–1247. [CrossRef]
148. Adegun, A.A.; Viriri, S. Deep Learning-Based System for Automatic Melanoma Detection. *IEEE Access* **2020**, *8*, 7160–7172. [CrossRef]
149. Azer, S.A. Challenges Facing the Detection of Colonic Polyps: What Can Deep Learning Do? *Medicina* **2019**, *55*, 473. [CrossRef]
150. Hamm, C.A.; Wang, C.J.; Savic, L.J.; Ferrante, M.; Schobert, I.; Schlachter, T.; Lin, M.; Duncan, J.S.; Weinreb, J.C.; Chapiro, J.; et al. Deep learning for liver tumor diagnosis part I: Development of a convolutional neural network classifier for multi-phasic MRI. *Eur. Radiol.* **2019**, *29*, 3338–3347. [CrossRef]

151. Yamakawa, M.; Shiina, T.; Nishida, N.; Kudo, M. Computer aided diagnosis system developed for ultrasound diagnosis of liver lesions using deep learning. In Proceedings of the 2019 IEEE International Ultrasonics Symposium (IUS), Glasgow, UK, 6–9 October 2019; pp. 2330–2333.
152. Kim, G.H.; Liang, P.S.; Bang, S.J.; Hwang, J.H. Screening and surveillance for gastric cancer in the United States: Is it needed? *Gastrointest. Endosc.* **2016**, *84*, 18–28. [CrossRef]
153. Lee, J.H.; Kim, Y.J.; Kim, Y.W.; Park, S.; Choi, Y.I.; Kim, Y.J.; Park, D.K.; Kim, K.G.; Chung, J.W. Spotting malignancies from gastric endoscopic images using deep learning. *Surg. Endosc.* **2019**, *33*, 3790–3797. [CrossRef]
154. Cho, B.J.; Bang, C.S.; Park, S.W.; Yang, Y.J.; Seo, S.I.; Lim, H.; Shin, W.G.; Hong, J.T.; Yoo, Y.T.; Hong, S.H.; et al. Automated classification of gastric neoplasms in endoscopic images using a convolutional neural network. *Endoscopy* **2019**, *51*, 1121–1129. [CrossRef] [PubMed]

Publisher's Note: MDPI stays neutral with regard to jurisdictional claims in published maps and institutional affiliations.

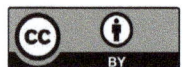

© 2020 by the authors. Licensee MDPI, Basel, Switzerland. This article is an open access article distributed under the terms and conditions of the Creative Commons Attribution (CC BY) license (http://creativecommons.org/licenses/by/4.0/).

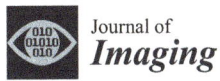

Review

Applications of Computational Methods in Biomedical Breast Cancer Imaging Diagnostics: A Review

Kehinde Aruleba [1], George Obaido [1], Blessing Ogbuokiri [1], Adewale Oluwaseun Fadaka [2,*], Ashwil Klein [2], Tayo Alex Adekiya [3] and Raphael Taiwo Aruleba [4,*]

[1] School of Computer Science and Applied Mathematics, University of the Witwatersrand, Johannesburg 2001, South Africa; arulebak@gmail.com (K.A.); rabeshi.george@gmail.com (G.O.); ogbuokiriblessing@gmail.com (B.O.)
[2] Department of Biotechnology, Faculty of Natural Sciences, University of the Western Cape, Private Bag X17, Bellville, Cape Town 7535, South Africa; aklein@uwc.ac.za
[3] Department of Pharmacy and Pharmacology, School of Therapeutic Science, Faculty of Health Sciences, University of the Witwatersrand, Johannesburg, 7 York Road, Parktown 2193, South Africa; adekiyatalex@gmail.com
[4] Department of Molecular and Cell Biology, Faculty of Science, University of Cape Town, Cape Town 7701, South Africa
* Correspondence: afadaka@uwc.ac.za (A.O.F.); arulebataiwo@yahoo.com (R.T.A.); Tel.: +27-835-569-614 (R.T.A.)

Received: 11 August 2020; Accepted: 14 September 2020; Published: 8 October 2020

Abstract: With the exponential increase in new cases coupled with an increased mortality rate, cancer has ranked as the second most prevalent cause of death in the world. Early detection is paramount for suitable diagnosis and effective treatment of different kinds of cancers, but this is limited to the accuracy and sensitivity of available diagnostic imaging methods. Breast cancer is the most widely diagnosed cancer among women across the globe with a high percentage of total cancer deaths requiring an intensive, accurate, and sensitive imaging approach. Indeed, it is treatable when detected at an early stage. Hence, the use of state of the art computational approaches has been proposed as a potential alternative approach for the design and development of novel diagnostic imaging methods for breast cancer. Thus, this review provides a concise overview of past and present conventional diagnostics approaches in breast cancer detection. Further, we gave an account of several computational models (machine learning, deep learning, and robotics), which have been developed and can serve as alternative techniques for breast cancer diagnostics imaging. This review will be helpful to academia, medical practitioners, and others for further study in this area to improve the biomedical breast cancer imaging diagnosis.

Keywords: cancer; breast cancer; diagnostics; imaging; computation; artificial intelligence

1. Introduction

Cancer is a non-communicable disease characterized by abnormal cell proliferation or cell division, with the ability to spread to other parts of the body [1]. Cancer continues to be a major public health problem and has been labeled as a global threat exacerbated by poor lifestyle choices and environmental factors [2,3]. Generally, cancer is classified according to the affected body part or tissue of origin. The most common cancer diseases include but are not limited to lung cancer, ovarian cancer, prostate cancer, head and neck cancer, breast cancer, etc. [4]. Indeed, breast cancer has been considered as one of the most common cancers diagnosed among women around the world. Breast cancer comprises 18% of the total cases of female cancer and approximately a million new cases are reported in the world every year [5]. Due to the ability of this type of cancer to metastasize to distant organs or lymph nodes, it has been considered to be the leading cause of mortality in females [5,6].

Due to the increase in the numbers of breast cancer over the years, there has been a rise in the number of computational models and algorithms for diagnosis and treatment to assist medical practitioners. A commonly, and frequently, used computational method is artificial intelligence (AI). Many AI related models have been developed for detecting and diagnosing diseases not only for breast cancer or mammography image analysis and classification [7] but for other diseases such as hycobacterium tuberculosis classification (MTC) [8], human immunodeficiency virus (HIV) therapy, screening, identification, and prediction [9], coronavirus disease 2019 (COVID-19) detection and diagnosis [10], etc. These AI models include machine learning, deep learning, and robotics. Rapid improvement in classification and learning algorithms is one of the main reasons these models have been widely used for these purposes with good and efficient results. Therefore, the contribution of this review is to provide a concise overview of past and present conventional diagnostics approaches in breast cancer detection and diagnosis. Further, we gave an account of several AI related computational models that have been developed and can serve as alternative models for breast cancer diagnosis. The remaining part of this paper is organized as follows: The types of biomedical imaging is presented in Section 2. The computational techniques used in breast cancer imaging diagnostics are outlined in Section 3. This section discusses the AI models used in breast cancer diagnosis. Finally, the paper is concluded in Section 4, where some points of future work are recommended.

2. Types of Biomedical Imaging

2.1. Mammography

Mammography is an excellent method used in primary breast imaging. It is used for early detection of abnormalities in the breast, especially those suspicious for breast cancer before it becomes apparent clinically, by using low-dose X-ray imaging to generate the images of the breast [11,12]. According to the United States of America preventive services task force (USPSTF), this type of breast imaging has been helpful in the earlier and better treatment for women over 40 years of age and has decreased breast cancer mortality by at least 30% [13]. Although this imaging approach remains the key for early breast cancer detection and screening, the overall accuracy of the test remains low and second-line accurate imaging techniques are required in some instances to lessen the number of unnecessary excisional biopsies [14,15].

Screening mammography is credited with the examination of an asymptomatic woman and decreases the risk of breast cancer-related death [16,17]. Conventional mammography has limitations in specificity and sensitivity, especially in dense breasts. The sensitivity of this type of imaging in breast cancer diagnostics is about 50 to 85%, depending on the density of the breast. Meanwhile, the sensitivity is below 50% in the dense breast due to tissue superposition; this is a major reason for the false-positive result, which leads to additional imagining and cost and false-negative results due to masking of true lesions [18–20].

In the breast, the normal internal mammary lymph node chain is usually below 5 mm in diameter. Metastases to this chain cannot be easily detected by mammography or ultrasonography clinical examination because they are normally covered by cartilaginous and bony structures of the chest wall [21,22]. The use of mammography in the detection of recurrent breast cancer is a challenging task due to changes in the architecture of the breast, mainly in fibrosis and scarring secondary to radiotherapy and surgery, resulting in difficulties to interpret mammograms. Breast compression is another major challenge faced by this modality due to accompanied pain which could lead to delayed diagnosis. Hence, considering all of the aforementioned mammography limitations, there is a call for alternative and more accurate methods that can resolve the imaging of dense breasts [19,20].

2.2. Tomosynthesis

Due to the limitations of mammography, breast tomosynthesis was introduced to the clinic because of its ability to produce three-dimensional information at a lower dose and its relative cost-effectiveness. Consequently, there has been an upsurge in interest in tomosynthesis. The Food and Drug Administration (FDA) has approved some products that are now in use and on the market [23]. This technique involves using X-ray projection images acquired over an arc to generate image slices for a partially 3D image [24]. Tomosynthesis allows for the generation of an arbitrary number of in-focus planes retrospectively from a series of radiograph projections obtained in a single motion of the X-ray tube [25]. Notably, a combination of tomosynthesis and digital mammography increases the brightness of invasive cancers while at the same time decreasing the likelihood of false-positive data [24]. Tomosynthesis has been applied to several clinical tasks, including dental imaging, angiography, breast imaging, bone imaging, and chest imaging [23]. In breast cancer, tomosynthesis increases the sensitivity of mammography, which could enhance the early detection of breast cancer due to the improved lesion margin conspicuity [25]. This is very beneficial to breast cancer patients, especially those with radiographically dense breasts. However, Poplack et al. [26] showed that breast tomosynthesis has a comparable or superior image when compared with diagnostic film-screen mammography in 89% of recruited subjects. More recently, this was supported by another study where one-view stand-alone digital breast tomosynthesis (DBT) detected more breast cancer than digital mammogram (DM) [27]. This suggests that the use of one-view DBT alone could be feasible in breast cancer screening. Although the acquisition procedures of tomosynthesis mimic standard mammography, the X-ray tube of tomosynthesis takes several low-dose exposures as it travels within a limited arc of motion unlike conventional mammography [26]. Sechopoulos [28] has written an excellent review of all aspects of tomosynthesis, including doses and reconstruction processes. When the overall dose used for visualization is constant, the quality of the image improves with a wider angular range [29]. However, the quality of image degenerates once the maximum is attained at a particular number of projections.

2.3. Ultrasound Imaging

Ultrasound (US) imaging diagnostics, otherwise known as sonography or ultrasound scanning, is a painless and safe approach. US makes use of 1 to 10 MHz sound waves to produce pictures that reveal the movement and structure of the breast, and other soft tissue [30,31]. It can also reveal the movements of blood and other materials within the blood vessels and body [31]. It is a cross-sectional technique that uses a small probe, known as a transducer, and gel that is directly placed on the breast/skin; it displays the tissues without overlap [31–33]. The high-frequency soundwaves travel from the probe via the gel into the body, and the probe receives the sounds that bounce back, which in turn produces an image on a computer. This type of imaging technique does not make use of radiation because it captures images in real-time [31–33].

In recent times, the development of high-resolution US technique has greatly improved the diagnosis of breast cancer because, in the past, US was thought to only be suitable for the diagnosis of cysts [34,35]. It has been shown to enhance the differential diagnosis of both benign and malignant lesions during guided interventional and local preoperative staging diagnosis. Due to the higher sensitivity of this type of imaging technique, it has been adopted as a complementary technique to mammography with limited sensitivity to identify early, node-negative cancer in dense breasts [36,37].

However, the use of US imaging techniques is diminishing due to the time and skill required to detect small tumors with hand-held imaging, and non-palpable cancers. The implementation of this imaging technique in breast cancer diagnostics has been hampered by limited numbers of qualified personnel and lack of uniformity in the results; this has caused low specificity that can lead to the generation of high numbers of false-positive results [38]. This assertion is corroborated by findings of some previous studies which revealed that US can identify and detect the presence of carcinoma in dense breasts. Some other studies have shown low detection of cancerous cells in dense breasts, but have proposed the addition of this imaging method to negate mammography which seems to have limited cost-efficiency and is controversial for women with dense breasts without any other major risk factors. In addition, due to the high scattering ability of the soundwaves at bone and air interfaces, various parts of the body are invisible, which limits the effectiveness of depth imaging in most organs to about 10 cm [39,40].

2.4. Dedicated Breast Computed Tomography

Dedicated breast computed tomography (DBCT) is a recently used and fastest-growing imaging technique that allows for true isotropic and provides three-dimensional (3D) information which can be reconstructed or rebuilt into several imaging planes. Although DBCT is comparable to breast magnetic resonance imaging (MRI), the process involved can be carried out without breast compression, and is not limited by breast implants or the density of the breast [41–43]. The radiation dose in this type of imaging technique is similar to that of a conventional two-view mammogram [42]. Boone et al. [44] investigated the feasibility of low dose radiation on the image quality of DBCT. The findings from their average glandular dose for 80-kVp breast CT study, when compared to two-view mammography, revealed that the breast CT dose for thicker breasts is approximately one-third lower than that of two-view mammography. For a typical breast of 5 cm 50% glandular, it was discovered that the maximum dose of mammography in 1 mm^3 voxel is far greater (20.0 mGy) than that of breast CT with 5.4 mGy. It was further stated that the CT images for 8 cm cadaveric breasts have an average glandular dose of 6.32 mGy, which is superior to the estimated dose of 5.06 mGy for the craniocaudal view, with an average glandular dose of 10.1 mGy for standard two-view mammography of the same specimen [44]. The invention, improvement, and development of DBCT with dedicated scanners with novel technology has been documented in the literature by Sarno et al. [45]. Studies further reported the development of low radiation dose scanners with improved spatial resolution and rapid image acquisition times, which is aimed at addressing the issue of imaging dense breasts and painful breast compression [41–43].

Kuzmiak et al. [42] investigated the confidence of radiology experts in the characterization of suspicious breast lesions with a DBCT system compared with the conventional diagnostics of two-dimensional (2D) digital mammography in terms of overall lesion visibility and dose. It was discovered that DBCT is superior in the characterization of the masses and radiologists' visualizations, although it is inferior to calcifications when diagnostic mammography is used. It was further averred that the DBCT application could help eliminate the 2D mammography drawback of overlapping tissue. Their study concluded that the technical challenges in breast imaging remain, but 3D DBCT could have a promising clinical application in breast cancer diagnosis or screening, however, this needs further investigation.

In 2008, Lindfors et al. [41] carried out a comparative study between the DBCT and screen-films mammograms where it was discovered, in the study of the selected group of women, that the visualization of breast lesions with both the DBCT and screen-film mammography is approximately the same. Although, DBCT was reported to be superior in the visualization of the masses, while in the imaging of microcalcification lesions screen-film mammography shows to be better. It was further deduced in their study that women are more comfortable with DBCT screening when compared to screen-film mammography. Hence, it was assumed that DBCT is a potential technology and may be a promising clinical application in diagnostic and screening for breast cancer investigation. Additionally, it was further presumed that DBCT is more accessible and could be a replacement for breast MRI or act as a control technique for tumor ablation procedures or robotic breast biopsy, all of this calls for further studies.

Recently, Shah et al. [43] investigated the characterization of computed tomography (CT). Hounsfield units were used in clinical settings for the purpose of tissue differentiation in a reconstructed CT image in 3D acquisition trajectories on a DBCT system. It was depicted in their statistical study that the approach has a better performance in the saddle orbit, mostly when close to the chest and the nipple areas of dense breast. It was further discovered that the saddle orbit functions significantly well and provides a tighter distribution of Hounsfield unit values in the reconstructed volumes. In addition, the study demonstrated the significance of the application of 3D acquisition for breast CT trajectories and other uses through the establishment of the robustness in Hounsfield unit values in the large reconstructed volumes.

2.5. Magnetic Resonance Imaging

Since the beginning of the third millennium, magnetic resonance imaging (MRI) has developed into a paramount tool in breast cancer screening, diagnosing, staging, and follow-up [46]. This imaging tool has played a vital role in the screening of high-risk breast cancer patients. Breast MRI uses an intravenous contrast agent such as gadolinium, which allows for the visualization of lesions. The sensitivity of this tool in breast cancer has been documented to be over 90% while the specificity is still about 72%; hence, the distinction between benign and malignant lesions is still challenging [46]. Although mammography is the basic imaging tool for breast tumor identification, it has been indicated that MRI has a higher sensitivity for detection of breast cancer, and the breast density does not affect it [47]. In most cases, the sensitivity of mammography in the detection of multiple malignant foci is below 50%. It is important to note that breast MRI is not meant to replace mammography particularly in ductal carcinoma in situ, which is not detectable by MRI but rather by mammography [48]. The MRI screening in women with genetic susceptibility to breast cancer has proved to be beneficial [49,50]. In a prospective cohort study, the sensitivity of MRI in women with a high risk of breast cancer but who were asymptomatic was between 93–100%, the 10-year survival was 95.3% [50]. Similarly, the sensitivity of MRI in contralateral breast tumor detection was documented to be 91%, and specificity was 88% [51]. In women with a known BRCA1/2 mutation, MRI surveillance detected breast cancer at early stages; encouragingly, there was no distant recurrence after 8.4 years follow-up since diagnosis [52]. This tool can be used in identifying the size and degree of the tumor towards achieving better surgery procedures. Nevertheless, the use of MRI before surgery continues to be controversial with extensive variations in the outcome; however, it helps in planning conservation in patients that respond to chemotherapy where feasible [46]. Despite the high sensitivity of this imaging tool in breast cancer, the cost involved in MRI makes it difficult to be employed in the general population. Conclusively, the invention and development of new imaging techniques such as diffusion-weighted imaging offer an added advantage in breast cancer management.

2.6. Diffusion-Weighted Imaging

Since the early years of the 21st century, diffusion-weighted imaging (DWI) has been at the forefront of cancer imaging attaining widespread recognition due to its ability in the diagnosis of stroke [53,54]. DWI is a noninvasive MRI technique that relies on the principle of random molecular motion of free water in tissues (Brownian movement). With the development of stronger diffusion gradients and application in whole-body imaging, DWI has attracted attention in oncology [55]. In breast cancer, Sinha et al. [56] demonstrated that DWI is reliable in a clinical setting with an echo-planar sequence and possesses potential in breast lesion characterization as either benign or malignant using apparent diffusion coefficient (ADC) values. Generally, breast lesions classified as malignant have a high-cellular level with limited water diffusion and lower ADC values when compared to benign lesions [57]. An earlier clinical study that recruited women with breast lesions stated that ADC values and the tumor biological aggressiveness correlate; hence, ADC is a promising factor in the evaluation and analysis of the degree of the malignancy [58]. In most clinical settings, DWI is interpreted in combination with dynamic contrast-enhanced (DCE)-MRI to increase the specificity. However, more recently, lesions in the breast (31 = malignant; 13 = benign) were analyzed using quantitative diffusion-weighted sequence on 3T MRI with b-values of 500 and 1000 s/mm^2 [59]. The ADC cut-off value for benign and malignant lesions was set to 1.21×10^{-3} mm^2/s for b = 500 s/mm^2 and 1.22×10^{-3} mm^2/s for b = 1000 s/mm^2, respectively. The sensitivity of DCE-MRI was 100% with a specificity of 66.7%, when DCE-MRI was combined with b = 1000 s/mm^2, 100% specificity was attained and sensitivity of 90.6%; there was no significant difference between the ADC and prognostic factors [59]. Non-contrast (NC)-MRI can be an alternative for DCE-MRI for breast cancer diagnosis, though its inferior lesion conspicuity and lower inter-reader agreement should be considered [60]. This study and many more have documented explanatory results for DWI as a tool for diagnosing breast lesion and aids the orthodox breast MRI procedures. Several pitfalls, which include but are not limited to motion artifacts, ADC value accuracy, image quality, and signal-to-noise ratio, are associated with DWI [61,62]. These challenges are bothersome and lay emphasis on the need to incorporate computer science into breast cancer diagnosis, for example, robotics could significantly decrease time in DWI MRI and create improved breast cancer detection.

2.7. Computed Tomography

CT scan is a method that exposes the pictures of cross-sections or 2D slices of the body's organs via a connected computer [63,64]. The use of a contrast solution (iodine), injected into the body via the arm, dramatically improves and aids in the visualization of the cancerous cells in organs. In 2003, the use of CT for breast cancer imaging was proposed by Suga et al. [65], after a surgical issue in patients, to obtain interstitial lymphography that can map and present sentinel lymph nodes of the breast. The use of CT in breast cancer has some advantages, which includes patient comfort and fast scanning time. However, CT has not been widely used in breast cancers due to the risks involved in radiation exposure and poor quality of the image produced.

Due to the dynamic technique of CT, it can be used in the detection and characterization of breast tumors, investigation of neoadjuvant chemotherapy effects, and local staging of cancerous cells in the breast. In 2015, Foo et al. [66] employed this imaging scan method to evaluate the staging of cancer cells in newly diagnosed breast cancer patients that are in a locally advanced stage. It was revealed that a limited number of patients involved in this study had some pelvic significance with relation to a patient who had peritoneal cancer with widespread metastasis, and a patient with a presumed gene carrier of a concurrent primary ovarian malignancy. It was further stated that 50% of all pelvic results required additional radiological examinations.

Although the CT scan technique in breast cancer examinations may not replace the conventional mammography routine, based on improvements carried out in some studies [67,68], it can be used to overcome several limitations associated with mammography such as detection of cancers in premenopausal, dysplastic, and dense breasts. The mean glandular dose of 8.2 ± 1.2 mGy has also been documented for different types of breast shapes and sizes [69]. As documented by Park et al. [68], in prone positions, low-dose perfusion CT is possible for imaging with regards to the quantification of tumor vascularity and radiation doses. CT can be used in the detection of unsuspected very small cancers in the breast that cannot be identified or seen by physical examinations or conventional mammography. It is useful in definitive diagnostic evaluation in a situation where physical examinations and mammography are inconclusive, and it can also be helpful in recognition of precancerous and high-risk lesions. More so, CT can be used in the discrimination of tumor tissue from normal tissue in breast cancer patients without the use of a contrast medium.

2.8. Near-Infrared (NIR) Fluorescence

During human surgery, X-ray fluoroscopy and ultrasound have been used widely. However, during X-ray fluoroscopy, patients and caregivers are exposed to ionizing radiation; in an ultrasound, only a thin surgical field-of-view is seen and requires direct contact with tissue, in this case, breast. Interestingly, none of the methods can be amended by target contrast agents to guide imaging during oncologic surgery due to the number of procedures required [70,71]. Thus, near-infrared (NIR) light, with a wavelength range of about 700 to 900 nm, has offered diverse significant advantages over some widely used tools including relatively high penetration of photon in and out of living tissue (breast) due to the reduction in the rate of absorbance and scatter. Owing to lower tissue autofluorescence, NIR has a higher signal-to-background ratio [71,72]. This technique has a great potential to interrogate deep tissues (breast) for molecular-based imaging. The NIR light is visible to the human eyes when conjugated with NIR excitable fluorophore or dyes. These are chemical compounds which convert light generated from one NIR wavelength into the NIR light of diverse wavelength. It has been recommended that the mapping of sentinel lymph nodes (SLN) is a standard approach for the management of breast cancer and care staging of the axilla [71].

NIR fluorescence imaging, which uses indocyanine green (ICG), has been shown to improve the procedure of the SLN mapping by facilitating percutaneous incisions and identifying the intraoperative ability of lymphatic channels and SLNs [71,72]. The safety and accuracy of NIR fluorescence imaging applications for identifying SLNs in patients suffering from breast cancer were demonstrated by Verbeek et al. [73]. The use of the Mini-FLARE camera system and 1.6 mL of 0.5 mM ICG showed the excellent identification of the SLN in patients with breast cancer. Although, the technique which should be used as the gold standard in future analyses, was raised as a question [73]. In a similar study by Mieog et al. [74], the clinical translation of a novel NIR fluorescence imaging system and the optimal ratio of ICG to the human serum albumin (HSA) dose for mapping of SLN in breast cancer was described. It was stated that 400 and 800 µM is the optimal dose of the injection ratio of ICG:HSA and this can be chosen based on the preferences of local preparation. For instance, a dose of 500 µM was depicted to be the most convenient in the United States due to the minimal requirement in the manipulation of albumin volumes. Other studies that have employed this approach in mapping SLNs in breast cancer patients include Sevick-Muraca et al. [75] which demonstrated the prospective feasibility in the use of the minimal dose of ICG in noninvasive optical imaging of lymph nodes in the breast cancer patients undergoing SLNs mapping. In 2008, Altınoğlu et al. [76]. demonstrated the synthesis and bioresorbable use of calcium phosphate nanoparticles (CPNPs) which incorporated the molecule of the NIR emitted fluorophore and ICG. In their study, the in vivo and ex vivo studies demonstrated the potentiality of the NIR CPNPs in diagnostic imaging of early breast solid tumors. Although, the result from their ex situ imaging of deep tissue showed that the depths of NIR CPNPs in porcine muscle tissue is 3 cm. Poellinger et al. [77] employed the use of NIR fluorescence imaging with the late and early enhancement of ICG, which corresponds to extravascular and vascular phases of contrast agent enhancement to distinguish between malignant and benign breast lesions as well as to detect breast cancer. Ke et al. [78] assessed the specificity of continuous-wave NIR fluorescence imaging by an intensified charge-coupled device (CDD) camera on a novel epidermal growth factor (EGF)-Cy5.5 to detect EGF receptors in breast cancer xenografts.

2.9. Single-Photon Emission Computed Tomography

Single-photon emission computed tomography (SPECT) is a medical imaging tool based on tomographic reconstruction protocols and routinely used in a clinical decision in cancer [79], coronary artery disease, left ventricular dysfunction [80], and Parkinson disease [81]. In fact, it is the most used tool in myocardial ischemia assessment. SPECT aims at getting a perfect 3D radioactivity distribution resulting from the uptake of a radiotracer in humans. One or more photons are released in random directions when a SPECT radioisotope decays [82]. However, collimators are used to focus the angle of the emitted photons that reach the detector because conventional lenses cannot restrict high-energy photons, and only 0.02% of the decay events is measured [82]. SPECT, coupled with CT, can be used when conventional images are complex to interpret, for example, suspicion of contamination [83]. Clinically, SPECT/CT provides more value in anatomical localization of sentinel nodes. This highlights a relevant role for this tool in the surgical approach and may improve staging [84]. The sentinel lymph node biopsy is a well-known procedure used in evaluating the status of the axillary lymph node in patients with early stages of breast cancer [85]. Markedly, SPECT/CT improved visualization from 84% to 92% in patients, but it only showed sentinel nodes in 11 out of 22 breast cancer patients (50%) with non-visualization on planar imaging [84]. Similarly, Lerman et al. [86] documented that the addition of SPECT/CT to lymphoscintigraphy enhances sentinel node identification in breast cancer patients who are overweight. Notably, SPECT/CT identified hot nodes in 91% of patients and sentinel nodes in 29 of 49 patients (59%) who were negative on planar imaging (planar lymphoscintigraphy) [86]. Hence, this technique is of high relevance in overweight breast cancer patients because intraoperative techniques have failed in the identification of draining nodes. Another SPECT/CT evaluation study demonstrated a sentinel node in 91.1% of breast cancer patients, and localization was more precise on SPECT/CT fusion images than on the planar views [87]. Mann et al. [88] documented that the use of dedicated SPECT identifies regions of interest at a global lower-level threshold within dense breast tissue without any negative effects, which in turn betters patient care. Additionally, dedicated breast positron emission tomography (PET)/CT can accurately visualize uncompressed breast suspected lesions in 3D [89]. However, this scanner was unable to generate a full quantitative image. Recently, Tornai et al. [90] developed a fully 3D CT in a hybrid SPECT/CT breast imaging system that facilitated complex trajectories, which improved the quality of the image when compared with simple circular breast CT acquisitions. The SPECT-subsystem allows viewing of the chest wall for pendant breast imaging [90]. Recently, it was shown that the hybrid SPECT/CT provides precise anatomical data that enables clear assessment of patients contaminated with radionuclide during the procedure [83]. Such precise data can assist surgeons towards a better surgical plan. Non-visualization of sentinel nodes, unexpected lymphatic drainage, and complicated planar imaging interpretation are challenges faced by these imaging techniques. However, this can be amended by incorporating AI, such as deep learning and machine learning algorithms, with currently available breast cancer imaging tools. Overall, such combinations will improve breast cancer diagnosis, predict treatment outcome and ultimately, improve the patient quality of life. The dose in the dedicated SPECT-CT system using both the geometric and anthropomorphic phantoms showed that the average doses absorbed in 100% fibroglandular-equivalent was 4.5 ± 0.4 mGy, while 100% adipose-equivalent tissues was 3.8 ± 0.2 mGy. More so, the dose measured in a cadaver breast using a radiochromic film in the same study yielded an average dose of 4.3 ± 0.3 mGY and 4.2 ± 0.3 mGy along two orthogonal planes [91].

3. Computational Techniques Used in Breast Cancer Imaging Diagnostics

A correct diagnosis of mammograms containing malignant tumors is a complex task for even the most experienced medical practitioner. To circumvent this complexity, several computational models have been developed to assist medical practitioners to distinguish between benign and malignant breast tumors. The models described in this paper are based on machine learning, deep learning, and robotics which have been shown to be useful in breast cancer diagnosis. In this section, we present some studies that have applied these models.

3.1. Machine Learning Algorithms

Several machine learning algorithms have been proposed for the detection and diagnosis of breast cancer. Despite this, the development of new algorithms and models for this purpose is still an active research area, especially in the detection of abnormalities in mammograms. In the following, we review machine learning models that have been used in diagnosing this type of cancer, such as artificial neural network (ANN) and support vector machine (SVM).

3.1.1. Support Vector Machines

SVMs are supervised learning models that aim at formulating a computationally effective approach of learning to separate hyperplanes in high-dimensional feature space [92]. It has been used and proven to be an efficient learning technique for several real-world problems such as image recognition [93], bioinformatics [94], and classification problems [95], among others. SVMs are one of the earliest machine learning techniques used for cancer diagnosis. Acharya et al. [96] focused on detecting breast abnormalities or cancer automatically by using infrared imaging. The approach used texture features and SVMs to detect breast cancer based on thermography. Texture features were obtained from a run-length matrix and co-occurrence matrix from 25 cancerous and 25 normal infra-red breast images. These features were then fed to an SVM for automatic classification and detection of malignant and normal breast conditions. A comparison of SVMs based classifiers with ANNs and Bayesian classifiers for the prognosis and diagnosis of breast cancer was done in Maglogiannis et al. [97]. The implementation of the comparison was performed on the Wisconsin prognostic breast cancer and the Wisconsin diagnostic breast cancer datasets. The expected result of the implementation was to predict a class that corresponds to a likely tumor recurrence in four-time intervals. The result also shows that SVM outperforms the other classifiers. Huang et al. [98] used SVM to evaluate several pathologically proven breast tumors. The study presented a computer-aided diagnosis (CAD) system with textural features for classifying malignant and benign breast tumors on medical ultrasound systems. The aim of the CAD is to assist medical practitioners and radiologists in identifying lesions and also to differentiate malignant lesions from benign lesions on the basis of medical images. The proposed SVM technique was able to identify solid breast nodules at very high accuracy. Recently, Wang et al. [7] proposed an approach to solving the limitations of machine learning models' performance in diagnosing breast cancer. The approach was based on an SVM-based ensemble learning algorithm; this approach reduces the diagnosis variance and increases diagnosis accuracy. In doing this, 12 different SVMs were hybrid using the proposed weight area under the receiver operating characteristics curve ensemble (WAUCE) approach.

3.1.2. Artificial Neural Network

ANN is a computational-intelligent model that uses different optimization tools to learn from the data available in the past and use that prior training to identify or predict new patterns or to classify new data. Several research works have applied ANN for medical purposes [99], such as cancer treatments [100]. The Memetic Pareto ANN (MPANN) approach was proposed by Abbass [101]. The approach was based on a pareto-differential evolution algorithm. This algorithm was augmented with a local search for the prediction and diagnosis of breast cancer. Tourassi et al. [102] proposed a new approach for breast cancer diagnosis based on the constraint satisfaction neural network (CSNN) technique using mammographic and breast cancer patient history findings. The main advantage of this technique is that it has a non-hierarchical architecture and flexibility that allows it to work as a predictive tool and as an analysis or data mining tool to discover the knowledge of association rules among clinical diagnosis and historical findings. In this work, the authors used two different datasets of breast cancer, each containing 250 patient cases. The CSNN was first used to train the first 250 datasets and the other 250 datasets were used to test the predictive strength of the CSNN. The result of the analysis was done based on the kind of mammographic lesions seen in each patient. The result of this study shows that CSNN is a very efficient CAD tool for predicting and diagnosing breast cancer from mammographic and historical findings. A study by Janghel et al. [103] implemented a model using ANN to assist medical practitioners in diagnosing breast cancer. The model has four phases, namely radial basis function networks (RBFN), back propagation algorithm (BPA), competitive learning network (CLN), and learning vector quantization (LVQ). The dataset used in this study consisted of 55 malignant cases and 184 benign cases. The result of the experiment showed that the LVQ output was the best result during testing then CLN, BPA, and RBFN in order. Figure 1 presents a simple ANN diagnosis for breast cancer.

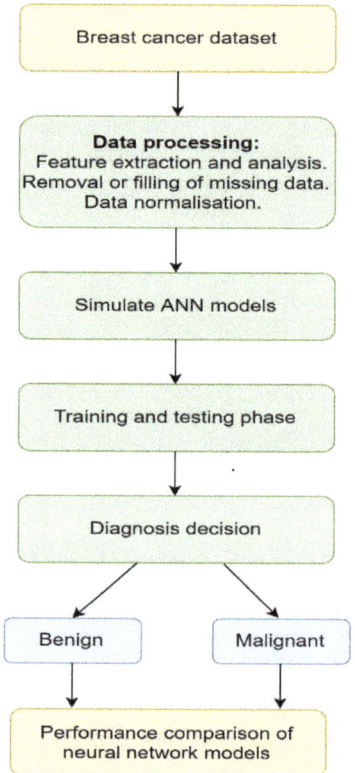

Figure 1. A simple artificial neural network (ANN) method on breast cancer [103].

Other works in the literature used data mining methods in diagnosing breast cancer [104,105]. Data mining is the process of extracting useful data from a larger set of raw data using one or more software. Çakır et al. [106] used Weka, a data mining tool to analyze 462 breast cancer patients data obtained from the Ankara Oncology Hospital. Classification algorithms are applied to each of the datasets and the outputs of the classification were compared to find the most effective treatment method. This work assists oncology doctors to suggest the best treatment method for a patient. Şahan et al. [107] proposed a hybrid system of a fuzzy-artificial immune system with the k-nearest neighbor (KNN) algorithm. This method was used to solve diagnosis problems through classifying the Wisconsin breast cancer dataset (WBCD). The system has a high classification accuracy on large datasets and can be used for any type of breast cancer diagnosis. Additionally, it can be used for other medical condition diagnoses. The Table 1 below presents an overview of machine learning (ML) techniques in breast cancer diagnosis that are explained in this section. The evaluation results presented in the table are the 50–50% training–test partition for the reference with three different training-test partitions.

Table 1. An overview of machine learning (ML) techniques in breast cancer diagnosis.

Reference	Computation Technique	Scope	Evaluation Results	Datasets
Acharya et al. [96]	Texture features + SVM	Breast cancer detection using thermal imaging	Accuracy = 88.10%, specificity = 90.48%, sensitivity = 85.71%	25 normal and 25 cancerous collected from Singapore General Hospital, Singapore
Maglogiannis et al. [97]	SVM	Diagnosis and prognosis	Accuracy = 96.91%, specificity = 97.67%, Sensitivity = 97.84%	Wisconsin prognostic breast cancer (WPBC)
Huang et al. [98]	SVM	Classifying benign and malignant	Accuracy = 94.4%, specificity = 94.4%, Sensitivity = 94.3%	250 images of benign breast tumors from 215 patients and carcinomas from 35 patients.
Wang et al. [7]	SVM	Reduce the diagnosis variance and increase the diagnostic accuracy of breast cancer	Variance = 97.89%, increase in accuracy by 33.34%	Wisconsin Breast Cancer, Wisconsin Diagnostic Breast Cancer, and the U.S. National Cancer Institute's Surveillance, Epidemiology, and End Results (SEER) program
Abbass [101]	EANN	Diagnosis	Average accuracy = 0.981 ± 0.005	Wisconsin
Bhardwaj et al. [108]	Genetically optimized neural network	Classification	Accuracy of 98.24%, 99.63% and 100% for 50–50, 60–40, 70–30 training–testing partition, respectively	WBCD
Tourassi et al. [102]	CSNN	Diagnosis	CSNN ROC area index = 0.84 ± 0.02	500 private images
Çakır et al. [106]	Weka	Treatment methods	Accuracy = 92%	462 patients data
Karabatak [109]	Weighted Naïve Bayesian	Detection	Sensitivity = 99.11%, specificity = 98.25%, accuracy = 98.54%	WBCD
Şahan et al. [107]	Fuzzy + KNN	Diagnosis	Accuracy = 99.14%	WBCD
Bagui et al. [110]	Rank nearest neighbor	Diagnosis	Accuracy = 98.1%	WBCD
Chen et al. [111]	Rough set_SVM	Distinguishing benign breast tumour from malignant one	Accuracy = 99.41%, Sensitivity = 100%, specificity = 100%	WBCD
Polat et al. [112]	Least square SVM	Classification	Accuracy = 94.87%, Sensitivity = 96.42%, specificity = 95.86%	WBCD

3.2. Deep Learning

In recent years, deep learning has set an exciting trend in the fields of machine learning and AI [113]. Deep learning techniques utilize computational models, composed of multiple processing layers that are used to learn data representations and applied to many real-world applications. These applications range from image recognition, object detection, power systems, breast cancer detection, speech recognition to drug discovery and genomics, etc. [114–117]. In the following sections, deep learning models for breast cancer diagnosis are presented.

3.2.1. Convolutional Neural Network

The convolutional neural network (CNN), often called ConvNet, is a type of deep learning model that has become dominant for many computer vision tasks, ranging from image classification, object tracking and detection to semantic segmentation [118,119]. CNN was designed to adaptively learn hierarchies of features, usually from low-level to high-level patterns [120]. Indolia et al. [121] explained that the CNN overcomes limitations as seen in traditional machine learning approaches; it has shown to be widely used for solving complex problems, especially in the medical imaging domain. Recent studies have adopted the CNN model for effective breast cancer diagnosis [122–124]. An example of CNN segmentation tasks for breast cancer diagnosis is presented in Figure 2.

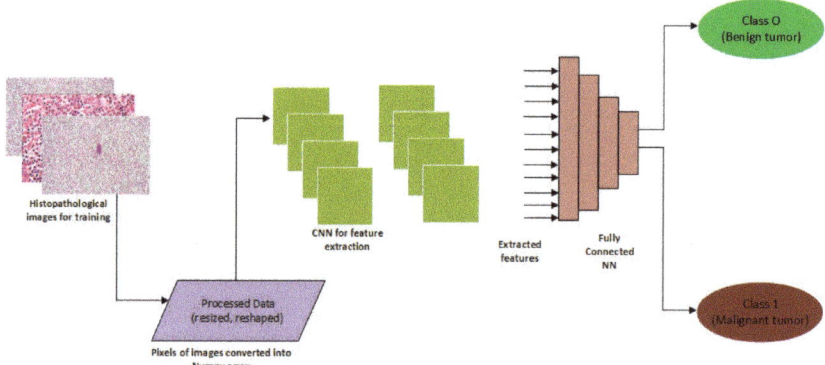

Figure 2. A convolutional neural network (CNN)-based approach for screening mammography [125].

For an improved diagnosis, Tan et al. [126] developed an imaging system called breast cancer detection using convolutional neural networks (BCDCNN) aimed at assisting medical practitioners to classify mammographic images into malignant or benign. The results showed that the BCDCNN system improved the accuracy of the classification tasks on the mini-Mammographic Image Analysis Society (mini-MIAS) database. Amit et al. [122] proposed an approach for dynamic contrast-enhanced (DCE) imaging that uses the CNN to correctly classify medical images and a pre-trained classifier to extract features in the images. The study showed that CNN outperformed the pre-trained classifier and accuracy improved significantly. In another study, Byra et al. [127] described a CAD approach that uses the Nakagami imaging method to train a CNN model, aimed at breast cancer diagnosis. The study was tested on 458 RF data matrices of breast lesions. The study showed that better area under the curve (AUC) results that amounts to 0.912 were obtained. Gao et al. [128] extended the use of CNN using the INbreast dataset to overcome the challenges faced with the contrast-enhanced digital mammography (CEDM), which is prone to a high false-positive rate. CNN was effective at differentiating benign cases from malignant lesions, which is the main challenge faced with a breast cancer diagnosis.

In a similar study, Wang et al. [129] explored a CAD method that utilizes feature fusion with CNN using a private dataset. The method uses CNN for feature extraction based on several image sub-regions. After the feature extraction tasks, the images were then classified into benign or malignant.

The study concluded that this task outperformed other existing methods. Murtaza et al. [124] applied the use of CNN on the BreakHis dataset to improve the detection of breast cancer. The study reported a high accuracy with the use of the CNN model. Other interesting areas of application of CNN to breast cancer diagnosis are found in the following references [126,130–136].

3.2.2. Generative Adversarial Networks

The advent of generative adversarial networks (GANs) by Goodfellow [137] has opened a new area of research within the image segmentation domain. According to Kazeminia et al. [138], GANs have been shown to generate realistic-looking images in the large, unlabelled corpus. One of the many challenges faced within the CV and medical image analysis (MIA) community is the heavy reliance on labelled training data, which can be a major limitation [7]. The communities have recognized the potential of GANs and have eagerly investigated in its efficacy to tackle many problems. Recently, a good deal of research has leveraged the use of GANs for image-to-image translation [139,140]. GANs have found many applications in generative modelling and distribution learning [139]. Furthermore, GANs unique generation and identification network is increasingly used for image segmentation and has achieved good results. GANs create outputs using its discriminator and generator [141]. Figure 3 shows the structure of GANs.

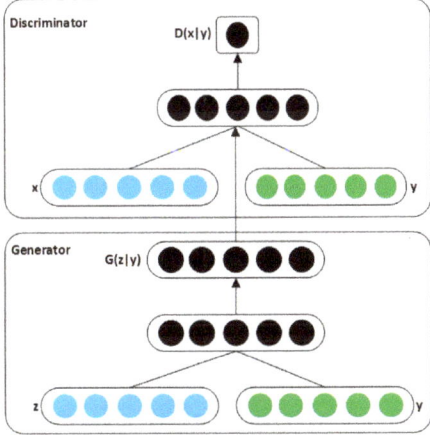

Figure 3. Structure of a generative adversarial networks (GANs) [142].

Shams et al. [143] developed DiaGRAM (deep GenerRAtive multi-task), which is based on GANs and CNN in a mammography study to detect early signs of breast cancer. The study concluded that feature learning with GANs led to high classification performance and an effective end-to-end scheme. A study by Singh et al. [144] applied GANs to segment mammographic images from regions of interests (ROIs) with varying length and sizes. GANs helped eliminate issues of overfitting on the datasets (INbreast and digital database for screening mammography (DDSM)) and showed effectiveness in the screening of cases. Wu et al. [145] addressed the issue of limited data and class imbalance for breast cancer classification using GANs. The classification performance of GANs was compared with other augmentation methods. The results showed that GANs improved the classification task. Guan et al. [146] applied GANs to generate synthetic images from a digital database for screening mammography. The authors opined that GANs performed better in augmenting the training dataset, which was useful for the study. Together, we have discussed the CNN and GANs approaches to breast cancer detection. Most of the works presented in this section are summarised in Table 2. In the table, we present the deep learning techniques, and scope of work that are used for breast cancer diagnosis. In addition, the performance metrics for each technique and the type of dataset used were presented.

Table 2. Summary of deep learning models in breast cancer diagnosis.

Reference	Deep Learning Technique	Scope	Evaluation Results	Datasets
Tan et al. [126]	CNN	Classification	Accuracy = 82%	mini-Mammographic Image Analysis Society (mini-MIAS)
Amit et al. [122]	CNN	Classification	Accuracy = 83%, Area under the curve = 0.91	ED (MRI)
Byra et al. [127]	CNN	Classification	Accuracy = 83%, Area under the curve = 0.912	ED (US, Nakagami)
Gao et al. [128]	CNN	Classification	Accuracy = 90% Area under the curve = 0.92	INbreast
Wang et al. [129]	CNN	Classification	Accuracy = 76.5%	Private
Tan et al. [126]	CNN	Classification	Accuracy = 95%, Area under the curve = 0.97	BreakHis
Litjens et al. [130]	CNN	Classification	Area under the curve = 0.99	Private
Araújo et al. [132]	CNN	Classification	Accuracy = 77.8% (four classes), Accuracy = 83.3% (two classes)	BICBH
Ragab et al. [135]	CNN with SVM	Feature extraction	Accuracy = 73%, Area under the curve = 0.94	Digital Database for Screening Mammography (DDSM), CBIS-DDSM
Acharya et al. [136]	CNN with K-means	Feature extraction	Accuracy = 97%	Private
Karthik et al. [147]	DNN	Classification	Accuracy = 98%	WBC
Yu et al. [134]	DNN + CNN	Classification	Accuracy = 81%, Area under the curve = 0.88	BCDR
Sun et al. [131]	CNN	Classification	Accuracy = 82.43%, Area under the curve = 0.8818	ED(Mg)
Hadad et al. [148]	CNN	Classification	Accuracy = 94%, Area under the curve = 0.98	ED(Mg, MRI)
Nahid et al. [123]	CNN	Classification	Accuracy = 91%	BreakHis
Shams et al. [143]	GANs	Classification	Area under the curve = 0.88, Area under the curve = 0.925	DDSM, INbreast
Singh et al. [144]	GANs + CNN	Classification	Accuracy = 72%	DDSM and Private
Wu et al. [149]	GANs	Classification	Accuracy = 89%	DDSM
Guan et al. [146]	GANs	Classification	Accuracy = 79.8%	DDSM

3.3. Robotics

With the improvements in medical robots' accuracy, robots in healthcare now assist by relieving medical practitioners from their routine tasks and also make medical procedures less costly and safer for patients [129]. These could be the reasons research into creating robots to detect and diagnose breast cancer in patients have been gaining popularity in the last decade. Robotics as a branch of AI, is developed based on some machine learning algorithms [129,150]. Such algorithms include but are not limited to reinforcement learning and deep reinforcement learning [150].

3.3.1. Reinforcement Learning

Reinforcement learning is an approach to machine learning that involves computational learning by interaction. It involves learning about what to do and how to map situations to actions to maximize a numerical solution. Unlike other machine learning approaches, reinforcement learning does not directly demonstrate how to perform a task but works through the problem on its own [129,150].

Examples of systems that are built based on the unsupervised learning approach of reinforcement learning are self-driving cars, a program playing chess (e.g., Alphago), etc. These systems interact with their environment, such that, when they complete a task successfully, they receive a reward state. Such tasks could be driving to a destination safely or winning a game. On the other hand, when the system does not complete a task successfully, they receive a penalty for performing incorrectly. Such a task could also be going off the road or being checkmated [150].

These systems, over time, make decisions to maximize their reward and minimize their penalty using dynamic programming. The advantage of this approach to AI is that it allows an AI program to learn without a programmer spelling out how a system should perform the task; this type of approach is popularly called unsupervised learning [150].

3.3.2. Robotic Tools for Breast Cancer Diagnosis

In the research reported by Kato et al. [151], a robotic system called WAPRO-4 was developed for the automatic palpation of breast cancer. The study aimed at palpating and diagnosing breast cancer without the assistance of medical personnel. The major objective was to aid the early detection of breast cancer. Additionally, WAPRO-4 consists of three parts which include the measuring instrument, the locomotion unit, and the microcomputer system [151]. The WAPRO-4 was constructed to detect tumors while ignoring breathing and the configuration of the chest wall. Kobayashi et al. [152] developed a palpation-based needle insertion method for diagnostic biopsy and treatment of breast cancer. The system locates cancerous tissues from force information and reduces tissue during needle insertion. Kobayashi et al. [152] compared the palpation-based needle insertion approach to the normal needle insertion approach using a numerical simulation of a breast tissue model. The outcome showed that palpation-based needle insertion had a smaller error which suggests that the procedure could be a safe and effective alternative [152].

Larson et al. [153] developed a robotic device to perform minimally invasive breast interventions with real-time MRI guidance for the early diagnosis and treatment of breast cancer. In this work, five computer-controlled degrees of freedom were used to perform minimally invasive interventions inside a closed MRI scanner. According to Larson et al. [153], the intervention consists of a biopsy of the suspicious lesion for diagnosis, which involves the therapies to destroy or remove malignant tissue in the breast. As a result, the procedure includes conditioning of the breast along with a prescribed orientation, the definition of an insertion vector by its height and pitch angle, and insertion into the breast. The entire device is made of materials compatible with an MRI machine, avoiding artefacts and distortion of the local magnetic field. This device was built to be remotely controlled via a graphical user interface.

Meanwhile, automated detection of breast lesions from DCE-MRI volumes was implemented based on deep reinforcement learning [154]. The method significantly reduces the inference time for lesion detection compared to an exhaustive search, while retaining state-of-the-art accuracy. The authors demonstrated their results on a dataset containing 117 DCE-MRI volumes, validating runtime and accuracy of lesion detection [154,155].

Moreover, Tsekos et al. [155] implemented a robotic device with haptic, tactile, and ultrasound capabilities, that can acquire and render the information of breast pathology remotely. In this work, the device is designed to screen for breast cancer by examination for the patient in a remote area without convenient access to medical personnel. The device was said to be more accurate than human medical personnel [155]. Further, a robotic based device designed to assist medical personnel in placing the instrument on the tumor location and automatically acquiring tumor images in real-time was implemented in [153,156]. This device has the potential to increase targeting accuracy while reducing the level of skill required to perform minimally invasive breast interventional procedures.

4. Conclusions

Breast cancer has shown to be one of the leading causes of female mortality in the world. Recent studies have shown that early diagnosis is the first step towards a successful treatment, which can help save many lives. This review presented a brief overview of past and present conventional diagnostics approaches as well as recent computational techniques that have contributed immensely to the diagnosis of breast cancer. Articles on breast cancer classification published from 2006 to 2020 were extensively reviewed. In total, 55 were carefully reviewed from different academic repositories. Several criteria were used for the review, such as conventional diagnostics approaches, the computational technique used, scope, evaluation results, and different types of datasets were used for these studies. We noticed that researchers preferred publicly available datasets over exclusive ones. For example, WBC and DDSM were seen to be popular among researchers. For computational approaches, we reviewed three areas: Machine learning, deep learning, and robotics. Out of these approaches, the deep learning techniques appear to be increasingly popular for most researchers. Among these techniques, we noticed that CNN was a popular choice, used for classification. Currently, GANs have shown to be a promising deep learning algorithm for breast cancer diagnosis due to its ability to give convincingly good results. Performance metrics such as AUC, accuracy, sensitivity, specificity, and measure were used for evaluating deep learning approaches.

Finally, this review provides a roadmap for future conversations about building better techniques for early detection, which could help save millions of lives. We believe that this comprehensive review will offer a better understanding of the breast cancer classification domain and provide valuable insights to researchers in this field.

Author Contributions: K.A., G.O., B.O., T.A.A., and R.T.A. conceived the idea; K.A., G.O., B.O., T.A.A., A.O.F., A.K., and R.T.A. designed and wrote the manuscript. All authors have read and agreed to the published version of the manuscript.

Funding: This research received no external funding

Conflicts of Interest: The authors declare no conflict of interest.

References

1. Adekiya, T.A.; Aruleba, R.T.; Khanyile, S.; Masamba, P.; Oyinloye, B.E.; Kappo, A.P. Structural analysis and epitope prediction of MHC class-1-chain related protein-a for cancer vaccine development. *Vaccines* **2018**, *6*, 1. [CrossRef]
2. Aruleba, R.T.; Adekiya, T.A.; Oyinloye, B.E.; Kappo, A.P. Structural studies of predicted ligand binding sites and molecular docking analysis of Slc2a4 as a therapeutic target for the treatment of cancer. *Int. J. Mol. Sci.* **2018**, *19*, 386. [CrossRef]
3. Oyinloye, B.E.; Adekiya, T.A.; Aruleba, R.T.; Ojo, O.A.; Ajiboye, B.O. Structure-Based Docking Studies of GLUT4 Towards Exploring Selected Phytochemicals from Solanum xanthocarpum as a Therapeutic Target for the Treatment of Cancer. *Curr. Drug Discov. Technol.* **2019**, *16*, 406–416. [CrossRef]
4. Shapiro, C.L. Cancer survivorship. *N. Engl. J. Med.* **2018**, *379*, 2438–2450. [CrossRef]
5. Akram, M.; Iqbal, M.; Daniyal, M.; Khan, A.U. Awareness and current knowledge of breast cancer. *Biol. Res.* **2017**, *50*, 33. [CrossRef]
6. Singh, S.K.; Singh, S.; Lillard, J.W., Jr.; Singh, R. Drug delivery approaches for breast cancer. *Int. J. Nanomed.* **2017**, *12*, 6205. [CrossRef]
7. Wang, H.; Zheng, B.; Yoon, S.W.; Ko, H.S. A support vector machine-based ensemble algorithm for breast cancer diagnosis. *Eur. J. Oper. Res.* **2018**, *267*, 687–699. [CrossRef]
8. Dande, P.; Samant, P. Acquaintance to artificial neural networks and use of artificial intelligence as a diagnostic tool for tuberculosis: A review. *Tuberculosis* **2018**, *108*, 1–9. [CrossRef]
9. Lengauer, T.; Sing, T. Bioinformatics-assisted anti-HIV therapy. *Nat. Rev. Genet.* **2006**, *4*, 790–797. [CrossRef]

10. Vaishya, R.; Javaid, M.; Khan, I.H.; Haleem, A. Artificial Intelligence (AI) applications for COVID-19 pandemic. *Diabet. Metab. Syndr. Clin. Res. Rev.* **2020**, *14*, 337–339. [CrossRef]
11. Nover, A.B.; Jagtap, S.; Anjum, W.; Yegingil, H.; Shih, W.Y.; Shih, W.-H.; Brooks, A.D. Modern breast cancer detection: A technological review. *Int. J. Biomed. Imaging* **2009**, *2009*, 1–14. [CrossRef] [PubMed]
12. Kolb, T.M.; Lichy, J.; Newhouse, J.H. Comparison of the performance of screening mammography, physical examination, and breast US and evaluation of factors that influence them: An analysis of 27825 patient evaluations. *Radiology* **2002**, *225*, 165–175. [CrossRef] [PubMed]
13. Nelson, H.D.; Tyne, K.; Naik, A.; Bougatsos, C.; Chan, B.K.; Humphrey, L. Screening for breast cancer: An update for the US Preventive Services Task Force. *Ann. Intern. Med.* **2009**, *151*, 727–737. [CrossRef] [PubMed]
14. Bagni, B.; Franceschetto, A.; Casolo, A.; De Santis, M.; Bagni, I.; Pansini, F.; Di Leo, C. Scintimammography with 99mTc-MIBI and magnetic resonance imaging in the evaluation of breast cancer. *Eur. J. Nucl. Med. Mol. Imaging* **2003**, *30*, 1383–1388. [CrossRef]
15. Lladó, X.; Oliver, A.; Freixenet, J.; Martí, R.; Martí, J. A textural approach for mass false positive reduction in mammography. *Comput. Med. Imaging Graph.* **2009**, *33*, 415–422. [CrossRef] [PubMed]
16. Aiken, L.S.; West, S.G.; Woodward, C.K.; Reno, R.R. Health beliefs and compliance with mammography-screening recommendations in asymptomatic women. *Health Psychol.* **1994**, *13*, 122. [CrossRef]
17. Kennedy, D.A.; Lee, T.; Seely, D. A comparative review of thermography as a breast cancer screening technique. *Integr. Cancer Ther.* **2009**, *8*, 9–16. [CrossRef]
18. Schillaci, O.; Buscombe, J.R. Breast scintigraphy today: Indications and limitations. *Eur. J. Nucl. Med. Mol. Imaging* **2004**, *31*, S35–S45. [CrossRef]
19. Cherel, P.; Hagay, C.; Benaim, B.; De Maulmont, C.; Engerand, S.; Langer, A.; Talma, V. Mammographic evaluation of dense breasts: Techniques and limits. *J. Radiol.* **2008**, *89*, 1156. [CrossRef]
20. Mori, M.; Akashi-Tanaka, S.; Suzuki, S.; Daniels, M.I.; Watanabe, C.; Hirose, M.; Nakamura, S. Diagnostic accuracy of contrast enhanced spectral mammography in comparison to conventional full-field digital mammography in a population of women with dense breasts. *Breast Cancer* **2017**, *24*, 104–110. [CrossRef]
21. Jung, J.I.; Kim, H.H.; Park, S.H.; Song, S.W.; Chung, M.H.; Kim, H.S.; Kim, K.J.; Ahn, M.I.; Seo, S.B.; Hahn, S.T. Thoracic manifestations of breast cancer and its therapy. *Radiographics* **2004**, *24*, 1269–1285. [CrossRef] [PubMed]
22. Savaridas, S.L.; Spratt, J.D.; Cox, J. Incidence and potential significance of internal mammary lymphadenopathy on computed tomography in patients with a diagnosis of primary breast cancer. *Breast Cancer Basic Clin. Res.* **2015**, *9*. [CrossRef] [PubMed]
23. Dobbins, J.T. Tomosynthesis imaging: At a translational crossroads. *Med. Phys.* **2009**, *36*, 1956–1967. [CrossRef] [PubMed]
24. Friedewald, S.M.; Rafferty, E.A.; Rose, S.L.; Durand, M.A.; Plecha, D.M.; Greenberg, J.S.; Hayes, M.K.; Copit, D.S.; Carlson, K.L.; Cink, T.M. Breast cancer screening using tomosynthesis in combination with digital mammography. *JAMA* **2014**, *311*, 2499–2507. [CrossRef] [PubMed]
25. Niklason, L.T.; Christian, B.T.; Niklason, L.E.; Kopans, D.B.; Castleberry, D.E.; Opsahl-Ong, B.; Landberg, C.E.; Slanetz, P.J.; Giardino, A.A.; Moore, R. Digital tomosynthesis in breast imaging. *Radiology* **1997**, *205*, 399–406. [CrossRef] [PubMed]
26. Poplack, S.P.; Tosteson, T.D.; Kogel, C.A.; Nagy, H.M. Digital breast tomosynthesis: Initial experience in 98 women with abnormal digital screening mammography. *Am. J. Roentgenol.* **2007**, *189*, 616–623. [CrossRef] [PubMed]
27. Lång, K.; Andersson, I.; Rosso, A.; Tingberg, A.; Timberg, P.; Zackrisson, S. Performance of one-view breast tomosynthesis as a stand-alone breast cancer screening modality: Results from the Malmö Breast Tomosynthesis Screening Trial, a population-based study. *Eur. Radiol.* **2016**, *26*, 184–190. [CrossRef]
28. Sechopoulos, I. A review of breast tomosynthesis. Part I. The image acquisition process. *Med. Phys.* **2013**, *40*, 014301. [CrossRef]
29. Van de Sompel, D.; Brady, M.; Boone, J. Task-based performance analysis of FBP, SART and ML for digital breast tomosynthesis using signal CNR and Channelised Hotelling Observers. *Med. Image Anal.* **2011**, *15*, 53–70. [CrossRef]
30. O'Brien, W.D., Jr. Ultrasound–biophysics mechanisms. *Prog. Biophys. Mol. Biol.* **2007**, *93*, 212–255.
31. Mason, T.J. Therapeutic ultrasound an overview. *Ultrason. Sonochem.* **2011**, *18*, 847–852. [CrossRef]

32. Dewall, R.J. Ultrasound elastography: Principles, techniques, and clinical applications. *Crit. Rev. Biomed. Eng.* **2013**, *41*, 1–19. [CrossRef] [PubMed]
33. Guo, R.; Lu, G.; Qin, B.; Fei, B. Ultrasound Imaging Technologies for Breast Cancer Detection and Management: A Review. *Ultrasound Med. Biol.* **2018**, *44*, 37–70. [CrossRef]
34. Thornton, G.D.; McPhail, M.J.W.; Nayagam, S.; Hewitt, M.J.; Vlavianos, P.; Monahan, K.J. Endoscopic ultrasound guided fine needle aspiration for the diagnosis of pancreatic cystic neoplasms: A meta-analysis. *Pancreatology* **2013**, *13*, 48–57. [CrossRef]
35. Liu, R.; Adler, D.G. Duplication cysts: Diagnosis, management, and the role of endoscopic ultrasound. *Endosc. Ultrasound* **2014**, *3*, 152–160. [CrossRef]
36. Park, M.K.; Jo, J.; Kwon, H.; Cho, J.H.; Oh, J.Y.; Noh, M.H.; Nam, K.J. Usefulness of acoustic radiation force impulse elastography in the differential diagnosis of benign and malignant solid pancreatic lesions. *Ultrasonography* **2014**, *33*, 26. [CrossRef] [PubMed]
37. Xie, X.-H.; Xu, H.-X.; Xie, X.-Y.; Lu, M.-D.; Kuang, M.; Xu, Z.-F.; Liu, G.-J.; Wang, Z.; Liang, J.-Y.; Chen, L.-D. Differential diagnosis between benign and malignant gallbladder diseases with real-time contrast-enhanced ultrasound. *Eur. Radiol.* **2010**, *20*, 239–248. [CrossRef] [PubMed]
38. Masroor, I.; Afzal, S.; Suffian, S.N. Imaging guided breast interventions. *J. Coll. Physicians Surg. Pak.* **2016**, *26*, 521–526.
39. Giuliano, V.; Giuliano, C. Improved breast cancer detection in asymptomatic women using 3D-automated breast ultrasound in mammographically dense breasts. *Clin. Imaging* **2013**, *37*, 480–486. [CrossRef]
40. Bachawal, S.V.; Jensen, K.C.; Lutz, A.M.; Gambhir, S.S.; Tranquart, F.; Tian, L.; Willmann, J.K. Earlier detection of breast cancer with ultrasound molecular imaging in a transgenic mouse model. *Cancer Res.* **2013**, *73*, 1689–1698. [CrossRef]
41. Lindfors, K.K.; Boone, J.M.; Nelson, T.R.; Yang, K.; Kwan, A.L.; Miller, D.F. Dedicated breast CT: Initial clinical experience. *Radiology* **2008**, *246*, 725–733. [CrossRef]
42. Kuzmiak, C.M.; Cole, E.B.; Zeng, D.; Tuttle, L.A.; Steed, D.; Pisano, E.D. Dedicated three-dimensional breast computed tomography: Lesion characteristic perception by radiologists. *J. Clin. Imaging Sci.* **2016**, *6*, 14. [CrossRef]
43. Shah, J.P.; Mann, S.D.; McKinley, R.L.; Tornai, M.P. Characterization of CT Hounsfield units for 3D acquisition trajectories on a dedicated breast CT system. *J. X-ray Sci. Technol.* **2018**, *26*, 535–551. [CrossRef]
44. Boone, J.M.; Nelson, T.R.; Lindfors, K.K.; Seibert, J.A. Dedicated breast CT: Radiation dose and image quality evaluation. *Radiology* **2001**, *221*, 657–667. [CrossRef]
45. Sarno, A.; Mettivier, G.; Russo, P. Dedicated breast computed tomography: Basic aspects. *Med. Phys.* **2015**, *42*, 2786–2804. [CrossRef]
46. Radhakrishna, S.; Agarwal, S.; Parikh, P.M.; Kaur, K.; Panwar, S.; Sharma, S.; Dey, A.; Saxena, K.; Chandra, M.; Sud, S. Role of magnetic resonance imaging in breast cancer management. *South Asian J. Cancer* **2018**, *7*, 69–71. [CrossRef]
47. Sardanelli, F.; Giuseppetti, G.M.; Panizza, P.; Bazzocchi, M.; Fausto, A.; Simonetti, G.; Lattanzio, V.; Del Maschio, A. Sensitivity of MRI versus mammography for detecting foci of multifocal, multicentric breast cancer in fatty and dense breasts using the whole-breast pathologic examination as a gold standard. *Am. J. Roentgenol.* **2004**, *183*, 1149–1157. [CrossRef]
48. Lee, C.H.; Dershaw, D.D.; Kopans, D.; Evans, P.; Monsees, B.; Monticciolo, D.; Brenner, R.J.; Bassett, L.; Berg, W.; Feig, S. Breast cancer screening with imaging: Recommendations from the Society of Breast Imaging and the ACR on the use of mammography, breast MRI, breast ultrasound, and other technologies for the detection of clinically occult breast cancer. *J. Am. Coll. Radiol.* **2010**, *7*, 18–27. [CrossRef]
49. Morrow, M.; Waters, J.; Morris, E. MRI for breast cancer screening, diagnosis, and treatment. *Lancet* **2011**, *378*, 1804–1811. [CrossRef]
50. Gareth, E.D.; Nisha, K.; Yit, L.; Soujanye, G.; Emma, H.; Massat, N.J.; Maxwell, A.J.; Sarah, I.; Rosalind, E.; Leach, M.O. MRI breast screening in high-risk women: Cancer detection and survival analysis. *Breast Cancer Res. Treat.* **2014**, *145*, 663–672. [CrossRef]
51. Lehman, C.D.; Gatsonis, C.; Kuhl, C.K.; Hendrick, R.E.; Pisano, E.D.; Hanna, L.; Peacock, S.; Smazal, S.F.; Maki, D.D.; Julian, T.B. MRI evaluation of the contralateral breast in women with recently diagnosed breast cancer. *N. Engl. J. Med.* **2007**, *356*, 1295–1303. [CrossRef] [PubMed]

52. Passaperuma, K.; Warner, E.; Causer, P.; Hill, K.; Messner, S.; Wong, J.; Jong, R.; Wright, F.; Yaffe, M.; Ramsay, E. Long-term results of screening with magnetic resonance imaging in women with BRCA mutations. *Br. J. Cancer* **2012**, *107*, 24–30. [CrossRef] [PubMed]
53. Bang, O.Y.; Li, W. Applications of diffusion-weighted imaging in diagnosis, evaluation, and treatment of acute ischemic stroke. *Precis. Future Med.* **2019**, *3*, 69–76. [CrossRef]
54. Chung, J.W.; Park, S.H.; Kim, N.; Kim, W.J.; Park, J.H.; Ko, Y.; Yang, M.H.; Jang, M.S.; Han, M.K.; Jung, C. Trial of ORG 10172 in Acute Stroke Treatment (TOAST) classification and vascular territory of ischemic stroke lesions diagnosed by diffusion-weighted imaging. *J. Am. Heart Assoc.* **2014**, *3*, e001119. [CrossRef] [PubMed]
55. Malayeri, A.A.; El Khouli, R.H.; Zaheer, A.; Jacobs, M.A.; Corona-Villalobos, C.P.; Kamel, I.R.; Macura, K.J. Principles and applications of diffusion-weighted imaging in cancer detection, staging, and treatment follow-up. *Radiographics* **2011**, *31*, 1773–1791. [CrossRef] [PubMed]
56. Sinha, S.; Lucas-Quesada, F.A.; Sinha, U.; De Bruhl, N.; Bassett, L.W. In vivo diffusion-weighted MRI of the breast: Potential for lesion characterization. *J. Magn. Reson. Imaging* **2002**, *15*, 693–704. [CrossRef]
57. Menezes, G.L.; Knuttel, F.M.; Stehouwer, B.L.; Pijnappel, R.M.; van den Bosch, M.A. Magnetic resonance imaging in breast cancer: A literature review and future perspectives. *World J. Clin. Oncol.* **2014**, *5*, 61. [CrossRef]
58. Costantini, M.; Belli, P.; Rinaldi, P.; Bufi, E.; Giardina, G.; Franceschini, G.; Petrone, G.; Bonomo, L. Diffusion-weighted imaging in breast cancer: Relationship between apparent diffusion coefficient and tumour aggressiveness. *Clin. Radiol.* **2010**, *65*, 1005–1012. [CrossRef]
59. Tan, S.; Rahmat, K.; Rozalli, F.; Mohd-Shah, M.; Aziz, Y.; Yip, C.; Vijayananthan, A.; Ng, K. Differentiation between benign and malignant breast lesions using quantitative diffusion-weighted sequence on 3 T MRI. *Clin. Radiol.* **2014**, *69*, 63–71. [CrossRef]
60. Baltzer, P.A.; Bickel, H.; Spick, C.; Wengert, G.; Woitek, R.; Kapetas, P.; Clauser, P.; Helbich, T.H.; Pinker, K. Potential of noncontrast magnetic resonance imaging with diffusion-weighted imaging in characterization of breast lesions: Intraindividual comparison with dynamic contrast-enhanced magnetic resonance imaging. *Investig. Radiol.* **2018**, *53*, 229–235. [CrossRef]
61. Chilla, G.S.; Tan, C.H.; Xu, C.; Poh, C.L. Diffusion weighted magnetic resonance imaging and its recent trend—A survey. *Quant. Imaging Med. Surg.* **2015**, *5*, 407. [PubMed]
62. Baliyan, V.; Das, C.J.; Sharma, R.; Gupta, A.K. Diffusion weighted imaging: Technique and applications. *World J. Radiol.* **2016**, *8*, 785. [CrossRef] [PubMed]
63. Scarfe, W.C.; Li, Z.; Aboelmaaty, W.; Scott, S.; Farman, A. Maxillofacial cone beam computed tomography: Essence, elements and steps to interpretation. *Aust. Dent. J.* **2012**, *57*, 46–60. [CrossRef] [PubMed]
64. Sun, W.; Lal, P. Recent development on computer aided tissue engineering—A review. *Comput. Methods Programs Biomed.* **2002**, *67*, 85–103. [CrossRef]
65. Suga, K.; Yuan, Y.; Ogasawara, N.; Okada, M.; Matsunaga, N. Localization of breast sentinel lymph nodes by MR lymphography with a conventional gadolinium contrast agent: Preliminary observations in dongs and humans. *Acta Radiol.* **2003**, *44*, 35–42. [CrossRef] [PubMed]
66. Foo, S.Y.; Gray, K. Computed tomography (CT) staging in breast cancer. *Clin. Radiol.* **2015**, *70*, S13. [CrossRef]
67. Okamura, Y.; Yoshizawa, N.; Yamaguchi, M.; Kashiwakura, I. Application of dual-energy computed tomography for breast cancer diagnosis. *Int. J. Med. Phys. Clin. Eng. Radiat. Oncol.* **2016**, *5*, 288–297. [CrossRef]
68. Park, E.K.; Seo, B.K.; Kwon, M.; Cho, K.R.; Woo, O.H.; Song, S.E.; Cha, J.; Lee, H.Y. Low-dose perfusion computed tomography for breast cancer to quantify tumor vascularity: Correlation with prognostic biomarkers. *Investig. Radiol.* **2019**, *54*, 273–281. [CrossRef] [PubMed]
69. Shah, J.P.; Mann, S.D.; McKinley, R.L.; Tornai, M.P. Three dimensional dose distribution comparison of simple and complex acquisition trajectories in dedicated breast CT. *Med. Phys.* **2015**, *42*, 4497–4510. [CrossRef]
70. Hawrysz, D.J.; Sevick-Muraca, E.M. Developments toward diagnostic breast cancer imaging using near-infrared optical measurements and fluorescent contrast agents1. *Neoplasia* **2000**, *2*, 388–417. [CrossRef]
71. Troyan, S.L.; Kianzad, V.; Gibbs-Strauss, S.L.; Gioux, S.; Matsui, A.; Oketokoun, R.; Ngo, L.; Khamene, A.; Azar, F.; Frangioni, J.V. The FLARE™ intraoperative near-infrared fluorescence imaging system: A first-in-human clinical trial in breast cancer sentinel lymph node mapping. *Ann. Surg. Oncol.* **2009**, *16*, 2943–2952. [CrossRef] [PubMed]

72. Tagaya, N.; Yamazaki, R.; Nakagawa, A.; Abe, A.; Hamada, K.; Kubota, K.; Oyama, T. Intraoperative identification of sentinel lymph nodes by near-infrared fluorescence imaging in patients with breast cancer. *Am. J. Surg.* **2008**, *195*, 850–853. [CrossRef] [PubMed]
73. Verbeek, F.P.; Troyan, S.L.; Mieog, J.S.D.; Liefers, G.-J.; Moffitt, L.A.; Rosenberg, M.; Hirshfield-Bartek, J.; Gioux, S.; van de Velde, C.J.; Vahrmeijer, A.L. Near-infrared fluorescence sentinel lymph node mapping in breast cancer: A multicenter experience. *Breast Cancer Res. Treat.* **2014**, *143*, 333–342. [CrossRef] [PubMed]
74. Mieog, J.S.D.; Troyan, S.L.; Hutteman, M.; Donohoe, K.J.; Van Der Vorst, J.R.; Stockdale, A.; Liefers, G.-J.; Choi, H.S.; Gibbs-Strauss, S.L.; Putter, H. Toward optimization of imaging system and lymphatic tracer for near-infrared fluorescent sentinel lymph node mapping in breast cancer. *Ann. Surg. Oncol.* **2011**, *18*, 2483–2491. [CrossRef] [PubMed]
75. Sevick-Muraca, E.M.; Sharma, R.; Rasmussen, J.C.; Marshall, M.V.; Wendt, J.A.; Pham, H.Q.; Bonefas, E.; Houston, J.P.; Sampath, L.; Adams, K.E. Imaging of lymph flow in breast cancer patients after microdose administration of a near-infrared fluorophore: Feasibility study. *Radiology* **2008**, *246*, 734–741. [CrossRef]
76. Altınoğlu, E.I.; Russin, T.J.; Kaiser, J.M.; Barth, B.M.; Eklund, P.C.; Kester, M.; Adair, J.H. Near-infrared emitting fluorophore-doped calcium phosphate nanoparticles for in vivo imaging of human breast cancer. *ACS Nano* **2008**, *2*, 2075–2084. [CrossRef] [PubMed]
77. Poellinger, A.; Burock, S.; Grosenick, D.; Hagen, A.; Lüdemann, L.; Diekmann, F.; Engelken, F.; Macdonald, R.; Rinneberg, H.; Schlag, P.-M. Breast cancer: Early-and late-fluorescence near-infrared imaging with indocyanine green—A preliminary study. *Radiology* **2011**, *258*, 409–416. [CrossRef]
78. Ke, S.; Wen, X.; Gurfinkel, M.; Charnsangavej, C.; Wallace, S.; Sevick-Muraca, E.M.; Li, C. Near-infrared optical imaging of epidermal growth factor receptor in breast cancer xenografts. *Cancer Res.* **2003**, *63*, 7870–7875.
79. Vallabhajosula, S.; Polack, B.D.; Babich, J.W. Molecular Imaging of Prostate Cancer: Radiopharmaceuticals for Positron Emission Tomography (PET) and Single-Photon Emission Computed Tomography (SPECT). In *Precision Molecular Pathology of Prostate Cancer*; Springer: Berlin/Heidelberg, Germany, 2018; pp. 475–501.
80. Pellikka, P.A.; She, L.; Holly, T.A.; Lin, G.; Varadarajan, P.; Pai, R.G.; Bonow, R.O.; Pohost, G.M.; Panza, J.A.; Berman, D.S. Variability in ejection fraction measured by echocardiography, gated single-photon emission computed tomography, and cardiac magnetic resonance in patients with coronary artery disease and left ventricular dysfunction. *JAMA Netw. Open* **2018**, *1*, e181456. [CrossRef]
81. Noyce, A.J.; Dickson, J.; Rees, R.N.; Bestwick, J.P.; Isaias, I.U.; Politis, M.; Giovannoni, G.; Warner, T.T.; Lees, A.J.; Schrag, A. Dopamine reuptake transporter-single-photon emission computed tomography and transcranial sonography as imaging markers of prediagnostic Parkinson's disease. *Mov. Disord.* **2018**, *33*, 478–482. [CrossRef]
82. Frangioni, J.V. New technologies for human cancer imaging. *J. Clin. Oncol.* **2008**, *26*, 4012. [CrossRef] [PubMed]
83. Koizumi, M.; Koyama, M. Comparison between single photon emission computed tomography with computed tomography and planar scintigraphy in sentinel node biopsy in breast cancer patients. *Ann. Nucl. Med.* **2019**, *33*, 160–168. [CrossRef] [PubMed]
84. Van der Ploeg, I.M.; Nieweg, O.E.; Kroon, B.B.; Rutgers, E.J.; Baas-Vrancken Peeters, M.J.; Vogel, W.V.; Hoefnagel, C.A.; Olmos, R.A. The yield of SPECT/CT for anatomical lymphatic mapping in patients with breast cancer. *Eur. J. Nucl. Med. Mol. Imaging* **2009**, *36*, 903–909. [CrossRef] [PubMed]
85. Maza, S.; Valencia, R.; Geworski, L.; Zander, A.; Guski, H.; Winzer, K.J.; Munz, D.L. Peritumoural versus subareolar administration of technetium-99m nanocolloid for sentinel lymph node detection in breast cancer: Preliminary results of a prospective intra-individual comparative study. *Eur. J. Nucl. Med. Mol. Imaging* **2003**, *30*, 651–656. [CrossRef] [PubMed]
86. Lerman, H.; Lievshitz, G.; Zak, O.; Metser, U.; Schneebaum, S.; Even-Sapir, E. Improved sentinel node identification by SPECT/CT in overweight patients with breast cancer. *J. Nucl. Med.* **2007**, *48*, 201–206.
87. Pecking, A.P.; Wartski, W.; Cluzan, R.; Bellet, D.; Albérini, J. SPECT–CT fusion imaging radionuclide lymphoscintigraphy: Potential for limb lymphedema assessment and sentinel node detection in breast cancer. In *Cancer Metastasis and the Lymphovascular System: Basis for Rational Therapy*; Springer: Berlin/Heidelberg, Germany, 2007; pp. 79–84.
88. Mann, S.D.; Perez, K.L.; McCracken, E.K.; Shah, J.P.; Wong, T.Z.; Tornai, M.P. Initial in vivo quantification of Tc-99m sestamibi uptake as a function of tissue type in healthy breasts using dedicated breast SPECT-CT. *J. Oncol.* **2012**, *2012*, 1–7. [CrossRef]

89. Bowen, S.L.; Wu, Y.; Chaudhari, A.J.; Fu, L.; Packard, N.J.; Burkett, G.W.; Yang, K.; Lindfors, K.K.; Shelton, D.K.; Hagge, R. Initial characterization of a dedicated breast PET/CT scanner during human imaging. *J. Nucl. Med.* **2009**, *50*, 1401–1408. [CrossRef]
90. Tornai, M.P.; Shah, J.P.; Mann, S.D.; McKinley, R.L. Development of Fully-3D CT in a Hybrid SPECT-CT Breast Imaging System. In Proceedings of the 13th International Workshop on Breast Imaging, Malmo, Sweden, 19–22 June 2016; pp. 567–575.
91. Crotty, D.J.; Brady, S.L.; Jackson, D.V.C.; Toncheva, G.I.; Anderson, C.E.; Yoshizumi, T.T.; Tornai, M.P. Evaluation of the absorbed dose to the breast using radiochromic film in a dedicated CT mammotomography system employing a quasi-monochromatic X-ray beam. *Med. Phys.* **2011**, *38*, 3232–3245. [CrossRef]
92. Suthaharan, S. Machine learning models and algorithms for big data classification. *Integr. Ser. Inf. Syst.* **2016**, *36*, 1–12.
93. Tsai, H.-H.; Chang, Y.-C. Facial expression recognition using a combination of multiple facial features and support vector machine. *Soft Comput.* **2018**, *22*, 4389–4405. [CrossRef]
94. Manavalan, B.; Shin, T.H.; Lee, G. PVP-SVM: Sequence-based prediction of phage virion proteins using a support vector machine. *Front. Microbiol.* **2018**, *9*, 476. [CrossRef]
95. Chen, S.; Wu, X.; Zhang, R. A novel twin support vector machine for binary classification problems. *Neural Process. Lett.* **2016**, *44*, 795–811. [CrossRef]
96. Acharya, U.R.; Ng, E.Y.-K.; Tan, J.-H.; Sree, S.V. Thermography based breast cancer detection using texture features and support vector machine. *J. Med. Syst.* **2012**, *36*, 1503–1510. [CrossRef]
97. Maglogiannis, I.; Zafiropoulos, E.; Anagnostopoulos, I. An intelligent system for automated breast cancer diagnosis and prognosis using SVM based classifiers. *Appl. Intell.* **2009**, *30*, 24–36. [CrossRef]
98. Huang, Y.-L.; Wang, K.-L.; Chen, D.-R. Diagnosis of breast tumors with ultrasonic texture analysis using support vector machines. *Neural Comput. Appl.* **2006**, *15*, 164–169. [CrossRef]
99. Abu-Elanien, A.E.; Salama, M.; Ibrahim, M. Determination of transformer health condition using artificial neural networks. In Proceedings of the 19th International Symposium on Innovations in Intelligent Systems and Applications, Warsaw, Poland, 28–30 June 2011; pp. 1–5.
100. Lisboa, P.J.; Taktak, A.F. The use of artificial neural networks in decision support in cancer: A systematic review. *Neural Netw.* **2006**, *19*, 408–415. [CrossRef] [PubMed]
101. Abbass, H.A. An evolutionary artificial neural networks approach for breast cancer diagnosis. *Artif. Intell. Med.* **2002**, *25*, 265–281. [CrossRef]
102. Tourassi, G.D.; Markey, M.K.; Lo, J.Y.; Floyd, C.E., Jr. A neural network approach to breast cancer diagnosis as a constraint satisfaction problem. *Med. Phys.* **2001**, *28*, 804–811. [CrossRef] [PubMed]
103. Janghel, R.; Shukla, A.; Tiwari, R.; Kala, R. Breast cancer diagnosis using artificial neural network models. In Proceedings of the 3rd International Conference on Information Sciences and Interaction Sciences, Chengdu, China, 23–25 June 2010; pp. 89–94.
104. Delen, D.; Walker, G.; Kadam, A. Predicting breast cancer survivability: A comparison of three data mining methods. *Artif. Intell. Med.* **2005**, *34*, 113–127. [CrossRef]
105. Sarvestani, A.S.; Safavi, A.; Parandeh, N.; Salehi, M. Predicting breast cancer survivability using data mining techniques. In Proceedings of the 2nd International Conference on Software Technology and Engineering, San Juan, PR, USA, 3–5 October 2010; p. V2-227.
106. Çakır, A.; Demirel, B. A software tool for determination of breast cancer treatment methods using data mining approach. *J. Med. Syst.* **2011**, *35*, 1503–1511. [CrossRef]
107. Şahan, S.; Polat, K.; Kodaz, H.; Güneş, S. A new hybrid method based on fuzzy-artificial immune system and k-nn algorithm for breast cancer diagnosis. *Comput. Biol. Med.* **2007**, *37*, 415–423. [CrossRef] [PubMed]
108. Bhardwaj, A.; Tiwari, A. Breast cancer diagnosis using genetically optimized neural network model. *Expert Syst. Appl.* **2015**, *42*, 4611–4620. [CrossRef]
109. Karabatak, M. A new classifier for breast cancer detection based on Naïve Bayesian. *Measurement* **2015**, *72*, 32–36. [CrossRef]
110. Bagui, S.C.; Bagui, S.; Pal, K.; Pal, N.R. Breast cancer detection using rank nearest neighbor classification rules. *Pattern Recognit.* **2003**, *36*, 25–34. [CrossRef]
111. Chen, H.-L.; Yang, B.; Liu, J.; Liu, D.-Y. A support vector machine classifier with rough set-based feature selection for breast cancer diagnosis. *Expert Syst. Appl.* **2011**, *38*, 9014–9022. [CrossRef]

112. Polat, K.; Güneş, S. Breast cancer diagnosis using least square support vector machine. *Digit. Signal Process.* **2007**, *17*, 694–701. [CrossRef]
113. Le Cun, Y.; Bengio, Y.; Hinton, G. Deep learning. *Nature* **2015**, *521*, 436–444. [CrossRef]
114. Zhao, R.; Yan, R.; Chen, Z.; Mao, K.; Wang, P.; Gao, R.X. Deep learning and its applications to machine health monitoring. *Mech. Syst. Signal Process.* **2019**, *115*, 213–237. [CrossRef]
115. Zou, J.; Huss, M.; Abid, A.; Mohammadi, P.; Torkamani, A.; Telenti, A. A primer on deep learning in genomics. *Nat. Genet.* **2019**, *51*, 12–18. [CrossRef]
116. Lee, S.M.; Seo, J.B.; Yun, J.; Cho, Y.-H.; Vogel-Claussen, J.; Schiebler, M.L.; Gefter, W.B.; Van Beek, E.J.; Goo, J.M.; Lee, K.S. Deep Learning Applications in Chest Radiography and Computed Tomography. *J. Thorac. Imaging* **2019**, *34*, 75–85. [CrossRef]
117. Mishra, S.; Glaws, A.; Palanisamy, P. Predictive Analytics in Future Power Systems: A Panorama and State-Of-The-Art of Deep Learning Applications. In *Optimization, Learning, and Control for Interdependent Complex Networks*; Springer: Berlin/Heidelberg, Germany, 2020; pp. 147–182.
118. Kalchbrenner, N.; Grefenstette, E.; Blunsom, P. A convolutional neural network for modelling sentences. *arXiv* **2014**, arXiv:1404.2188.
119. Cong, I.; Choi, S.; Lukin, M.D. Quantum convolutional neural networks. *Nat. Phys.* **2019**, *15*, 1273–1278. [CrossRef]
120. Coley, C.W.; Jin, W.; Rogers, L.; Jamison, T.F.; Jaakkola, T.S.; Green, W.H.; Barzilay, R.; Jensen, K.F. A graph-convolutional neural network model for the prediction of chemical reactivity. *Chem. Sci.* **2019**, *10*, 370–377. [CrossRef] [PubMed]
121. Indolia, S.; Goswami, A.K.; Mishra, S.; Asopa, P. Conceptual understanding of convolutional neural network-a deep learning approach. *Procedia Comput. Sci.* **2018**, *132*, 679–688. [CrossRef]
122. Amit, G.; Ben-Ari, R.; Hadad, O.; Monovich, E.; Granot, N.; Hashoul, S. Classification of breast MRI lesions using small-size training sets: Comparison of deep learning approaches. In Proceedings of the Medical Imaging: Computer-Aided Diagnosis Conference, Orlando, FL, USA, 11–16 February 2017; p. 101341H.
123. Nahid, A.-A.; Mehrabi, M.A.; Kong, Y. Histopathological breast cancer image classification by deep neural network techniques guided by local clustering. *BioMed Res. Int.* **2018**. [CrossRef] [PubMed]
124. Murtaza, G.; Shuib, L.; Mujtaba, G.; Raza, G. Breast cancer multi-classification through deep neural network and hierarchical classification approach. *Multimed. Tools Appl.* **2019**. [CrossRef]
125. Dabeer, S.; Khan, M.M.; Islam, S. Cancer diagnosis in histopathological image: CNN based approach. *Inform. Med. Unlocked* **2019**, *16*, 100231. [CrossRef]
126. Tan, Y.; Sim, K.; Ting, F. Breast cancer detection using convolutional neural networks for mammogram imaging system. In Proceedings of the 27th International Conference on Robotics, Automation and Sciences (ICORAS), Melaka, Malaysia, 27–29 November 2017; pp. 1–5.
127. Byra, M.; Piotrzkowska-Wróblewska, H.; Dobruch-Sobczak, K.; Nowicki, A. Combining Nakagami imaging and convolutional neural network for breast lesion classification. In Proceedings of the 2017 IEEE International Ultrasonics Symposium (IUS), Washington, DC, USA, 6–9 September 2017; pp. 1–4.
128. Gao, F.; Wu, T.; Li, J.; Zheng, B.; Ruan, L.; Shang, D.; Patel, B. SD-CNN: A shallow-deep CNN for improved breast cancer diagnosis. *Comput. Med. Imaging Graph.* **2018**, *70*, 53–62. [CrossRef]
129. Wang, Z.; Li, M.; Wang, H.; Jiang, H.; Yao, Y.; Zhang, H.; Xin, J. Breast cancer detection using extreme learning machine based on feature fusion with CNN deep features. *IEEE Access* **2019**, *7*, 105146–105158. [CrossRef]
130. Litjens, G.; Sánchez, C.I.; Timofeeva, N.; Hermsen, M.; Nagtegaal, I.; Kovacs, I.; Hulsbergen-Van De Kaa, C.; Bult, P.; Van Ginneken, B.; Van Der Laak, J. Deep learning as a tool for increased accuracy and efficiency of histopathological diagnosis. *Sci. Rep.* **2016**, *6*, 26286. [CrossRef]
131. Sun, W.; Tseng, T.-L.B.; Zhang, J.; Qian, W. Enhancing deep convolutional neural network scheme for breast cancer diagnosis with unlabeled data. *Comput. Med. Imaging Graph.* **2017**, *57*, 4–9. [CrossRef] [PubMed]
132. Araújo, T.; Aresta, G.; Castro, E.; Rouco, J.; Aguiar, P.; Eloy, C.; Polónia, A.; Campilho, A. Classification of breast cancer histology images using convolutional neural networks. *PLoS ONE* **2017**, *12*, e0177544. [CrossRef] [PubMed]
133. Hernández-Julio, Y.F.; Prieto-Guevara, M.J.; Nieto-Bernal, W.; Meriño-Fuentes, I.; Guerrero-Avendaño, A. Framework for the development of data-driven Mamdani-type fuzzy clinical decision support systems. *Diagnostics* **2019**, *9*, 52. [CrossRef] [PubMed]

134. Yu, S.; Liu, L.; Wang, Z.; Dai, G.; Xie, Y. Transferring deep neural networks for the differentiation of mammographic breast lesions. *Sci. China Technol. Sci.* **2019**, *62*, 441–447. [CrossRef]
135. Ragab, D.A.; Sharkas, M.; Marshall, S.; Ren, J. Breast cancer detection using deep convolutional neural networks and support vector machines. *PeerJ* **2019**, *7*, e6201. [CrossRef]
136. Acharya, S.; Alsadoon, A.; Prasad, P.; Abdullah, S.; Deva, A. Deep convolutional network for breast cancer classification: Enhanced loss function (ELF). *J. Supercomput.* **2020**. [CrossRef]
137. Goodfellow, I.J. On distinguishability criteria for estimating generative models. *arXiv* **2014**, arXiv:1412.6515.
138. Kazeminia, S.; Baur, C.; Kuijper, A.; van Ginneken, B.; Navab, N.; Albarqouni, S.; Mukhopadhyay, A. GANs for medical image analysis. *Artif. Intell. Med.* **2020**. [CrossRef]
139. Odena, A.; Olah, C.; Shlens, J. Conditional image synthesis with auxiliary classifier gans. In Proceedings of the 34th International Conference on Machine Learning (ICML), Sydney, Australia, 6–11 August 2017; pp. 2642–2651.
140. Son, J.; Park, S.J.; Jung, K.-H. Retinal vessel segmentation in fundoscopic images with generative adversarial networks. *arXiv* **2017**, arXiv:1706.09318.
141. Pan, Z.; Yu, W.; Yi, X.; Khan, A.; Yuan, F.; Zheng, Y. Recent progress on generative adversarial networks (GANs): A survey. *IEEE Access* **2019**, *7*, 36322–36333. [CrossRef]
142. Mirza, M.; Osindero, S. Conditional generative adversarial nets. *arXiv* **2014**, arXiv:1411.1784.
143. Shams, S.; Platania, R.; Zhang, J.; Kim, J.; Lee, K.; Park, S.-J. Deep generative breast cancer screening and diagnosis. In Proceedings of the 21st International Conference on Medical Image Computing and Computer-Assisted Intervention, Granada, Spain, 16–20 September 2018; pp. 859–867.
144. Singh, V.K.; Romani, S.; Rashwan, H.A.; Akram, F.; Pandey, N.; Sarker, M.M.K.; Abdulwahab, S.; Torrents-Barrena, J.; Saleh, A.; Arquez, M. Conditional generative adversarial and convolutional networks for X-ray breast mass segmentation and shape classification. In Proceedings of the 21st International Conference on Medical Image Computing and Computer-Assisted Intervention, Granada, Spain, 16–20 September 2018; pp. 833–840.
145. Wu, E.; Wu, K.; Cox, D.; Lotter, W. Conditional infilling GANs for data augmentation in mammogram classification. In *Image Analysis for Moving Organ, Breast, and Thoracic Images*; Springer: Berlin/Heidelberg, Germany, 2018; pp. 98–106.
146. Guan, S.; Loew, M. Breast cancer detection using synthetic mammograms from generative adversarial networks in convolutional neural networks. *J. Med. Imaging* **2019**, *6*, 031411. [CrossRef] [PubMed]
147. Karthik, S.; Perumal, R.S.; Mouli, P.C. Breast cancer classification using deep neural networks. In *Knowledge Computing and Its Applications*; Springer: Berlin/Heidelberg, Germany, 2018; pp. 227–241.
148. Hadad, O.; Bakalo, R.; Ben-Ari, R.; Hashoul, S.; Amit, G. Classification of breast lesions using cross-modal deep learning. In Proceedings of the IEEE 14th International Symposium on Biomedical Imaging (ISBI 2017), Melbourne, Australia, 18–21 April 2017; pp. 109–112.
149. Wu, E.; Wu, K.; Lotter, W. Synthesizing lesions using contextual GANs improves breast cancer classification on mammograms. *arXiv* **2020**, arXiv:2006.00086.
150. Sutton, S.R.; Barto, G.A. Reinforcement Learning: An Introduction. In *A Bradford Book*; The MIT Press: Cambridge, MA, USA, 2015.
151. Kato, I.; Koganezawa, K.; Takanishi, A. Automatic breast cancer palpation robot: WAPRO-4. *Adv. Robot.* **1988**, *3*, 251–261. [CrossRef]
152. Kobayashi, Y.; Suzuki, M.; Kato, A.; Konishi, K.; Hashizume, M.; Fujie, M.G. A robotic palpation-based needle insertion method for diagnostic biopsy and treatment of breast cancer. In Proceedings of the IEEE/RSJ International Conference on Intelligent Robots and Systems, St Louis, MO, USA, 11–15 October 2009; pp. 5534–5539.
153. Larson, B.T.; Tsekos, N.V.; Erdman, A.G. A robotic device for minimally invasive breast interventions with real-time MRI guidance. In Proceedings of the Third IEEE Symposium on Bioinformatics and Bioengineering, Bethesda, MD, USA, 10–12 March 2003; pp. 190–197.
154. Maicas, G.; Carneiro, G.; Bradley, A.P.; Nascimento, J.C.; Reid, I. Deep reinforcement learning for active breast lesion detection from DCE-MRI. In Proceedings of the 20th International Conference on Medical Image Computing and Computer-Assisted Intervention, Quebec City, QC, Canada, 10–14 September 2017; pp. 665–673.

155. Tsekos, N.V.; Shudy, J.; Yacoub, E.; Tsekos, P.V.; Koutlas, I.G. Development of a robotic device for MRI-guided interventions in the breast. In Proceedings of the 2nd Annual IEEE International Symposium on Bioinformatics and Bioengineering (BIBE 2001), Bethesda, MD, USA, 4–6 November 2001; pp. 201–208.
156. Mallapragada, V.; Sarkar, N.; Podder, T.K. Toward a robot-assisted breast intervention system. *IEEE/ASME Trans. Mechatron.* **2010**, *16*, 1011–1020. [CrossRef]

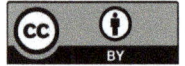

© 2020 by the authors. Licensee MDPI, Basel, Switzerland. This article is an open access article distributed under the terms and conditions of the Creative Commons Attribution (CC BY) license (http://creativecommons.org/licenses/by/4.0/).

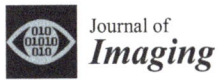

Review

Explainable Deep Learning Models in Medical Image Analysis

Amitojdeep Singh [1,2,*], Sourya Sengupta [1,2] and Vasudevan Lakshminarayanan [1,2]

1. Theoretical and Experimental Epistemology Laboratory, School of Optometry and Vision Science, University of Waterloo, Waterloo, ON N2L 3G1, Canada; sourya.sengupta@uwaterloo.ca (S.S.); vengulak@uwaterloo.ca (V.L.)
2. Department of Systems Design Engineering, University of Waterloo, Waterloo, ON N2L 3G1, Canada
* Correspondence: amitojdeep.singh@uwaterloo.ca

Received: 28 May 2020; Accepted: 17 June 2020; Published: 20 June 2020

Abstract: Deep learning methods have been very effective for a variety of medical diagnostic tasks and have even outperformed human experts on some of those. However, the black-box nature of the algorithms has restricted their clinical use. Recent explainability studies aim to show the features that influence the decision of a model the most. The majority of literature reviews of this area have focused on taxonomy, ethics, and the need for explanations. A review of the current applications of explainable deep learning for different medical imaging tasks is presented here. The various approaches, challenges for clinical deployment, and the areas requiring further research are discussed here from a practical standpoint of a deep learning researcher designing a system for the clinical end-users.

Keywords: explainability; explainable AI; XAI; deep learning; medical imaging; diagnosis

1. Introduction

Computer-aided diagnostics (CAD) using artificial intelligence (AI) provides a promising way to make the diagnosis process more efficient and available to the masses. Deep learning is the leading artificial intelligence (AI) method for a wide range of tasks including medical imaging problems. It is the state of the art for several computer vision tasks and has been used for medical imaging tasks like the classification of Alzheimer's [1], lung cancer detection [2], retinal disease detection [3,4], etc. Despite achieving remarkable results in the medical domain, AI-based methods have not achieved a significant deployment in the clinics. This is due to the underlying black-box nature of the deep learning algorithms along with other reasons like computational costs. It arises from the fact that, despite having the underlying statistical principles, there is a lack of ability to explicitly represent the knowledge for a given task performed by a deep neural network. Simpler AI methods like linear regression and decision trees are self-explanatory as the decision boundary used for classification can be visualized in a few dimensions using the model parameters. However, these lack the complexity required for tasks such as classification of 3D and most 2D medical images. The lack of tools to inspect the behavior of black-box models affects the use of deep learning in all domains including finance and autonomous driving where explainability and reliability are the key elements for trust by the end-user. A schematic explaining the relationship between deep learning and the need for explanations is shown in Figure 1.

A medical diagnosis system needs to be transparent, understandable, and explainable to gain the trust of physicians, regulators as well as the patients. Ideally, it should be able to explain the complete logic of making a certain decision to all the parties involved. Newer regulations like the European General Data Protection Regulation (GDPR) are making it harder for the use of black-box models in all businesses including healthcare because retraceability of the decisions is now a requirement [5].

An artificial intelligence (AI) system to complement medical professionals should have a certain amount of explainability and allow the human expert to retrace the decisions and use their judgment. Some researchers also emphasize that even humans are not always able to or even willing to explain their decisions [5]. Explainability is the key to safe, ethical, fair, and trust-able use of artificial intelligence (AI) and a key enabler for its deployment in the real world. Breaking myths about artificial intelligence (AI) by showing what a model looked at while making the decision can inculcate trust among the end-users. It is even more important to show the domain-specific features used in the decision for non-deep learning users like most medical professionals.

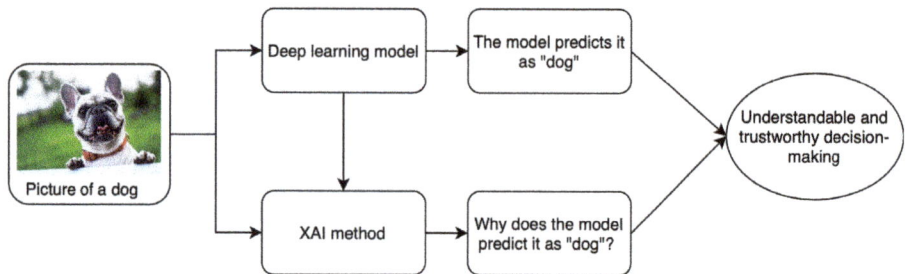

Figure 1. A brief schematic of basics of XAI methods.

The terms explainability and interpretability are often used interchangeably in the literature. A distinction between these was provided in [6] where interpretation was defined as mapping an abstract concept like the output class into a domain example, while explanation was defined as a set of domain features such as pixels of an image the contribute to the output decision of the model. A related term to this concept is the uncertainty associated with the decision of a model. Deep learning classifiers are usually not able to say "I don't know" in situations with ambiguity and instead return the class with the highest probability, even if by a narrow margin, making uncertainty a crucial topic. Lately, uncertainty has been analyzed along with the problem of explainability in many studies to highlight the cases where a model is unsure and in turn, make the models more acceptable to non-deep learning users. There have been studies about the uncertainty of machine learning algorithms which include those for endoscopic videos [7] and tissue parameter estimation [8]. We limit the scope of this paper to explainability methods and discuss uncertainty if a study used it along with explainability. The topic of uncertainty in deep learning models can be itself a subject of a future review. As noted earlier, deep learning models are considered as non-transparent as the weights of the neurons can not be understood as knowledge directly. [9] showed that neither the magnitude or the selectivity of the activations, nor the impact on network decisions is sufficient for deciding the importance of a neuron for a given task. A detailed analysis of the terminologies, concepts and, use cases of explainable artificial intelligence (AI) is provided in [10].

This paper describes the studies related to the explainability of deep learning models in the context of medical imaging. A general taxonomy of explainability approaches is described briefly in the next section and a comparison of various attribution based methods is performed in Section 3. Section 4 reviews various explainability methods applied to different medical imaging modalities. The analysis is broken down into Sections 4.1 and 4.2 depending upon the use of attributions or other methods of explainability. The evolution, current trends, and some future possibilities of the explainable deep learning models in medical image analysis are summarized in Section 5.

2. Taxonomy of Explainability Approaches

Several taxonomies have been proposed in the literature to classify different explainability methods [11,12]. Generally, the classification techniques are not absolute, it can vary widely depending upon the characteristics of the methods and can be classified into many overlapping or non-overlapping classes simultaneously. Different kinds of taxonomies and classification methods are discussed briefly here and a detailed analysis of the taxonomies can be found in [10,11] and a flow chart for them is shown in Figure 2.

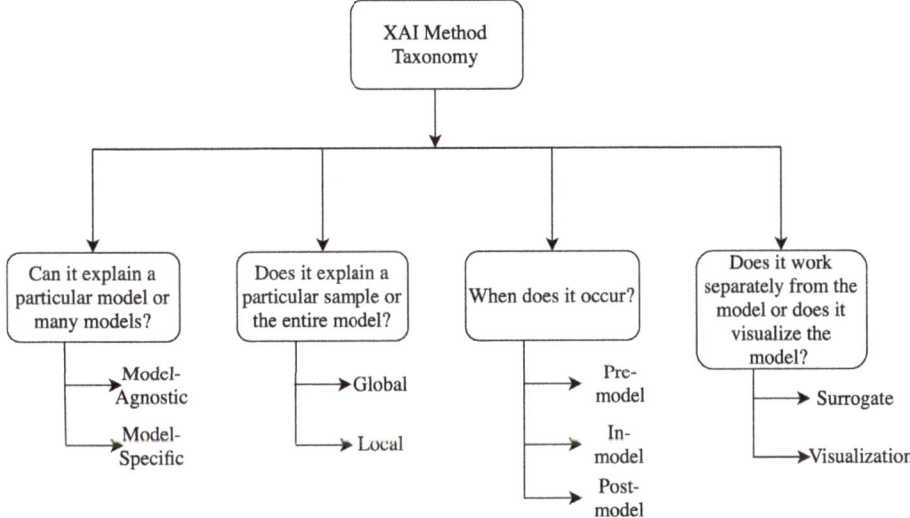

Figure 2. Taxonomy of XAI methods.

2.1. Model Specific vs. Model Agnostic

Model-specific interpretation methods are based on the parameters of the individual models. The graph neural network explainer (GNNExplainer) [13] is a special type of model-specific interpretability where the complexity of data representation needs specifically the graph neural network (GNN). Model Agnostic methods are mainly applicable in post-hoc analysis and not limited to specified model architecture. These methods do not have direct access to the internal model weights or structural parameters.

2.2. Global Methods vs. Local Methods

Local interpretable methods are applicable to a single outcome of the model. This can be done by designing methods that can explain the reason for a particular prediction or outcome. For example, it is interested in specific features and their characteristics. On the contrary, global methods concentrate on the inside of a model by exploiting the overall knowledge about the model, the training, and the associated data. It tries to explain the behavior of the model in general. Feature importance is a good example of this method, which tries to figure out the features which are in general responsible for better performance of the model among all different features.

2.3. Pre-Model vs. In-Model vs. Post-Model

Pre-model methods are independent and do not depend on a particular model architecture to use it on. Principal component analysis (PCA) [14], t-Distributed Stochastic Neighbor Embedding (t-SNE) [15] are some common examples of these methods. Interpretability methods, integrated into the model itself, are called as in-model methods. Some methods are implemented after building a model and hence these methods are termed as post model and these methods can potentially develop meaningful insights about what exactly a model learned during the training.

2.4. Surrogate Methods vs. Visualization Methods

Surrogate methods consist of different models as an ensemble which are used to analyze other black-box models. The black box models can be understood better by interpreting the surrogate model's decisions by comparing the black-box model's decision and surrogate model's decision. The decision tree [16] is an example of surrogate methods. The visualization methods are not a different model, but it helps to explain some parts of the models by visual understanding like activation maps.

It is to be noted that these classification methods are non-exclusive, these are built upon different logical intuitions and hence have significant overlaps. For example, most of the post-hoc models like attributions can also be seen as model agnostic as these methods are typically not dependent upon the structure of a model. However, some requirements regarding the limitations on model layers or the activation functions do exist for some of the attribution methods. The next section describes the basic concept and subtle difference between various attribution methods to facilitate a comparative discussion of the applications in Section 4.

3. Explainability Methods—Attribution Based

There are broadly two types of approaches to explain the results of deep neural networks (DNN) in medical imaging—those using standard attribution based methods and those using novel, often architecture, or domain-specific techniques. A majority of the papers for explaining deep learning in medical image diagnosis use attribution based methods. Their model agnostic plug and play nature along with readily available open-source implementations make them a convenient solution. The deep learning practitioners can, therefore, focus on designing a model optimal for a given task and use these easy to generate explanations for understanding the model better. Since attribution based studies are a majority (with many of them using multiple attribution based methods), we discuss them beforehand. The applications for those methods are ordered according to the anatomical districts, i.e., organ groups for the diagnosed diseases in Section 4.1. Other methods are used in only a few studies each which typically uses a single method and are hence discussed along with their applications in Section 4.2 which is ordered by the explainability method used.

The problem of assigning an attribution value or contribution or relevance to each input feature of a network led to the development of several attribution methods. The goal of an attribution method is to determine the contribution of an input feature to the target neuron which is usually the output neuron of the correct class for a classification problem. The arrangement of the attributions of all the input features in the shape of the input sample forms heatmaps known as the attribution maps. Some examples of attribution maps for different images are shown in Figure 3. The features with a positive contribution to the activation of the target neuron are typically marked in red while those negatively affecting the activation are marked in blue. These are the features or pixels in case of images providing positive and negative evidence of different magnitudes, respectively.

The commonly used attribution methods are discussed in this section and the applications in the next section. It must be noted that some of the approaches like DeepTaylor [17] provide only positive evidence and can be useful for a certain set of tasks. The attribution methods can be applied on a black box convolutional neural network (CNN) without any modification to the underlying architecture making them a convenient yet powerful XAI tool. An empirical comparison of some of the methods discussed in this section and a unified framework called DeepExplain is available in [18]. Most of the methods discussed here apart from the newer Deep Learning Important FeaTures (LIFT) and Deep SHapley Additive exPlanations (SHAP) are implemented in the iNNvestigate toolbox [19].

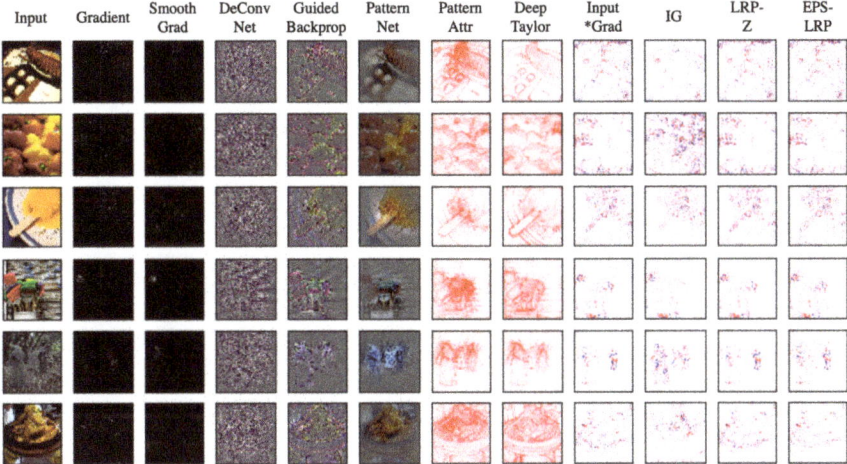

Figure 3. Attributions of VGG-16 with images from Imagenet using the methods implemented in [19].

3.1. Perturbation Based Methods—Occlusion

Perturbation is the simplest way to analyze the effect of changing the input features on the output of an AI model. This can be implemented by removing, masking, or modifying certain input features, and running the forward pass (output computation), and measuring the difference from the original output. This is similar to the sensitivity analysis performed in parametric control system models. The input features affecting the output the most are ranked as the most important. It is computationally expensive as a forward pass needs to be run after perturbing each group of features of the input. In the case of image data the perturbation is performed by covering parts of an image with a grey patch and hence occluding them from the system's view. It can provide both positive and negative evidence by highlighting the responsible features.

This technique was applied by Zeiler and Fergus [20] to the convolutional neural network (CNN) for the image classification task. Occlusion is the benchmark for any attribution study as it is a simple to perform model agnostic approach which reveals the feature importance of a model. It can reveal if a model is overfitting and learning irrelevant features as in the case of adversarial examples [21]. The adversarial examples are the inputs designed to cause the model to make a false decision and are like optical illusions for the models. In that case, the model misclassifies the image (say a cat as a dog) despite the presence of discriminating feature

Occluding all features (pixels) one-by-one and running the forward pass each time can be computationally expensive and can take several hours per image [18]. It is common to use patches of sizes such as 5×5, 10×10, or even larger depending on the size of the target features and computational resources available.

Another perturbation based approach is Shapley value sampling which computes approximate Shapely Values by taking each input feature for a sample number of times. It a method from the coalitional game theory which describes the fair distribution of the gains and losses among the input features. It was originally proposed for the analysis of regression [22]. It is slower than all other approaches as the network has to be run samples × number of features times. As a result it is not a practical method in its original form but has led to the development of game theory-based methods like Deep SHapley Additive exPlanations (SHAP) as discussed in the next subsection.

3.2. Backpropagation Based Methods

These methods compute the attribution for all the input features with a single forward and backward pass through the network. In some of the methods these steps need to be repeated multiple times but it is independent of the number of input features and much lower than for perturbation-based methods. The faster run-time comes at the expense of a weaker relationship between the outcome and the variation of the output. Various backpropagation based attribution methods are described in Table 1. It must be noted that some of these methods provide only positive evidence while others provide both positive and negative evidence. The methods providing both positive and negative evidence tend to have high-frequency noise which can make the results seem spurious. [18].

Table 1. Backpropagation based attribution methods.

Method	Description	Notes
Gradient	Computes the gradient of the output of the **target neuron** with respect to the input.	The **simplest** approach but is usually not the most effective.
DeConvNet [20]	Applies the **ReLU to the gradient computation instead of** the gradient of a neuron with ReLU activation.	Used to **visualize the features** learned by the layers. **Limited** to CNN models with **ReLU activation**.
Saliency Maps [23]	Takes the **absolute value of the partial derivative** of the target output neuron with respect to the input features to find the features which affect the output the most with least perturbation.	**Can't distinguish between positive and negative** evidence due to absolute values.
Guided backpropagation (GBP) [24]	Applies the **ReLU to the gradient computation in addition to** the gradient of a neuron with ReLU activation.	Like DeConvNet, it is textbflimited to CNN models with **ReLU activation**.
LRP [25]	**Redistributes the prediction score** layer by layer with a backward pass on the network using a particular rule like the ϵ-rule while ensuring numerical stability	There are alternative stability rules and **limited** to CNN models with **ReLU activation** when all activations are ReLU.
Gradient × input [26]	Initially proposed as a method to **improve sharpness of attribution maps** and is computed by multiplying the signed partial derivative of the output with the input.	It **can approximate occlusion** better than other methods in certain cases like multi layer perceptron (MLP) with Tanh on MNIST data [18] while being instant to compute.
GradCAM [27]	Produces **gradient-weighted class activation maps** using the gradients of the target concept as it flows to the final convolutional layer	Applicable to **only CNN** including those with fully connected layers, structured output (like captions) and reinforcement learning.
IG [28]	Computes the **average gradient** as the input is varied from the **baseline** (often zero) to the actual input value unlike the Gradient × input which uses a single derivative at the input.	It is **highly correlated with the rescale rule of** DeepLIFT discussed below which can act as a good and faster approximation.
DeepTaylor [17]	Finds a rootpoint near each neuron with a value close to the input but with output as 0 and uses it to recursively estimate the attribution of each neuron using **Taylor decomposition**	Provides **sparser explanations**, i.e., focuses on key features but provides **no negative evidence** due to its assumptions of only positive effect.
PatternNet [29]	Estimates the input signal of the output neuron using an **objective function**.	Proposed to counter the incorrect attributions of other methods on **linear systems** and generalized to deep networks.
Pattern Attribution [29]	Applies Deep Taylor decomposition by searching the **rootpoints in the signal direction** for each neuron	Proposed along with **PatternNet** and uses decomposition instead of signal visualization
DeepLIFT [30]	Uses a reference input and computes the reference values of all hidden units using a forward pass and then proceeds backward **like LRP**. It has two variants—**Rescale rule** and the one introduced later called **RevealCancel** which treats positive and negative contributions to a neuron separately.	Rescale is strongly related to and **equivalent in some cases to ϵ-LRP** but is **not applicable** to models involving **multiplicative rules**. RevealCancel handles such cases and using RevealCancel for convolutional and Rescale for fully connected layers reduces noise.
SmoothGrad [31]	An improvement on the gradient method which averages the gradient over multiple inputs with additional noise	Designed to visually sharpen the attributions produced by gradient method using class score function.
Deep SHAP [32]	It is a fast **approximation** algorithm to compute the game theory based **SHAP values**. It is connected to DeepLIFT and uses **multiple background samples** instead of one baseline.	Finds attributions for **non neural net models** like trees, support vector machines (SVM) and **ensemble** of those with a neural net using various tools in the the SHAP library.

An important property of attribution methods known as completeness was introduced in the DeepLIFT [30] paper. It states that the attributions for a given input add up to the target output minus the target output at the baseline input. It is satisfied by integrated gradients, DeepTaylor and Deep SHAP but not by DeepLIFT in its rescale rule. A measure generalizing this property is proposed in [18] for a quantitative comparison of various attribution methods. It is called sensitivity-n and involves comparing the sum of the attributions and the variation in the target output in terms of PCC. Occlusion is found to have a higher PCC than other methods as it finds a direct relationship between the variation in the input and that in the output.

The evaluation of attribution methods is complex as it is challenging to discern between the errors of the model and the attribution method explaining it. Measures like sensitivity-n reward the methods designed to reflect the network behavior closely. However, a more practically relevant measure of an attribution method is the similarity of attributions to a human observer's expectation. It needs to be performed with a human expert for a given task and carries an observer bias as the methods closer to the observer expectation can be favored at the cost of those explaining the model behavior. We underscore the argument that the ratings of different attribution methods by experts of a specific domain are potentially useful to develop explainable models which are more likely to be trusted by the end users and hence should be a critical part of the development of an XAI system.

4. Applications

The applications of explainability in medical imaging are reviewed here by categorizing them into two types—those using pre-existing attribution based methods and those using other, often specific methods. The methods are discussed according to the explainability method and the medical imaging application. Table 2 provides a brief overview of the methods.

4.1. Attribution Based

A majority of the medical imaging literature that studied interpretability of deep learning methods used attribution based methods due to their ease of use. Researchers can train a suitable neural network architecture without the added complexity of making it inherently explainable and use a readily available attribution model. This allows the use of either a pre-existing deep learning model or one with a custom architecture for the best performance on the given task. The former makes the implementation easier and allows one to leverage techniques like transfer learning [33,34] while the latter can be used to focus on specific data and avoid overfitting by using fewer parameters. Both approaches are beneficial for medical imaging datasets which tend to be relatively smaller than computer vision benchmarks like ImageNet [35].

Post-model analysis using attributions can reveal if the model is learning relevant features or if it is overfitting to the input by learning spurious features. This allows researchers to adjust the model architecture and hyperparameters to achieve better results on the test data and in turn a potential real-world setting. In this subsection, some recent studies using attribution methods across different medical imaging modalities are reviewed in the order of the anatomical districts from top to bottom of the human body. The reviewed tasks include explanations of deep learning for diagnosing conditions from brain MRI, retinal imaging, breast imaging, CT scans, chest X-ray as well as skin imaging.

4.1.1. Brain Imaging

A study comparing the robustness of various attribution based methods for convolutional neural network (CNN) in Alzheimer's classification using brain MRI [36] performed a quantitative analysis of different methods. Gradient × input, Guided backpropagation (GBP), LRP, and occlusion were the compared methods. The L2 norm between the average attribution maps of multiple runs for the same model to check the repeatability of heatmaps for identically trained models. It was found to be an order of magnitude lower for the first three methods compared to the baseline occlusion since occlusion covers a larger area. LRP performed the best overall indicating the superiority of a completely attribution based method over function and signal-based methods. The similarity between the sum, density, and gain (sum/density) for the top 10 regions of the attributions across the runs was also the highest for LRP. In another study [37] GradCAM and Guided backpropagation (GBP) were used to analyze the clinical coherence of the features learned by a CNN for automated grading of brain tumor from MRI. For the correctly graded cases, both the methods had the most activation in the tumor region while also activating the surrounding ventricles which can indicate malignancy as well. In some cases, this focus on non-tumor regions and some spurious patterns in Guided backpropagation (GBP) maps lead to errors indicating unreliability of the features.

4.1.2. Retinal Imaging

A system producing IG heatmaps along with model predictions was explored as a tool to assist diabetic retinopathy (DR) grading by ophthalmologists [38]. This assistance was found to increase the accuracy of the grading compared to that of an unassisted expert or with the model predictions alone. Initially, the system increased the grading time but with the user's experience, the grading time decreased and the grading confidence increased, especially when both predictions and heatmaps were used. Notably, the accuracy did reduce for patients without DR when model assistance was used and an option to toggle the assistance was provided. An extension of IG called Expressive gradients (EG) was proposed in [39] for weakly supervised segmentation of lesions for Age-related macular degeneration (AMD) diagnosis. A convolutional neural network (CNN) with a compact architecture outperformed larger existing convolutional neural network (CNN)s and Expressive gradients (EG) highlighted the regions of interest better than conventional IG and Guided backpropagation (GBP) methods. Expressive gradients (EG) extends IG by enriching input-level attribution map with high-level attribution maps. A comparative analysis of various explainability models including DeepDeep Learning Important FeaTures (LIFT), DeepSHapley Additive exPlanations (SHAP), IG, etc. was performed for on a model for detection of choroidal neovascularization (CNV), diabetic macular edema (DME), and drusens from optical coherence tomography (OCT) scans [40]. Figure 4 highlights better localization achieved by newer methods (e.g., DeepSHAP) in contrast to noisy results from older methods (e.g., saliency maps).

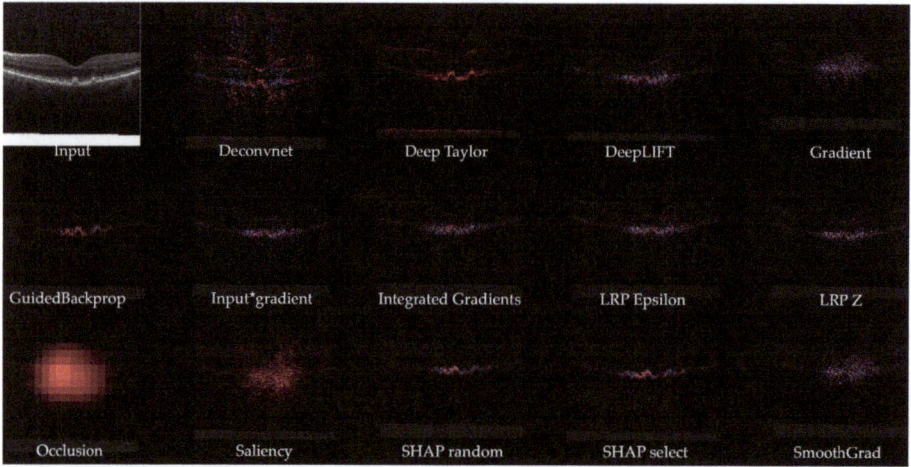

Figure 4. Example of heat maps from a retinal OCT image [40].

4.1.3. Breast Imaging

IG and SmoothGrad were used to visualize the features of a convolutional neural network (CNN) used for classifying estrogen receptor status from breast MRI [41]. The model was observed to have learned relevant features in both spatial and dynamic domains with different contributions from both. The visualizations revealed the learning of certain irrelevant features resulting from pre-processing artifacts. These observations led to changes in the pre-processing and training approaches. An earlier study for breast mass classification from mammograms [42] using two different convolutional neural network (CNN)s—AlexNet [43] and GoogleNet [44]—employed saliency maps to visualize the image features. Both the convolutional neural network (CNN)s were seen to learn the edges of the mass which are the main clinical criteria, while also being sensitive to the context.

4.1.4. CT Imaging

A DeepDreams [45] inspired attribution method was presented in [46] for explaining the segmentation of tumor from liver CT images. This novel method formulated using the concepts of DeapDreams, an image generation algorithm can be applied to a black-box neural network like other attribution methods discussed in Section 3. It performed a sensitivity analysis of the features by maximizing the activation of the target neuron by performing gradient ascent, i.e., finding the steepest slope of the function. A comparison between networks trained on real tumors and synthetic tumors revealed that the former was more sensitive to clinically relevant features and the latter was focusing on other features too. The network was found to be sensitive to intensity as well as sphericity in coherence with domain knowledge.

4.1.5. X-ray Imaging

In a recent study for detection of COVID-19 from chest X-ray images [47], a method called GSInquire was used to produce heatmaps for verifying the features learned by the proposed COVID-net model. GSInquire [48] was developed as an attribution method that outperformed prior methods like SHAP and Expected gradients in terms of the proposed new metrics—impact score and impact coverage. The impact score was defined as the percentage of features which impacted the model decision or confidence strongly. While impact coverage was defined in the context of the coverage of adversarially impacted factors in the input. Another study performed the analysis of uncertainty and interpretability for COVID-19 detection using chest X-rays. The heatmaps of the sample inputs for the trained model were generated using saliency maps, Guided GradCAM, GBP, and Class activation maps (CAM).

4.1.6. Skin Imaging

The features of a suite of 30 CNN models trained for melanoma detection [49] were compared using GradCAM and Kernel SHapley Additive exPlanations (SHAP). It was shown that even the models with high accuracy would occasionally focus on the features that were irrelevant for the diagnosis. There were differences in the explanations of the models that produced similar accuracy which was highlighted by the attribution maps of both the methods. This showed that distinct neural network architectures tend to learn different features. Another study [50] visualized the convolutional neural network (CNN) features for skin lesion classification. The features for the last two layers were visualized by rescaling the feature maps of the activations to the input size. The layers were observed to be looking at indicators like lesion borders and non-uniformity in color as well as risk factors like lighter skin color or pink texture. However, spurious features like artifacts and hair which have no significance were also learned indicating some extent of overfitting.

There are other studies using attribution based methods for diagnosis in addition to the more common imaging modalities discussed above. For example, a study performed uncertainty and interpretability analysis on CNNs for semantic segmentation of colorectal polyps, a precursor of rectal cancers [51]. Using GBP for heatmaps the convolutional neural network (CNN)s were found to be utilizing the edge and shape information to make predictions. Moreover, the uncertainty analysis revealed higher uncertainty in misclassified samples. There is plenty of opportunity for applying the explainability of deep learning methods to other modalities like laparoscopy and endoscopy e.g., [52]. An explainable model using SHapley Additive exPlanations (SHAP) attributions for hypoxemia, i.e., low blood oxygen tension prediction during surgery was presented in [53]. The study was performed for analyzing preoperative factors as well as in-surgery parameters. The resulting attributions were in line with known factors like BMI, physical status (ASA), tidal volume, inspired oxygen, etc.

The attribution based methods were one of the initial ways of visualizing neural networks and have since then evolved from simple class activation map and gradient-based methods to advanced techniques like Deep SHapley Additive exPlanations (SHAP). The better visualizations of these methods show that the models were learning relevant features in most of the cases. Any presence of spurious features was scrutinized, flagged to the readers, and brought adjustments to the model training methods. Smaller and task-specific models like [39] along with custom variants of the attribution methods can improve the identification of relevant features.

4.2. Non-Attribution Based

The studies discussed in this subsection approached the problem of explainability by developing a methodology and validating it on a given problem rather than performing a separate analysis using pre-existing attributions based methods like those previously discussed. These used approaches like attention maps, concept vectors, returning a similar image, text justifications, expert knowledge, generative modeling, combination with other machine learning methods, etc. It must be noted that the majority of these are still post-model but their implementation usually needs specific changes to the model structure such as in the attention maps or the addition of expert knowledge in case of rule-based methods. In this section, the studies are grouped by the explainability approach they took. Figure 5 shows a schematic of these methods according to the taxonomy discussed in Section 2. These are characterized in a hierarchical way using multiple taxonomies for a finer classification.

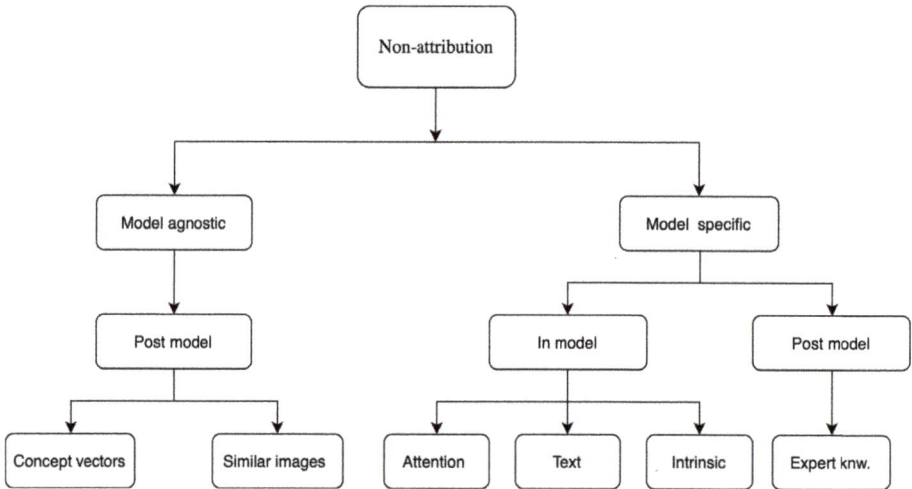

Figure 5. Classification of explainability methods that are not attribution based.

4.2.1. Attention Based

Attention is a popular and useful concept in deep learning. The basic idea of attention is inspired by the way humans pay attention to different parts of an image or other data sources to analyze them. More details about attention mechanisms in neural networks are discussed in [54]. An example of attention in medical diagnosis is given in [55]. Here, we discuss how attention-based methods can be used as an explainable deep learning tool for medical image analysis.

A network called MDNet was proposed [56] to perform a direct mapping between medical images and corresponding diagnostic reports. With an image model and a language model in it, the method used attention mechanisms to visualize the detection process. Using that attention mechanism, the language model found predominant and discriminatory features to learn the mapping between images and the diagnostic reports. This was the first work that exploited the attention mechanism to get insightful information from medical image dataset.

In [57] an interpretable version of U-Net [58] called SAUNet was proposed. It added a parallel secondary shape stream to capture important shape-based information along with the regular texture features of the images. The architecture used an attention module in the decoder part of the U-Net. The spatial and shape attention maps were generated using SmoothGrad to visualize the high activation region of the images.

4.2.2. Concept Vectors

A novel method called TCAV was proposed in [59] to explain the features learned by different layers to the domain experts without any deep learning expertise in terms of human-understandable concepts. It took the directional derivative of the network in the concept space much like that in the input feature space for saliency maps. It was tested to explain the predictions of diabetic retinopathy (DR) levels where it successfully detected the presence of microaneurysms and aneurysms in the retina. This provided justifications that were readily interpretable for the medical practitioners in terms of presence or absence of a given concept or physical structure in the image. However, many clinical concepts like the texture or the shape of a structure cannot be sufficiently described in terms of the presence or absence and need a continuous scale of measurement.

An extension of TCAV, which used the presence or absence of concepts, using Regression Concept Vectors (RCV) in the activation space of a layer was used to detect continuous concepts [60]. The task of the network was to detect tumors from breast lymph node samples. It was found that most of the relevant features like area and contrast were present in the early layers of the model. A further improvement over the TCAV used a new metric called Uniform unit Ball surface Sampling (UBS) [61] to provide layer-agnostic explanations for continuous and high dimensional features. It could explain high dimensional radiomics concepts across multiple layers which were validated using mammographic images. The model produced variations amongst the important concepts which were found to be lower across the layers of the SqueezeNet [62] compared to a baseline CNN with 3 dense layers explaining the better performance of the SqueezeNet.

4.2.3. Expert Knowledge

A vast majority of the research discussed in this review tried to correlate model features with expert knowledge using different approaches. Another approach was to use domain-specific knowledge to craft rules for prediction and explanation. An example of using task-specific knowledge to improve the results as well as the explanations were provided in [63] for brain midline shift (MLS) estimation using U-Net [58] based architecture and keypoints. It was reduced to the problem of detecting a midline using the model under domain constraints. The original midline was obtained using the endpoints and hence the shift from the predicted one was computed. The model also provided confidence intervals of the predictions making them more trustworthy for the end-user. Another study [64] used guidelines for rule-based segmentation of lung nodules followed by a perturbation analysis to compute the importance of features in each region. The explanations provided in terms of the regions already marked using rules were found to be more understandable for the users and showed the bias in data for improving the model. This method was then used to provide explanations at a global level for the entire dataset providing an overview of the relevant features.

4.2.4. Similar Images

Some studies provided similarly labeled images to the user as a reason for making a prediction for a given test image. A study [6] proposed analysis of layers of a 3D-convolutional neural network (CNN) using Gaussian mixture model (GMM) and binary encoding of training and test images based on their Gaussian mixture model (GMM) components for returning similar 3D images as explanations. The system returned activation wise similar training images using atlas as a clarification for its decision. It was demonstrated on 3D MNIST and an MRI dataset where it returned images with similar atrophy conditions. However, it was found that the activation similarity depended on the spatial orientation of images in certain cases which could affect the choice of the returned images.

In a study on dermoscopic images, a triplet-loss and k nearest neighbors (kNN) search-based learning strategy was used to learn convolutional neural network (CNN) feature embeddings for interpretable classification [65]. The evidence was provided as nearest neighbors and local image regions responsible for the lowest distance between the test image and those neighbors. Another approach used monotonic constraints to explain the predictions in terms of style and depth two datasets—dermoscopy images and post-surgical breast aesthetics [66]. It concatenated input streams with constrained monotonic convolutional neural network (CNN) and unconstrained convolutional neural network (CNN) to produce the predictions along with their explanations in terms of similar images as well as complementary images. The system was designed for only binary classification.

4.2.5. Textual Justification

A model that can explain its decision in terms of sentences or phrases giving the reasoning can directly communicate with both expert and general users. A justification model that took inputs from the visual features of a classifier, as well as embeddings of the predictions, was used to generate a diagnostic sentence and visual heatmaps for breast mass classification [67]. A visual word constraint loss was applied in the training of the justification generator to produce justifications in the presence of only a limited number of medical reports. Such multimodal explanations can be used to obtain greater user confidence due to a similarity with the usual workflow and learning process.

4.2.6. Intrinsic Explainability

Intrinsic explainability refers to the ability of a model to explain its decisions in terms of human observable decision boundaries or features. These usually include relatively simpler models like regression, decision trees, and support vector machines (SVM) for a few dimensions where the decision boundaries can be observed. Recent studies to make deep learning model intrinsically explainable using different methods such as a hybrid with machine learning classifiers and visualizing the features in a segmentation space.

An example of the latter was presented in [68] using the latent space of the features of a variational autoencoder for classification and segmentation of the brain MRI of Alzheimer's patients. The classification was performed in a two-dimensional latent space using an multi layer perceptron (MLP). The segmentation was performed in a three-dimensional latent space in terms of the anatomical variability encoded in the discriminating features. This led to the visualization of the features of the classifier as global and local anatomical characteristics which were usually used for clinical decisions. A study for detection of autism pectrum disorder (ASD) from functional magnetic resonance imaging (fMRI) used a hybrid of deep learning and support vector machines (SVM) to perform explainable classification [69]. The support vector machines (SVM) was used as a classifier on the features of a deep learning model and the visualization of the decision boundary explained the model.

This subsection discussed a variety of non-attribution explainability methods but the list is not exhaustive as newer methods are published frequently due to high interest in the area. The design of these methods is more involved than the application of attribution based methods on the inputs of a trained model. Specific elements like concept vectors, expert-based rules, image retrieval methods need to be integrated often at a model training level. This added complexity can potentially provide more domain-specific explanations at the expense of higher design effort. Notably, a majority of these techniques are still a post-hoc step but for a specific architecture or domain. Moreover, we have limited our scope to medical imaging as that is the dominant approach for automated diagnosis because of the detailed information presented by the images. However, patient records also provide rich information for diagnosis and there were studies discussing their explainability. For example, in [70] a gated recurrent unit (GRU)-based recurrent neural network (RNN) for mortality prediction from diagnostic codes from electronic healthcare record (EHR) was presented. It used hierarchical attention in the network for interpretability and visualization of the results.

Table 2. Applications of explainability in medical imaging.

Method	Algorithm	Model	Application	Modality
Attribution	Gradient*I/P, GBP, LRP, occlusion [36]	3D CNN	Alzheimer's detection	Brain MRI
	GradCAM, GBP [37]	Custom CNN	Grading brain tumor	Brain MRI
	IG [38]	Inception-v4	DR grading	Fundus images
	EG [39]	Custom CNN	Lesion segmentation for AMD	Retinal OCT
	IG, SmoothGrad [41]	AlexNet	Estrogen receptor status	Breast MRI
	Saliency maps [42]	AlexNet	Breast mass classification	Breast MRI
	GradCAM, SHAP [49]	Inception	Melanoma detection	Skin images
	Activation maps [50]	Custom CNN	Lesion classification	Skin images
	DeepDreams [46]	Custom CNN	Segmentation of tumor from liver	CT imaging
	GSInquire, GBP, activation maps [47]	COVIDNet CNN	COVID-19 detection	X-ray images
Attention	Mapping between image to reports [56]	CNN & LSTM	Bladder cancer	Tissue images
	U-Net with shape attention stream [57]	U-net based	Cardiac volume estimation	Cardiac MRI
Concept vectors	TCAV [59]	Inception	DR detection	Fundus images
	TCAV with RCV [60]	ResNet101	Breast tumor detection	Breast lymph node images
	UBS [61]	SqueezeNet	Breast mass classification	Mammography images
Expert knowledge	Domain constraints [63]	U-net	Brain MLS estimation	Brain MRI
	Rule-based segmentation, perturbation [64]	VGG16	Lung nodule segmentation	Lung CT
Similar images	GMM and atlas [6]	3D CNN	MRI classification	3D MNIST, Brain MRI
	Triplet loss, kNN [65]	AlexNet based with shared weights	Melanoma	Dermoscopy images
	Monotonic constraints [66]	DNN with two streams	Melanoma detection	Dermoscopy images
Textual justification	LSTM, visual word constraint [67]	Breast mass classification	CNN	Mammography images
Intrinsic explainability	Deep Hierarchical Generative Models [68]	Auto-encoders	Classification and segmentation for Alzheimer's	Brain MRI
	SVM margin [69]	Hybrid of CNN & SVM	ASD detection	Brain fMRI

5. Discussion

There has been significant progress in explaining the decisions of deep learning models, especially those used for medical diagnosis. Understanding the features responsible for a certain decision is useful for the model designers to iron out reliability concerns for the end-users to gain trust and make better judgments. Almost all of these methods target local explainability, i.e., explaining the decisions for a single example. This then is extrapolated to a global level by averaging the highlighted features, especially in cases where the images have the same spatial orientation. However, emerging methods like concept vectors (Section 4.2.2) provide a more global view of the decisions for each class in terms of domain concepts.

It is important to analyze the features of a black-box which can make the right decision due to the wrong reason. It is a major issue that can affect performance when the system is deployed in the real world. Most of the methods, especially the attribution based are available as open-source implementations. However, some methods like GSInquire [48] which show higher performance on some metrics are proprietary. There is an increasing commercial interest in explainability, and specifically the attribution methods which can be leveraged for a variety of business use cases.

The explainability methods have two different but overlapping objectives for the two different user groups. Deep learning practitioners can use them to design better systems by analyzing the model features and understanding the interactions between the model and the data. The clinical end-users can be provided with the explanations as a reasoning for the model decision and hence build confidence and trust in the model decision and also help identify potentially questionable decisions. A recent study compared the understanding of explanations amongst data scientists [71]. In this study common issues like missing data and redundant features were introduced and the data scientists were provided explanations of the trained models in order to identify the problems. The study reported over trust on the models as they tried to justify the issues as meaningful features. This is contrary to lower trust and acceptance from end-users who are wary of the black-box nature. It is notable that the experienced data scientists were able to use them effectively for understanding model and data issues.

Studies analyzing the effect of explanations on the decisions of the clinical end-users show in general positive outcomes [38]. There are studies comparing explainability methods quantitatively [36,39] which are discussed previously. The quantitative analysis focuses on theoretical correctness and robustness while missing out on actual clinical usefulness. There is a pertinent need to perform end-user based qualitative comparison of explanations for medical imaging applications. This can help to identify the most relevant techniques for explaining decisions to the clinicians. Such studies can be performed using expert agreement where a panel of experts can be asked to rate the explanations. A similar approach was used for deep learning based methods in [72] and for clinical diagnosis in [73]. We are currently working on a quantitative and qualitative analysis of various XAI methods in the diagnosis of retinal disease. The explanations will have quantitative comparisons along with qualitative evaluation by expert clinicians rating the explanations. This would also help to evaluate the overlap between the clinical knowledge acquired through clinical training and experience and the model features acquired for the pattern recognition task for a given dataset.

Studies have extended existing explainability methods to better suit the challenges of the medical imaging domain. For example, [39] proposed Expressive gradients (EG), an extension of commonly used IG to cover the retinal lesions better while [60] extended concept vectors from [59] for continuous concepts like texture and shape. Such studies lead to the advancement of the explainability domain and provided customization without designing new methods from scratch. Despite all these advances, there is still a need to make the explainability methods more holistic and interwoven with uncertainty methods. Expert feedback must be incorporated into the design of such explainability methods to tailor the feedback for their needs. Initially, any clinical application of such explainable deep learning methods is likely to be a human-in-the-loop (HITL) hybrid keeping the clinical expert in the control of the process. It can be considered analogous to driving aids like adaptive cruise control or lane keep assistance in cars where the driver is still in control and responsible for the final decisions but with a reduced workload and an added safety net.

Another direction of work can be to use multiple modalities like medical images and patients' records together in the decision-making process and attribute the model decisions to each of them. This can simulate the diagnostic workflow of a clinician where both images and physical parameters of a patient are used to make a decision. This can potentially improve accuracy as well as explain the phenomena more comprehensively. To sum up, explainable diagnosis is making convincing strides but there is still some way to go to meet the expectations of end-users, regulators, and the general public.

Funding: This work is supported by an NSERC Discovery Grant and NVIDIA Titan V GPU Grant to V.L. This research was enabled in part by Compute Canada (www.computecanada.ca).

Conflicts of Interest: The authors declare no conflict of interest.

Acronyms

AI	artificial intelligence
AMD	Age-related macular degeneration
ASD	autism pectrum disorder
CAD	Computer-aided diagnostics
CAM	Class activation maps
CNN	convolutional neural network
CNV	choroidal neovascularization
CT	computerized tomography
DME	diabetic macular edema
DNN	deep neural networks
DR	diabetic retinopathy
EG	Expressive gradients
EHR	electronic healthcare record
fMRI	functional magnetic resonance imaging
GBP	Guided backpropagation
GDPR	General Data Protection Regulation
GMM	Gaussian mixture model
GradCAM	Gradient weighted class activation mapping
GRU	gated recurrent unit
HITL	human-in-the-loop
IG	Integrated gradients
kNN	k nearest neighbors
LIFT	Deep Learning Important FeaTures
LRP	Layer wise relevance propagation
MLP	multi layer perceptron
MLS	midline shift
MRI	magnetic resonance imaging
OCT	optical coherence tomography
PCC	Pearson's correlation coefficient
RCV	Regression Concept Vectors
ReLU	rectified linear unit
RNN	recurrent neural network
SHAP	SHapley Additive exPlanations
SVM	support vector machines
TCAV	Testing Concept Activation Vectors
UBS	Uniform unit Ball surface Sampling

References

1. Jo, T.; Nho, K.; Saykin, A.J. Deep learning in Alzheimer's disease: Diagnostic classification and prognostic prediction using neuroimaging data. *Front. Aging Neurosci.* **2019**, *11*, 220. [CrossRef]
2. Hua, K.L.; Hsu, C.H.; Hidayati, S.C.; Cheng, W.H.; Chen, Y.J. Computer-aided classification of lung nodules on computed tomography images via deep learning technique. *OncoTargets Ther.* **2015**, *8*, 2015–2022.
3. Sengupta, S.; Singh, A.; Leopold, H.A.; Gulati, T.; Lakshminarayanan, V. Ophthalmic diagnosis using deep learning with fundus images–A critical review. *Artif. Intell. Med.* **2020**, *102*, 101758. [CrossRef] [PubMed]
4. Leopold, H.; Singh, A.; Sengupta, S.; Zelek, J.; Lakshminarayanan, V., Recent Advances in Deep Learning Applications for Retinal Diagnosis using OCT. In *State of the Art in Neural Networks*; El-Baz, A.S., Ed.; Elsevier: New York, NY, USA, 2020; in press.
5. Holzinger, A.; Biemann, C.; Pattichis, C.S.; Kell, D.B. What do we need to build explainable AI systems for the medical domain? *arXiv* **2017**, arXiv:1712.09923.
6. Stano, M.; Benesova, W.; Martak, L.S. Explainable 3D convolutional neural network using GMM encoding. In Proceedings of the Twelfth International Conference on Machine Vision, Amsterdam, The Netherlands, 16–18 November 2019; Volume 11433, p. 114331U.
7. Moccia, S.; Wirkert, S.J.; Kenngott, H.; Vemuri, A.S.; Apitz, M.; Mayer, B.; De Momi, E.; Mattos, L.S.; Maier-Hein, L. Uncertainty-aware organ classification for surgical data science applications in laparoscopy. *IEEE Trans. Biomed. Eng.* **2018**, *65*, 2649–2659. [CrossRef] [PubMed]
8. Adler, T.J.; Ardizzone, L.; Vemuri, A.; Ayala, L.; Gröhl, J.; Kirchner, T.; Wirkert, S.; Kruse, J.; Rother, C.; Köthe, U.; et al. Uncertainty-aware performance assessment of optical imaging modalities with invertible neural networks. *Int. J. Comput. Assist. Radiol. Surg.* **2019**, *14*, 997–1007. [CrossRef]
9. Meyes, R.; de Puiseau, C.W.; Posada-Moreno, A.; Meisen, T. Under the Hood of Neural Networks: Characterizing Learned Representations by Functional Neuron Populations and Network Ablations. *arXiv* **2020**, arXiv:2004.01254.
10. Arrieta, A.B.; Díaz-Rodríguez, N.; Del Ser, J.; Bennetot, A.; Tabik, S.; Barbado, A.; García, S.; Gil-López, S.; Molina, D.; Benjamins, R.; et al. Explainable Artificial Intelligence (XAI): Concepts, taxonomies, opportunities and challenges toward responsible AI. *Inf. Fusion* **2020**, *58*, 82–115. [CrossRef]
11. Stiglic, G.; Kocbek, P.; Fijacko, N.; Zitnik, M.; Verbert, K.; Cilar, L. Interpretability of machine learning based prediction models in healthcare. *arXiv* **2020**, arXiv:2002.08596.
12. Arya, V.; Bellamy, R.K.; Chen, P.Y.; Dhurandhar, A.; Hind, M.; Hoffman, S.C.; Houde, S.; Liao, Q.V.; Luss, R.; Mojsilović, A.; et al. One explanation does not fit all: A toolkit and taxonomy of ai explainability techniques. *arXiv* **2019**, arXiv:1909.03012.
13. Ying, Z.; Bourgeois, D.; You, J.; Zitnik, M.; Leskovec, J. Gnnexplainer: Generating explanations for graph neural networks. In Proceedings of the Advances in Neural Information Processing Systems 32, Vancouver, BC, Canada, 8–14 December 2019; Volume 32, pp. 9240–9251.
14. Wold, S.; Esbensen, K.; Geladi, P. Principal component analysis. *Chemom. Intell. Lab. Syst.* **1987**, *2*, 37–52. [CrossRef]
15. Maaten, L.V.D.; Hinton, G. Visualizing data using t-SNE. *J. Mach. Learn. Res.* **2008**, *9*, 2579–2605.
16. Safavian, S.R.; Landgrebe, D. A survey of decision tree classifier methodology. *IEEE Trans. Syst. Man Cybern.* **1991**, *21*, 660–674. [CrossRef]
17. Montavon, G.; Lapuschkin, S.; Binder, A.; Samek, W.; Müller, K.R. Explaining nonlinear classification decisions with deep taylor decomposition. *Pattern Recognit.* **2017**, *65*, 211–222. [CrossRef]
18. Ancona, M.; Ceolini, E.; Öztireli, C.; Gross, M. Towards better understanding of gradient-based attribution methods for deep neural networks. *arXiv* **2017**, arXiv:1711.06104.
19. Alber, M.; Lapuschkin, S.; Seegerer, P.; Hägele, M.; Schütt, K.T.; Montavon, G.; Samek, W.; Müller, K.R.; Dähne, S.; Kindermans, P.J. iNNvestigate neural networks. *J. Mach. Learn. Res.* **2019**, *20*, 1–8.
20. Zeiler, M.D.; Fergus, R. Visualizing and understanding convolutional networks. In Proceedings of the European Conference on Computer Vision, Zurich, Switzerland, 6–12 September 2014; Springer: Cham, Switzerland; pp. 818–833.
21. Goodfellow, I.J.; Shlens, J.; Szegedy, C. Explaining and harnessing adversarial examples. *arXiv* **2014**, arXiv:1412.6572.

22. Lipovetsky, S.; Conklin, M. Analysis of regression in game theory approach. *Appl. Stoch. Model. Bus. Ind.* **2001**, *17*, 319–330. [CrossRef]
23. Simonyan, K.; Vedaldi, A.; Zisserman, A. Deep inside convolutional networks: Visualising image classification models and saliency maps. *arXiv* **2013**, arXiv:1312.6034.
24. Springenberg, J.T.; Dosovitskiy, A.; Brox, T.; Riedmiller, M. Striving for simplicity: The all convolutional net. *arXiv* **2014**, arXiv:1412.6806.
25. Bach, S.; Binder, A.; Montavon, G.; Klauschen, F.; Müller, K.R.; Samek, W. On pixel-wise explanations for non-linear classifier decisions by layer-wise relevance propagation. *PLoS ONE* **2015**, *10*. [CrossRef] [PubMed]
26. Shrikumar, A.; Greenside, P.; Shcherbina, A.; Kundaje, A. Not just a black box: Learning important features through propagating activation differences. *arXiv* **2016**, arXiv:1605.01713.
27. Selvaraju, R.R.; Cogswell, M.; Das, A.; Vedantam, R.; Parikh, D.; Batra, D. Grad-cam: Visual explanations from deep networks via gradient-based localization. In Proceedings of the IEEE International Conference on Computer Vision, Venice, Italy, 22–29 October 2017; pp. 618–626. [CrossRef]
28. Sundararajan, M.; Taly, A.; Yan, Q. Axiomatic attribution for deep networks. In Proceedings of the 34th International Conference on Machine Learning, Sydney, Australia, 6–11 August 2017; Voume 70, pp. 3319–3328.
29. Kindermans, P.J.; Schütt, K.T.; Alber, M.; Müller, K.R.; Erhan, D.; Kim, B.; Dähne, S. Learning how to explain neural networks: Patternnet and patternattribution. *arXiv* **2017**, arXiv:1705.05598.
30. Shrikumar, A.; Greenside, P.; Kundaje, A. Learning important features through propagating activation differences. In Proceedings of the 34th International Conference on Machine Learning, Sydney, Australia, 6–11 August 2017; Voume 70, pp. 3145–3153.
31. Smilkov, D.; Thorat, N.; Kim, B.; Viégas, F.; Wattenberg, M. Smoothgrad: Removing noise by adding noise. *arXiv* **2017**, arXiv:1706.03825.
32. Chen, H.; Lundberg, S.; Lee, S.I. Explaining Models by Propagating Shapley Values of Local Components. *arXiv* **2019**, arXiv:1911.11888.
33. Yosinski, J.; Clune, J.; Bengio, Y.; Lipson, H. How transferable are features in deep neural networks? In Proceedings of the Advances in Neural Information Processing Systems, Montreal, QC, USA, 8–13 December 2014; pp. 3320–3328.
34. Singh, A.; Sengupta, S.; Lakshminarayanan, V. Glaucoma diagnosis using transfer learning methods. In *Proceedings of the Applications of Machine Learning*; International Society for Optics and Photonics (SPIE): Bellingham, WA, USA, 2019; Volume 11139, p. 111390U.
35. Deng, J.; Dong, W.; Socher, R.; Li, L.J.; Li, K.; Fei-Fei, L. Imagenet: A large-scale hierarchical image database. In Proceedings of the 2009 IEEE Conference on Computer Vision and Pattern Recognition, Miami, FL, USA, 20–25 June 2009; pp. 248–255.
36. Eitel, F.; Ritter, K.; Alzheimer's Disease Neuroimaging Initiative (ADNI). Testing the Robustness of Attribution Methods for Convolutional Neural Networks in MRI-Based Alzheimer's Disease Classification. In *Interpretability of Machine Intelligence in Medical Image Computing and Multimodal Learning for Clinical Decision Support, ML-CDS 2019, IMIMIC 2019*; Lecture Notes in Computer Science; Suzuki, K., et al., Eds.; Springer: Cham, Switzerland, 2019; Volume 11797. [CrossRef]
37. Pereira, S.; Meier, R.; Alves, V.; Reyes, M.; Silva, C.A. Automatic brain tumor grading from MRI data using convolutional neural networks and quality assessment. In *Understanding and Interpreting Machine Learning in Medical Image Computing Applications*; Springer: Cham, Switzerland, 2018; pp. 106–114.
38. Sayres, R.; Taly, A.; Rahimy, E.; Blumer, K.; Coz, D.; Hammel, N.; Krause, J.; Narayanaswamy, A.; Rastegar, Z.; Wu, D.; et al. Using a deep learning algorithm and integrated gradients explanation to assist grading for diabetic retinopathy. *Ophthalmology* **2019**, *126*, 552–564. [CrossRef]
39. Yang, H.L.; Kim, J.J.; Kim, J.H.; Kang, Y.K.; Park, D.H.; Park, H.S.; Kim, H.K.; Kim, M.S. Weakly supervised lesion localization for age-related macular degeneration detection using optical coherence tomography images. *PLoS ONE* **2019**, *14*, e0215076. [CrossRef]
40. Singh, A.; Sengupta, S.; Lakshminarayanan, V. Interpretation of deep learning using attributions: Application to ophthalmic diagnosis. In *Proceedings of the Applications of Machine Learning*; International Society for Optics and Photonics (SPIE): Bellingham, WA, USA, 2020; in press.

41. Papanastasopoulos, Z.; Samala, R.K.; Chan, H.P.; Hadjiiski, L.; Paramagul, C.; Helvie, M.A.; Neal, C.H. Explainable AI for medical imaging: Deep-learning CNN ensemble for classification of estrogen receptor status from breast MRI. In *Proceedings of the SPIE Medical Imaging 2020: Computer-Aided Diagnosis*; International Society for Optics and Photonics: Bellingham, WA, USA, 2020; Volume 11314, p. 113140Z.
42. Lévy, D.; Jain, A. Breast mass classification from mammograms using deep convolutional neural networks. *arXiv* **2016**, arXiv:1612.00542.
43. Szegedy, C.; Liu, W.; Jia, Y.; Sermanet, P.; Reed, S.; Anguelov, D.; Erhan, D.; Vanhoucke, V.; Rabinovich, A. Going deeper with convolutions. In Proceedings of the 2015 IEEE Conference on Computer Vision and Pattern Recognition (CVPR), Boston, MA, USA, 7–12 June 2015; pp. 1–9.
44. Krizhevsky, A.; Sutskever, I.; Hinton, G.E. Imagenet classification with deep convolutional neural networks. In Proceedings of the Advances in Neural Information Processing Systems, Lake Tahoe, NV, USA, 3–6 December 2012; pp. 1097–1105.
45. Mordvintsev, A.; Olah, C.; Tyka, M. Inceptionism: Going Deeper into Neural Networks. Google AI Blog. 2015. Available online: https://ai.googleblog.com/2015/06/inceptionism-going-deeper-into-neural.html (accessed on 23 May 2020)
46. Couteaux, V.; Nempont, O.; Pizaine, G.; Bloch, I. Towards Interpretability of Segmentation Networks by Analyzing DeepDreams. In *Interpretability of Machine Intelligence in Medical Image Computing and Multimodal Learning for Clinical Decision Support*; Springer: Cham, Switzerland, 2019; pp. 56–63.
47. Wang, L.; Wong, A. COVID-Net: A tailored deep convolutional neural network design for detection of COVID-19 cases from chest radiography images. *arXiv* **2020**, arXiv:2003.09871.
48. Lin, Z.Q.; Shafiee, M.J.; Bochkarev, S.; Jules, M.S.; Wang, X.Y.; Wong, A. Explaining with Impact: A Machine-centric Strategy to Quantify the Performance of Explainability Algorithms. *arXiv* **2019**, arXiv:1910.07387.
49. Young, K.; Booth, G.; Simpson, B.; Dutton, R.; Shrapnel, S. Deep neural network or dermatologist? In *Interpretability of Machine Intelligence in Medical Image Computing and Multimodal Learning for Clinical Decision Support*; Springer: Cham, Switzerland, 2019; pp. 48–55.
50. Van Molle, P.; De Strooper, M.; Verbelen, T.; Vankeirsbilck, B.; Simoens, P.; Dhoedt, B. Visualizing convolutional neural networks to improve decision support for skin lesion classification. In *Understanding and Interpreting Machine Learning in Medical Image Computing Applications*; Springer: Cham, Switzerland, 2018; pp. 115–123.
51. Wickstrøm, K.; Kampffmeyer, M.; Jenssen, R. Uncertainty and interpretability in convolutional neural networks for semantic segmentation of colorectal polyps. *Med Image Anal.* **2020**, *60*, 101619. [CrossRef] [PubMed]
52. Moccia, S.; De Momi, E.; Guarnaschelli, M.; Savazzi, M.; Laborai, A.; Guastini, L.; Peretti, G.; Mattos, L.S. Confident texture-based laryngeal tissue classification for early stage diagnosis support. *J. Med Imaging* **2017**, *4*, 034502. [CrossRef] [PubMed]
53. Lundberg, S.M.; Nair, B.; Vavilala, M.S.; Horibe, M.; Eisses, M.J.; Adams, T.; Liston, D.E.; Low, D.K.W.; Newman, S.F.; Kim, J.; et al. Explainable machine-learning predictions for the prevention of hypoxaemia during surgery. *Nat. Biomed. Eng.* **2018**, *2*, 749–760. [CrossRef]
54. Vaswani, A.; Shazeer, N.; Parmar, N.; Uszkoreit, J.; Jones, L.; Gomez, A.N.; Kaiser, Ł.; Polosukhin, I. Attention is all you need. In Proceedings of the Advances in Neural Information Processing Systems, Long Beach, CA, USA, 4–9 December 2017; pp. 5998–6008.
55. Bamba, U.; Pandey, D.; Lakshminarayanan, V. Classification of brain lesions from MRI images using a novel neural network. In *Multimodal Biomedical Imaging XV*; International Society for Optics and Photonics: Bellingham, WA, USA, 2020; Volume 11232, p. 112320K.
56. Zhang, Z.; Xie, Y.; Xing, F.; McGough, M.; Yang, L. Mdnet: A semantically and visually interpretable medical image diagnosis network. In Proceedings of the IEEE Conference on Computer Vision and Pattern Recognition, Honolulu, HI, USA, 21–26 July 2017; pp. 6428–6436.
57. Sun, J.; Darbeha, F.; Zaidi, M.; Wang, B. SAUNet: Shape Attentive U-Net for Interpretable Medical Image Segmentation. *arXiv* **2020**, arXiv:2001.07645.
58. Ronneberger, O.; Fischer, P.; Brox, T. U-net: Convolutional networks for biomedical image segmentation. In Proceedings of the International Conference on Medical Image Computing and Computer-Assisted Intervention, Munich, Germany, 5–9 October 2015; Springer: Cham, Switzerland; pp. 234–241.

59. Kim, B.; Wattenberg, M.; Gilmer, J.; Cai, C.; Wexler, J.; Viegas, F.; Sayres, R. Interpretability beyond feature attribution: Quantitative testing with concept activation vectors (tcav). *arXiv* **2017**, arXiv:1711.11279.
60. Graziani, M.; Andrearczyk, V.; Müller, H. Regression concept vectors for bidirectional explanations in histopathology. In *Understanding and Interpreting Machine Learning in Medical Image Computing Applications*; Springer: Cham, Switzerland, 2018; pp. 124–132.
61. Yeche, H.; Harrison, J.; Berthier, T. UBS: A Dimension-Agnostic Metric for Concept Vector Interpretability Applied to Radiomics. In *Interpretability of Machine Intelligence in Medical Image Computing and Multimodal Learning for Clinical Decision Support*; Springer: Cham, Switzerland, 2019; pp. 12–20.
62. Iandola, F.N.; Han, S.; Moskewicz, M.W.; Ashraf, K.; Dally, W.J.; Keutzer, K. SqueezeNet: AlexNet-level accuracy with 50x fewer parameters and <0.5 MB model size. *arXiv* **2016**, arXiv:1602.07360.
63. Pisov, M.; Goncharov, M.; Kurochkina, N.; Morozov, S.; Gombolevsky, V.; Chernina, V.; Vladzymyrskyy, A.; Zamyatina, K.; Cheskova, A.; Pronin, I.; et al. Incorporating Task-Specific Structural Knowledge into CNNs for Brain Midline Shift Detection. In *Interpretability of Machine Intelligence in Medical Image Computing and Multimodal Learning for Clinical Decision Support*; Springer: Cham, Switzerland, 2019; pp. 30–38.
64. Zhu, P.; Ogino, M. Guideline-Based Additive Explanation for Computer-Aided Diagnosis of Lung Nodules. In *Interpretability of Machine Intelligence in Medical Image Computing and Multimodal Learning for Clinical Decision Support*; Springer: Cham, Switzerland, 2019; pp. 39–47.
65. Codella, N.C.; Lin, C.C.; Halpern, A.; Hind, M.; Feris, R.; Smith, J.R. Collaborative Human-AI (CHAI): Evidence-based interpretable melanoma classification in dermoscopic images. In *Understanding and Interpreting Machine Learning in Medical Image Computing Applications*; Springer: Cham, Switzerland, 2018; pp. 97–105.
66. Silva, W.; Fernandes, K.; Cardoso, M.J.; Cardoso, J.S. Towards complementary explanations using deep neural networks. In *Understanding and Interpreting Machine Learning in Medical Image Computing Applications*; Springer: Cham, Switzerland, 2018; pp. 133–140.
67. Lee, H.; Kim, S.T.; Ro, Y.M. Generation of Multimodal Justification Using Visual Word Constraint Model for Explainable Computer Aided Diagnosis. In *Interpretability of Machine Intelligence in Medical Image Computing and Multimodal Learning for Clinical Decision Support*; Springer: Cham, Switzerland, 2019; pp. 21–29.
68. Biffi, C.; Cerrolaza, J.J.; Tarroni, G.; Bai, W.; De Marvao, A.; Oktay, O.; Ledig, C.; Le Folgoc, L.; Kamnitsas, K.; Doumou, G.; et al. Explainable Anatomical Shape Analysis through Deep Hierarchical Generative Models. *IEEE Trans. Med. Imaging* **2020**. [CrossRef]
69. Eslami, T.; Raiker, J.S.; Saeed, F. Explainable and Scalable Machine-Learning Algorithms for Detection of Autism Spectrum Disorder using fMRI Data. *arXiv* **2020**, arXiv:2003.01541.
70. Sha, Y.; Wang, M.D. Interpretable predictions of clinical outcomes with an attention-based recurrent neural network. In Proceedings of the 8th ACM International Conference on Bioinformatics, Computational Biology, and Health Informatics, Boston, MA, USA, 20–23 August 2017; pp. 233–240.
71. Kaur, H.; Nori, H.; Jenkins, S.; Caruana, R.; Wallach, H.; Wortman Vaughan, J. Interpreting Interpretability: Understanding Data Scientists' Use of Interpretability Tools for Machine Learning. In Proceedings of the CHI Conference on Human Factors in Computing Systems, Honolulu, HI, USA, 25–30 April 2020; pp. 1–14. [CrossRef]
72. Arbabshirani, M.R.; Fornwalt, B.K.; Mongelluzzo, G.J.; Suever, J.D.; Geise, B.D.; Patel, A.A.; Moore, G.J. Advanced machine learning in action: Identification of intracranial hemorrhage on computed tomography scans of the head with clinical workflow integration. *NPJ Digit. Med.* **2018**, *1*, 1–7. [CrossRef]
73. Almazroa, A.; Alodhayb, S.; Osman, E.; Ramadan, E.; Hummadi, M.; Dlaim, M.; Alkatee, M.; Raahemifar, K.; Lakshminarayanan, V. Agreement among ophthalmologists in marking the optic disc and optic cup in fundus images. *Int. Ophthalmol.* **2017**, *37*, 701–717. [CrossRef]

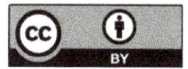

© 2020 by the authors. Licensee MDPI, Basel, Switzerland. This article is an open access article distributed under the terms and conditions of the Creative Commons Attribution (CC BY) license (http://creativecommons.org/licenses/by/4.0/).

MDPI
St. Alban-Anlage 66
4052 Basel
Switzerland
Tel. +41 61 683 77 34
Fax +41 61 302 89 18
www.mdpi.com

Journal of Imaging Editorial Office
E-mail: jimaging@mdpi.com
www.mdpi.com/journal/jimaging

www.ingramcontent.com/pod-product-compliance
Lightning Source LLC
LaVergne TN
LVHW070126100526
838202LV00016B/2236